Radiology Illustrated: Chest Radiology

Kyung Soo Lee • Joungho Han • Man Pyo Chung
Yeon Joo Jeong

# Radiology Illustrated: Chest Radiology

Springer

Kyung Soo Lee
Department of Radiology
Samsung Medical Center
Sungkyunkwan University School of Medicine
Seoul
Korea, Republic of (South Korea)

Joungho Han
Department of Pathology
Samsung Medical Center
Sungkyunkwan University School of Medicine
Seoul
Korea, Republic of (South Korea)

Man Pyo Chung
Department of Medicine
Division of Pulmonary and Critical Care
Samsung Medical Center
Sungkyunkwan University School of Medicine
Seoul
Korea, Republic of (South Korea)

Yeon Joo Jeong
Department of Radiology
Pusan National University Hospital
Busan
Korea, Republic of (South Korea)

ISSN 2196-114X eISSN 2196-1158
ISBN 978-3-662-51287-6 ISBN 978-3-642-37096-0 (eBook)
DOI 10.1007/978-3-642-37096-0
Springer Heidelberg New York Dordrecht London


Softcover reprint of the hardcover 1st edition 2014


Printed on acid-free paper

Springer is part of Springer Science+Business Media (www.springer.com)

*To our spouses and children:*
*Kyung Sook Yi and Joo Hwang and Joo Young*
*Young Hee Chon and Seung Hwan and Jae Won*
*Seoun Min Ahn and Seung Hwan and You Seoun*
*Youseock Jeong and Yean and Jian*

# Preface

Multidetector CT images of the state-of-the-art quality are increasingly produced in thoracic imaging, and in the near future, the CT imaging is expected to substitute chest radiography especially in outpatient clinic and may be ordered as a routine admission battery examination.

In MEDLINE or other search engines, writing down several keywords regarding lung diseases with correct MeSH (Medical Subject Headings) words would promptly bring you several diseases among which you may choose correct diagnosis of pulmonary diseases in consideration of most compatible patient symptoms and signs. Likewise, we authors would like to publish a book that will guide readers to correct diagnosis, when they use correct MeSH words or keywords for describing lung lesion patterns identified on chest CT images. When readers encounter similar patterns or distribution of lung abnormalities at CT, they may need to enumerate many diseases as potential differential diagnoses. This book provides the imaging algorithms based on patterns and distributions of lung lesions and the most relevant differential diagnoses. Because all diseases could not be enlisted as potential diagnostic possibilities, we tried to enumerate as many as common diseases that appear with similar patterns and distribution. Thus, familiarity with correct glossary of terms of lung lesion description is basic prerequisite for effective and helpful reading of this book and for making a correct diagnosis seen on chest CT scans.

After enlisting the diseases showing such pattern and distribution, the text provides the key points for differential diagnosis based on clinical and imaging features and tables that outline the classic manifestations of the various diseases. For each disease, succinct description of histopathology, clinical symptoms and signs, CT–pathology correlation, and patient prognosis has been given. Thus, this book is expected to be a shepherd for imaging diagnosis of lung diseases to radiology residents, fellows for thoracic imaging, chest physicians, and general practitioners. Moreover, as many cases are illustrated with their corresponding pathology, lung pathologists may also like to read this book. Like a cherishing substance, by keeping this handy book nearby and by comparing CT images of your patients with illustrated cases shown on this book, you may narrow differential diagnoses of your cases seen in patients of your references.

In mobile web and smartphone era, such automatic diagnosis App devices are expected to be developed such that taking a photograph of representative CT image of your patient CT might bring you an easy and automatic diagnosis of the lung disease of your patient. This approach may be feasible by pattern approach using cumulative image database. We wish that this book would be a cornerstone for such App (application) in the near future.

Last but not least, we should thank Young Joo Moon for her enthusiastic editorial help and Springer people, Dr. Ute Heilmann and Ms. Lauren Kim, for encouraging us to write this precious book.

Gangnam-gu, Seoul and Seo-gu, Pusan in Korea, August 2013

Kyung Soo Lee
Joungho Han
Man Pyo Chung
Yeon Joo Jeong

# Contents

# Pattern Approach for Lung Imaging

Flowcharts “Focal involvement” and “Diffuse involvement” see following pages.

## Focal Involvement

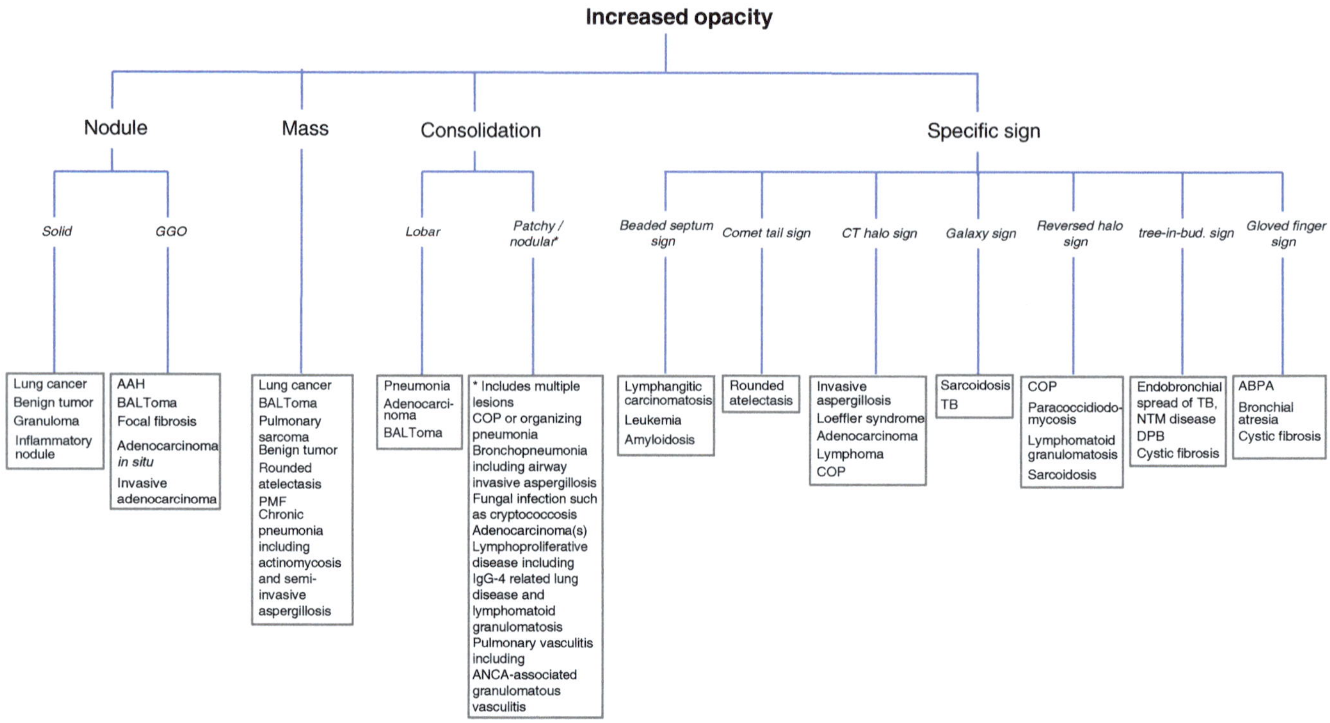


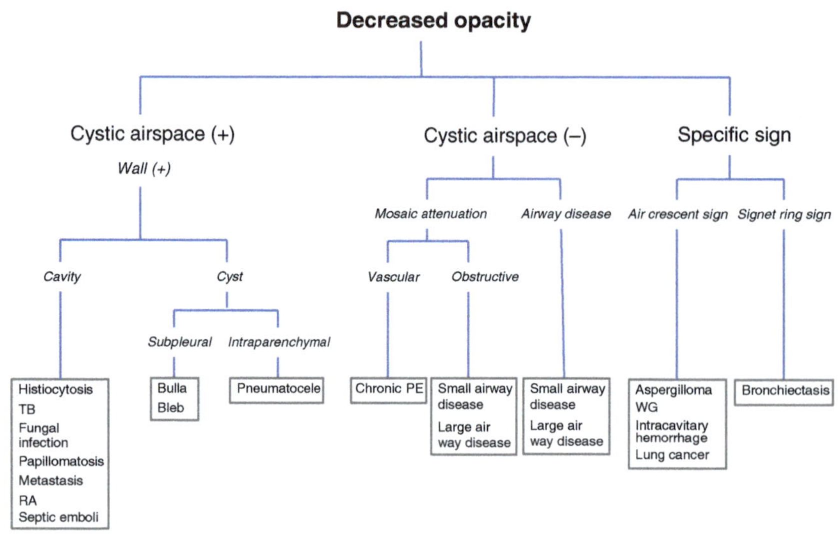

## Diffuse Involvement

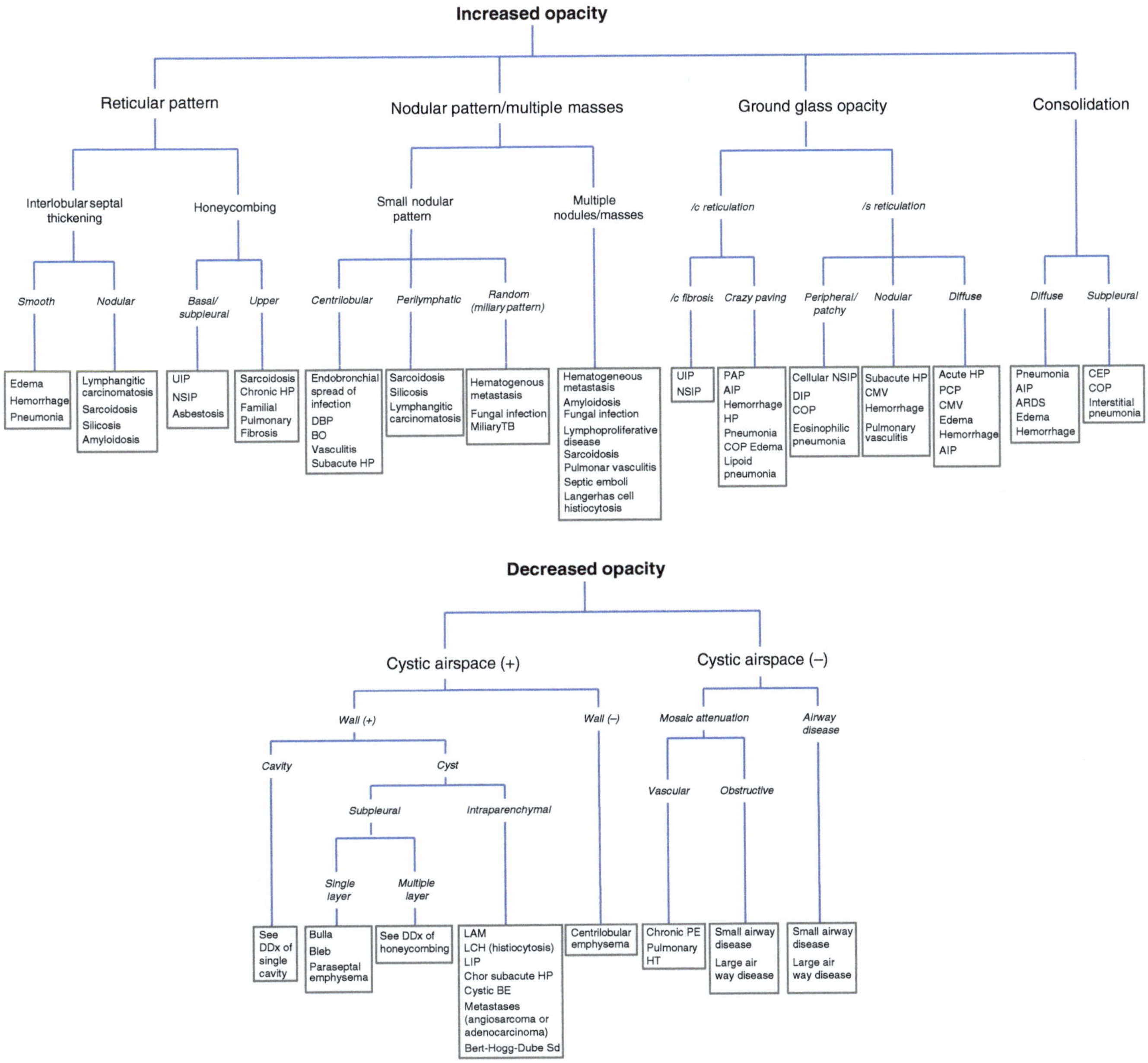

# Part I

# Focal Lung Diseases

# Nodule

1

## Solitary Pulmonary Nodule (SPN), Solid

### Definition

Solitary pulmonary nodules (SPNs) are defined as focal, round, or oval areas of increased opacity in the lung with diameters of ≤3 cm [1] (Fig. 1.1). The lesion is not associated with pneumonia, atelectasis, or lymphadenopathy.

Particularly when the nodule is less than 10 mm in diameter, it may be called small nodule (Fig. 1.2). With its diameter less than 3 mm, it may be called micronodule [2].

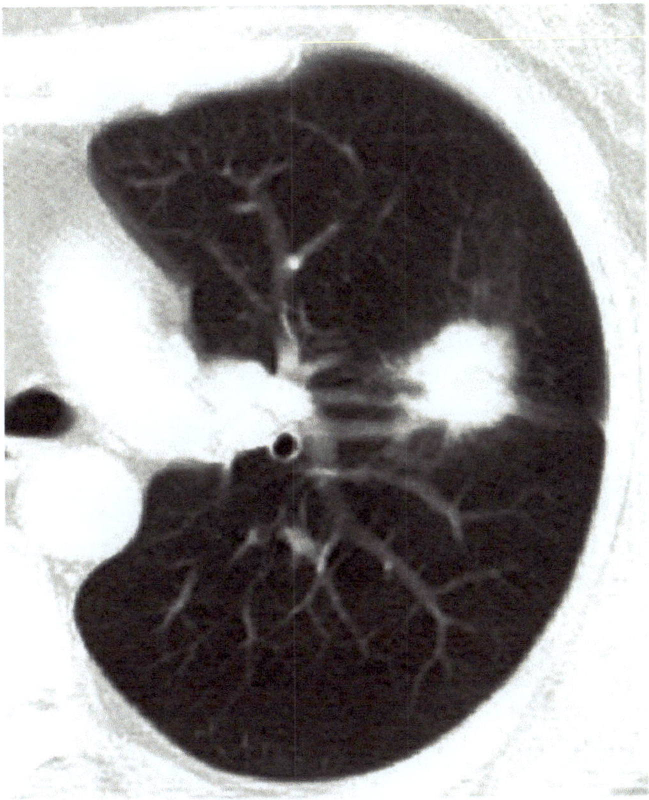

**Fig. 1.1** A lung nodule representing lung adenocarcinoma with acinar- and papillary-predominant subtypes in a 52-year-old woman. Thin-section (2.5-mm section thickness) CT scan obtained at level of tracheal carina shows a 22-mm-sized nodule with lobulated and spiculated margin in the left upper lobe

### Diseases Causing the Pattern

The most common cause is malignant tumor including *lung cancer* (Fig. 1.3), *carcinoid* (Fig. 1.4), *bronchus-associated lymphoid tissue* (*BALT*) *lymphoma* (Fig. 1.5), and a solitary metastasis to the lung. Benign tumors are *granuloma* (Fig. 1.6), *hamartoma* (Fig. 1.7), *sclerosing hemangiomas* (Fig. 1.8), *inflammatory myofibroblastic tumor* (*IMT, inflammatory pseudotumor*) (Fig. 1.9), rheumatoid nodule (Fig. 1.2), parasitic infection (*Paragonimus westermani*), and *nodule in antineutrophil cytoplasmic antibody* (*ANCA*)-*associated granulomatous vasculitis* (*former Wegener's granulomatosis*) (Fig. 1.10) (Table 1.1).

### Distribution

Likelihood ratio for malignancy in upper and middle lobe nodule is 1.22 as compared with 0.66 in lower lobe nodule [3].

### Clinical Considerations

The hierarchy of radiologic and clinical likelihood ratios for malignancy includes, in decreasing rank, a cavity of 16 mm in thickness, irregular or speculated margin on CT scans, patient complaints of hemoptysis, a patient history of malignancy, patient age >70 years, nodule size of 21–30 mm in diameter, nodule growth rate of 7–464 days, an ill-defined nodule on chest radiographs, a currently smoking patient, and nodules with indeterminate calcification on CT scans [3].

K.S. Lee et al., *Radiology Illustrated: Chest Radiology*, Radiology Illustrated,
DOI 10.1007/978-3-642-37096-0_1, © Springer-Verlag Berlin Heidelberg 2014

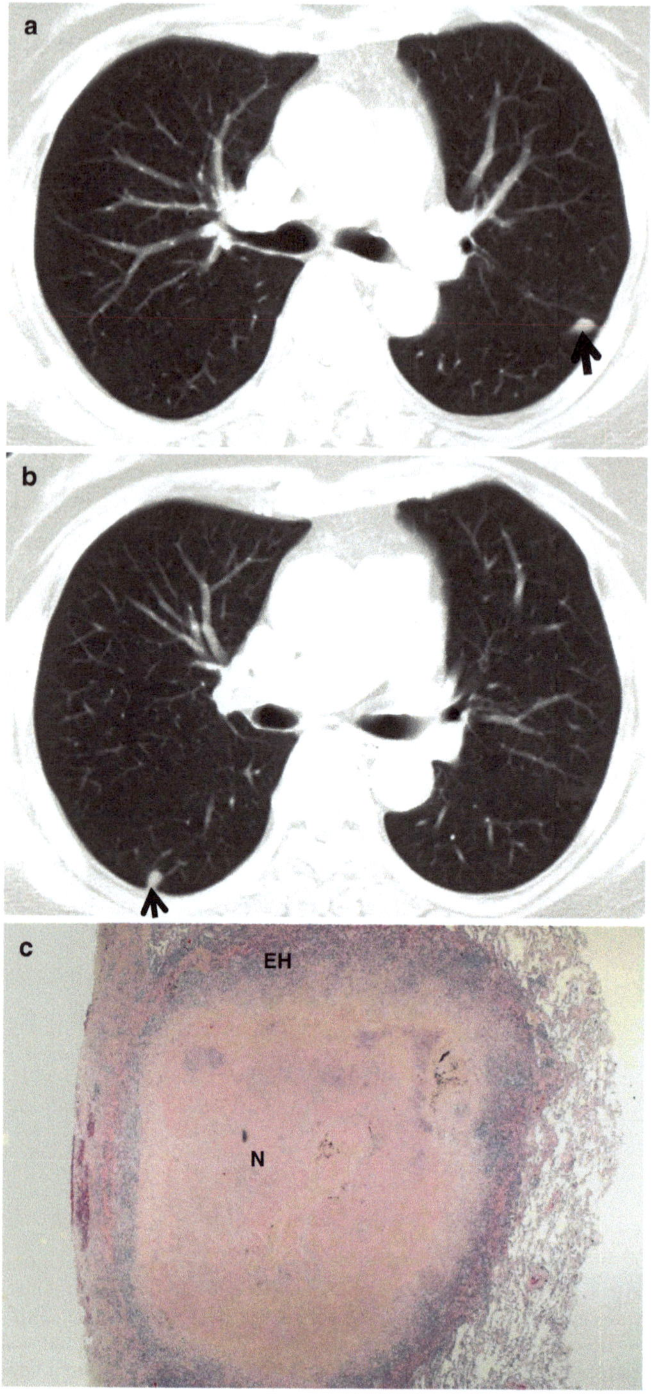


**Fig. 1.2** Small nodules representing rheumatoid nodules in a 70-year-old woman with rheumatoid arthritis. (**a**, **b**) CT scans (5.0-mm section thickness) obtained at levels of main bronchi (**a**) and bronchus intermedius (**b**), respectively, show subcentimeter nodules (*arrows*) in the left upper lobe and right lower lobe. (**c**) Low-magnification (×2) photomicrograph of biopsy specimen obtained from right lower lobe nodule demonstrates central necrosis (*N*) area surrounded by a rim of epithelioid histiocytes (*EH*) and fibrous tissue

**Key Points for Differential Diagnosis**

1. The growth rate of small nodules should be assessed using serial volume measurements rather than diameter. Computer-aided 3D quantitative volume-measurement methods have been developed and applied clinically [4–6].
2. On multivariate analysis, lobulated or spiculated margin and the absence of a satellite nodule appear to be independently associated with malignant nodule with high odd ratio [7].
3. Diffuse, laminated, central nodular, and popcorn-like calcifications within nodules suggest benignity; on the other hand, eccentric or stippled calcifications have been described in malignant nodules [1].
4. Fat or calcification may be observed in up to 30–50 % of pulmonary hamartoma [8].
5. Evaluation based on analyses of wash-in values (>25 HU) plus morphologic features (lobulated or spiculated margin and absence of a satellite nodule) on dynamic CT appears to be the most efficient method for characterizing an SPN [9].
6. By rendering both morphologic and metabolic information, $^{18}$fluorine fluorodeoxyglucose (FDG) PET–CT allows significantly better specificity than CT alone or PET alone, and both PET–CT and PET alone provide more confidence than CT alone for the characterization of SPNs [10]. But due to expensive cost and high radiation dose, it may be selectively used to characterize SPNs when dynamic CT shows inconsistent results between morphologic and hemodynamic nodule characteristics [1].
7. Specifically for small nodules less than 10 mm in diameter, serial volume measurements of nodules are regarded as the most reliable technique for their characterization [1].

## Lung Cancer (Solid Adenocarcinoma)

### Pathology and Pathogenesis

Adenocarcinoma is the most common histologic type of lung cancer in many countries. Adenocarcinoma is a malignant epithelial tumor with glandular differentiation or mucin production, showing lepidic, acinar, papillary, solid, and micropapillary pattern or a mixture of these patterns [11] (Figs. 1.1 and 1.3).

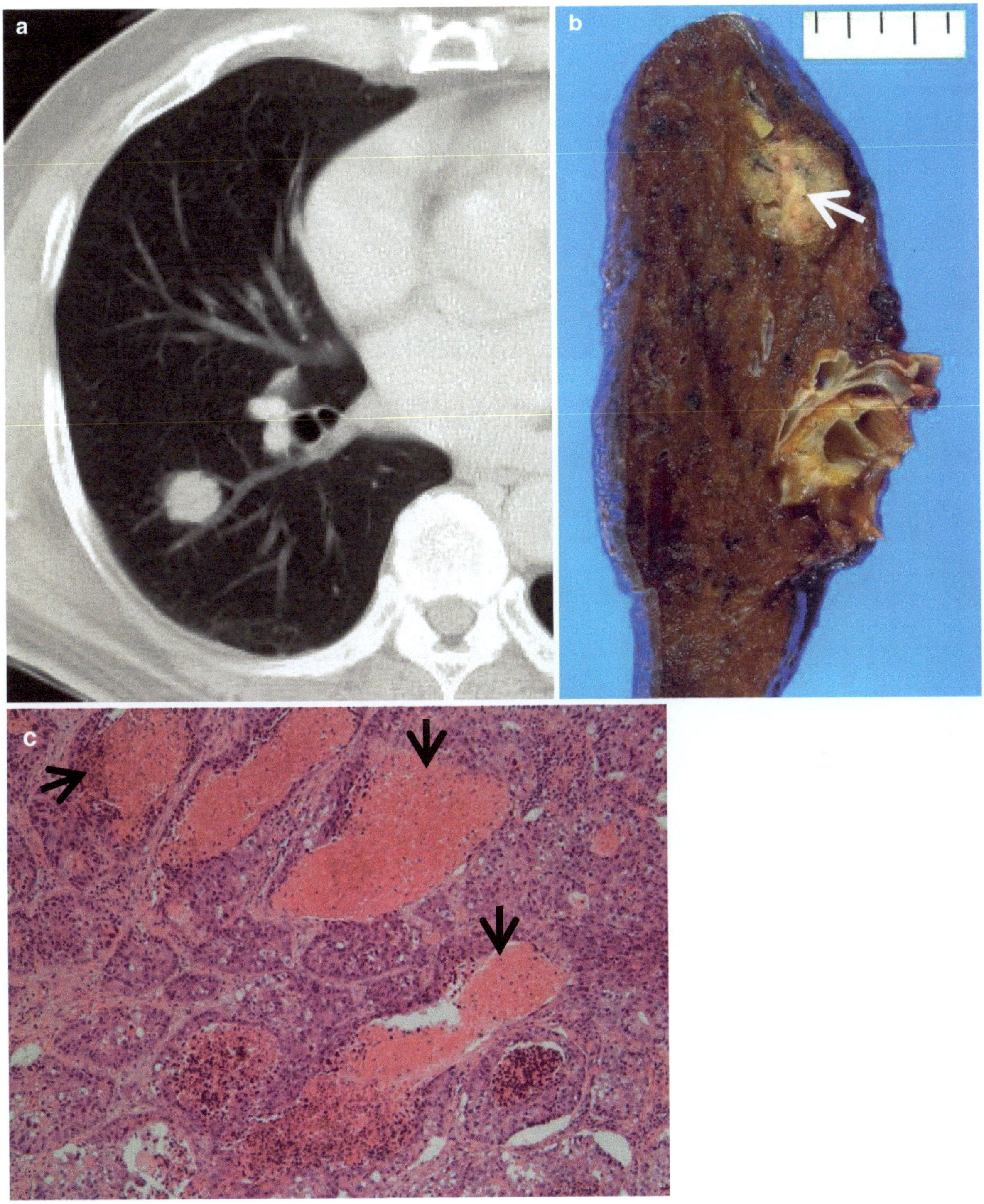


**Fig. 1.3** High-grade lung adenocarcinoma simulating a metastatic nodule from a colon cancer in a 65-year-old man. (**a**) CT scan (5.0-mm section thickness) obtained at level of truncus basalis shows a 21-mm-sized nodule in superior segment of the right lower lobe. (**b**) Gross pathologic specimen demonstrates a yellowish-gray round nodule with yellow necrotic spots (*arrow*). (**c**) High-magnification (×200) photomicrograph discloses high-grade, enteric-type lung adenocarcinoma showing glandular structures with multifocal dirty necrosis (*arrows*) simulating metastatic colon adenocarcinoma

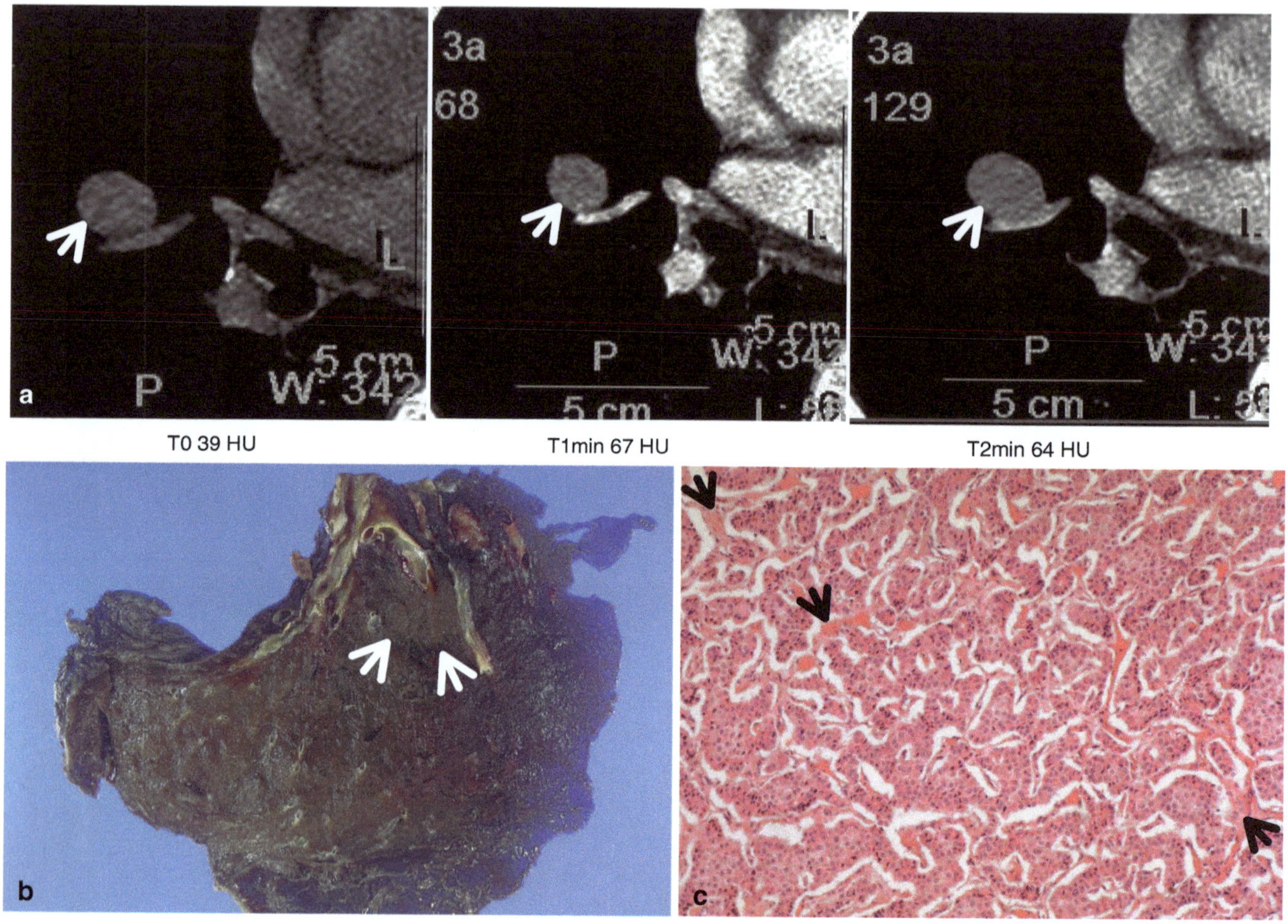


**Fig. 1.4** Typical carcinoid tumor showing high and early enhancement in a 58-year-old man. (**a**) Dynamic CT scans obtained at level of right middle lobar bronchus takeoff show an 18-mm-sized well-defined nodule (*arrows*) in the right middle lobe. Nodule depicts high enhancement (39 HU, 67 HU, and 64 HU; before, at 1 min, and at 2 min after contrast-medium injection, respectively). (**b**) Gross pathologic specimen demonstrates a well-defined nodule (*arrows*) in the right middle lobe adjacent to the segmental bronchus. (**c**) High-magnification (×100) photomicrograph of right lower lobectomy specimen discloses neoplastic cells grouped in small nests separated by numerous thin-walled vascular stroma (*arrows*)

## Symptoms and Signs

Patients with lung cancer presenting with an SPN are usually asymptomatic. Physical examination shows no specific abnormality. In most cases, the SPN is detected by routine chest imaging.

## CT Findings

The characteristic CT finding of solid adenocarcinoma consists of a solitary nodule or mass with a lobulated or spiculated margin. On multivariate analysis, lobulated or spiculated margin and the absence of a satellite nodule appear to be independently associated with malignant nodule with high odd ratio [7]. The nodules enhance following intravenous administration of contrast medium. The enhancement of >25 HU plus morphologic malignant features on dynamic CT appears to be the most efficient method for characterizing a malignant SPN [9].

## CT–Pathology Comparisons

The histopathologic correlation of spiculated margin is variable and may correspond to the strands of fibrous tissue that extend from the tumor margin into the lung, to the direct infiltration of tumor into the adjacent parenchyma, to the

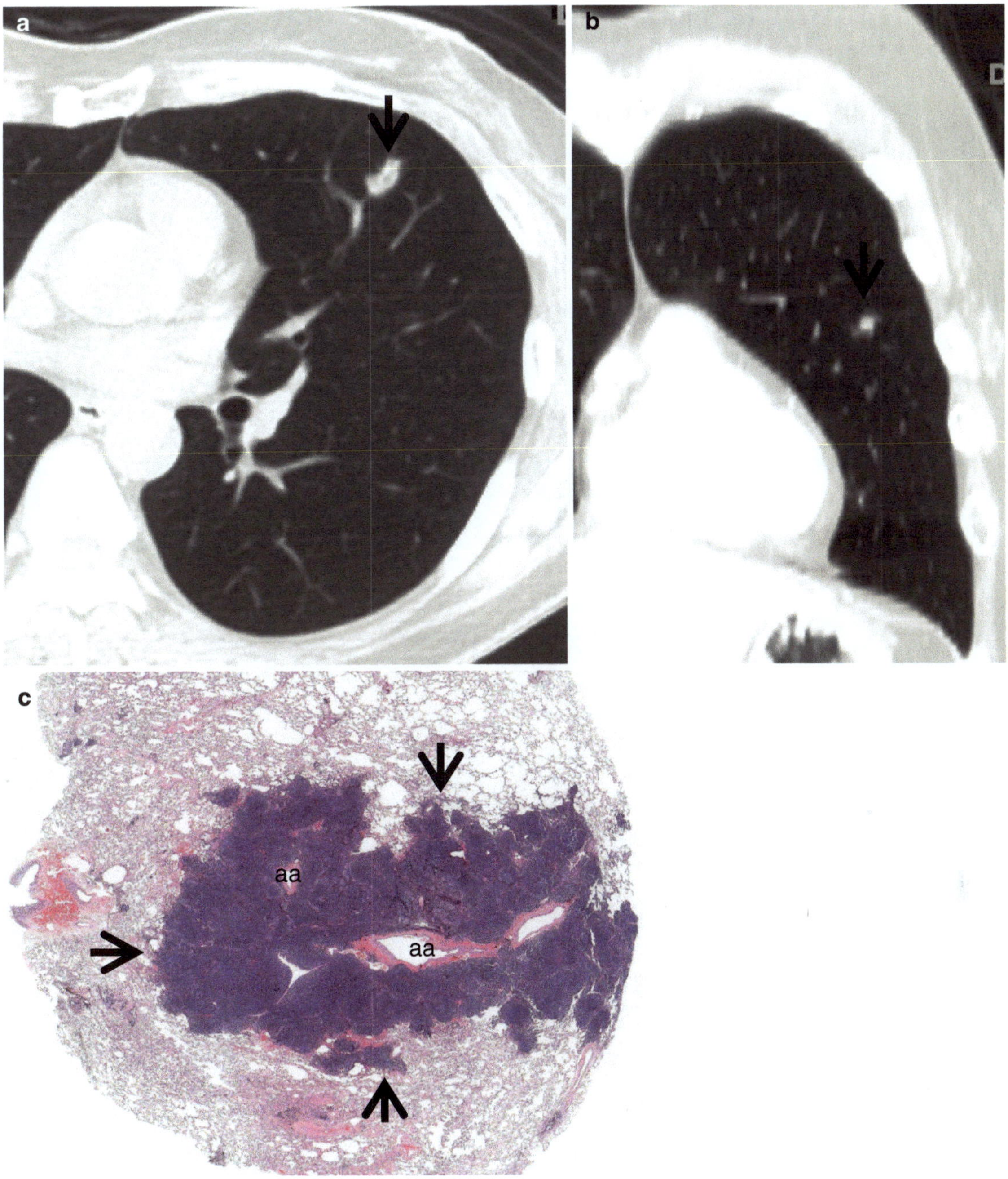


**Fig. 1.5** Bronchus-associated lymphoid tissue (BALT) lymphoma in a 51-year-old woman. (**a**, **b**) Transverse (**a**, 2.5-mm section thickness) and coronal reformatted (**b**) CT scans, respectively, show a 13-mm-sized polygonal nodule (*arrows*) in lingular division of the left upper lobe. Lesion has internal CT air-bronchogram sign. (**c**) Low-magnification (×2) photomicrograph of biopsy specimen obtained from left upper lobe nodule demonstrates lymphoepithelial lesions (*arrows*) surrounding the pulmonary arteries (*aa*) and their accompanying bronchi (lumina have been compressed and collapsed)

small foci of parenchymal collapse as a result of bronchiolar obstruction by the expanding tumor, or to the spread of tumor cells into the lymphatic channels and interstitial tissue of adjacent vessels, airways, or the interlobular septa [12]. The enhancement of nodules presumably reflects the vascular stroma of the tumor [13].

## Patient Prognosis

In solitary adenocarcinomas with part-solid and solid nodule, the prognosis depends on nodal and distant metastasis. Solid tumors exhibit more malignant behavior and have a poorer prognosis than part-solid tumors [14].

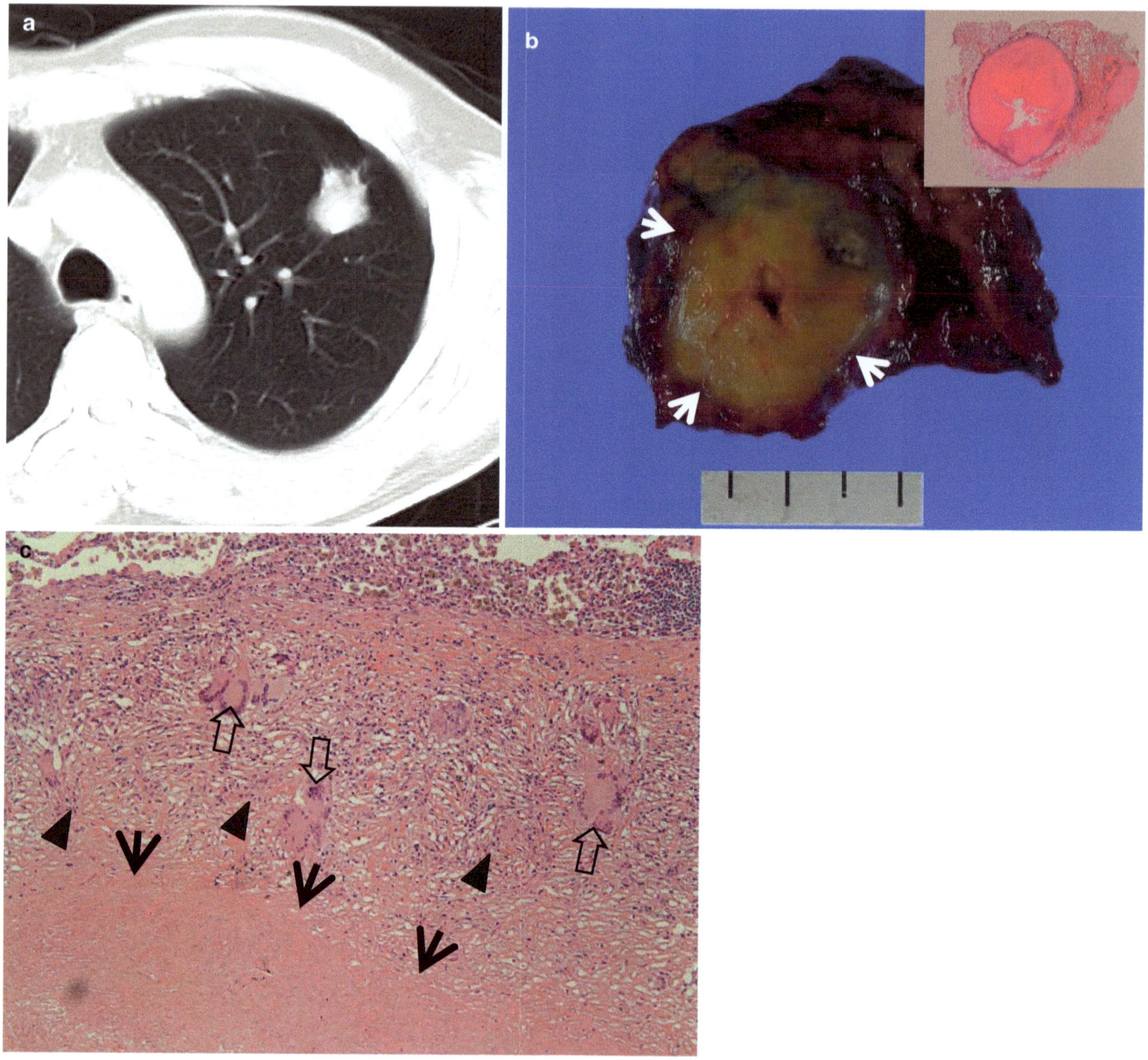


**Fig. 1.6** Tuberculoma in a 47-year-old woman. (**a**) CT scan (5.0-mm section thickness) obtained at level of aortic arch shows a 27-mm-sized nodule in anterior segment of the left upper lobe. (**b**) Gross pathologic specimen demonstrates a well-defined round nodule (*arrows*). *Inset*: central caseation necrosis and peripheral epithelioid histiocytes, multinuclear giant cells, and collagenous tissue. (**c**) High-magnification (×100) photomicrograph discloses a focus of a necrotic lung (*arrows*) surrounded by a layer of epithelioid histiocytes (*arrowheads*) and scattered giant cells (*open arrows*). Numerous lymphocytes and collagenous tissues are seen adjacent to granulomatous inflammation

## Carcinoid or Atypical Carcinoid

### Pathology and Pathogenesis

Carcinoids are slow-growing neuroendocrine tumors characterized by their growth patterns (organoid, trabecular, insular, palisading, ribbon, rosette-like arrangements). They consist of typical carcinoids and atypical carcinoids according to mitotic count or presence of necrosis. Carcinoid is a distinct disease entity, discriminated from other pulmonary neuroendocrine tumors such as large cell neuroendocrine carcinoma or small cell carcinoma [15] (Fig. 1.4).

### Symptoms and Signs

Typical carcinoid may be accompanied with hormone-related manifestations. Fewer than 5 % have the carcinoid syndrome (cutaneous flushing, bronchospasm, diarrhea). Cushing's syndrome can also occur. Atypical carcinoid, one

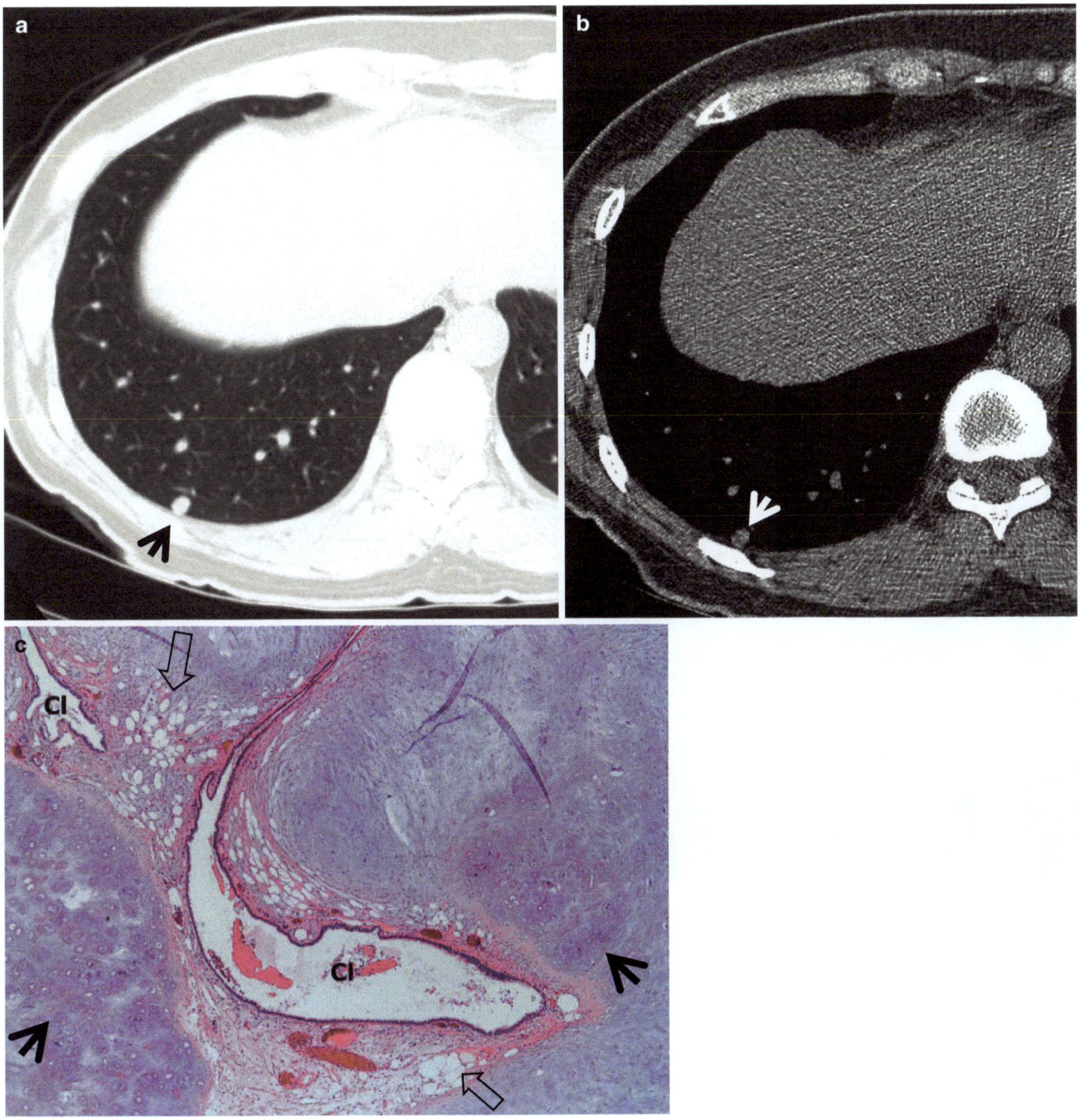


Fig. 1.7 Chondroid hamartoma in a 40-year-old woman. (**a**, **b**) Lung (**a**) and mediastinal (**b**) window images of CT scan (5.0-mm section thickness) obtained at level of lover dome show an 8-mm-sized well-defined nodule (*arrows*) in posterior basal segment of the right lower lobe. Please note fat and calcification attenuation areas within nodule. (**c**) Low-magnification (×10) photomicrograph of wedge resection from the right lower lobe demonstrates islands of mature chondroid (*arrows*) and adipocytic (*open arrows*) tissues. Also note entrapped bronchiolar epithelial cleft (*Cl*) within lesion

on the contrary, may cause lymph node and distant metastasis in half of the cases.

## CT Findings

The most common imaging finding of carcinoid is a lung nodule or a mass. The CT features of a peripheral carcinoid presenting as SPN include a lobulated nodule of high attenuation on contrast-enhanced CT; nodule that densely enhances with IV contrast-medium administration; the presence of calcification (approximately 30 % of cases have calcification on CT) (Fig. 1.4); subsegmental airway involvement on thin-section analysis; and nodules associated with distal hyperlucency, bronchiectasis, or atelectasis [16]. Typical carcinoid tends to be smaller (average diameter 2 cm) than atypical

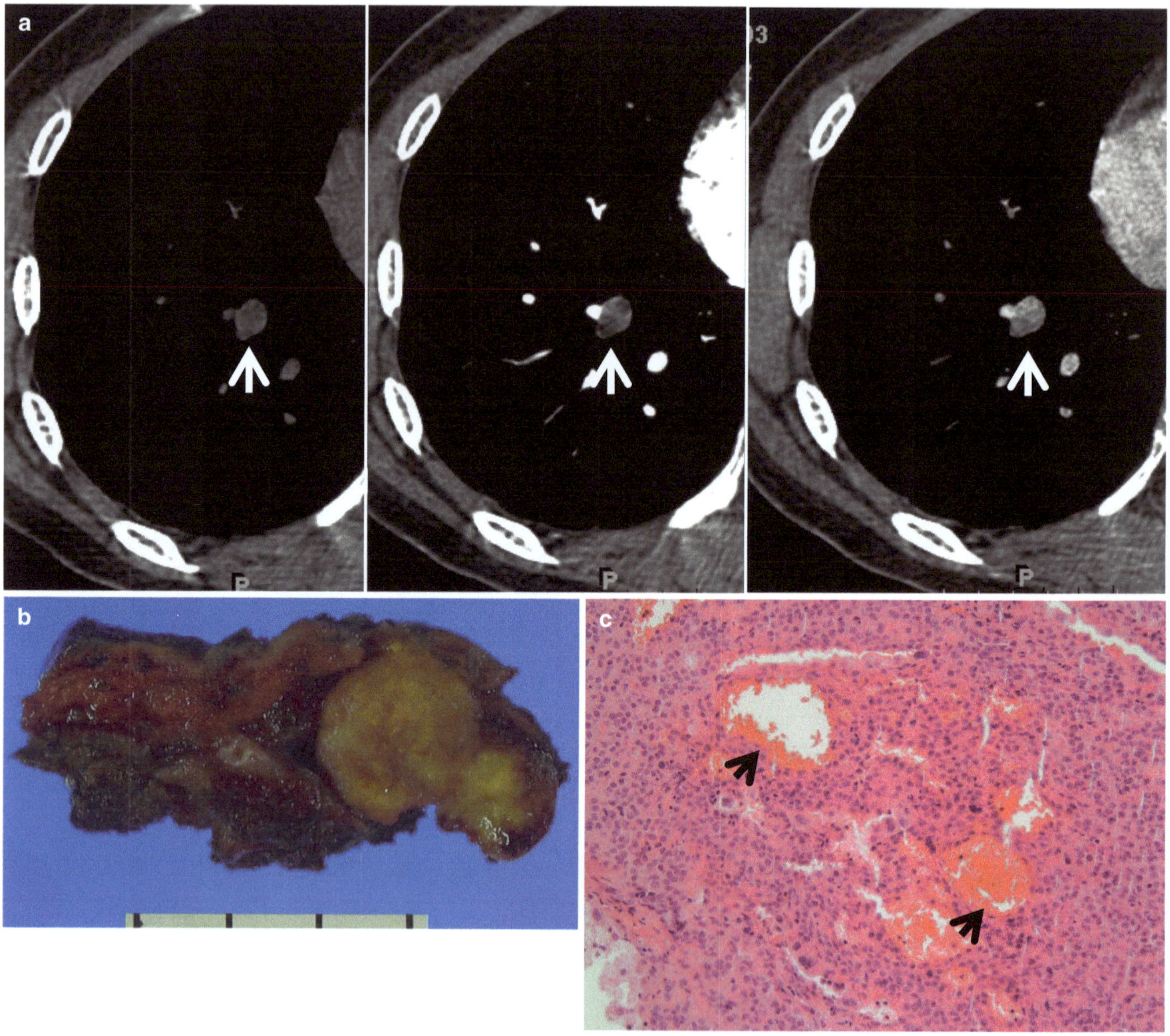


Fig. 1.8 Sclerosing pneumocytoma (hemangiomas) showing high and early enhancement in a 50-year-old woman. (**a**) Dynamic CT scans obtained at level of suprahepatic inferior vena cava (IVC) show a 16-mm-sized well-defined nodule (*arrows*) in the right lower lobe. Nodule depicts high enhancement (19 HU, 38 HU, and 69 HU; before, at 1 min, and at 2 min after contrast-medium injection, respectively). (**b**) Gross pathologic specimen obtained with wedge tumor resection demonstrates a well-defined yellowish round nodule. (**c**) High-magnification (×200) photomicrograph discloses solid growth of polygonal cells with internal hemorrhagic spaces (*arrows*)

carcinoid (average diameter 4 cm) [17]. Secondary effects on distal lung parenchyma such as distal hyperlucency are uncommon in atypical carcinoids.

## CT–Pathology Comparisons

The neoplastic cells of carcinoids are grouped in small nests or trabeculae separated by a prominent vascular stroma (Fig. 1.4). Because of their vascular stroma, most carcinoids show marked enhancement following intravenous administration of contrast [18]. Segmental or lobar atelectasis, obstructive pneumonitis, and segmental oligemia are related to complete or partial obstruction of airway.

## Patient Prognosis

Since typical carcinoids are extremely slow growing, the long-term prognosis is excellent if completely resected.

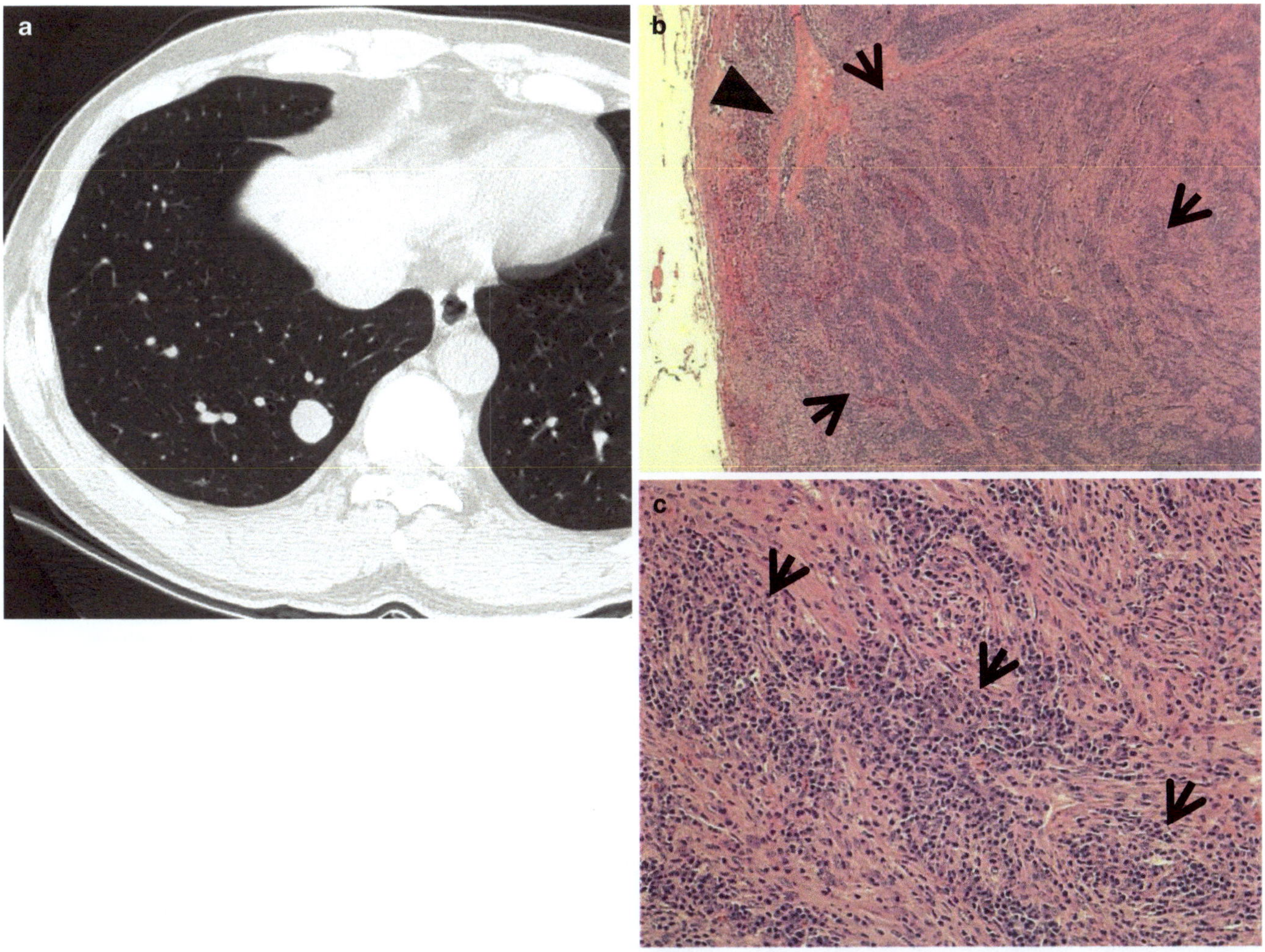


**Fig. 1.9** Inflammatory myofibroblastic tumor in a 29-year-old man. (**a**) Thin-section (2.5-mm section thickness) CT scan obtained at level of suprahepatic inferior vena cava (IVC) shows a 19-mm-sized well-defined nodule in the right lower lobe. (**b**) Low-magnification (×2) photomicrograph of wedge resection of tumor from the right lower lobe demonstrates areas of inflammatory cell infiltration (*arrows*; mainly composed of plasma cells) and fibrosis (*arrowhead*). (**c**) High-magnification (×100) photomicrograph discloses fascicular spindle cell proliferation and admixed areas of lymphocytes and plasma cells (*arrows*)

However, all carcinoids are malignant although indolent. Nodal involvement clearly affects survival [19]. The 5-year survival of patients with atypical carcinoids is only 57 %.

## BALT Lymphoma

### Pathology and Pathogenesis

Pulmonary marginal zone B-cell lymphoma of bronchus-associated lymphoid tissue (BALT) is an extranodal lymphoma, which is thought to arise in acquired MALT secondary to inflammatory or autoimmune processes. The neoplastic cells infiltrate the bronchiolar epithelium, forming lymphoepithelial lesion [20] (Fig. 1.5).

### Symptoms and Signs

BALT lymphoma of SPN rarely causes pulmonary symptoms. Weight loss and night sweating may be found. Extrapulmonary symptoms and signs of connective tissue diseases such as Sjögren's syndrome, systemic lupus erythematosus, and rheumatoid arthritis may occur.

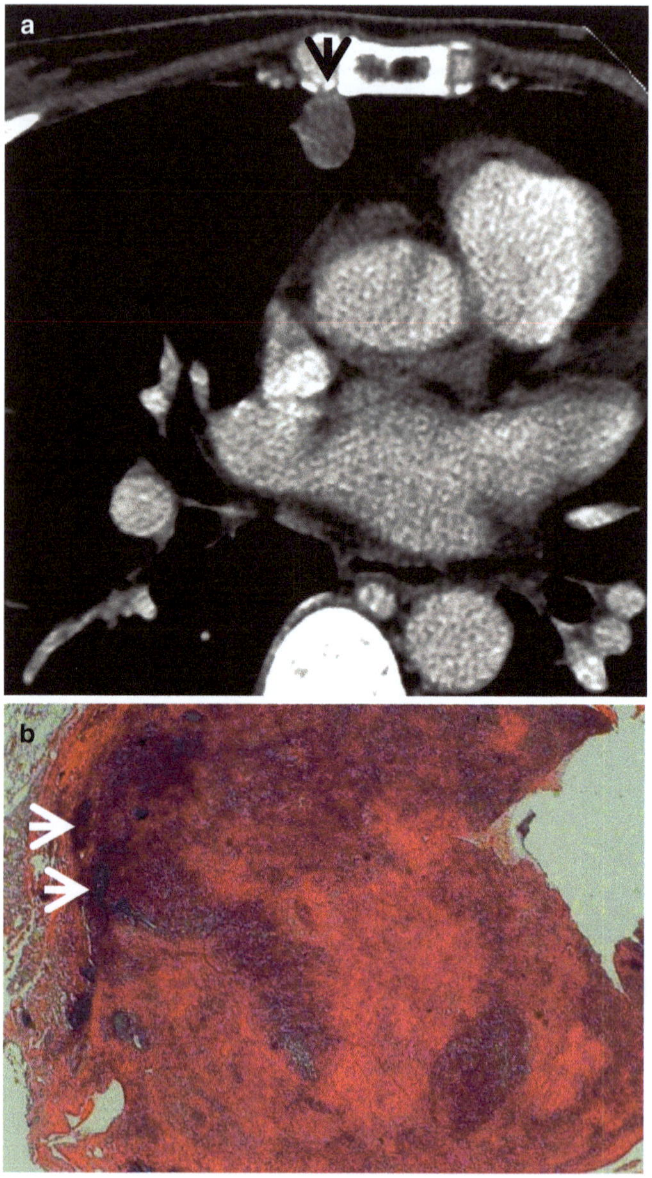


**Fig. 1.10** ANCA (antineutrophil cytoplasmic antibody)-associated granulomatous vasculitis (former Wegener's granulomatosis) manifesting as a solitary pulmonary nodule in a 51-year-old woman. (**a**) Mediastinal window image of CT scan (5.0-mm section thickness) obtained at level of the right middle lobar bronchus shows a 13-mm-sized nodule (*arrow*) in the right middle lobe. (**b**) Low-magnification (×40) photomicrograph of wedge resection of tumor from the right middle lobe demonstrates basophilic inflammatory nodule containing geographic necrotic areas (*arrows*)

## CT Findings

Typical CT findings of BALT lymphoma include solitary (Fig. 1.5) or multifocal nodules or masses and areas of airspace consolidation with an air bronchogram [20, 21]. Less common findings include ground-glass opacity (GGO) lesion, interlobular septal thickening, centrilobular nodules, and bronchial wall thickening and pleural effusion.

**Table 1.1** Common diseases manifesting as solitary pulmonary nodule

| Disease | Key points for differential diagnosis |
|---|---|
| Malignant nodule | |
| Lung cancer | Wash-in values of >25 HU, lobulated or spiculated margin, and absence of a satellite nodule |
| Carcinoid | Lobulated nodule with dense enhancement |
| BALT lymphoma | Consolidation or nodules with air bronchograms |
| Solitary metastasis | |
| Benign nodule | |
| Granuloma | No or little enhancement, satellite nodules |
| Hamartoma | Focal areas of fat or calcification, septal or cleft-like enhancement |
| Sclerosing hemangioma | Subpleural homogeneous mass, rapid and strong enhancement |
| Inflammatory myofibroblastic tumor | |
| Rheumatoid nodule | |
| Parasitic infection (PW) | Cavitary nodules or masses in the subpleural or subfissural areas |
| ANCA-associated granulomatous vasculitis | Multiple, bilateral, subpleural nodules or masses |

*Note*: *HU* Hounsfield unit, *BALT* bronchus-associated lymphoid tissue, *PW* *Paragonimus westermani*, *ANCA* antineutrophil cytoplasmic antibody

## CT–Pathology Comparisons

CT findings of BALT lymphoma showing solitary or multifocal nodules or masses and areas of airspace consolidation are related to proliferation of tumor cells within the interstitium such that the alveolar airspaces and transitional airways are obliterated [22] (Fig. 1.5). Because the bronchi and membranous bronchioles tend to be unaffected, an air bronchogram is common. Interlobular septal thickening, centrilobular nodules, and bronchial wall thickening on CT images are related to perilymphatic interstitial infiltration of tumor cells.

## Patient Prognosis

BALT lymphoma shows the indolent clinical course. The estimated 5- and 10-year overall survival rates have been reported to be 90 and 72 %, respectively [23]. Age and performance status are the prognostic factors.

## Tuberculoma

### Pathology and Pathogenesis

Tuberculoma is a parenchymal nodular histologic reaction which is primarily granulomatous and necrotizing with frequent cavitation. The granulomas may have palisading histiocytes, prominent epithelioid cells, or Langerhans-type giant cells. These necrotizing granulomas can progress to fibrosis and calcification [24] (Fig. 1.6).

### Symptoms and Signs

In active tuberculoma, constitutional symptoms (fever, malaise, night sweating, weight loss, and anorexia) as well as respiratory symptoms (cough, blood-tinged sputum) occur infrequently. Most patients with inactive tuberculoma are asymptomatic.

### CT Findings

Tuberculoma is seen as a sharply marginated round or oval lesion measuring 0.5–4.0 cm in diameter [10, 25]. However, fibrosis related to vessels, interlobular septa, or lung parenchyma adjacent to the nodule may result in a spiculated margin. Calcification within the nodule is present in 20–30 % of cases. Satellite nodules around the tuberculoma may present in as many as 80 % of cases [26]. Following intravenous administration of contrast medium, tuberculomas usually show no or little enhancement although sometimes show ringlike enhancement [27] (Fig. 1.6).

### CT–Pathology Comparisons

The central part of tuberculoma consists of caseous material and the periphery of epithelioid histiocytes and multinucleated giant cells and a variable amount of collagen. Ringlike enhancement corresponds histologically to the granulomatous inflammatory tissue capsule, whereas the non-enhancing area corresponds to the central necrotic material [27].

### Patient Prognosis

It has been reported that a majority of pulmonary tuberculomas show decrease in size with antituberculous treatment. Over 15 % did not show a decrease in size even after the medical treatment [28].

## Hamartoma

### Pathology and Pathogenesis

Hamartomas are benign neoplasms composed of varying proportions of mesenchymal tissues, such as cartilage, fat, smooth muscle, and connective tissue, typically combined with entrapped respiratory epithelium. Genetic studies indicate a neoplastic rather than hamartomatous origin [29] (Fig. 1.7).

### Symptoms and Signs

Pulmonary hamartomas are usually asymptomatic and found incidentally when imaging the chest for other reasons. It can occasionally present with hemoptysis, bronchial obstruction, and cough (especially endobronchial types) [30].

### CT Findings

The characteristic CT findings of hamartomas are comprised of a lesion of 2.5 cm or smaller in diameter, of a smooth margin, and of focal areas of fat (CT attenuation values between −40 and −120 HU) or calcification [8]. However, these findings are present in only 30–50 % of the tumors (Fig. 1.7). Recent MRI and dynamic CT studies demonstrate septal or cleft-like enhancements of pulmonary hamartomas [31, 32].

### CT–Pathology Comparisons

Hamartomas are composed of mature cartilage and fat, which are often surrounded by a thin layer of loose mesenchymal tissue. Recent MRI and dynamic CT studies demonstrated septal or cleft-like enhancement of pulmonary hamartomas [31, 32]. Pathologically, these structures were found to represent variable mesenchymal tissue components arrayed along respiratory epithelial cells lining the cleft and show richer vascularity than main cartilaginous portion of pulmonary hamartoma.

### Patient Prognosis

Surgical resection is curative. Recurrence or malignant transformation is rare.

## Sclerosing Hemangioma

### Pathology and Pathogenesis

Although sclerosing hemangiomas (SHs) were originally termed as a variant of hemangiomas, now there is a consensus that they are epithelial tumors. SH comprises a mixture of four histologic patterns, such as papillary, sclerotic, solid, and hemorrhagic [33] (Fig. 1.8).

### Symptoms and Signs

Most patients are asymptomatic at the time of diagnosis.

### CT Findings

On CT scans, SH appears as a well-defined, round- or oval-shaped, homogeneous mass with smooth margin in subpleural area [34]. On dynamic CT, it has strong and rapid enhancement [35] (Fig. 1.8). Unusual manifestations of SH include mediastinal mass, tumor with a cystic appearance, air trapping around the tumor, multiple tumors, or a tumor surrounded by multiple daughter nodules in the same lobe; it can also be accompanied by hilar lymph node metastasis [36–40].

### CT–Pathology Comparisons

On CT–pathology comparisons, dynamic characteristics of sclerosing hemangioma depend on the levels of hemangiomatous or papillary (early and strong enhancement) and solid or sclerotic (slow and persistent enhancement and little washout) components present [35] (Fig. 1.8).

### Patient Prognosis

Regardless of surgical resection, the prognosis of patients with sclerosing hemangioma is excellent in cases manifesting as SPN.

## Inflammatory Myofibroblastic Tumor

### Pathology and Pathogenesis

Inflammatory myofibroblastic tumor (IMT) is a proliferation of cells showing myofibroblastic differentiation, and IMT is a subgroup of the broad category of inflammatory pseudotumors and is composed of a variable mixture of collagen, inflammatory cells, and bland spindle cells showing myofibroblastic differentiation [41] (Fig. 1.9).

### Symptoms and Signs

Most patients are asymptomatic.

### CT Findings

On CT, IMT usually is seen as a well-circumscribed, solitary, peripheral pulmonary nodule or mass with a variable degree of contrast enhancement [41, 42] (Fig. 1.9). The lesion may be homogeneous or heterogeneous after contrast enhancement. Intratumoral calcification has been identified in about 15 % of cases. Endoluminal airway involvement has been known to occur in 10–80 % cases.

### CT–Pathology Comparisons

According to the recent theory on the pathogenesis of IMT, the tumor appears to originate from fibroblasts in the connective tissue of the airway [43]. In one series on the studies of CT–pathology correlation of IMT, a much higher incidence of airway involvement (80 %) was noted [41]. Peripheral solitary nodules seen on CT were also related to an adjacent bronchiole on histopathologic examinations (Fig. 1.9). Therefore, when a well-defined polypoid endobronchial nodule or a well-defined peripheral SPN related to an adjacent airway is seen on CT, IMT should be included in the differential diagnosis.

### Patient Prognosis

Since incomplete resection is related to a substantial risk of recurrence and locally aggressive behavior, complete surgical resection is the only treatment to prevent recurrence.

## ANCA-Associated Granulomatous Vasculitis (Former Wegener's Granulomatosis) Manifesting as a Solitary Pulmonary Nodule

### Pathology and Pathogenesis

The classic pattern of pulmonary involvement of ANCA-associated granulomatous vasculitis is that of multiple nodules with frequent cavitation. Solid nodular zones of consolidation with foci of punctate or geographic necrosis, associated with granulomatous inflammation and vasculitis, are often seen [44] (Fig. 1.10).

## Symptoms and Signs

When detected as SPN, systemic symptoms are usually absent. Patients may have cough or blood-tinged sputum.

## CT Findings

The most common pattern on CT images at the initial presentation is the presence of nodules or masses in 90 % of cases [45] (Fig. 1.10). The distribution of nodules or masses seen on CT is multiple in 85 % of patients, bilateral in 67 %, subpleural in 89 %, and peribronchovascular in 41 %. Airway involvements are also common with segmental or subsegmental bronchial wall thickening in 70 % of patients and large airway abnormality in 30 % of patients. Another common manifestation is airspace consolidation and GGO with random or patchy distribution, seen in 25–50 % of cases. Centrilobular nodules and a tree-in-bud sign pattern may be seen in up to 10 % of patients, usually mixed with other changes.

## CT–Pathology Comparisons

The most common imaging findings of pulmonary involvement of ANCA-associated granulomatous vasculitis are multiple bilateral pulmonary nodules with frequent cavitation which are histologically corresponded to large areas of parenchymal necrosis, granulomatous inflammation, and vasculitis [45]. Airspace consolidation and GGO with random or patchy distribution are regarded to diffuse alveolar hemorrhage caused by necrotizing capillaritis. Centrilobular nodules and the tree-in-bud sign may result from bronchiolar inflammatory changes rather than from vasculitis.

## Patient Prognosis

Solitary nodular form of ANCA-associated granulomatous vasculitis may have a better prognosis [46]. With the introduction of the use of cyclophosphamide in immunosuppressive therapy, complete remission has been achieved in 70–90 % of patients, but relapses are common. A poor prognosis is associated with DAH, severe azotemia, an advanced age, and positivity for proteinase 3 ANCA [47].

# Ground-Glass Opacity Nodule

## Definition

Ground-glass opacity nodules (GGNs, or subsolid nodules) are further divided into nonsolid pure GGNs and part-solid nodules; the former nodules have no patch of parenchyma that are completely obscured with soft tissue structures (Fig. 1.11), whereas the latter nodules harbor such patches [48, 49] (Fig. 1.12).

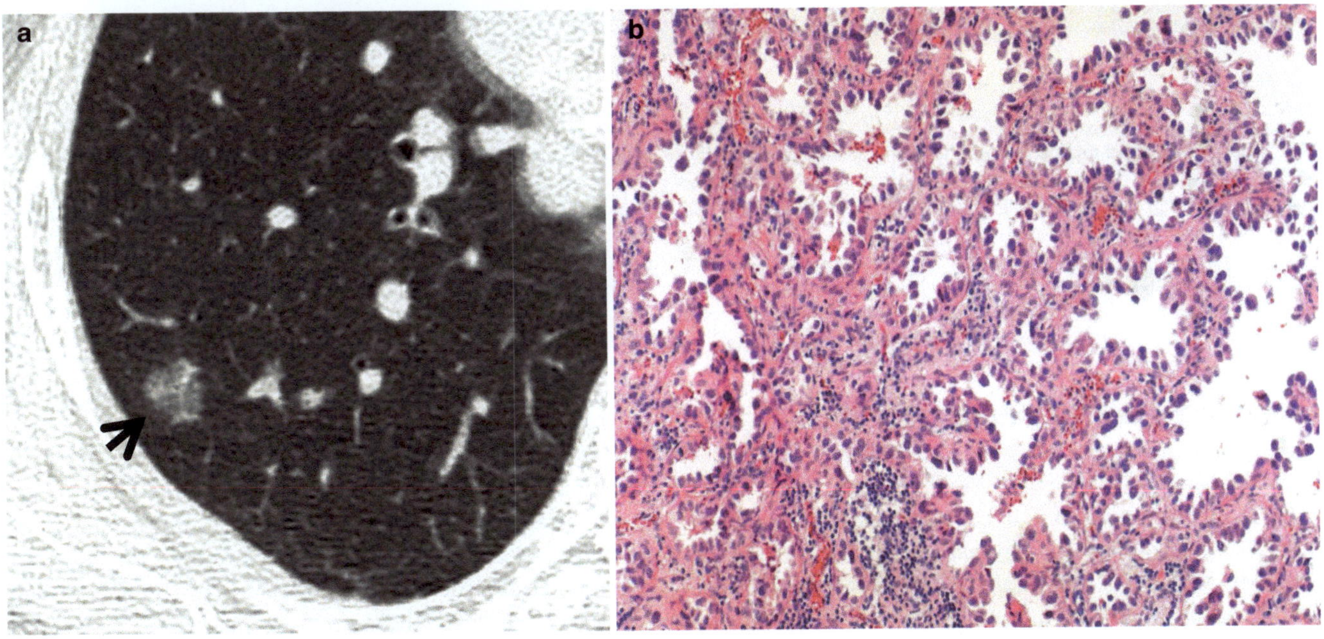


**Fig. 1.11** Pure ground-glass opacity nodule representing adenocarcinoma in situ (AIS, former bronchioloalveolar carcinoma) in a 45-year-old woman. (**a**) Targeted view of thin-section (1.5-mm section thickness) CT scan obtained at the basal segmental bronchi shows a 13-mm-sized ground-glass opacity nodule (*arrow*) in superior segment of the right lower lobe. (**b**) High-magnification photomicrograph shows spread of neoplastic cells on airspace surface with preservation of underlying architecture (so-called lepidic growth). Note thickened alveolar walls

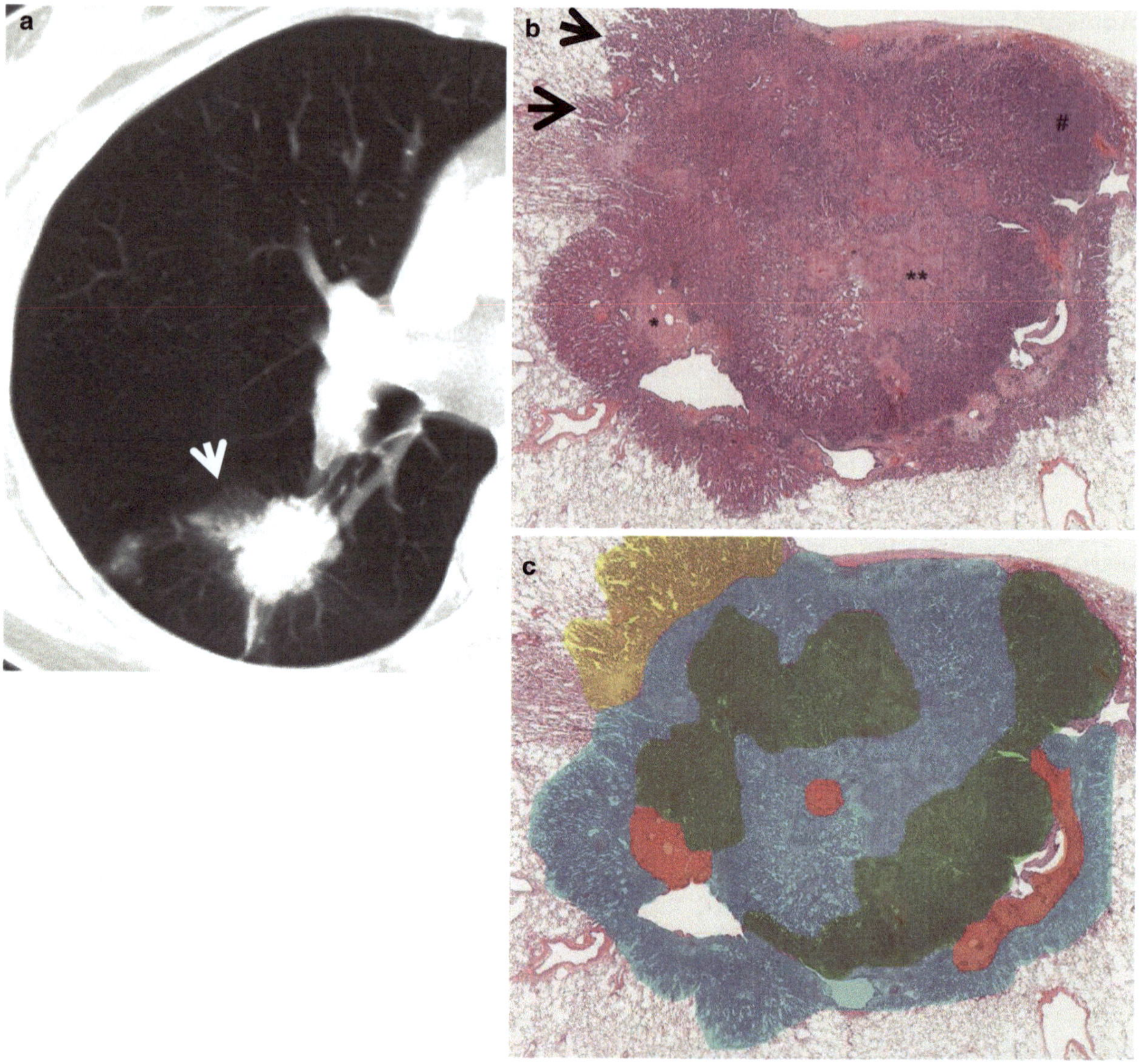


**Fig. 1.12** A part-solid nodule representing lung adenocarcinoma in a 67-year-old woman. (**a**) Targeted view of thin-section (2.5-mm section thickness) CT scan obtained at superior segmental bronchus level of the right lower lobe shows a 25-mm-sized part-solid nodule (*arrow*) in superior segment of the right lower lobe. (**b**) Low-magnification (×10) photomicrograph (H & E stain) demonstrates internal scar tissue (*), surrounding areas of acinar (**) and solid (#) adenocarcinoma patterns, and lepidic pattern (*arrows*, uniform cuboid cellular proliferation along alveolar walls) only at tumor periphery. (**c**) In a schematic drawing of tumor components, percentages of lepidic growth pattern (*yellow area*), acinar pattern (*blue area*), solid pattern (*green area*), and central fibrosis (*red area*) are estimated as 10, 50, 30, and 10 %, respectively (Reprinted from Lee et al. [70] with permission)

## Diseases Causing the Pattern

The persistent presence of a GGN at thin-section CT (TSCT), in more than 80 % of cases, suggests the diagnosis of *atypical adenomatous hyperplasia (AAH)*, *adenocarcinoma in situ (AIS)*, *minimally invasive adenocarcinoma (MIA)*, or invasive lung adenocarcinomas [48]. AAH and AIS are collectively called preinvasive adenocarcinoma [11] (Figs. 1.13 and 1.14). Among lung cancer screening-detected nodules, malignancy rates of GGNs (34 %, subsolid nodules) are higher than that of solid nodules (7 %); in particular, the rates of part-solid nodules and pure GGNs (nonsolid nodules) were 64 and 18 %, respectively [50]. Bronchus-associated lymphoid tissue (BALT) lymphoma may also appear as GGN [20]. Pulmonary non-hemorrhagic or hemorrhagic metastases from extrathoracic malignant melanoma, choriocarcinoma, or renal cell carcinoma may also be seen as a GGN [51].

Subsolid nodules can be seen in nontumorous conditions including *Loeffler's syndrome* (*pulmonary infiltration with eosinophilia* [*PIE*] *syndrome*), invasive pulmonary aspergillosis, and organizing pneumonia [52] (Table 1.2).

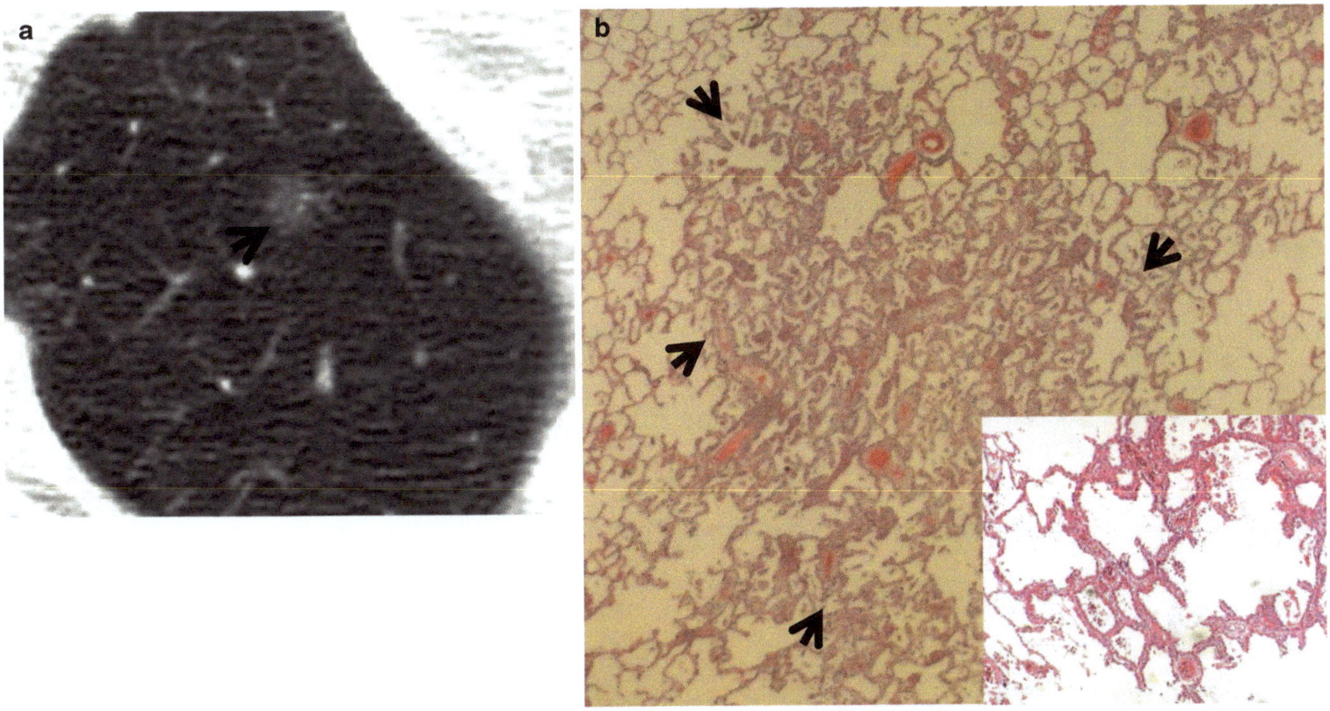


Fig. 1.13 Atypical adenomatous hyperplasia in a 44-year-old man. (**a**) Targeted view of thin-section (2.5-mm section thickness) CT scan obtained throughout the right upper lobe shows a 9-mm-sized ground-glass opacity nodule (*arrow*) in the right upper lobe. (**b**) Low-magnification (×10) photomicrograph (H & E stain) demonstrates atypical epithelial cell proliferation along alveolar septa in atypical adenomatous hyperplasia (*arrows*). *Inset*: no attendant stromal thickening and harbors more airspaces and fewer cellular components histopathologically than adenocarcinoma in situ

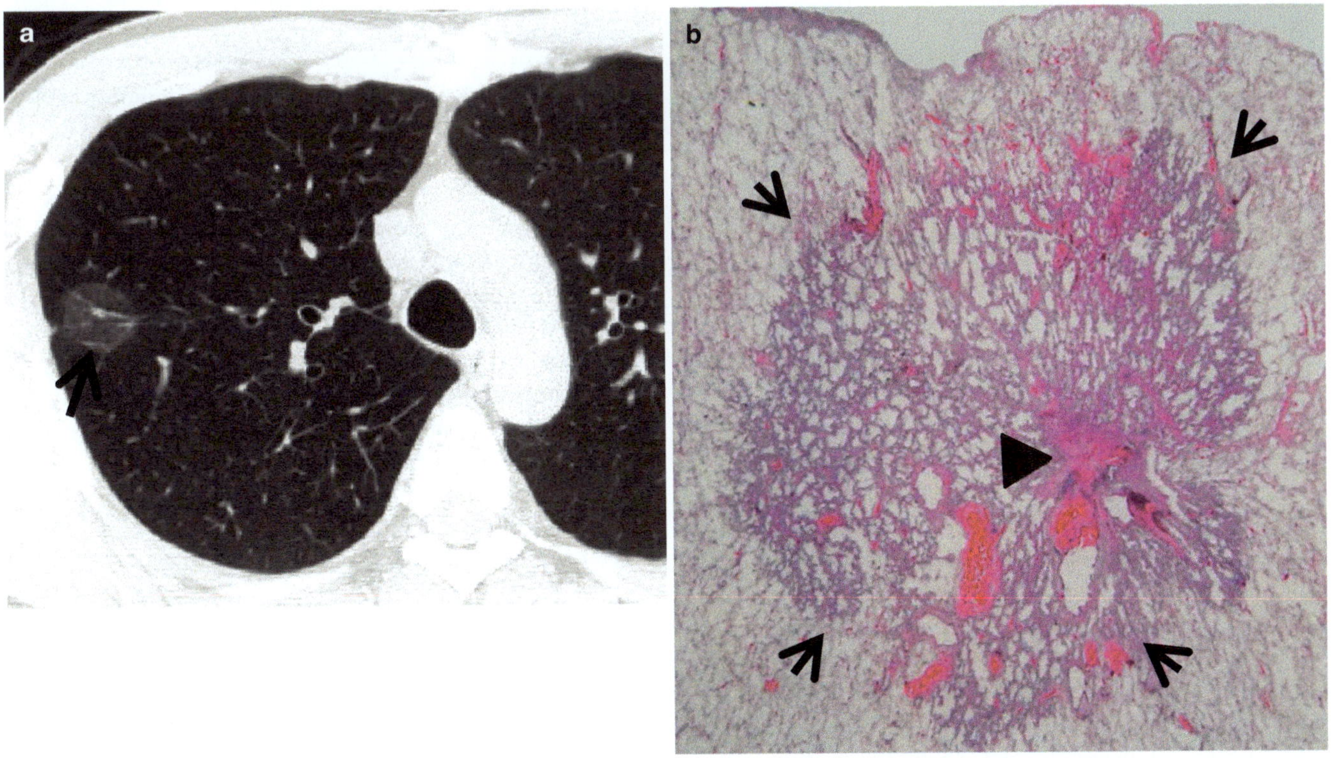


Fig. 1.14 Adenocarcinoma in situ (former bronchioloalveolar carcinoma) in a 56-year-old man. (**a**) Lung window image of thin-section (1.5-mm section thickness) CT scan obtained at level of the azygos arch shows a 19-mm-sized ground-glass opacity nodule (*arrow*) in the right upper lobe. (**b**) Low-magnification (×10) photomicrograph (H & E stain) demonstrates lepidic tumor growth along alveolar walls (*arrows*). Please note maintained alveolar architecture. *Arrowhead* indicates scar tissue within tumor

## Distribution

Likelihood ratio for malignancy in upper and middle lobe nodule is 1.22 as compared with 0.66 in lower lobe nodule [3].

## Clinical Considerations

Fleeting or transient and migratory nature of GGNs favors the diagnosis of an inflammatory condition such as Loeffler's syndrome, whereas persistent presence suggests the diagnosis of preinvasive, minimally invasive, and invasive lung adenocarcinomas or BALT lymphoma [48, 52].

**Table 1.2** Common diseases manifesting as ground-glass opacity nodule

| Disease | Key points for differential diagnosis |
|---|---|
| Tumorous condition | |
| AAH | Faint pure GGN usually < 5 mm |
| Nonmucinous AIS | Pure GGN |
| MIA | Part-solid nodule for nonmucinous MIA, solid or part-solid nodule for mucinous MIA |
| BALT lymphoma | Consolidation or nodules with air bronchograms |
| Metastasis from melanoma or RCC | |
| Nontumorous condition | |
| Loeffler's syndrome | Transient, migrating periphery GGO or consolidation |
| Invasive pulmonary aspergillosis | Nodules with a GGO, wedge-shaped pleural-based areas of consolidation |
| Organizing pneumonia | |

*Note*: *AAH* atypical adenomatous hyperplasia, *AIS* adenocarcinoma in situ, *MIA* minimally invasive adenocarcinoma, *BALT* bronchus-associated lymphoid tissue, *RCC* renal cell carcinoma, *GGN* ground-glass nodule, *GGO* ground-glass opacity

**Table 1.3** IASLC/ATS/ERS classification of lung adenocarcinoma in resection specimens

| |
|---|
| Preinvasive lesions |
| Atypical adenomatous hyperplasia |
| Adenocarcinoma in situ (≤3 cm, former BAC) |
| Nonmucinous |
| Mucinous |
| Mixed mucinous/nonmucinous |
| Minimally invasive adenocarcinoma (≤3-cm lepidic predominant tumor with ≤5-mm invasion) |
| Nonmucinous |
| Mucinous |
| Mixed mucinous/nonmucinous |
| Invasive adenocarcinoma |
| Lepidic predominant (former nonmucinous BAC pattern, with >5-mm invasion) |
| Acinar predominant |
| Papillary predominant |
| Micropapillary predominant |
| Solid predominant with mucin production |
| Variants of invasive adenocarcinoma |
| Invasive mucinous adenocarcinoma (former mucinous BAC) |
| Colloid |
| Fetal (low and high grade) |
| Enteric |

*Note*: *IASLC* International Association for the Study of Lung Cancer, *ATS* American Thoracic Society, *ERS* European Respiratory Society, *BAC* bronchioloalveolar carcinoma

**Key Points for Differential Diagnosis**

1. New lung adenocarcinoma classifications have been put forth by the International Association for the Study of Lung Cancer/American Thoracic Society/European Respiratory Society. The principal changes are as follows: (1) an end to the use of the term bronchioloalveolar carcinoma (BAC; the term is replaced by adenocarcinoma in situ [AIS]), (2) the addition of a new category of minimally invasive adenocarcinoma (e.g., patients with a 2-cm or smaller AIS with an invasive area measuring ≤5 mm in thickness), (3) elimination of the category of mixed subtype adenocarcinoma, and (4) renaming of what was formerly referred to as mucinous BAC as mucinous adenocarcinoma [11] (Table 1.3).
2. Although the maximum diameter (8 mm ± 3.8) of AAH tended to be smaller than that of AIS or invasive adenocarcinoma with predominantly lepidic pattern (13 mm ± 6.9), there was no significant difference in morphologic findings at TSCT between AAH and AIS or invasive adenocarcinoma [48].
3. According to a study [53], (1) the size >16.4 mm in diameter in pure GGNs is associated with invasive adenocarcinoma and the size is closely correlated with the mass (nodule volume × attenuation) of a nodule, (2) the mass is significantly larger in invasive adenocarcinoma (mean attenuation value, −507 HU) than no (mean attenuation value, −620) or minimally invasive (mean attenuation value, −636 HU) adenocarcinoma in both uni- and multivariate analyses, (3) the presence of air bronchogram favors the diagnosis of invasive adenocarcinomas in univariate analysis and had very close correlation with nodule size, and finally (4) none with pure GGNs had tumor recurrence or metastasis at 3- or 5-year follow-up study.

## Atypical Adenomatous Hyperplasia (AAH)

### Pathology and Pathogenesis

AAH is a localized, small (usually 0.5 cm or less) proliferation of mildly to moderately atypical type II pneumocytes or Clara cells lining alveolar walls and sometimes respiratory bronchioles (Fig. 1.13). There is a continuum of morphologic changes between AAH and AIS. A spectrum of cellularity and atypia occurs in AAH [11].

### Symptoms and Signs

Since AAHs are incidentally detected in the lungs resected for adenocarcinoma or by screening chest CT, patients with AAH are asymptomatic.

### CT Findings

On CT, AAH is characteristically shown as a small pure ground-glass nodule (GGN) usually measuring <5 mm [54]. However, no significant difference in the maximum diameter of GGN of AAH and AIS on TSCT was found [48]. The ground-glass opacities (GGOs) of AAH observed on TSCT are typically very faint [49]. AAH can be either single or multiple [55].

### CT–Pathology Comparisons

AAH generally exhibits no attendant stromal thickening and harbors more airspaces and fewer cellular components histopathologically than AIS. Therefore, the GGOs of AAH observed on TSCT are typically very faint [49].

### Patient Prognosis

AAHs have been proposed as possible precursors of peripheral adenocarcinoma although this hypothesis has yet to be confirmed [56].

## Adenocarcinoma in Situ (AIS)

### Pathology and Pathogenesis

AIS (one of the lesions formerly known as BAC) is a localized small (≤3 cm) adenocarcinoma with growth restricted to neoplastic cells along preexisting alveolar structures (lepidic growth), lacking stromal, vascular, or pleural invasion. Papillary or micropapillary patterns and intra-alveolar tumor cells are absent (Fig. 1.14). AIS is subdivided into nonmucinous and mucinous variants. Virtually, all cases of AIS are nonmucinous [11].

### Symptoms and Signs

AIS, owing to its small size and peripheral location, rarely causes symptoms or signs.

### CT Findings

On CT, nonmucinous AIS appears typically as a pure GGN. Mucinous AIS can appear as a solid nodule or as a part-solid nodule [57]. Mean maximum diameter of AIS is 13 mm ± 6.9 [48]. The pure GGN of AIS usually appears on TSCT as slightly higher attenuation compared with the very faint GGN of AAH [49]. AIS also can be either single or multiple.

### CT–Pathology Comparisons

The GGOs of AIS generally manifest as regions of slightly higher attenuation relative to the very faint opacities of AAH. This difference in GGN attenuation is probably due to histopathologic dissimilarity in the amount of alveolar airspace and cellular components contained within the nodule [58] (Fig. 1.14). The solid or part-solid nodular features of mucinous AIS may be histopathologically related to (1) a prominent central scar, (2) compact tumor cells surrounded by abundant mucin, and (3) alveolar spaces filled with mucin and mononuclear cells and alveolar walls lined with mucin-containing tumor cells [57].

### Patient Prognosis

Patients with AIS will have 100 % disease-specific survival if they undergo complete resection [59, 60].

## Minimally Invasive Adenocarcinoma (MIA)

### Pathology and Pathogenesis

MIA is a small, solitary adenocarcinoma (≤3 cm), with a predominantly lepidic pattern and ≤5-mm invasion in greatest dimension in any one focus (Fig. 1.15). MIA is usually nonmucinous but rarely may be mucinous. MIA is, by definition, solitary and discrete. The criteria for MIA can be applied in the setting of multiple tumors, only if the other tumors are regarded as synchronous primaries rather than intrapulmonary metastases. The invasive component to be

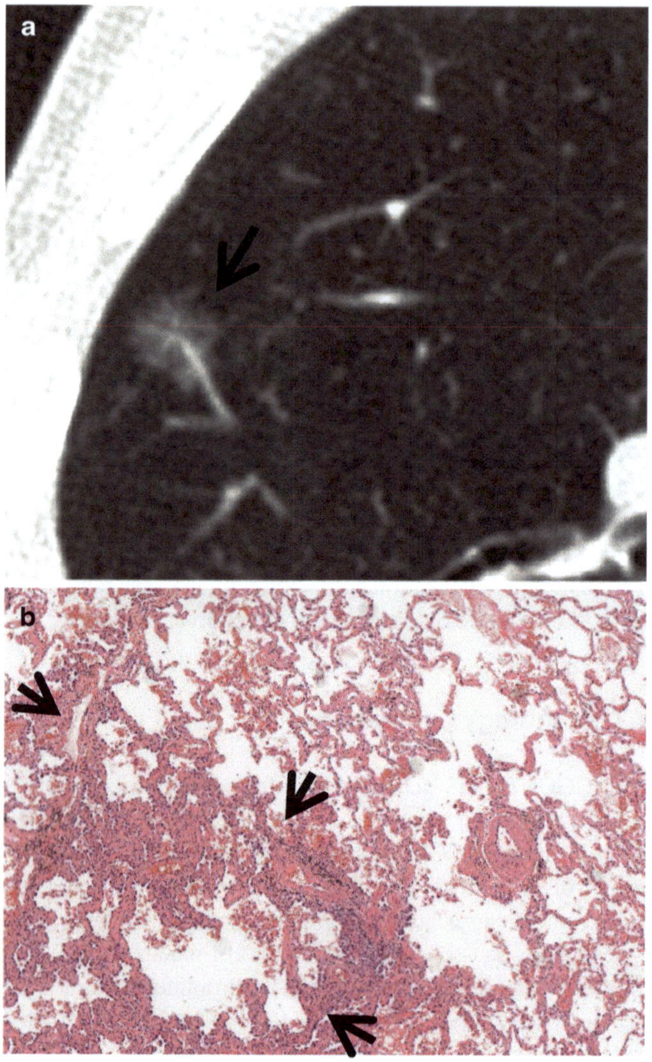


**Fig. 1.15** Minimally invasive adenocarcinoma (MIA) in a 64-year-old woman. (**a**) Targeted view of thin-section (2.0-mm section thickness) CT scan obtained throughout the right upper lobe shows a 12-mm-sized ground-glass opacity nodule (*arrow*) in the right upper lobe. (**b**) High-magnification (×100) photomicrograph demonstrates tumor consisting of predominant background lepidic subtype and mixed area (*arrows*) of invasive acinar subtype (less than 5 mm in thickness, thus so-called minimally invasive adenocarcinoma)

measured in MIA is defined as histologic subtypes other than a lepidic pattern or tumor cells infiltrating myofibroblastic stroma. MIA is excluded if the tumor invades lymphatics, blood vessels, or pleura or contains tumor necrosis. If multiple microinvasive areas are found in one tumor, the size of the largest invasive area should be measured in the largest dimension, and it should be ≤5 mm in size [61].

### Symptoms and Signs

As in the case of AIS, patients with MIA are usually asymptomatic.

### CT Findings

Imaging features of MIA are as yet not fully described. A provisional description of nonmucinous MIA on TSCT is a part-solid nodule consisting of a predominant ground-glass component and a small solid component measuring 5 mm or less [61, 62]. Mucinous MIA can appear as a solid or part-solid nodule [63]. MIA is, by definition, solitary and discrete. For nonsolid nodules, shape does not appear to be a differentiating criterion between AIS and MIA.

### CT–Pathology Comparisons

Invasive component of MIA has been thought to be characteristically solid at CT, and the noninvasive lepidic component is hazy and nonsolid (GGO) at thin-section CT [64]. Because the histopathologic components of small adenocarcinomas can include alveolar collapse, inflammatory cells, fibroblasts, fibrosis, as well as invasive adenocarcinoma, the size of the solid component may be larger at CT than the size of the actual invasive adenocarcinoma component [62]. However, because the invasive component in MIA is defined histopathologically [11], the invasive component (≤5 mm in its greatest dimension) does not contribute much to increase CT attenuation and appears as a pure GGN of 10 mm or greater in diameter, not differently from AIS or invasive adenocarcinoma of greater than 16.4 mm in diameter [53]. For the mucinous MIA, the mucin may contribute to a solid or part-solid appearance of tumor at CT.

### Patient Prognosis

Patients with nonmucinous MIA (predominantly lepidic growth pattern and invasive components of acinar, papillary, or micropapillary pattern) have shown near 100 % disease-specific or very favorable overall survival, if completely resected [65–67]. There is very limited data regarding mucinous MIA. A recent series of surgically resected solitary mucinous BAC in eight patients had 100 % overall 5-year survival rates [68].

## Loeffler's Syndrome

### Pathology and Pathogenesis

The lung in Loeffler's syndrome shows intra-alveolar eosinophils and macrophages with proteinaceous exudate. Charcot–Leyden crystals, interstitial eosinophilic infiltrate, organizing pneumonia, or eosinophilic microabscess or granuloma may be present [69] (Fig. 1.16).

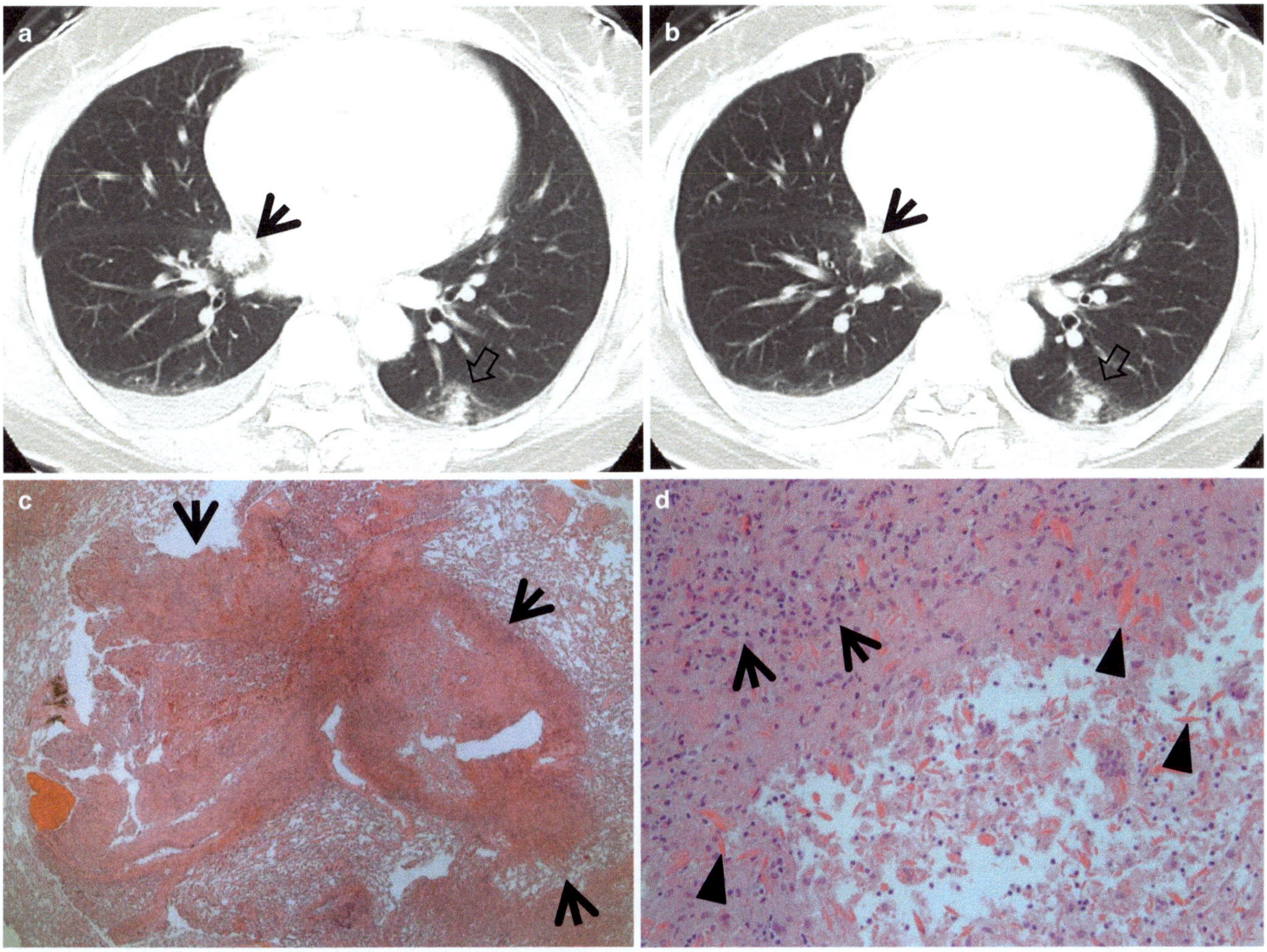


**Fig. 1.16** Loeffler's (pulmonary infiltration with eosinophilia, PIE) syndrome in a 50-year-old woman. (**a**, **b**) Lung window of consecutive CT scans (5.0-mm section thickness) obtained at levels of the inferior pulmonary veins shows a nodule (*arrows* in **a** and **b**) in medial basal segment of the right lower lobe and a nodule and halo sign (*open arrows* in **a** and **b**) in superior segment of the left lower lobe. (**c**) Low-magnification (×40) photomicrograph (H & E stain) demonstrates an inflammatory nodule mainly composed of eosinophilic abscesses (*arrows*). (**d**) High-magnification (×200) photomicrograph discloses eosinophilic abscess containing granulomas (*arrows*) due to foreign-body reaction. Also note Charcot–Leyden crystals (*arrowheads*)

## Symptoms and Signs

Patients are usually asymptomatic. Respiratory symptoms are minimal or absent. Malaise, fever, and cough may be present. A careful search for parasitic infection or drug reaction should be pursued.

## CT Findings

TSCT findings of Loeffler's syndrome consist of GGO or airspace consolidation, usually transient and migratory, involving mainly the peripheral regions of the middle and upper lung zones, as well as single or multiple airspace nodules with surrounding GGO [35, 36] (Fig. 1.16).

## CT–Pathology Comparisons

TSCT findings showing GGO or airspace consolidation involving the peripheral lung regions are histopathologically related to edema and accumulation of eosinophils in alveolar septa and interstitium [37]. A halo of GGO results histopathologically from pulmonary infiltrations of eosinophils and other inflammatory cells [52].

## Patient Prognosis

By definition, this infiltration resolves spontaneously within 4 weeks. Complete resolution is the rule.

## References


1. Jeong YJ, Yi CA, Lee KS. Solitary pulmonary nodules: detection, characterization, and guidance for further diagnostic workup and treatment. AJR Am J Roentgenol. 2007;188:57–68.
2. Hansell DM, Bankier AA, MacMahon H, McLoud TC, Muller NL, Remy J. Fleischner Society: glossary of terms for thoracic imaging. Radiology. 2008;246:697–722.
3. Gurney JW. Determining the likelihood of malignancy in solitary pulmonary nodules with Bayesian analysis. Part I. Theory. Radiology. 1993;186:405–13.
4. Yankelevitz DF, Reeves AP, Kostis WJ, Zhao B, Henschke CI. Small pulmonary nodules: volumetrically determined growth rates based on CT evaluation. Radiology. 2000;217:251–6.
5. Revel MP, Lefort C, Bissery A, et al. Pulmonary nodules: preliminary experience with three-dimensional evaluation. Radiology. 2004;231:459–66.
6. Marchiano A, Calabro E, Civelli E, et al. Pulmonary nodules: volume repeatability at multidetector CT lung cancer screening. Radiology. 2009;251:919–25.
7. Jeong YJ, Lee KS, Jeong SY, et al. Solitary pulmonary nodule: characterization with combined wash-in and washout features at dynamic multi-detector row CT. Radiology. 2005;237:675–83.
8. Siegelman SS, Khouri NF, Scott Jr WW, et al. Pulmonary hamartoma: CT findings. Radiology. 1986;160:313–7.
9. Lee KS, Yi CA, Jeong SY, et al. Solid or partly solid solitary pulmonary nodules: their characterization using contrast wash-in and morphologic features at helical CT. Chest. 2007;131:1516–25.
10. Jeong YJ, Lee KS. Pulmonary tuberculosis: up-to-date imaging and management. AJR Am J Roentgenol. 2008;191:834–44.
11. Travis WD, Brambilla E, Noguchi M, et al. International Association for the Study of Lung Cancer/American Thoracic Society/European Respiratory Society International Multidisciplinary Classification of Lung Adenocarcinoma. J Thorac Oncol. 2011;6:244–85.
12. Zwirewich CV, Vedal S, Miller RR, Muller NL. Solitary pulmonary nodule: high-resolution CT and radiologic-pathologic correlation. Radiology. 1991;179:469–76.
13. Yi CA, Lee KS, Kim EA, et al. Solitary pulmonary nodules: dynamic enhanced multi-detector row CT study and comparison with vascular endothelial growth factor and microvessel density. Radiology. 2004;233:191–9.
14. Godoy MC, Naidich DP. Overview and strategic management of subsolid pulmonary nodules. J Thorac Imaging. 2012;27:240–8.
15. Travis WD, Rush W, Flieder DB, et al. Survival analysis of 200 pulmonary neuroendocrine tumors with clarification of criteria for atypical carcinoid and its separation from typical carcinoid. Am J Surg Pathol. 1998;22:934–44.
16. Meisinger QC, Klein JS, Butnor KJ, Gentchos G, Leavitt BJ. CT features of peripheral pulmonary carcinoid tumors. AJR Am J Roentgenol. 2011;197:1073–80.
17. Chong S, Lee KS, Chung MJ, Han J, Kwon OJ, Kim TS. Neuroendocrine tumors of the lung: clinical, pathologic, and imaging findings. Radiographics. 2006;26:41–57; discussion 57–8.
18. Forster BB, Muller NL, Miller RR, Nelems B, Evans KG. Neuroendocrine carcinomas of the lung: clinical, radiologic, and pathologic correlation. Radiology. 1989;170:441–5.
19. Detterbeck FC. Management of carcinoid tumors. Ann Thorac Surg. 2010;89:998–1005.
20. Bae YA, Lee KS, Han J, et al. Marginal zone B-cell lymphoma of bronchus-associated lymphoid tissue: imaging findings in 21 patients. Chest. 2008;133:433–40.
21. Lee DK, Im JG, Lee KS, et al. B-cell lymphoma of bronchus-associated lymphoid tissue (BALT): CT features in 10 patients. J Comput Assist Tomogr. 2000;24:30–4.
22. Wislez M, Cadranel J, Antoine M, et al. Lymphoma of pulmonary mucosa-associated lymphoid tissue: CT scan findings and pathological correlations. Eur Respir J. 1999;14:423–9.
23. Borie R, Wislez M, Thabut G, et al. Clinical characteristics and prognostic factors of pulmonary MALT lymphoma. Eur Respir J. 2009;34:1408–16.
24. Lee JY, Lee KS, Jung KJ, et al. Pulmonary tuberculosis: CT and pathologic correlation. J Comput Assist Tomogr. 2000;24:691–8.
25. Lee KS, Im JG. CT in adults with tuberculosis of the chest: characteristic findings and role in management. AJR Am J Roentgenol. 1995;164:1361–7.
26. Sochocky S. Tuberculoma of the lung. Am Rev Tuberc. 1958;78:403–10.
27. Murayama S, Murakami J, Hashimoto S, Torii Y, Masuda K. Noncalcified pulmonary tuberculomas: CT enhancement patterns with histological correlation. J Thorac Imaging. 1995;10:91–5.
28. Lee HS, Oh JY, Lee JH, et al. Response of pulmonary tuberculomas to anti-tuberculous treatment. Eur Respir J. 2004;23:452–5.
29. Rogalla P, Lemke I, Kazmierczak B, Bullerdiek J. An identical HMGIC-LPP fusion transcript is consistently expressed in pulmonary chondroid hamartomas with t(3;12)(q27-28;q14-15). Genes Chromosomes Cancer. 2000;29:363–6.
30. Thomas JW, Staerkel GA, Whitman GJ. Pulmonary hamartoma. AJR Am J Roentgenol. 1999;172:1643.
31. Park KY, Kim SJ, Noh TW, et al. Diagnostic efficacy and characteristic feature of MRI in pulmonary hamartoma: comparison with CT, specimen MRI, and pathology. J Comput Assist Tomogr. 2008;32:919–25.
32. Potente G, Macori F, Caimi M, Mingazzini P, Volpino P. Noncalcified pulmonary hamartomas: computed tomography enhancement patterns with histologic correlation. J Thorac Imaging. 1999;14:101–4.
33. Kim GY, Kim J, Choi YS, Kim HJ, Ahn G, Han J. Sixteen cases of sclerosing hemangioma of the lung including unusual presentations. J Korean Med Sci. 2004;19:352–8.
34. Im JG, Kim WH, Han MC, et al. Sclerosing hemangiomas of the lung and interlobar fissures: CT findings. J Comput Assist Tomogr. 1994;18:34–8.
35. Chung MJ, Lee KS, Han J, Sung YM, Chong S, Kwon OJ. Pulmonary sclerosing hemangioma presenting as solitary pulmonary nodule: dynamic CT findings and histopathologic comparisons. AJR Am J Roentgenol. 2006;187:430–7.
36. Kitagawa H, Goto A, Minami M, Nakajima J, Niki T, Fukayama M. Sclerosing hemangioma of the lung with cystic appearance. Jpn J Clin Oncol. 2003;33:360–3.
37. Lee ST, Lee YC, Hsu CY, Lin CC. Bilateral multiple sclerosing hemangiomas of the lung. Chest. 1992;101:572–3.
38. Nam JE, Ryu YH, Cho SH, et al. Air-trapping zone surrounding sclerosing hemangioma of the lung. J Comput Assist Tomogr. 2002;26:358–61.
39. Sakamoto K, Okita M, Kumagiri H, Kawamura S, Takeuchi K, Mikami R. Sclerosing hemangioma isolated to the mediastinum. Ann Thorac Surg. 2003;75:1021–3.
40. Shimosato Y. Lung tumors of uncertain histogenesis. Semin Diagn Pathol. 1995;12:185–92.
41. Kim TS, Han J, Kim GY, Lee KS, Kim H, Kim J. Pulmonary inflammatory pseudotumor (inflammatory myofibroblastic tumor): CT features with pathologic correlation. J Comput Assist Tomogr. 2005;29:633–9.
42. Agrons GA, Rosado-de-Christenson ML, Kirejczyk WM, Conran RM, Stocker JT. Pulmonary inflammatory pseudotumor: radiologic features. Radiology. 1998;206:511–8.
43. Eyden B. Electron microscopy in the study of myofibroblastic lesions. Semin Diagn Pathol. 2003;20:13–24.

44. Travis WD, Hoffman GS, Leavitt RY, Pass HI, Fauci AS. Surgical pathology of the lung in Wegener's granulomatosis. Review of 87 open lung biopsies from 67 patients. Am J Surg Pathol. 1991;15:315–33.
45. Lee KS, Kim TS, Fujimoto K, et al. Thoracic manifestation of Wegener's granulomatosis: CT findings in 30 patients. Eur Radiol. 2003;13:43–51.
46. Cassan SM, Coles DT, Harrison Jr EG. The concept of limited forms of Wegener's granulomatosis. Am J Med. 1970;49:366–79.
47. Lamprecht P, Gross WL. Wegener's granulomatosis. Herz. 2004;29:47–56.
48. Kim HY, Shim YM, Lee KS, Han J, Yi CA, Kim YK. Persistent pulmonary nodular ground-glass opacity at thin-section CT: histopathologic comparisons. Radiology. 2007;245:267–75.
49. Lee HY, Lee KS. Ground-glass opacity nodules: histopathology, imaging evaluation, and clinical implications. J Thorac Imaging. 2011;26:106–18.
50. Henschke CI, Yankelevitz DF, Mirtcheva R, et al. CT screening for lung cancer: frequency and significance of part-solid and nonsolid nodules. AJR Am J Roentgenol. 2002;178:1053–7.
51. Park CM, Goo JM, Kim TJ, et al. Pulmonary nodular ground-glass opacities in patients with extrapulmonary cancers: what is their clinical significance and how can we determine whether they are malignant or benign lesions? Chest. 2008;133:1402–9.
52. Kim Y, Lee KS, Jung KJ, Han J, Kim JS, Suh JS. Halo sign on high resolution CT: findings in spectrum of pulmonary diseases with pathologic correlation. J Comput Assist Tomogr. 1999; 23:622–6.
53. Lim H, Ahn S, Lee KS, et al. Persistent pure ground-glass opacity lung nodules >10 mm in diameter at CT: histopathologic comparisons and prognostic implications. Chest 2013;144:1291–9.
54. Lee HJ, Goo JM, Lee CH, et al. Predictive CT findings of malignancy in ground-glass nodules on thin-section chest CT: the effects on radiologist performance. Eur Radiol. 2009;19:552–60.
55. Kim TJ, Goo JM, Lee KW, Park CM, Lee HJ. Clinical, pathological and thin-section CT features of persistent multiple ground-glass opacity nodules: comparison with solitary ground-glass opacity nodule. Lung Cancer. 2009;64:171–8.
56. Ullmann R, Bongiovanni M, Halbwedl I, et al. Is high-grade adenomatous hyperplasia an early bronchioloalveolar adenocarcinoma? J Pathol. 2003;201:371–6.
57. Lee HY, Lee KS, Han J, et al. Mucinous versus nonmucinous solitary pulmonary nodular bronchioloalveolar carcinoma: CT and FDG PET findings and pathologic comparisons. Lung Cancer. 2009;65:170–5.
58. Ikeda K, Awai K, Mori T, Kawanaka K, Yamashita Y, Nomori H. Differential diagnosis of ground-glass opacity nodules: CT number analysis by three-dimensional computerized quantification. Chest. 2007;132:984–90.
59. Yoshida J, Nagai K, Yokose T, et al. Limited resection trial for pulmonary ground-glass opacity nodules: fifty-case experience. J Thorac Cardiovasc Surg. 2005;129:991–6.
60. Koike T, Togashi K, Shirato T, et al. Limited resection for noninvasive bronchioloalveolar carcinoma diagnosed by intraoperative pathologic examination. Ann Thorac Surg. 2009;88:1106–11.
61. Travis WD, Garg K, Franklin WA, et al. Evolving concepts in the pathology and computed tomography imaging of lung adenocarcinoma and bronchioloalveolar carcinoma. J Clin Oncol. 2005;23:3279–87.
62. Austin JH, Garg K, Aberle D, et al. Radiologic implications of the 2011 classification of adenocarcinoma of the lung. Radiology. 2013;266:62–71.
63. Suzuki K, Kusumoto M, Watanabe S, Tsuchiya R, Asamura H. Radiologic classification of small adenocarcinoma of the lung: radiologic-pathologic correlation and its prognostic impact. Ann Thorac Surg. 2006;81:413–9.
64. Johkoh T, Muller NL, Akira M, et al. Eosinophilic lung diseases: diagnostic accuracy of thin-section CT in 111 patients. Radiology. 2000;216:773–80.
65. Noguchi M, Morikawa A, Kawasaki M, et al. Small adenocarcinoma of the lung. Histologic characteristics and prognosis. Cancer. 1995;75:2844–52.
66. Borczuk AC, Qian F, Kazeros A, et al. Invasive size is an independent predictor of survival in pulmonary adenocarcinoma. Am J Surg Pathol. 2009;33:462–9.
67. Yim J, Zhu LC, Chiriboga L, Watson HN, Goldberg JD, Moreira AL. Histologic features are important prognostic indicators in early stages lung adenocarcinomas. Mod Pathol. 2007;20:233–41.
68. Oka S, Hanagiri T, Uramoto H, et al. Surgical resection for patients with mucinous bronchioloalveolar carcinoma. Asian J Surg. 2010;33:89–93.
69. Bhatt NY, Allen JN. Update on eosinophilic lung diseases. Semin Respir Crit Care Med. 2012;33:555–71.
70. Lee HY, Jeong JY, Lee KS, et al. Solitary pulmonary nodular lung adenocarcinoma: correlation of histopathologic scoring and patient survival with imaging biomarkers. Radiology. 2012;264:884–93.

# 2 Mass

## Definition

A lung mass is any pulmonary lesion seen as an opacity greater than 30 mm in diameter irrespective of its contour, border, or attenuation characteristics. The mass usually implies a solid or partly solid opacity. CT allows more exact evaluation of size, location, and attenuation [1] (Figs. 2.1 and 2.2).

## Diseases Causing the Pattern

The most common cause is malignant tumor including lung cancer (Figs. 2.1 and 2.2), bronchus-associated lymphoid tissue (BALT) lymphoma, and *pulmonary sarcoma* [2] (Fig. 2.3). Benign condition such as benign tumor, rounded atelectasis [3, 4], and *progressive massive fibrosis* [5] (Fig. 2.4) may present with a lung mass. Chronic pneumonia including *actinomycosis* [6] (Fig. 2.5) and semi-invasive aspergillosis (chronic necrotizing pulmonary aspergillosis) [7] may also manifest a mass lesion (Table 2.1).

## Distribution

Likelihood ratio for malignancy in upper and middle lobe nodule or mass is 1.22 as compared with 0.66 in lower lobe nodule [8]. Otherwise, there is no central-subpleural or bronchovascular predominance.

## Clinical Considerations

Rounded atelectasis is seen in patients with asbestos exposure, while progressive massive fibrosis (PMF) is seen in patients with silicosis or coal workers' pneumoconiosis [5]. Pulmonary actinomycosis is usually seen in immunocompetent patients with respiratory disorders (emphysema and chronic bronchitis), poor oral hygiene, alcoholism, and chronic debilitating diseases [9]. Semi-invasive aspergillosis usually occur in patients with underlying illness such as diabetes, pulmonary tuberculosis, or chronic alcoholism [7].

**Key Points for Differential Diagnosis**

1. Pulmonary sarcomas are rare and account for 0.5 % of all primary malignant lung disease [10]. Histologic types include malignant fibrous histiocytoma, pleuropulmonary synovial sarcoma, malignant nerve sheath tumor, leiomyosarcoma, fibrosarcoma, and hemangiopericytoma [2, 11].
2. The signal intensity manifested on T2-weighted images provides a clue for the differentiation of lung cancer from progressive massive fibrosis. When a mass lesion is depicted with high signal intensity on T2-weighted MR images, the finding is highly suggestive of lung cancer. Progressive massive fibrosis appears as a low- or black-signal-intensity abnormality on T2-wighted MR images [12].
3. Rounded atelectasis appears on CT as a rounded mass abutting a thickened pleural surface in the lung periphery. The margin closest to the hilum is blurred by the entering vessels. Typically, bronchi and vessels curve into the mass at its hilar pole, giving the so-called comet tail sign [3, 4].
4. Dense consolidation or a mass is the main pattern of pulmonary actinomycosis and semi-invasive aspergillosis.
5. The presence of geographic central low-attenuation area (microabscesses with sulfur granule) within the lesion and peripheral enhancement are suggestive of pulmonary actinomycosis [6].

K.S. Lee et al., *Radiology Illustrated: Chest Radiology*, Radiology Illustrated,
DOI 10.1007/978-3-642-37096-0_2, © Springer-Verlag Berlin Heidelberg 2014

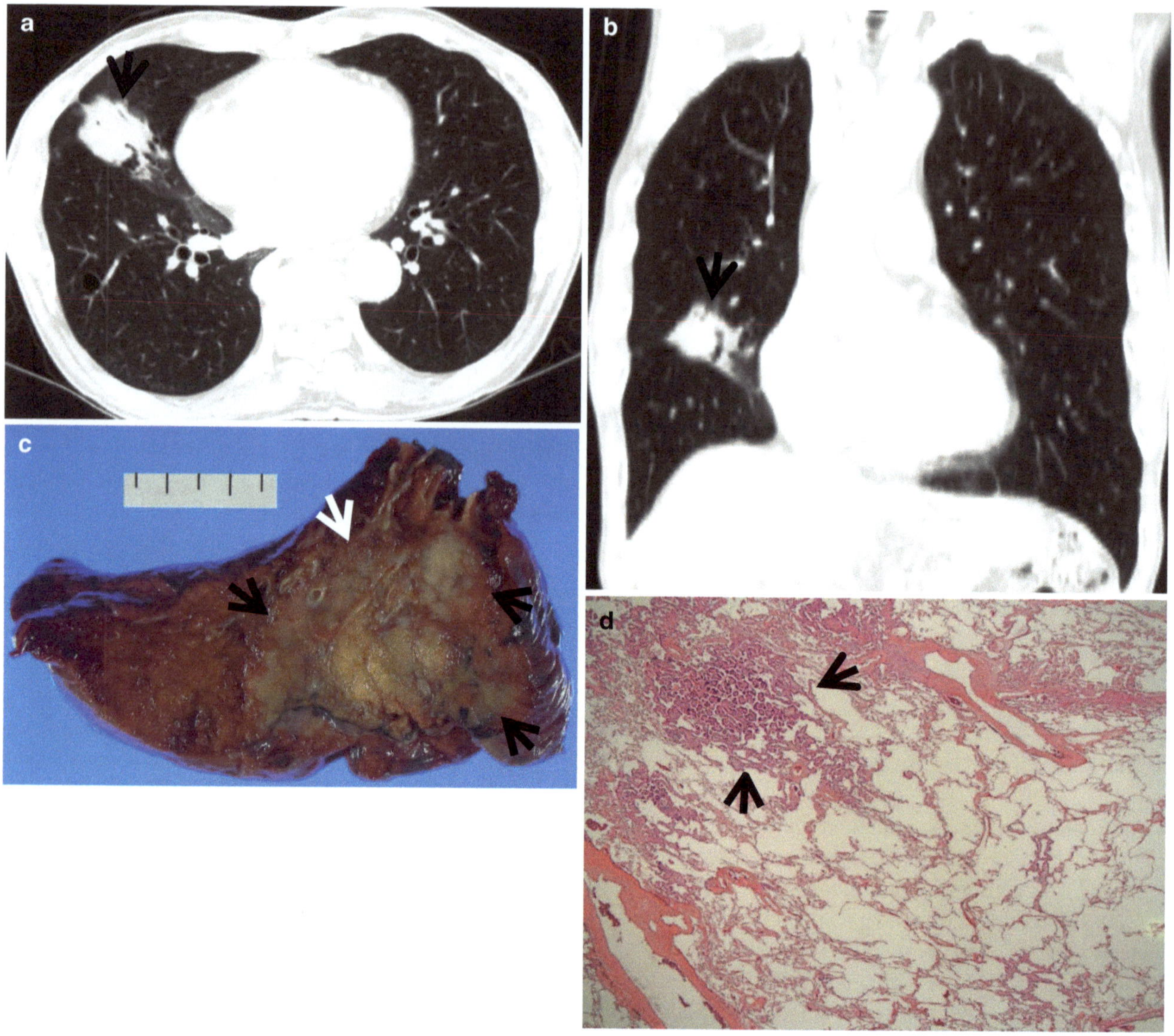


**Fig. 2.1** Lung mass representing a lung adenocarcinoma in a 75-year-old man. (**a**, **b**) Lung window of transverse and coronal reformatted images of CT scans shows a 42-mm-sized mass (*arrows* in **a** and **b**) in the right middle lobe. (**c**) Gross specimen obtained with right middle lobectomy demonstrates variable appearances of tumor, namely, white and yellow areas, respectively, with lobulated margin (*arrows*). This is due to heterogeneous subtypes of adenocarcinoma. (**d**) Low-magnification (×40) photomicrograph discloses papillary pattern of tumor growth (*arrows*) with background of lepidic growth pattern

## Pulmonary Sarcoma

### Pathology and Pathogenesis

True primary sarcomas of the lung are rare, and they include Kaposi sarcoma, fibrosarcoma, leiomyosarcoma, epithelioid hemangioendothelioma, malignant fibrous histiocytoma, rhabdomyosarcoma, chondrosarcoma, synovial sarcoma, and pulmonary artery sarcoma.

### Symptoms and Signs

In patients with primary pulmonary sarcoma, clinical symptoms are nonspecific. Cough, dyspnea, chest pain, and hemoptysis may develop, depending on the size and the location of the lesions.

### CT Findings

Primary pulmonary sarcomas usually manifest as large and heterogeneous masses on CT (Fig. 2.3), and the different histologic types of sarcomas are frequently indistinguishable at imaging analysis. Malignant fibrous histiocytoma originates from the muscles of the chest wall and seldom from the lungs, mediastinum, or pleura. They appear as well-defined, smooth or lobulated soft tissue masses with heterogeneous enhancement and rarely contain calcifications [13]. Pleuropulmonary synovial sarcoma often demonstrates a

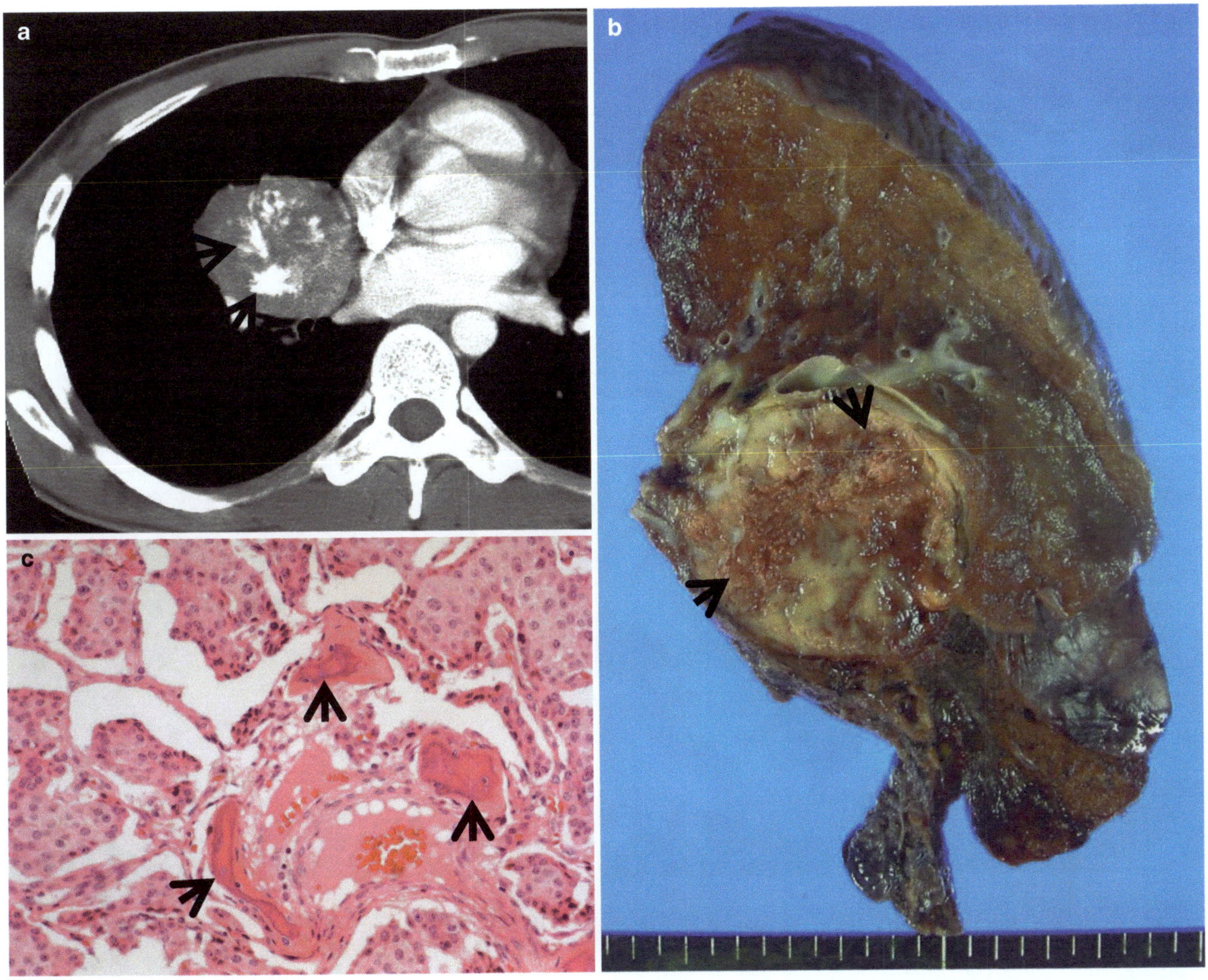


**Fig. 2.2** Lung mass representing a typical carcinoid in a 24-year-old man. (**a**) Enhanced CT scan (5.0-mm section thickness) obtained at level of the inferior pulmonary veins shows a 60-mm-sized enhancing mass in the right middle lobe. Also note internal ossifications (*arrows*). (**b**) Gross specimen obtained with right middle lobectomy demonstrates well-marginated mass growing with compressive rather than infiltrative manner to adjacent lung parenchyma. Also note internal ossifications (*arrows*). (**c**) High-magnification (×200) photomicrograph displays trabeculae of uniform tumor cells separated by numerous vascular septa. Also note connective tissue containing the bones (*arrows*)

well-defined mass with patchy low attenuation on unenhanced CT images and heterogeneous enhancement on contrast-enhanced CT images [14]. Calcification is a common finding in synovial sarcoma at para-articular sites but a rare finding in pleuropulmonary synovial sarcoma.

## CT–Pathology Comparisons

Most pulmonary sarcomas derive from smooth muscle or fibrous tissue; therefore, they show mild or marked enhancement on contrast-enhanced CT. On CT–pathology correlations of pleuropulmonary synovial sarcoma, patchy low-density areas on unenhanced CT are correlated with the myxoid or collagenous elements, and heterogeneous enhancement on contrast-enhanced CT is correlated with areas of hemorrhage, necrosis, and cystic change [14].

## Patient Prognosis

Surgery is the most effective treatment. Chemoradiation therapy may be the best treatment option in unresectable case. Prognosis mainly depends on whether complete surgical resection is accomplished. Therefore, early diagnosis is the most important prognosis-determining factor. Overall 5-year survival has been reported to be 40–50 % [15, 16].

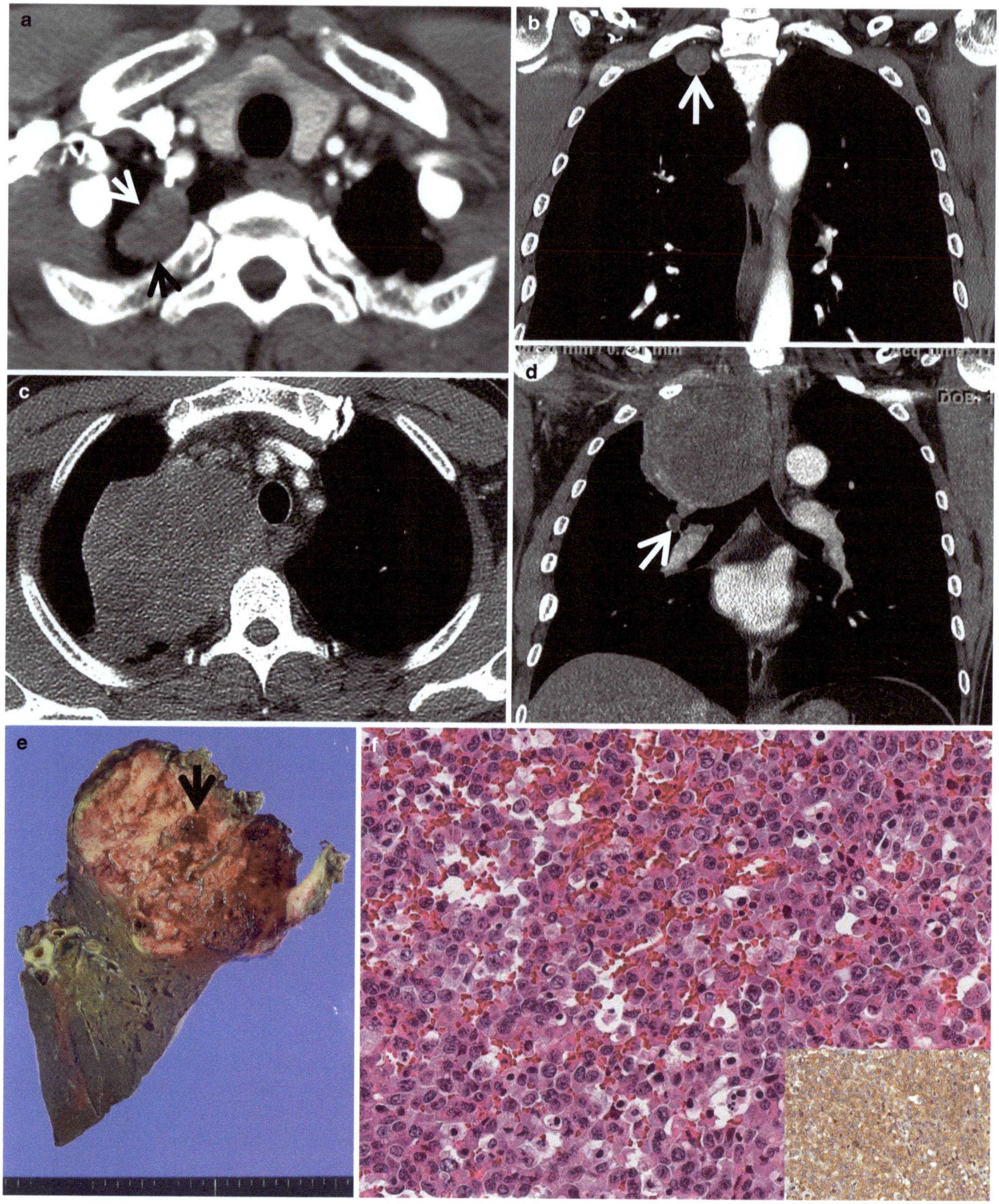


**Fig. 2.3** Lung mass proved to be an undifferentiated pulmonary sarcoma in a 49-year-old man. (**a**, **b**) Mediastinal window of transverse (**a**) and coronal (**b**) reformatted images of CT scans shows a 28-mm-sized nodule (*arrows* in **a** and **b**) in right apical area. Initially nodule was interpreted as a neurogenic tumor. (**c**, **d**) CT scans obtained 7 months after **a** and **b** demonstrate markedly enlarged mass measuring 90 mm in diameter at this time. Also note tumor embolus (*arrow* in **d**) in a branch of the right superior pulmonary vein. (**e**) Gross pathologic specimen obtained with right upper lobectomy discloses a large mass containing necrotic area (*arrow*) in apex of lobe. (**f**) High-magnification (×200) photomicrography discloses tumor cells showing round shape with high pleomorphism and marked mitotic activity. *Inset*: positive staging for CD99

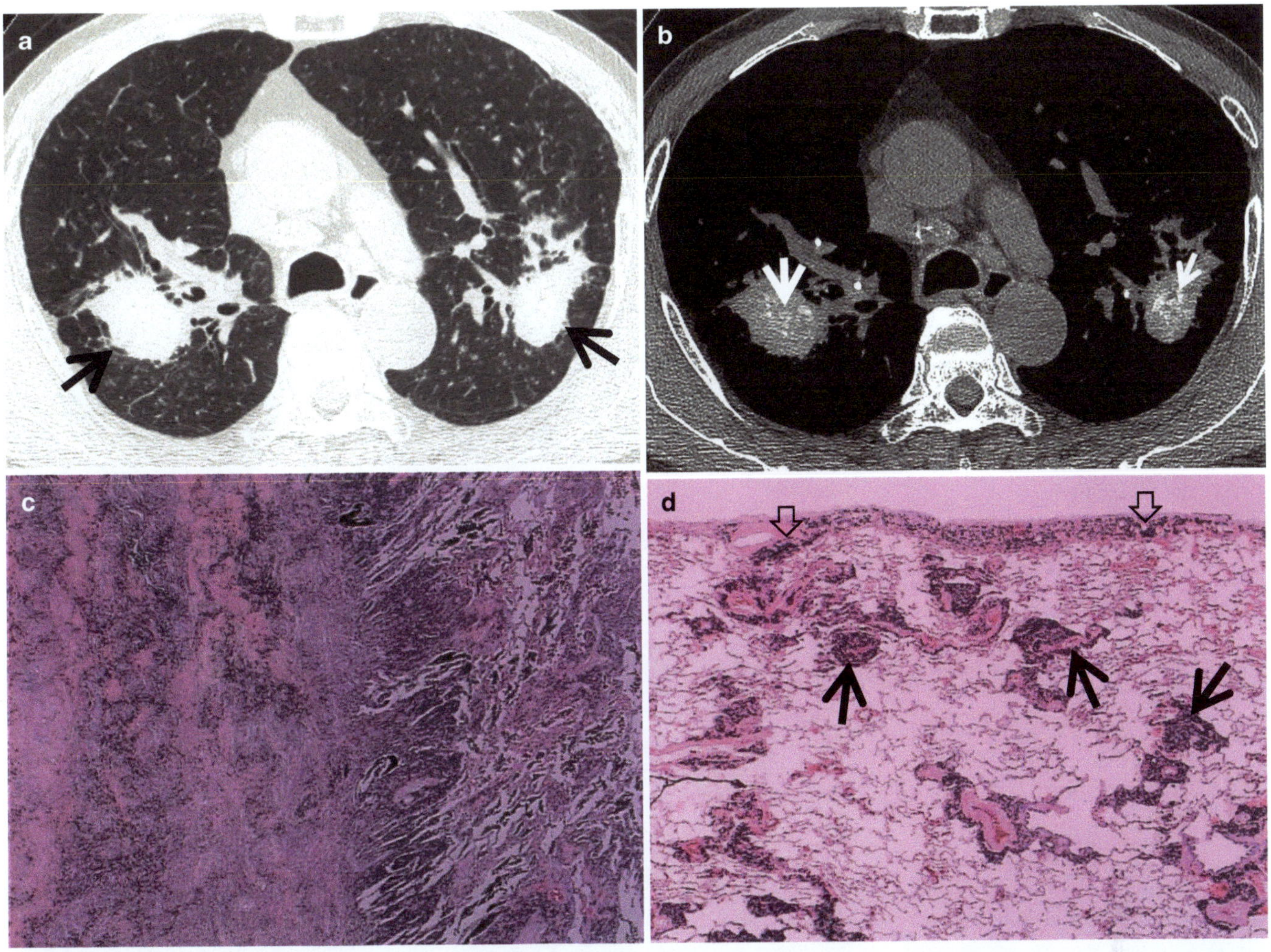


**Fig. 2.4** Lung masses as progressive mass fibrosis in a 73-year-old man. (**a**) Lung window of thin-section (1.5-mm section thickness) CT scan obtained at level of the azygos arch shows two masses (*arrows*) in posterior aspect of both upper lobes. Also note small nodules in both lungs. Combined findings of two large masses and surrounding small nodules in upper lung zones are suggestive of progressive massive fibrosis and pneumoconiotic small nodules. (**b**) Mediastinal window image demonstrates internal calcifications (*arrows*) within progressive massive fibrosis. Also note calcified lymph nodes in the mediastinum. (**c**) Low-magnification (×10) photomicrograph of biopsy specimen obtained from different patient with progressive massive fibrosis discloses large amount of fibrous tissue containing black pigments (anthracosis). (**d**) Low-magnification (×40) photomicrograph shows numerous well-circumscribed black nodules (*arrows*) mainly in centrilobular location along bronchovascular bundles. Pigmented fibrosis (*open arrows*) adjacent to pleura may be seen as pleural-based small nodule at thin-section CT

## Progressive Massive Fibrosis

### Pathology and Pathogenesis

PMF develops in a background of simple coal worker's pneumoconiosis (CWP) (Fig. 2.4). PMF is identified as zones of pigmented fibrosis that tend to be bilateral and distributed in the upper lobes posteriorly. There is replacement of lung tissue by fibrosis, with interspersed, abundant, pigmented coal dusts.

### Symptoms and Signs

Shortness of breath is the main symptom of PMF. Cough, sputum, and wheezing sound are often present. Symptoms and signs of right heart failure are found in severe advanced cases. Acute exacerbation by asthmatic airway narrowing or superimposed pneumonia may develop.

### CT Findings

PMF appears as a mass usually with irregular margins and associated with adjacent paracicatricial emphysema and lung parenchymal architectural distortion [5, 17]. They are usually bilateral and symmetric (Fig. 2.4). When present, calcification may be punctate, curvilinear, or massive (Fig. 2.4). Cavitation also can occur as the result of ischemia or superimposed mycobacterial infection. On MR images, PMF appears as a low signal intensity on T2-weighted image,

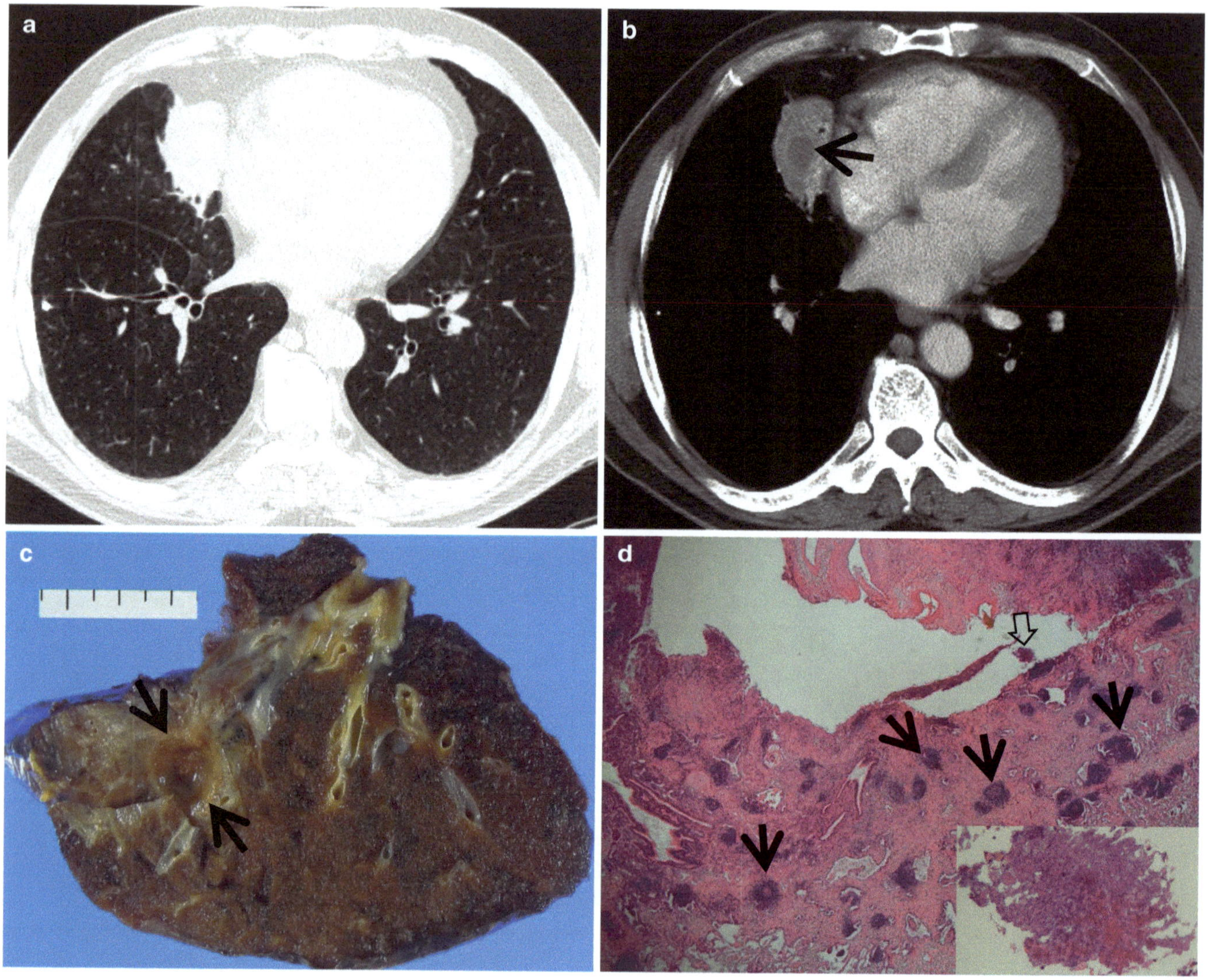


**Fig. 2.5** Lung mass representing actinomycosis in a 60-year-old man. (**a**) Lung window of thin-section (1.5-mm section thickness) CT scan obtained at level of inferior pulmonary veins shows a 42-mm-sized fusiform mass in the right middle lobe. (**b**) Mediastinal window image shows a geographic central necrotic area (*arrow*) within lesion. (**c**) Gross pathologic specimen obtained with right middle lobectomy displays area of pneumonic consolidation harboring internal round necrotic cavity (*arrows*). (**d**) Low-magnification (×40) photomicrograph discloses parenchymal lesion of chronic inflammation and fibrosis with many lymphoid follicles (*arrows*). Within abscess cavity, a basophilic material (*open arrow*) is noted. *Inset*: magnified view of basophilic material, consistent with a sulfur granule

which provides a clue for the differentiation of lung cancer from PMF [12].

## CT–Pathology Comparisons

PMF is usually associated with an increased amount of fibrous tissue and foci of necrosis (Fig. 2.4). Because of fibrous tissue within PMF, most lesions appear as a low-signal-intensity lesion on T2-weighted image. Necrosis within PMF appears as a focal hyperintense area within PMF on T2-weighted image and low-attenuation area on CT. On enhanced MR images, rim enhancement is present in more than half of cases, which is caused by collapsed alveoli secondary to emphysema. The remaining lesions do not enhance. This lack of enhancement is thought to reflect the hypovascular nature of the hyaline collagenous tissue of PMF lesion [12].

## Patient Prognosis

Since lung fibrosis is irreversible, prognosis is grave. Patients should be removed from further exposure. Improvement of lung function by bronchodilators and prevention of pneumonia are very important in the management of patients with PMF [18].

**Table 2.1** Common diseases manifesting as lung mass

| Disease | Key points for differential diagnosis |
|---|---|
| Malignant condition | |
| Lung caner | Wash-in values of >25 HU, lobulated or spiculated margin, and absence of a satellite nodule |
| BALT lymphoma | Consolidation or nodule with air bronchograms |
| Pulmonary sarcoma | Large mass with heterogeneous enhancement |
| Nontumorous condition | |
| Benign tumor | |
| Rounded atelectasis | Round mass abutting a thickened pleura, comet tail sign |
| Progressive massive fibrosis | Mass with irregular margin and associated paracicatricial emphysema, low SI on T2WI |
| Actinomycosis | Consolidation or mass containing central low attenuation and peripheral enhancement |
| Semi-invasive aspergillosis | |

*Note*: *BALT* bronchus-associated lymphoid tissue, *HU* Hounsfield unit, *SI* signal intensity, *T2WI* T2-weighted images

## Pulmonary Actinomycosis

### Pathology and Pathogenesis

Actinomycosis is an infection caused by the anaerobic filamentous bacteria *Actinomyces* species. Acute bronchopneumonia with abscess formation is the initial reaction, and the process typically progresses to fibrosis. The process is often associated with localized interlobular septal and pleural thickening. In rare cases, infection can cause an endobronchial infection. The endobronchial form reflects actinomycosis colonization of preexisting obstructive broncholiths or endobronchial foreign bodies, which causes the inflammation of the adjacent airway and results in distal obstructive pneumonia. Broncholiths are formed by erosion of calcified lymph nodes into the airway as a result of a granulomatous process [19].

### Symptoms and Signs

Patients with small nodule or mass-like consolidation are often asymptomatic. The most frequent respiratory symptom is chronic cough. Constitutional symptoms of low-grade fever, weight loss, and fatigue may be the main complaints prior to the detection of lung lesion, which mimic the clinical features of malignancy, tuberculosis, and fungal infection. As disease progresses, most patients develop productive cough and pleuritic chest pain. In more advanced case, discharge of characteristic "sulfur granule" from the fistula tract on the chest wall from the pleural cavity can be found.

### CT Findings

In acute disease, actinomycosis manifests as a small, poorly defined, and peripheral pulmonary nodule with or without interlobular septal thickening on CT. With progression of infection, the pulmonary nodule gradually increases in extent to manifest as an airspace consolidation or a mass. Typically, consolidation or mass contains central areas of low attenuation with peripheral enhancement [6] (Fig. 2.5). Other CT findings include hilar or mediastinal lymphadenopathy, localized pleural thickening, or pleural effusion.

### CT–Pathology Comparisons

Pulmonary parenchymal infection is characterized pathologically by bronchopneumonia with focal or multifocal abscess formation. The low-attenuation areas on contrast-enhanced CT represent abscesses or dilated bronchi containing inflammatory exudate; the enhancing rim corresponds to vascular granulation tissue in the abscess wall or hyperplastic bronchial vessels in the mucosa of draining airways [6].

### Patient Prognosis

Pulmonary actinomycosis responds well to prolonged antibiotic treatment. Standard treatment is initial parenteral antibiotic administration for 4–6 weeks followed by at least 6 months of oral antibiotic therapy. In mild case, treatment duration can be shortened [20]. Adjunctive surgical resection may be necessary in the case with severe pleural and chest wall involvement.

## References


1. Hansell DM, Bankier AA, MacMahon H, McLoud TC, Muller NL, Remy J. Fleischner Society: glossary of terms for thoracic imaging. Radiology. 2008;246:697–722.
2. Magne N, Porsin B, Pivot X, et al. Primary lung sarcomas: long survivors obtained with iterative complete surgery. Lung Cancer. 2001;31:241–5.
3. Doyle TC, Lawler GA. CT features of rounded atelectasis of the lung. AJR Am J Roentgenol. 1984;143:225–8.
4. McHugh K, Blaquiere RM. CT features of rounded atelectasis. AJR Am J Roentgenol. 1989;153:257–60.
5. Chong S, Lee KS, Chung MJ, Han J, Kwon OJ, Kim TS. Pneumoconiosis: comparison of imaging and pathologic findings. Radiographics. 2006;26:59–77.
6. Cheon JE, Im JG, Kim MY, Lee JS, Choi GM, Yeon KM. Thoracic actinomycosis: CT findings. Radiology. 1998;209:229–33.
7. Kim SY, Lee KS, Han J, et al. Semiinvasive pulmonary aspergillosis: CT and pathologic findings in six patients. AJR Am J Roentgenol. 2000;174:795–8.
8. Gurney JW. Determining the likelihood of malignancy in solitary pulmonary nodules with Bayesian analysis. Part I. Theory. Radiology. 1993;186:405–13.

9. Han JY, Lee KN, Lee JK, et al. An overview of thoracic actinomycosis: CT features. Insights Imaging. 2013;4:245–52.
10. Nascimento AG, Unni KK, Bernatz PE. Sarcomas of the lung. Mayo Clin Proc. 1982;57:355–9.
11. Keel SB, Bacha E, Mark EJ, Nielsen GP, Rosenberg AE. Primary pulmonary sarcoma: a clinicopathologic study of 26 cases. Mod Pathol. 1999;12:1124–31.
12. Matsumoto S, Miyake H, Oga M, Takaki H, Mori H. Diagnosis of lung cancer in a patient with pneumoconiosis and progressive massive fibrosis using MRI. Eur Radiol. 1998;8:615–7.
13. Gladish GW, Sabloff BM, Munden RF, Truong MT, Erasmus JJ, Chasen MH. Primary thoracic sarcomas. Radiographics. 2002;22:621–37.
14. Zhang WD, Guan YB, Chen YF, Li CX. CT imaging of primary pleuropulmonary synovial sarcoma. Clin Radiol. 2012;67: 884–8.
15. Porte HL, Metois DG, Leroy X, Conti M, Gosselin B, Wurtz A. Surgical treatment of primary sarcoma of the lung. Eur J Cardiothorac Surg. 2000;18:136–42.
16. Janssen JP, Mulder JJ, Wagenaar SS, Elbers HR, van den Bosch JM. Primary sarcoma of the lung: a clinical study with long-term follow-up. Ann Thorac Surg. 1994;58:1151–5.
17. Begin R, Bergeron D, Samson L, Boctor M, Cantin A. CT assessment of silicosis in exposed workers. AJR Am J Roentgenol. 1987;148:509–14.
18. Leung CC, Yu IT, Chen W. Silicosis. Lancet. 2012;379:2008–18.
19. Kim TS, Han J, Koh WJ, et al. Thoracic actinomycosis: CT features with histopathologic correlation. AJR Am J Roentgenol. 2006;186:225–31.
20. Choi J, Koh WJ, Kim TS, et al. Optimal duration of IV and oral antibiotics in the treatment of thoracic actinomycosis. Chest. 2005;128:2211–7.

# 3 Consolidation

## Lobar Consolidation

### Definition

Consolidation on CT scans refers to a pattern of pulmonary abnormality that appears as a homogeneous increase in lung parenchymal attenuation that obscures the margins of vessels and airway walls. Air-bronchogram sign may be present within the lesion [1] (Fig. 3.1). Pathologically, the consolidation consists of an exudate or other product of disease that replaces alveolar air, rendering the lung solid (as in infective pneumonia) [2].

### Diseases Causing the Pattern

Lobar consolidation is the representative pattern of lobar pneumonia. The *lobar pneumonia* is one of the two morphologic classifications of pneumonia (the other being bronchopneumonia) (Figs. 3.1 and 3.2). The most common organisms causing lobar pneumonia are *Streptococcus* (*Pneumococcus*) *pneumoniae*, *Hemophilus influenzae*, and *Moraxella catarrhalis*. *Mycobacterium tuberculosis* may also cause lobar pneumonia [3] (Table 3.1).

Tumorous conditions such as *invasive mucinous adenocarcinoma* [4] (Figs. 3.3 and 3.4) and *bronchus-associated lymphoid tissue lymphoma* [5] (Fig. 3.5) also occur with lobar consolidation.

The lobar consolidation may also be associated with obstructive pneumonia, cicatricial or passive atelectasis, and *pulmonary infarction* [6] (Fig. 3.6).

### Distribution

Lobar consolidation in lobar pneumonia tends to be located at the middle and outer thirds of the lung. In contrast, atypical pneumonia frequently shows centrilobular nodules or acinar opacity and lobular consolidation or lobular ground-glass opacity and tends to be distributed at the inner third of the lung in addition to the middle and outer thirds [7].

### Clinical Considerations

The presence of acute pneumonia symptoms and signs favors the diagnosis of lobar pneumonia. Also the rapid development of symptoms and signs may help diagnose acute lobar pneumonia.

MRI examination with ultrafast "water-sensitive" sequence depicts bright signal, the so-called MR white lung sign, from lung consolidative lesions in patients with mucinous adenocarcinoma [8].

**Key Points for Differential Diagnosis**

1. The presence of acute pneumonia symptoms and signs and their development speed help diagnose acute lobar pneumonia.
2. Stretching, squeezing, and widening of the branching angle of CT air-bronchogram sign and bulging of the surrounding interlobar fissure suggest the diagnosis of lobar mucinous adenocarcinoma [4].
3. Indolent and slow progressive nature of consolidative lesion may help make a diagnosis of bronchus-associated lymphoid tissue lymphoma [5].
4. When mucinous adenocarcinoma is suspected, MR imaging may be conducted to see whether or not the so-called MR white lung sign is present [6, 8].
5. Central lucencies in peripheral consolidations on lung window images (a kind of reversed halo sign) are highly suggestive of pulmonary infarction [9, 10].

K.S. Lee et al., *Radiology Illustrated: Chest Radiology*, Radiology Illustrated,
DOI 10.1007/978-3-642-37096-0_3, © Springer-Verlag Berlin Heidelberg 2014

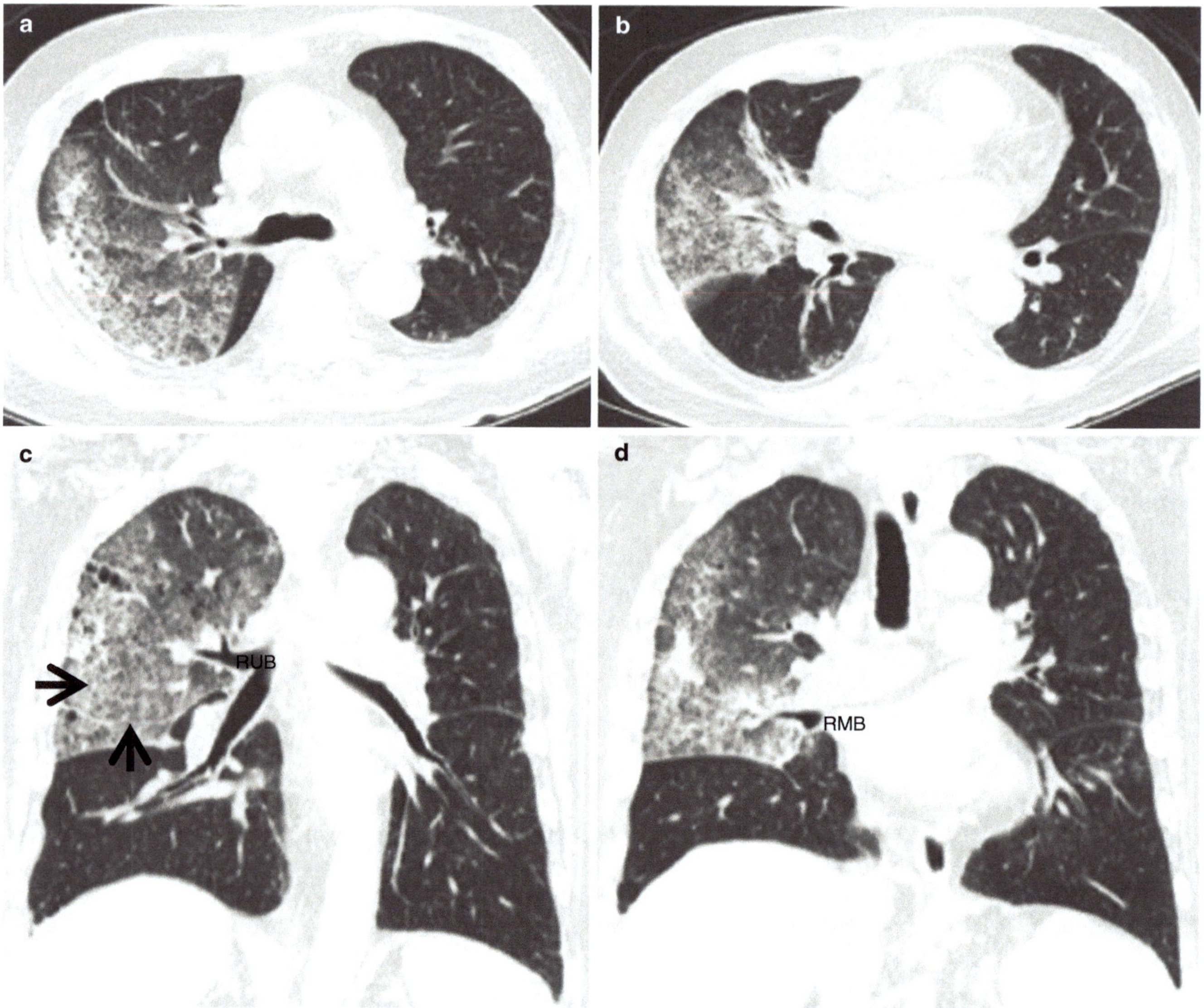


**Fig. 3.1** Lobar pneumonia in a 74-year-old man with acute myeloid leukemia and neutropenic fever. Urine culture disclosed gram-positive cocci. (**a, b**) Thin-section (2.5-mm section thickness) CT scans at levels of the right upper (**a**) and middle lobar (**b**) bronchi, respectively, show lobar parenchymal opacity involving the right upper and middle lobes. (**c, d**) Coronal reformatted images at levels showing the right upper lobar bronchus (RUB) (**c**) and right middle lobar bronchus (RMB) (**d**), respectively, demonstrate parenchymal opacity in the right upper and middle lobes. Also note crazy-paving appearance (*arrows* in **c**) within parenchymal opacity lesion

## Lobar Pneumonia

### Pathology and Pathogenesis

Fibrinosuppurative consolidation of a large portion of a lobe, or of entire lobe, is the dominant characteristic of lobar pneumonia, while patchy consolidation defines bronchopneumonia. There are four stages of the inflammatory response: congestion (vascular engorgement, intra-alveolar fluid with few neutrophils), red hepatization (massive confluent exudation with neutrophils and red blood cells, filling alveolar spaces), gray hepatization (progressive disintegration of red blood cells), and resolution (organized by fibroblasts growing into it) [11].

### Symptoms and Signs

Acute development of fever and purulent sputum is the classic manifestation of lobar pneumonia. Dyspnea, pleuritic chest pain, and hemoptysis may be present. Leukocytosis is often found, suggesting acute inflammatory process. In older debilitated or immunosuppressed patients, it may be mild or absent. Inspiratory crackle is heard on chest auscultation.

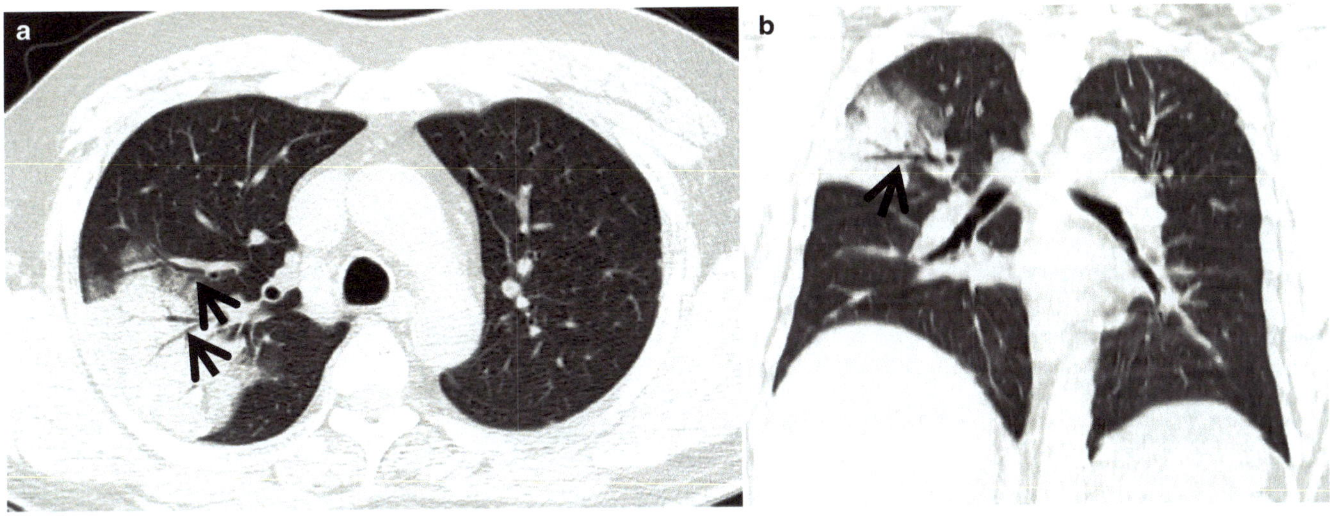


**Fig. 3.2** Segmental pneumonia as community-acquired pneumonia in a 38-year-old man. (**a**, **b**) Transverse (**a**, 2.5-mm section thickness) and coronal (**b**, 2.0-mm section thickness) reformatted CT images show segmental consolidation in posterior segment of the right upper lobe. Please note CT air-bronchogram signs (*arrows*). Patient proved to have *Streptococcus pneumoniae* pneumonia

**Table 3.1** Common diseases manifesting as lobar consolidation

| Disease | Key points for differential diagnosis |
|---|---|
| Lobar pneumonia | Acute pneumonia symptoms, homogeneous airspace consolidation with air bronchograms |
| Mucinous adenocarcinoma | Consolidation; stretching, squeezing, and widening of the branching angle of CT air-bronchogram sign and bulging of the surrounding interlobar fissure; MRI white lung sign |
| BALT lymphoma | Indolent and slow progressive nature of consolidative lesion |
| Pulmonary infarction | Peripheral wedge-shaped consolidation with central lucencies |

*Note*: *BALT* bronchus-associated lymphoid tissue

## CT Findings

On CT, homogeneous airspace consolidation involving adjacent segments of a lobe is the predominant finding of lobar pneumonia [7] (Figs. 3.1 and 3.2). Areas of ground-glass attenuation can be seen adjacent to the airspace consolidation. The consolidation typically extends across lobular and segmental boundaries. Air bronchograms are usually seen.

## CT–Pathology Comparisons

Lobar pneumonia is characterized histologically by filling of alveolar airspaces by an exudate of edema fluid and neutrophils. This filling usually begins at the periphery of the lung adjacent to the visceral pleura and spreads via interalveolar pores and small airways centripetally, resulting in a homogeneous area of consolidation. Incomplete filling of alveoli can be seen as areas of ground-glass opacity. The bronchi remain filled with gas and become surrounded by the expanding inflammatory exudates and thus are often seen as air bronchograms on CT scans (Figs. 3.1 and 3.2).

## Patient Prognosis

Prognosis depends on the severity of pneumonia. Pneumonia severity index (PSI) is a point scoring system to assess the risk of death due to pneumonia, including age, comorbid illnesses, physical examination findings, and laboratory findings [12]. CURB-65 is another useful scoring system [13]. Early adequate antibiotic administration and management stratification according to the scoring system are essential in the treatment of pneumonia.

# Invasive Mucinous Adenocarcinoma

## Pathology and Pathogenesis

Invasive mucinous adenocarcinoma (formerly mucinous BAC) has a distinctive histologic appearance with tumor cells having a goblet or columnar cell morphology with abundant intracytoplasmic mucin (Figs. 3.3 and 3.4). There is a strong tendency for multicentric, multilobar, and bilateral lung involvement, which may reflect aerogenous spread. They show frequent KRAS mutation [14].

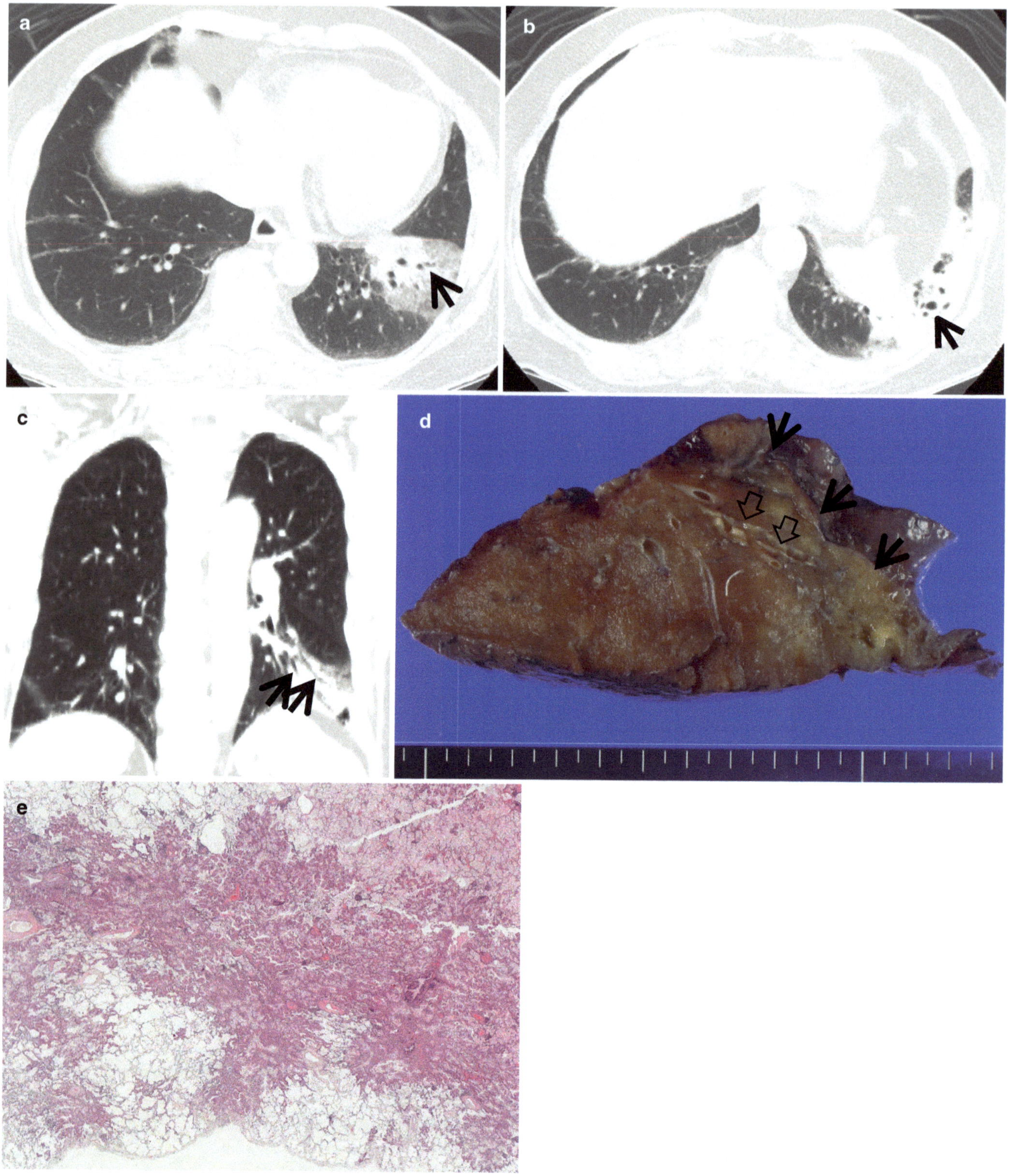


**Fig. 3.3** Lobar mucinous adenocarcinoma in a 75-year-old woman. (**a**, **b**) Transverse CT scans (5.0-mm section thickness) obtained at levels of liver (**a**) and splenic (**b**) domes, respectively, show non-segmental parenchymal consolidation and internal CT air-bronchogram signs (*arrows*) in the left lower lobe. Also note decreased lobar volume in the same lobe. (**c**) Coronal reformatted image shows parenchymal consolidation in the left lower lobe with CT air-bronchogram signs (*arrows*). (**d**) Gross pathologic specimen obtained with left lower lobectomy demonstrates a yellow-to-brown and somewhat myxoid tumor (*arrows*) in the left lower lobe. Also note the dilated bronchus with wall destruction (*open arrows*) within tumor. (**e**) High-magnification (×100) photomicrograph shows lack of circumscribed border with permeative tumor spread to adjacent lung parenchyma. Alveolar spaces often contain mucin. Tumor has a distinctive appearance with neoplastic cells having a goblet or columnar morphology with abundant intracytoplasmic mucin

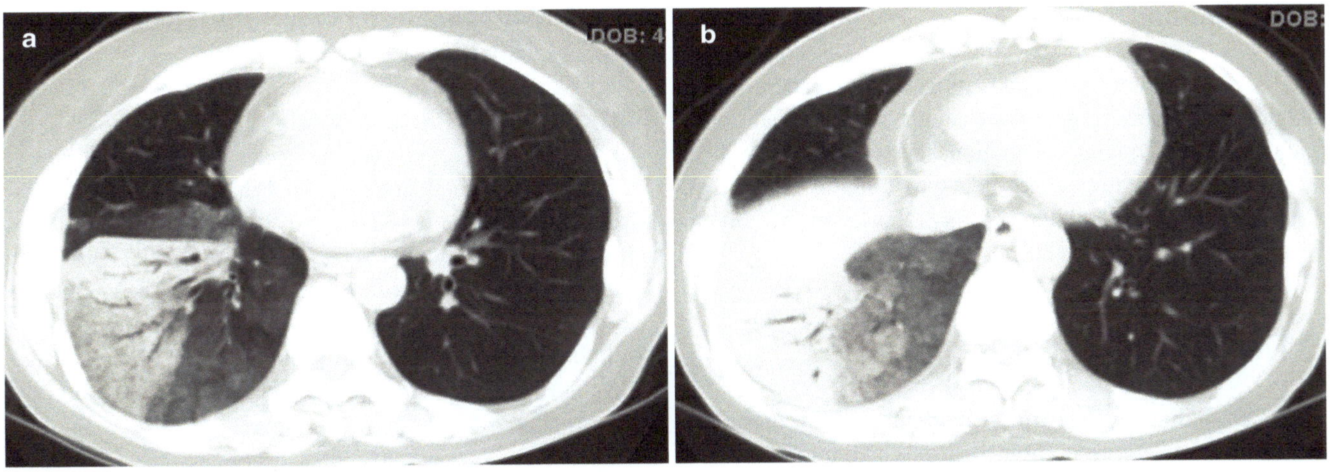


**Fig. 3.4** Diffuse adenocarcinoma in a 57-year-old woman. (**a**, **b**) CT scans (5.0-mm section thickness) obtained at levels of the basal segmental bronchi (**a**) and suprahepatic inferior vena cava (**b**), respectively, show parenchymal opacity (consolidation and ground-glass opacity) in the right lower lobe and in a portion of the right middle lobe. Also note CT air-bronchogram signs within lesions. Biopsy specimen obtained from the right lower lobe disclosed adenocarcinoma of moderate differentiation with tumor pleural invasion

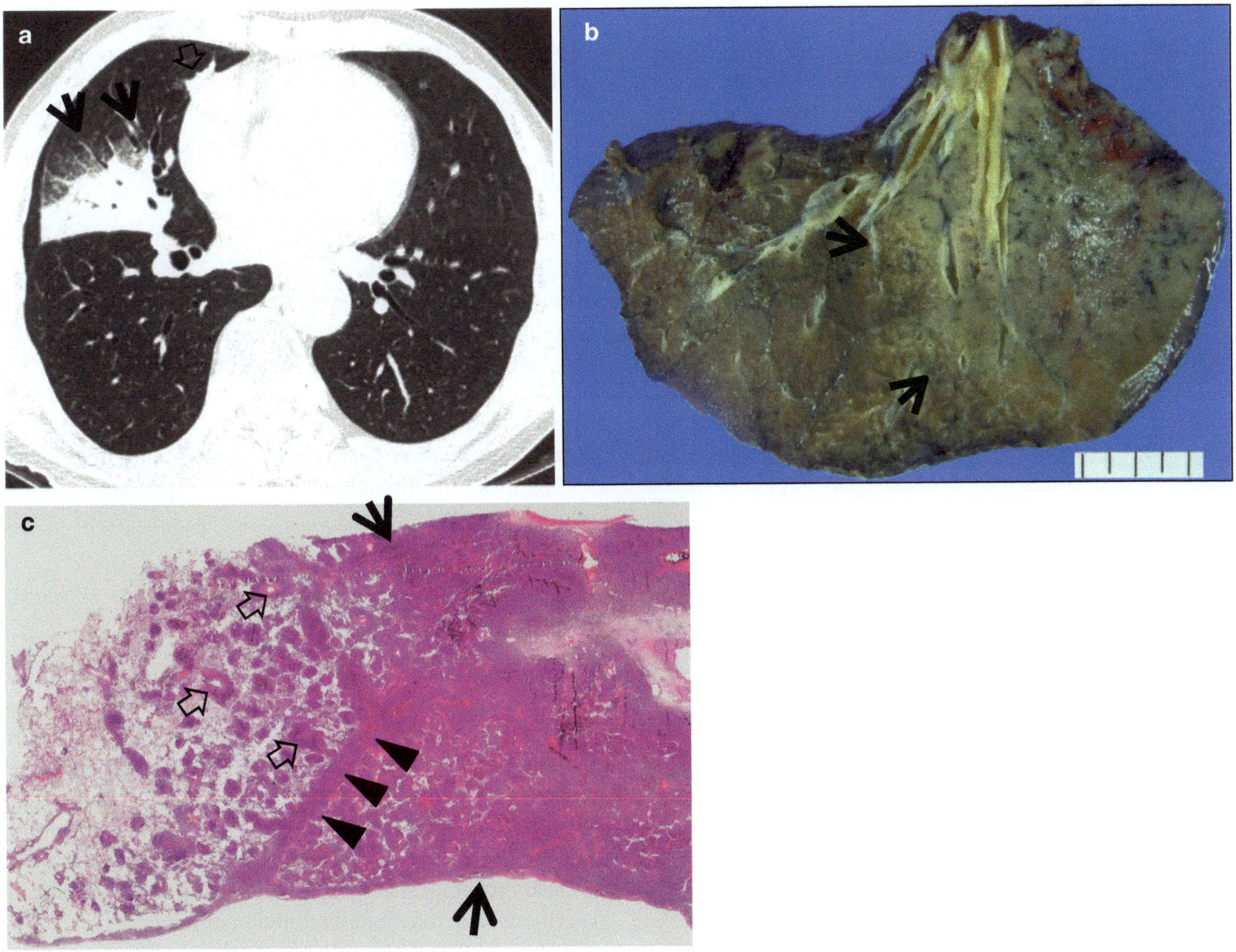


**Fig. 3.5** Bronchus-associated lymphoid tissue lymphoma in a 60-year-old man. (**a**) Thin-section (1.5-mm section thickness) CT scan obtained at level of the inferior pulmonary veins shows parenchymal consolidation and ground-glass opacity (*arrows*) in lateral segment of the right middle lobe. Also note small rectangular consolidative lesion (*open arrow*) in medial segment of the same lobe. (**b**) Cut surface of gross pathologic specimen obtained with right middle lobectomy demonstrates ill-defined gray-tan consolidative lesion (*arrows*). Please note central solid area. (**c**) Low-magnification (×5) photomicrograph discloses tumor expansion from bronchovascular interstitium to alveolar space to form consolidative lesion (*arrows*) in the right half of specimen. In the left half, tumor cells are confined to bronchovascular interstitium only to appear as small centrilobular nodules (*open arrows*). Also note thickened interlobular septa and venules (*arrowheads*) with tumor cell infiltration

### Symptoms and Signs

Due to abundant mucin production of the cancer cells, patients with invasive mucinous adenocarcinoma can complain of copious amount of sputum, the so-called bronchorrhea. Otherwise, patients may be asymptomatic. As disease progresses to the bilateral lung, shortness of breath develops.

### CT Findings

The CT findings of invasive mucinous adenocarcinoma include consolidations, air bronchograms, and multifocal and sometimes multilobar solid and subsolid nodules or masses, which tend to be centrilobular or bronchocentric [15, 16]. Stretching, squeezing, and widening of the branching angle of CT air-bronchogram sign and bulging of the surrounding interlobar fissure may be helpful in the diagnosis of lobar mucinous adenocarcinoma [4] (Figs. 3.3 and 3.4). MRI white lung sign (bright high signal intensity on water-sensitive sequences) is also useful in the differential diagnosis between mucinous adenocarcinoma and infectious pneumonia [8].

### CT–Pathology Comparisons

The CT features of invasive mucinous adenocarcinoma showing airspace consolidation and air bronchograms are caused by tumor growth along the alveolar wall (lepidic growth) combined with secretion of mucin [17, 18] (Figs. 3.3 and 3.4). As the tumor fills the alveolar spaces and infiltrates the alveolar septa and bronchial walls, the bronchus becomes stretched, squeezed, and rigid [4]. Production of mucin may result in expansion of the lobe, leading to bulging of interlobar fissures. MRI white lung sign is related to the high intratumoral content of mucin.

### Patient Prognosis

Invasive mucinous adenocarcinoma has a strong tendency for multifocal, multilobar, and bilateral lung involvement, which may reflect aerogenous spread. Even if surgically resected in the localized stage, it frequently recurs in the remaining lung. Mucinous adenocarcinoma is essentially insensitive to *EGFR*-targeted therapy [19]. The overall prognosis for patients with invasive mucinous adenocarcinoma is worse than for those with the nonmucinous adenocarcinoma.

## Bronchus-Associated Lymphoid Tissue (BALT) Lymphoma

### Pathology and Pathogenesis

Pulmonary marginal zone B-cell lymphoma of bronchus-associated lymphoid tissue (BALT) is an extranodal lymphoma, which is thought to arise in acquired BALT secondary to inflammatory or autoimmune processes. The neoplastic cells infiltrate the bronchiolar epithelium, forming lymphoepithelial lesion. They typically show a yellow-gray consolidative mass and appear as diffuse infiltrate of small lymphoid cells [5] (Fig. 3.5).

### Symptoms and Signs

In BALT lymphoma of lobar consolidation type, constitutional symptoms such as weight loss, night sweating, and fever are more common than respiratory symptoms. Chronic cough and dyspnea are the main respiratory symptoms.

### CT Findings

The main CT findings of BALT lymphoma are airspace consolidation or nodules containing air bronchograms within the lesions [5]. The lesions are usually multiple and bilateral (Fig. 3.5). Other findings include single nodule (also note section “Solitary Pulmonary Nodule (SPN), Solid” in Chap. 1), bronchiectasis and bronchiolitis, and diffuse interstitial lung disease pattern. Indolent and slow progressive nature of consolidative lesion may help make a diagnosis of bronchus-associated lymphoid tissue lymphoma.

### CT–Pathology Comparisons

CT findings of BALT lymphoma showing solitary or multifocal nodules or masses and areas of airspace consolidation are related to proliferation of tumor cells within the interstitium such that the alveolar airspaces and transitional airways are obliterated [20] (Fig. 3.5). Because the bronchi and membranous bronchioles tend to be unaffected, an air bronchogram is common. Interlobular septal thickening, centrilobular nodules, and bronchial wall thickening on CT images are related to perilymphatic interstitial infiltration of tumor cells.

## Patient Prognosis

BALT lymphoma shows the indolent clinical course. The estimated 5- and 10-year overall survival rates have been reported to be 90 and 72 %, respectively [21]. Age and performance status are the prognostic factors.

# Pulmonary Infarction

## Pathology and Pathogenesis

Infarction in the lungs is generally wedge-shaped and commonly multiple. An occluded pulmonary artery is found at the apex of the infarct; the base of the infarct is on the pleura. Any part of the lung may be affected but infarction is most common at the lung bases. It is classically hemorrhagic and appears as a red-blue area in early stage and becomes paler and red-brown due to hemosiderin deposition. With passage of time, fibrinous replacement begins and eventually converts the infarct into contracted scar. In thromboembolism, alternatively, the embolus may result in pulmonary infarction, which is indicated clinically by an attack of localized pleural pain, dyspnea, and hemoptysis. Often there is more than one embolic episode [11].

## Symptoms and Signs

Acute development of more severe dyspnea, pleuritic chest pain, and blood-tinged sputum are the cardinal symptoms of pulmonary infarction. Purulent sputum is absent. Tachypnea, tachycardia, and hypoxia are found. Lower leg swelling and positive Homan's sign can be detected, reflecting deep venous thrombosis.

## CT Findings

A peripheral wedge-shaped area of consolidation on CT is suggestive of pulmonary infarction [22]. Internal morphologic characteristics of this consolidation include the presence of central lucencies and the absence of air bronchograms [9] (Fig. 3.6). A slight and continuous FDG uptake at the border of a peripheral lung consolidation (rim sign) can be seen at FDG PET–CT [23]. Cavitation can occur within the central portion of the consolidation.

## CT–Pathology Comparisons

The consolidation in pulmonary infarction is mainly caused by central blood alveolar filling or central necrosis with a peripheral inflammatory reaction [24]. Central lucencies within consolidation are related to areas of central necrosis surrounded by an inflammatory reaction [9]. A rim of FDG uptake in a pulmonary infarction is related to peripheral inflammatory reaction [23].

## Patient Prognosis

Early detection and administration of anticoagulation or thrombolytic therapy is the most important for the management of pulmonary infarction. Pulmonary infarction occurs in approximately 20–30 % of patients with significant cardiac or pulmonary disease, the overall prognosis of pulmonary infarction is worse than pulmonary embolism without infarction.

# Patchy and Nodular Consolidation

## Definition

Lung parenchymal lesions of opacification (consolidation, poorly defined nodules, or ground-glass opacity), with ill-defined margin, are occasionally observed in unilateral or bilateral lungs. The lung abnormalities are spotty, inconsistent, or not uniform (patchy) in distribution. They may appear as multifocal lesions of a single pattern or as a simultaneous combination of various patterns of consolidation, poorly defined nodules, and ground-glass opacity. They may involve a single lung (Fig. 3.7) or both lungs.

When the lesions of opacification appear with discrete margin, we call them multiple nodules or masses (please note Chap. 19).

## Diseases Causing the Pattern

This pattern of lung abnormalities can be observed in cryptogenic organizing pneumonia or organizing stage of acute pneumonias [10, 25], extensive bronchopneumonia including *airway-invasive pulmonary aspergillosis* [26] (Fig. 3.8), fungal infection such as *cryptococcosis* [27] (Figs. 3.7 and 3.9), diffuse form of adenocarcinoma(s) [18],

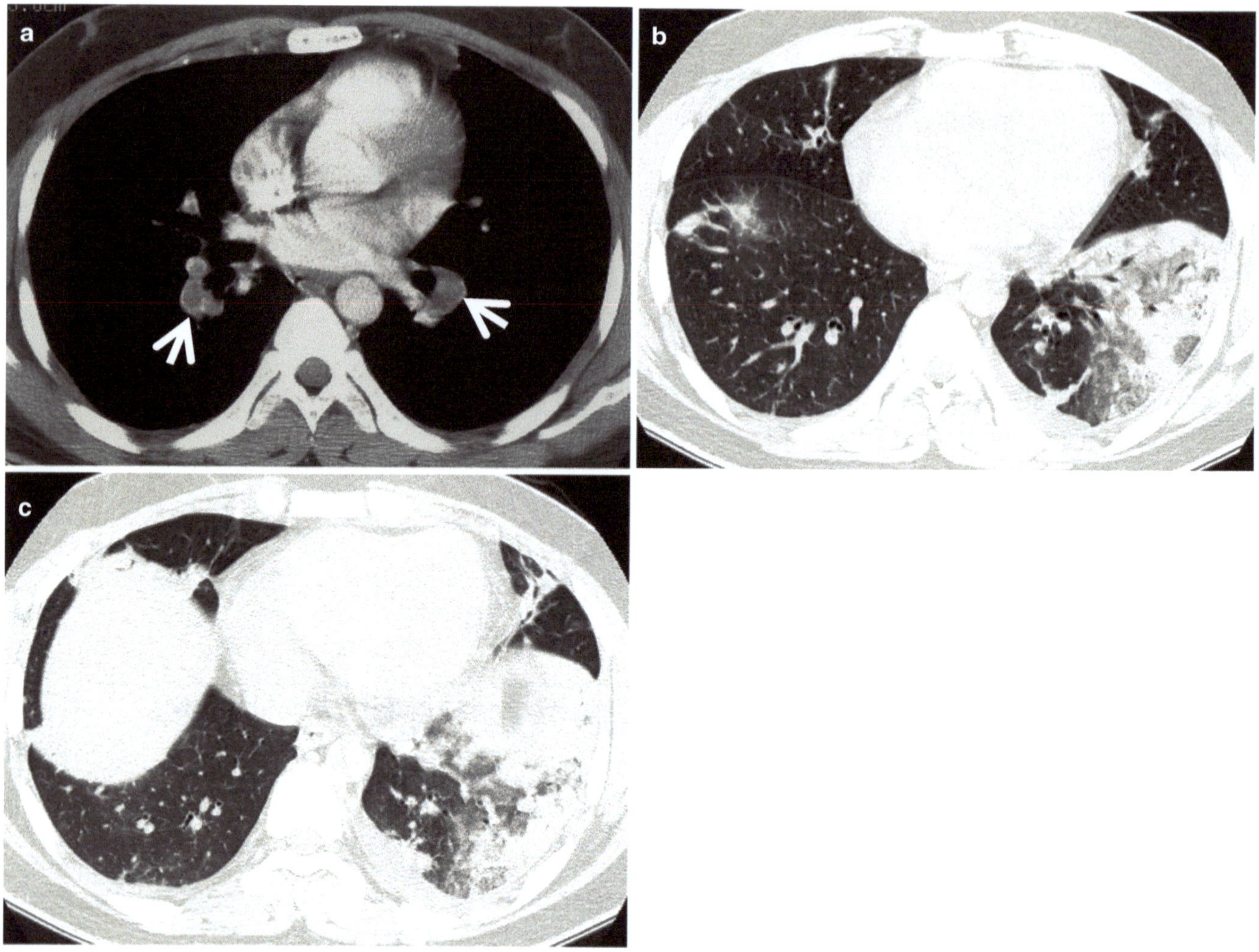


**Fig. 3.6** Pulmonary embolism and consequent lung infarction in a 32-year-old man with chronic liver disease and deep vein thrombosis. (**a**) Enhanced CT scan (5.0-mm section thickness) obtained at level of basal trunks shows filling defects (*arrows*, embolism) in the bilateral lower lobar pulmonary arteries. (**b**, **c**) Lung window images of CT scans (2.5-mm section thickness) obtained at levels of the cardiac ventricle (**b**) and liver dome (**c**), respectively, demonstrate parenchymal opacity in both lower lobes, particularly in the left lower lobe. Consolidative lesions have disappeared after resolution of pulmonary embolism

lymphoproliferative disease including *IgG4-related lung disease* [5, 28] (Fig. 3.10) and *lymphomatoid granulomatosis* [29] (Fig. 3.11), and pulmonary vasculitis including antineutrophil cytoplasmic antibody (ANCA)-associated granulomatous vasculitis (former Wegener's granulomatosis) [30] (Table 3.2).

## Distribution

Lesions in the above-mentioned diseases show spotty, inconsistent, or not uniform distribution. The abnormalities may depict their distribution along the bronchovascular bundles.

## Clinical Considerations

Airway-invasive pulmonary aspergillosis is a disease in immunocompromised patients (those who have hematologic malignancy and who underwent hematopoietic stem cell transplantation) particularly whose peripheral blood absolute neutrophil count is <500 cells/μL (neutropenia). Cryptococcosis is an indolent lung infection in mildly immunocompromised patients [27]. Generalized symptoms and signs, such as diffuse alveolar hemorrhage, acute glomerulonephritis, chronic refractory sinusitis or rhinorrhea, imaging findings of nodules or cavities, and multisystemic disease, precede typical imaging findings in pulmonary vasculitis [31].

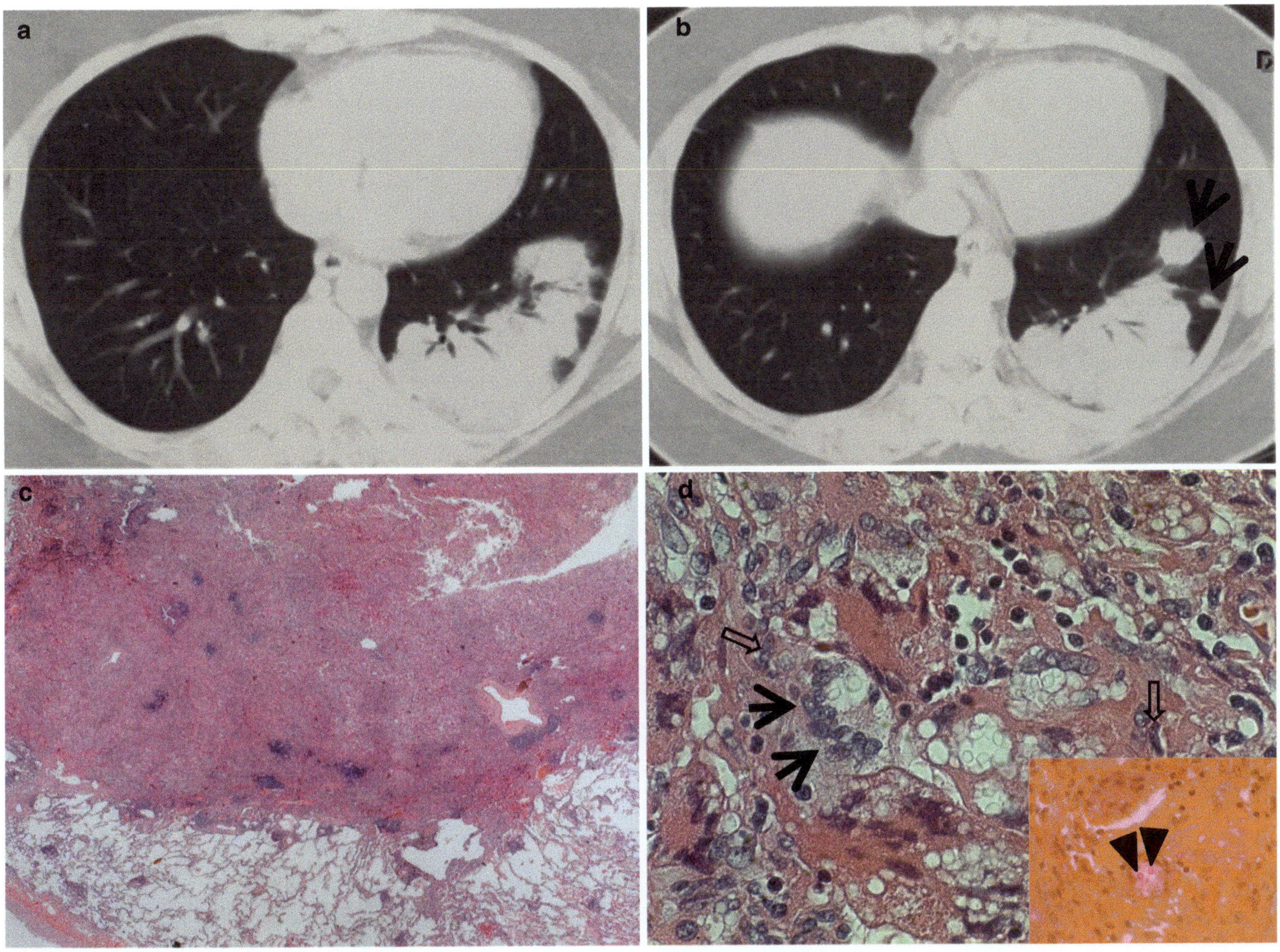


**Fig. 3.7** Pulmonary cryptococcosis appearing as localized consolidation or nodule in a 34-year-old immunocompetent woman. (**a, b**) Lung window images of CT scans (5.0-mm section thickness) obtained at levels of the cardiac ventricle (**a**) and liver dome (**b**), respectively, show large area of consolidation and several poorly defined nodules (*arrows* in **b**) in the left lower lobe. (**c**) Low-magnification (×5) photomicrograph demonstrates relatively well-defined, homogeneous consolidation lesion without necrotic portion. (**d**) High-magnification (×200) photomicrograph displays foreign-body-type giant cells (*arrows*) and histiocytes (*open arrows*). *Inset*: mucicarmine staining highlighting yeast-form organisms (*arrowheads*)

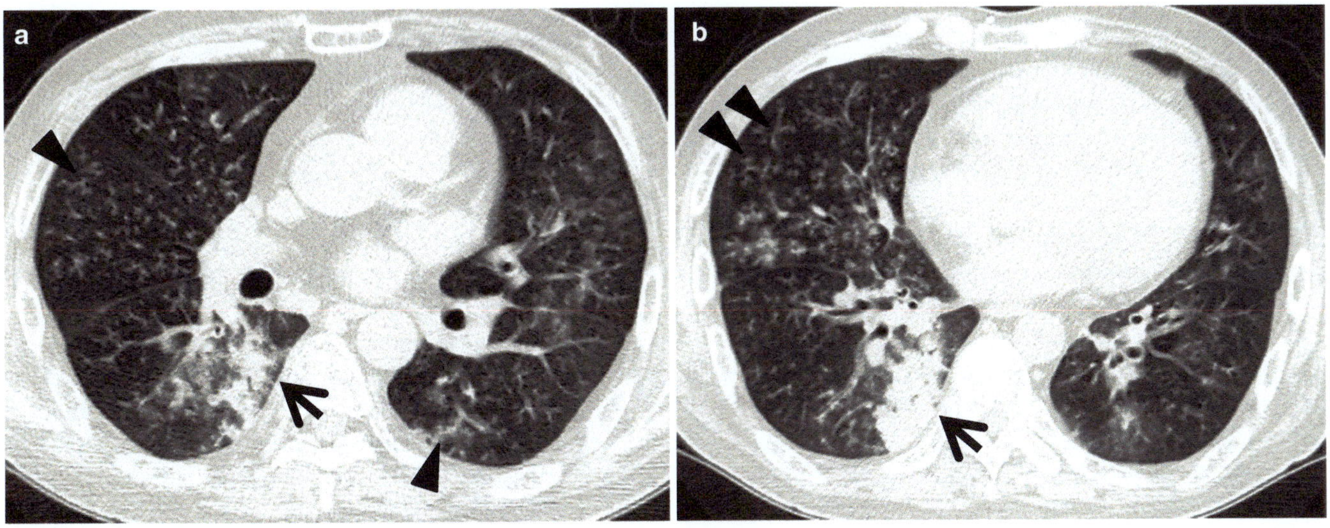


**Fig. 3.8** Airway-invasive pulmonary aspergillosis presenting as multifocal areas of consolidation and branching small nodular lesions in a 46-year-old man who had brain tumor and who received corticosteroid therapy. (**a, b**) Thin-section (1.0-mm section thickness) CT scans obtained at levels of the bronchus intermedius (**a**) and basal segmental bronchi (**b**), respectively, show patchy areas of consolidation (*arrows*) and extensive areas of cellular bronchiolitis with tree-in-bud signs (*arrowheads*) in both lungs. Patient had positive antigen for *Aspergillus* from his serum. Lesions showed improvement after antifungal therapy

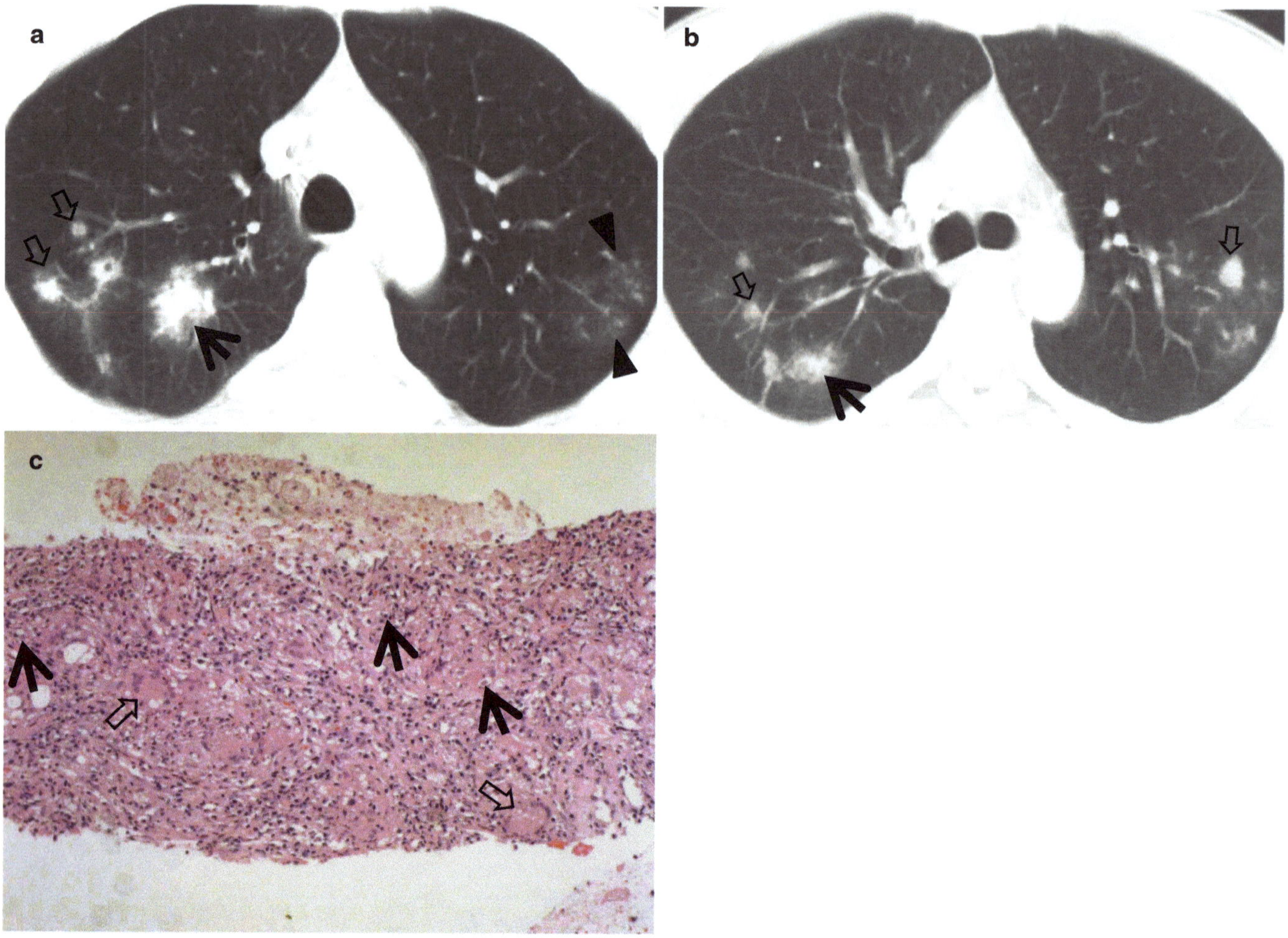


Fig. 3.9 Pulmonary cryptococcosis appearing as patchy areas of consolidation, poorly defined nodules, or nodular branching lesions in both lungs in a 37-year-old man. (**a**, **b**) Lung window images of CT scans (5.0-mm section thickness) obtained at levels of the aortic arch (**a**) and main bronchi (**b**), respectively, show patchy areas of poorly defined nodules (*arrows*), areas of consolidation (*open arrows*), and tree-in-bud signs (*arrowheads*) in both lungs. (**c**) Low-magnification (×5) photomicrograph demonstrates interstitial pneumonitis and alveolar inflammation. Alveolar spaces are filled with numerous macrophages (*arrows*) and giant cells (*open arrows*) containing small, cyst-like spaces. Both Gomori methenamine silver and mucicarmine staining disclosed yeast-form organisms within the cells

**Key Points for Differential Diagnosis**

1. In cryptogenic organizing pneumonia or organizing stage of acute pneumonia, consolidation or poorly defined nodules are characteristically distributed along the bronchovascular bundles or the subpleural lungs. The areas of consolidation or nodules may show reversed halo sign [10].
2. Pulmonary cryptococcosis most commonly presents as clustered nodules but also as solitary nodular, scattered nodular, or bronchopneumonic lesion and is a slowly progressive and slowly resolving pulmonary infection [27].
3. Lymphoproliferative disease and IgG4-related lung disease manifest diverse patterns of lung abnormality on CT scans, including a single nodular or consolidative pattern, multiple nodular or areas of consolidation, bronchiectasis and bronchiolitis, and diffuse interstitial lung disease pattern [5, 28].
4. Central necrotic low attenuation within a mass or a nodule, peripheral rim-like enhancement and surrounding ground-glass halo are important characteristic findings that may help suggest the diagnosis of pulmonary lymphomatoid granulomatosis [29]. Likewise, in ANCA-associated granulomatous vasculitis, central necrosis, rim enhancement, and halo are also seen, and the necrosis is mainly associated with underlying histopathology of neutrophilic microabscesses or a large zone of geographic necrosis that usually appears deeply basophilic due to the presence of nuclear debris of neutrophils [30, 31]. In both the diseases, there may be cavitation within lesions with airway communication and excavation of the central necrotic portion [29–31].

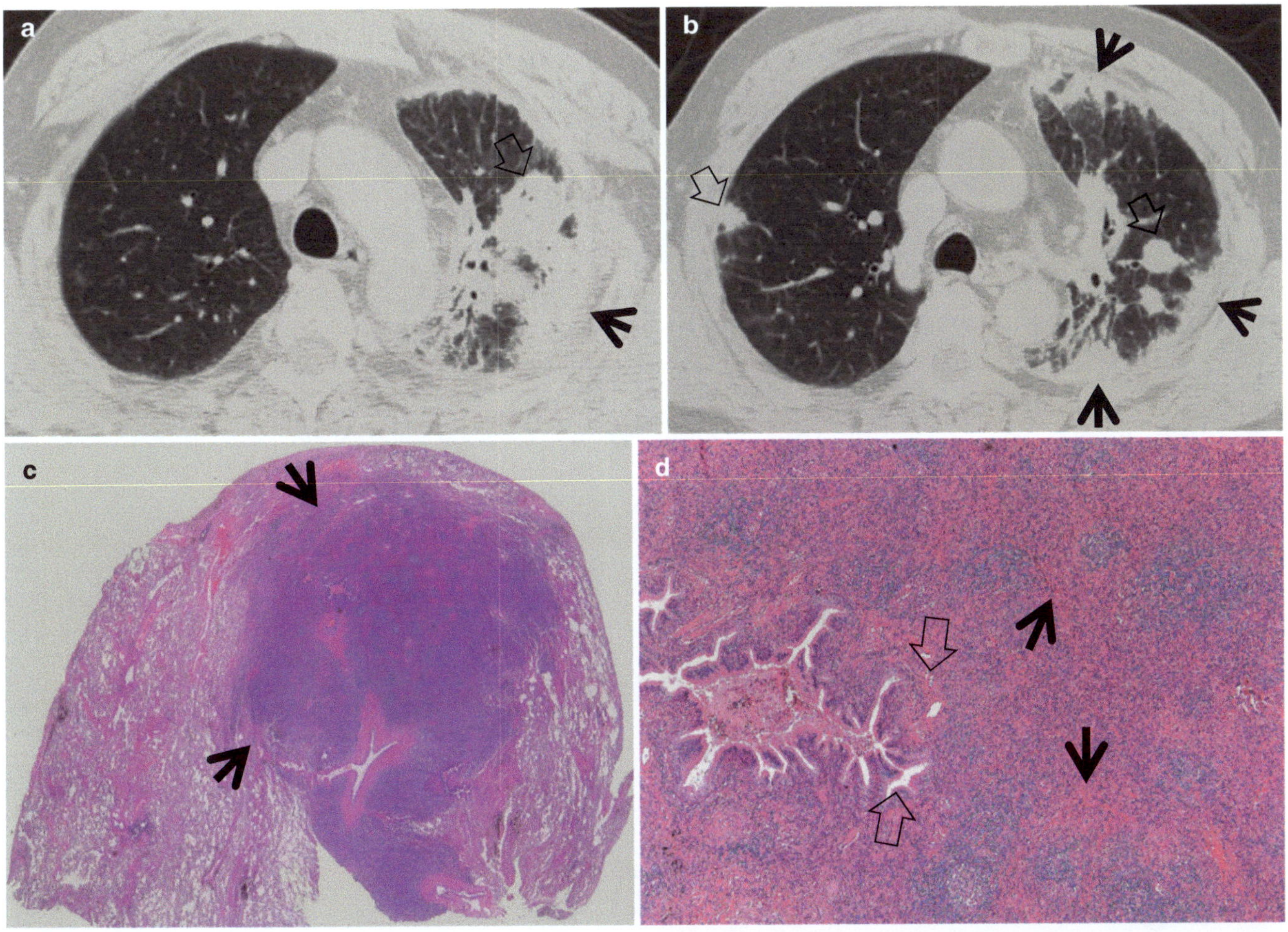


**Fig. 3.10** IgG4-related lung disease manifesting as multifocal areas of consolidation and nodules in both lungs in a 51-year-old man. (**a**, **b**) Lung window images of CT scans (5.0-mm section thickness) obtained at levels of the aortic (**a**) and azygos (**b**) arches, respectively, show patchy areas of consolidation (*arrows*) and nodules (*open arrows*) in both lungs. Axial and peripheral interstitial thickening is also observed in the left lung. (**c**) Low-magnification (×2) photomicrograph of pathologic specimen obtained from a nodule in the right upper lobe demonstrates a relatively well-defined subpleural nodule (*arrows*). (**d**) Low-magnification (×8) photomicrograph discloses lymphoplasmacytic infiltration along with irregular fibrosis (*arrows*) and obliterated vascular structure (*open arrows*). IgG4 and CD43 immunohistologic staining depicted positive results

## Airway-Invasive Pulmonary Aspergillosis

### Pathology and Pathogenesis

Airway-invasive pulmonary aspergillosis is characterized histologically by liquefaction necrosis and neutrophilic infiltrate, which is centered at membranous and respiratory bronchioles. Vascular infiltration and coagulative necrosis are usually absent or minimal in extent [26] (Fig. 3.8).

### Symptoms and Signs

Airway-invasive pulmonary aspergillosis predominantly affects severely immunocompromised patients, particularly those with AIDS, heart–lung or lung transplantation, and hematologic malignancy. While most patients with lung transplantation are asymptomatic, those with AIDS and hematologic malignancy are usually symptomatic with dyspnea, inspiratory wheezes, fever, and nonproductive cough. Airway obstruction may result in atelectasis and severe respiratory failure [32].

### CT Findings

HRCT demonstrates centrilobular nodules, tree-in-bud signs, and patchy areas of consolidation, often in a peribronchial distribution [26] (Fig. 3.8). Wall thickening of the trachea or the bronchi may be seen in tracheobronchitis.

### CT–Pathology Comparisons

CT findings of centrilobular small nodules, tree-in-bud signs, and patchy areas of consolidation correspond to the foci of

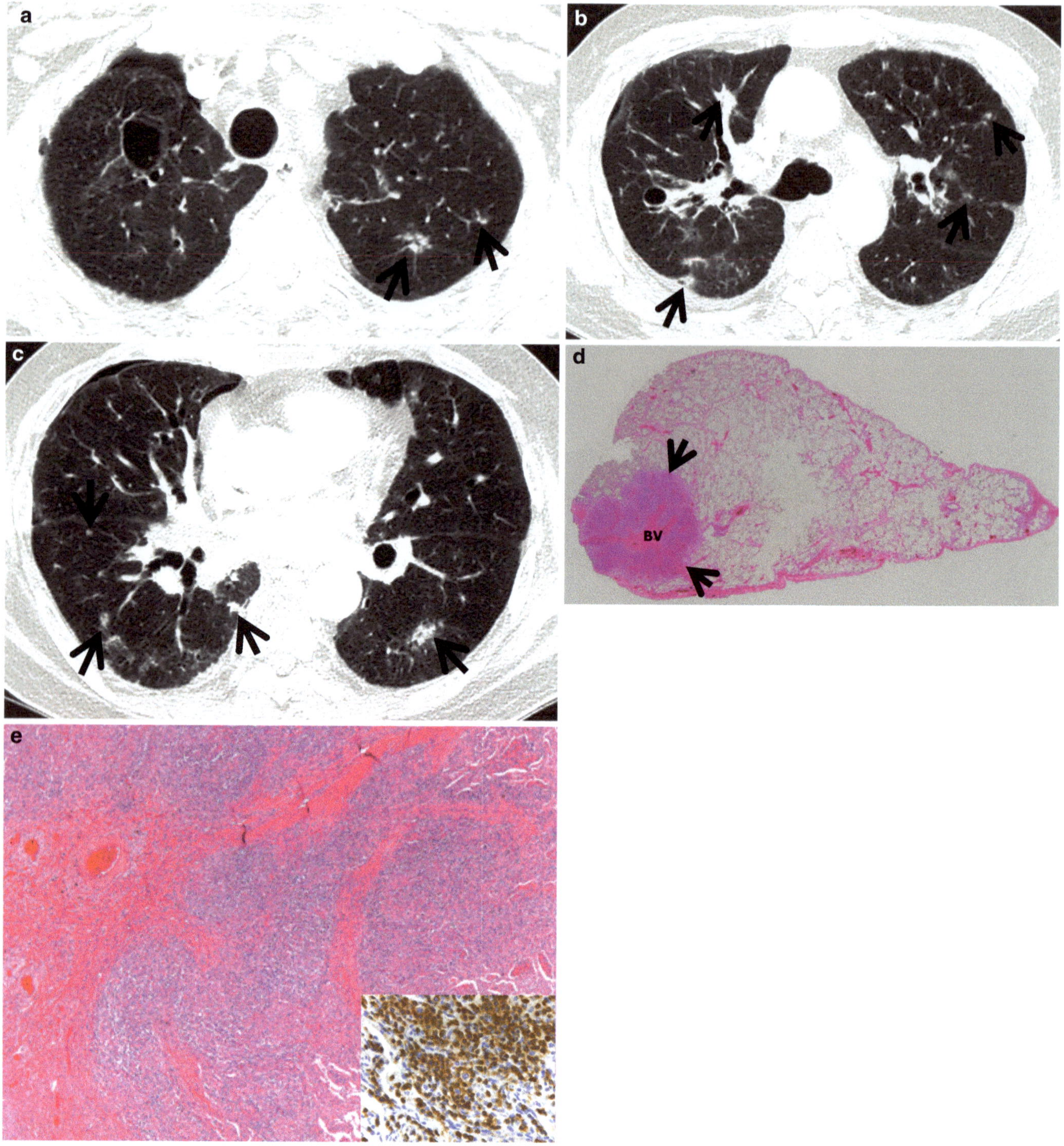


**Fig. 3.11** Lymphomatoid granulomatosis appearing as patchy areas of consolidation or nodules in both lungs in a 70-year-old man. (**a–c**) Lung window images of thin-section (1.5-mm section thickness) CT scans obtained at levels of the great vessel takeoff (**a**), aortic arch (**b**), and lower lobar branch (**c**), respectively, show patchy areas of nodules or variable size and morphology (*arrows*) in both lungs. Also note air-filled cysts in the right upper lobe and pneumothorax, small in amount and in right pleural space, due to previous lung biopsy. (**d**) Low-magnification (×2) photomicrograph of pathologic specimen obtained from a nodule in the left lower lobe demonstrates a relatively well-defined subpleural nodule (*arrows*) surrounding central bronchovascular structures (*BV*). (**e**) Low-magnification (×10) photomicrograph discloses. *Inset*: positive staining for $CD3^+$

**Table 3.2** Common diseases manifesting as patchy and nodular consolidation

| Disease | Key points for differential diagnosis |
|---|---|
| Cryptogenic organizing pneumonia | Consolidation or poorly defined nodules with peribronchovascular and subpleural distribution |
| Extensive bronchopneumonia | |
| Cryptococcosis | Multiple clustered-nodular patterns, single nodular or scattered nodular lesion, mass-like consolidation, bronchopneumonia pattern |
| Diffuse form of adenocarcinoma | |
| IgG4-related lung disease | Solitary large nodular lesion, round-shaped GGO, thickening of bronchovascular bundles and interlobular septa, bronchiectasis |
| Lymphomatoid granulomatosis | Pulmonary nodules and masses with central low attenuation and peripheral rim enhancement and ground-glass opacity halo |
| ANCA-associated granulomatous vasculitis | Multiple, bilateral, subpleural nodules or masses |

*Note*: *GGO* ground-glass opacity, *ANCA* antineutrophil cytoplasmic antibody

necrotizing bronchitis and bronchiolitis, typically associated with a neutrophilic inflammatory reaction [26].

### Patient Prognosis

Early diagnosis by bronchoscopic examination and aggressive antifungal therapy is the most important step to improve the prognosis. Mortality rate of the patients with lung transplantation is 24 %. However, the prognosis in those with hematologic malignancy or hematopoietic stem cell transplantation is significantly worse, showing 72 % of mortality [32].

## Pulmonary Cryptococcosis

### Pathology and Pathogenesis

Pulmonary cryptococcal lesions usually show solitary or multiple relatively well-defined, yellow-to-brown, and oval nodular mass or patchy consolidation. Microscopically, aggregates of foamy histiocytes containing cytoplasmic fungi of 6–25 um in size are found. They were stained with GMS, PAS, and mucicarmine [33] (Fig. 3.7).

### Symptoms and Signs

The clinical presentation of pulmonary cryptococcosis varies from asymptomatic infection to severe pneumonia with respiratory failure [34]. Symptoms are nonspecific, characterized by cough, fever, dyspnea, pleuritic chest pain, hemoptysis, and malaise. Acute respiratory failure with rapid progression has been reported [35].

### CT Findings

Pulmonary cryptococcosis in non-AIDS patients appears with various patterns of lung lesions and indolent course. The most common CT findings are multiple clustered-nodular patterns, localized to a lung lobe [26]. Other findings include single nodular or scattered nodular lesion, mass-like consolidation, and bronchopneumonia pattern. Diffuse involvement including miliary pattern, lymph node enlargement, and cavitation is seen most commonly in immunocompromised patient [36] (Figs. 3.7 and 3.9).

### CT–Pathology Comparisons

Nodular pulmonary cryptococcosis (cryptococcomas) histopathologically consists of central zone of necrosis surrounded by a thick fibrous capsule. At the interface of the nodule and the parenchyma, the alveolar septa are widened by mononuclear inflammatory cells, granulomas, or reactive lymphoid follicles. The airspaces contain foamy macrophages and proteinaceous eosinophilic fluid collections. These histopathologic findings corresponded to the area of a rim of ground-glass opacity around the nodule [37].

### Patient Prognosis

Immune status of the patient, severity of pulmonary involvement, and presence of meningoencephalitis determine the treatment regimen for pulmonary cryptococcosis. With the introduction of new less toxic and more effective antifungal drugs, treatment outcome is favorable [38].

## IgG4-Related Lung Disease

### Pathology and Pathogenesis

Immunoglobulin G4 (IgG4)-related sclerosing disease is characterized clinicopathologically by an elevated serum IgG4 level, fibrotic inflammation with numerous IgG4-positive plasma cells, and a response to steroid therapy. In lung IgG4-related disease, pathology demonstrates a great variety of pulmonary and pleural lesions, and it is important to know the morphologic variety and clinicopathologic characteristics of this disorder [39, 40] (Fig. 3.10).

## Symptoms and Signs

Respiratory symptoms including cough, exertional dyspnea, and chest pain have been described in one-half of the patients with IgG4-related lung disease, while the remaining patients were asymptomatic [41]. Constitutional symptoms such as fever and weight loss can occur. Symptoms related to the extrapulmonary organ involvement (pancreas) may be present. Elevated serum IgG4 level is found in 70–90 % of the patients.

## CT Findings

IgG4-related lung disease can be categorized into four types on the basis of the predominant CT findings: a solitary large nodular lesion including a mass, round-shaped ground-glass opacity, the thickening of bronchovascular bundles and interlobular septa, and bronchiectasis [28] (Fig. 3.10).

## CT–Pathology Comparisons

Large nodules on CT histopathologically consist of diffuse lymphoplasmacytic infiltration with fibrosis [28]. Sclerosing inflammation extends along the interlobular septa and alveolar walls, and these findings correspond to the CT findings of spiculation around a nodule. Small nodules histologically correspond to the areas of sclerosing inflammation in the peribronchiolar area. Thickened bronchovascular bundles or interlobular septa at CT histologically correspond to lymphoplasmacytic infiltration with stromal fibrosis. Bronchi or bronchioles involved in the lesions are slightly dilated.

## Patient Prognosis

In general, IgG4-related lung disease responds well to corticosteroid therapy. The optimal dose and duration of corticosteroid therapy remains to be determined. The relapse is not uncommon when corticosteroid administration is discontinued.

# Lymphomatoid Granulomatosis

## Pathology and Pathogenesis

Lymphomatoid granulomatosis is an extranodal angiocentric and angio-destructive lymphoproliferative disorder, composed of a polymorphous infiltrate of atypical B cells (Fig. 3.11), which are infected by Epstein–Barr virus (EBV), and more abundant reactive T cells. They show a spectrum of grade, which is related to the proportion of EBV-positive B cells. They may progress to an EBV-positive diffuse large B-cell lymphoma [42].

## Symptoms and Signs

The most common symptoms include fever, persistent productive cough, dyspnea, and chest tightness [43]. The presentation is typically insidious, and lung lesions may wax and wane. Constitutional symptoms such as weight loss, malaise, and fatigue may be present. Symptoms related to the other organ involvement of the skin, central nervous system, and kidney can occur.

## CT Findings

Characteristic CT findings are pulmonary nodules and masses with central low attenuation and peripheral rim enhancement and ground-glass opacity halo. The nodules and masses are lower lobe predominant with a peribronchovascular or subpleural distribution [29] (Fig. 3.11). Coarse irregular opacities and small thin-walled cysts are also seen [44].

## CT–Pathology Comparisons

Pulmonary nodules and masses are histologically caused by intravascular and perivascular infiltration of atypical lymphoid cells [44]. A low attenuation center corresponds to the histologic findings of central necrosis, and peripheral rim enhancement of the nodules is related to the angioinvasive and angio-destructive nature of lymphomatoid granulomatosis [29].

## Patient Prognosis

Lymphomatoid granulomatosis is usually an EBV-driven lymphoproliferative disease in immunocompromised patients; thus, immunosuppressive agents should be discontinued if at all. Specific therapy with corticosteroids, anti-CD20 monoclonal antibodies such as rituximab, interferon-alpha-2b, and combination chemotherapy have showed a variable success rate [43].

# References

1. Leung AN, Miller RR, Muller NL. Parenchymal opacification in chronic infiltrative lung diseases: CT-pathologic correlation. Radiology. 1993;188:209–14.
2. Hansell DM, Bankier AA, MacMahon H, McLoud TC, Muller NL, Remy J. Fleischner Society: glossary of terms for thoracic imaging. Radiology. 2008;246:697–722.
3. Jeong YJ, Lee KS. Pulmonary tuberculosis: up-to-date imaging and management. AJR Am J Roentgenol. 2008;191:834–44.
4. Jung JI, Kim H, Park SH, et al. CT differentiation of pneumonic-type bronchioloalveolar cell carcinoma and infectious pneumonia. Br J Radiol. 2001;74:490–4.

5. Bae YA, Lee KS, Han J, et al. Marginal zone B-cell lymphoma of bronchus-associated lymphoid tissue: imaging findings in 21 patients. Chest. 2008;133:433–40.
6. Gaeta M, Minutoli F, Ascenti G, et al. MR white lung sign: incidence and significance in pulmonary consolidations. J Comput Assist Tomogr. 2001;25:890–6.
7. Tanaka N, Matsumoto T, Kuramitsu T, et al. High resolution CT findings in community-acquired pneumonia. J Comput Assist Tomogr. 1996;20:600–8.
8. Gaeta M, Ascenti G, Mazziotti S, Contiguglia R, Barone M, Mileto A. MRI differentiation of pneumonia-like mucinous adenocarcinoma and infectious pneumonia. Eur J Radiol. 2012;81: 3587–91.
9. Revel MP, Triki R, Chatellier G, et al. Is it possible to recognize pulmonary infarction on multisection CT images? Radiology. 2007;244:875–82.
10. Kim SJ, Lee KS, Ryu YH, et al. Reversed halo sign on high-resolution CT of cryptogenic organizing pneumonia: diagnostic implications. AJR Am J Roentgenol. 2003;180:1251–4.
11. Husain AN. Chapter 15. The lung. In: Maitra A, Kumar V, editors. Robbins and Cotran pathologic basis of disease. International edition, 8th ed. Philadelphia: Elsevier/Saunders; 2010. p. 706.
12. Chan SS, Yuen EH, Kew J, Cheung WL, Cocks RA. Community-acquired pneumonia–implementation of a prediction rule to guide selection of patients for outpatient treatment. Eur J Emerg Med. 2001;8:279–86.
13. British Thoracic Society Standards of Care Committee. BTS guidelines for the management of community acquired pneumonia in adults. Thorax. 2001;56 Suppl 4:IV1–64.
14. Travis WD, Brambilla E, Noguchi M, et al. International Association for the Study of Lung Cancer/American Thoracic Society/European Respiratory Society International Multidisciplinary Classification of Lung Adenocarcinoma. J Thorac Oncol. 2011;6:244–85.
15. Akira M, Atagi S, Kawahara M, Iuchi K, Johkoh T. High-resolution CT findings of diffuse bronchioloalveolar carcinoma in 38 patients. AJR Am J Roentgenol. 1999;173:1623–9.
16. Austin JH, Garg K, Aberle D, et al. Radiologic implications of the 2011 classification of adenocarcinoma of the lung. Radiology. 2013;266:62–71.
17. Shah RM, Balsara G, Webster M, Friedman AC. Bronchioloalveolar cell carcinoma: impact of histology on dominant CT pattern. J Thorac Imaging. 2000;15:180–6.
18. Lee KS, Kim Y, Han J, Ko EJ, Park CK, Primack SL. Bronchioloalveolar carcinoma: clinical, histopathologic, and radiologic findings. Radiographics. 1997;17:1345–57.
19. Erman M, Grunenwald D, Penault-Llorca F, et al. Epidermal growth factor receptor, HER-2/neu and related pathways in lung adenocarcinomas with bronchioloalveolar features. Lung Cancer. 2005;47:315–23.
20. Wislez M, Cadranel J, Antoine M, et al. Lymphoma of pulmonary mucosa-associated lymphoid tissue: CT scan findings and pathological correlations. Eur Respir J. 1999;14:423–9.
21. Borie R, Wislez M, Thabut G, et al. Clinical characteristics and prognostic factors of pulmonary MALT lymphoma. Eur Respir J. 2009;34:1408–16.
22. Chintapalli K, Thorsen MK, Olson DL, Goodman LR, Gurney J. Computed tomography of pulmonary thromboembolism and infarction. J Comput Assist Tomogr. 1988;12:553–9.
23. Soussan M, Rust E, Pop G, Morere JF, Brillet PY, Eder V. The rim sign: FDG-PET/CT pattern of pulmonary infarction. Insights Imaging. 2012;3:629–33.
24. Balakrishnan J, Meziane MA, Siegelman SS, Fishman EK. Pulmonary infarction: CT appearance with pathologic correlation. J Comput Assist Tomogr. 1989;13:941–5.
25. Lee KS, Kullnig P, Hartman TE, Muller NL. Cryptogenic organizing pneumonia: CT findings in 43 patients. AJR Am J Roentgenol. 1994;162:543–6.
26. Logan PM, Primack SL, Miller RR, Muller NL. Invasive aspergillosis of the airways: radiographic, CT, and pathologic findings. Radiology. 1994;193:383–8.
27. Song KD, Lee KS, Chung MP, et al. Pulmonary cryptococcosis: imaging findings in 23 non-AIDS patients. Korean J Radiol. 2010;11:407–16.
28. Inoue D, Zen Y, Abo H, et al. Immunoglobulin G4-related lung disease: CT findings with pathologic correlations. Radiology. 2009;251:260–70.
29. Chung JH, Wu CC, Gilman MD, Palmer EL, Hasserjian RP, Shepard JA. Lymphomatoid granulomatosis: CT and FDG-PET findings. Korean J Radiol. 2011;12:671–8.
30. Lee KS, Kim TS, Fujimoto K, et al. Thoracic manifestation of Wegener's granulomatosis: CT findings in 30 patients. Eur Radiol. 2003;13:43–51.
31. Chung MP, Yi CA, Lee HY, Han J, Lee KS. Imaging of pulmonary vasculitis. Radiology. 2010;255:322–41.
32. Krenke R, Grabczak EM. Tracheobronchial manifestations of Aspergillus infections. Sci World J. 2011;11:2310–29.
33. Kim NR, Ha SY, Chung DH, et al. Isolated pulmonary cryptococcosis: report of six cases and review of the Korean cases. Korean J Pathol. 2003;37:193–8.
34. Brizendine KD, Baddley JW, Pappas PG. Pulmonary cryptococcosis. Semin Respir Crit Care Med. 2011;32:727–34.
35. Lee KH, Chang UI, Kim HW, et al. Acute respiratory failure associated with cryptococcal pneumonia and disseminated cryptococcosis in an AIDS patient. Korean J Intern Med. 2006; 21:39–42.
36. Patz Jr EF, Goodman PC. Pulmonary cryptococcosis. J Thorac Imaging. 1992;7:51–5.
37. Zinck SE, Leung AN, Frost M, Berry GJ, Muller NL. Pulmonary cryptococcosis: CT and pathologic findings. J Comput Assist Tomogr. 2002;26:330–4.
38. Limper AH, Knox KS, Sarosi GA, et al. An official American Thoracic Society statement: treatment of fungal infections in adult pulmonary and critical care patients. Am J Respir Crit Care Med. 2011;183:96–128.
39. Zen Y, Inoue D, Kitao A, et al. IgG4-related lung and pleural disease: a clinicopathologic study of 21 cases. Am J Surg Pathol. 2009;33:1886–93.
40. Park HY, Han J, Kang G, Yi CA, Chung MP. IgG4-related lung disease presenting as a consolidative mass: a case report. J Lung Cancer. 2010;9:103–5.
41. Ryu JH, Sekiguchi H, Yi ES. Pulmonary manifestations of immunoglobulin G4-related sclerosing disease. Eur Respir J. 2012;39: 180–6.
42. Guinee Jr DG, Perkins SL, Travis WD, Holden JA, Tripp SR, Koss MN. Proliferation and cellular phenotype in lymphomatoid granulomatosis: implications of a higher proliferation index in B cells. Am J Surg Pathol. 1998;22:1093–100.
43. Roschewski M, Wilson WH. Lymphomatoid granulomatosis. Cancer J. 2012;18:469–74.
44. Lee JS, Tuder R, Lynch DA. Lymphomatoid granulomatosis: radiologic features and pathologic correlations. AJR Am J Roentgenol. 2000;175:1335–9.

# 4 Beaded Septum Sign

## Definition

The sign consists of irregular and nodular thickening of interlobular septa reminiscent of a row of beads [1] (Fig. 4.1).

## Diseases Causing the Sign

It may be seen as a localized disease in pulmonary lymphangitic carcinomatosis (PLC) and less often in sarcoidosis [2] (Fig. 4.2). In sarcoidosis, the thickened interlobular septa are usually smooth rather than beaded [3, 4].

## Distribution

Pulmonary lymphangitic metastasis may be localized as a focal disease or diffuse in a generalized disease [5].

## Clinical Considerations

Please refer to sections "Nodular Septal Thickening" in Chap. 16 and "Small Nodules with Perilymphatic Distribution" in Chap. 18.

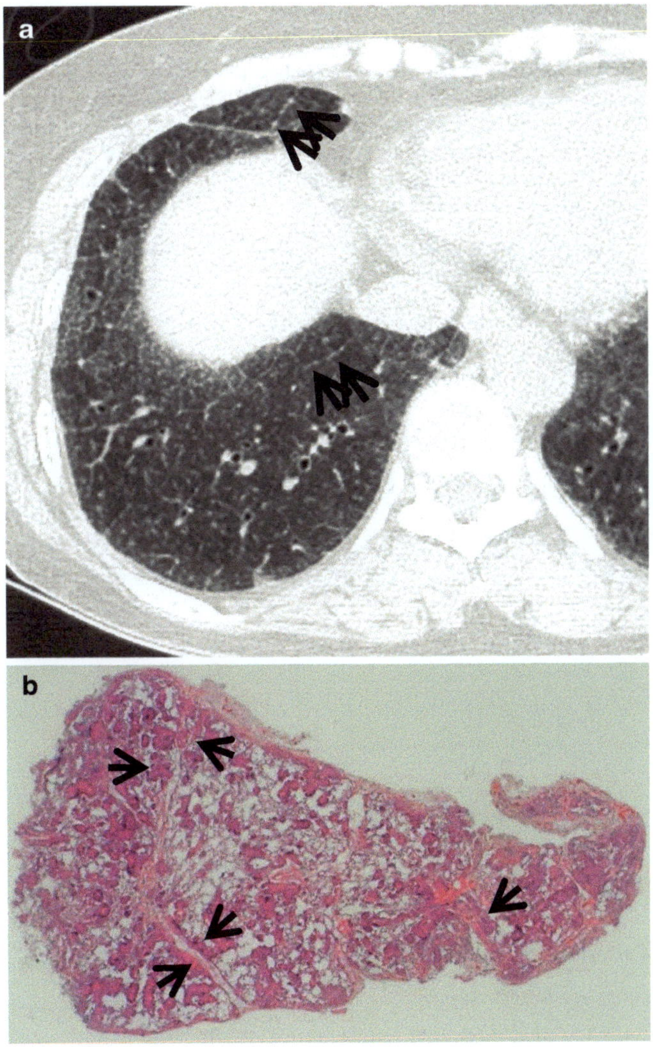

**Fig. 4.1** Pulmonary sarcoidosis showing beaded septum sign in a 57-year-old woman with Sjögren's syndrome. (**a**) Targeted view of thin-section (2.5-mm section thickness) scan obtained at level of liver dome shows thickened interlobular septa (*arrows*) with string of bead appearance. Also note diffuse ground-glass opacity in both lungs. (**b**) Low magnification (×10) photomicrograph of biopsy specimen demonstrates non-caseating granulomas distributed along pleura, bronchovascular bundles, alveolar walls, and interlobular septa (*arrows*) as well. Granulomatous nodules along interlobular septa have caused beaded septum sign on CT

K.S. Lee et al., *Radiology Illustrated: Chest Radiology*, Radiology Illustrated,
DOI 10.1007/978-3-642-37096-0_4, © Springer-Verlag Berlin Heidelberg 2014

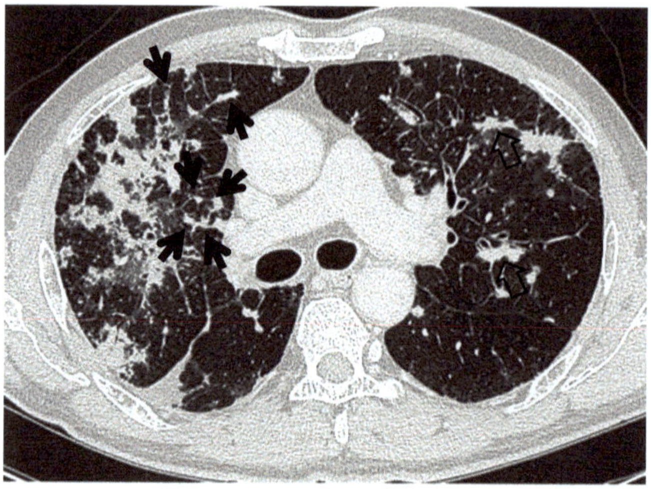

**Fig. 4.2** Lung adenocarcinoma and pulmonary lymphangitic carcinomatosis in a 65-year-old man. Thin-section (1.5-mm section thickness) CT scan obtained at subcarinal level shows multiple variable-sized, poorly or well-defined nodules in both lungs. Nodular or band-like interlobular septal thickening (*arrows*) is seen in the right lung. Also note thickened axial interstitium (*open arrows*)

## References


1. Hansell DM, Bankier AA, MacMahon H, McLoud TC, Muller NL, Remy J. Fleischner Society: glossary of terms for thoracic imaging. Radiology. 2008;246:697–722.
2. Ren H, Hruban RH, Kuhlman JE, et al. Computed tomography of inflation-fixed lungs: the beaded septum sign of pulmonary metastases. J Comput Assist Tomogr. 1989;13:411–6.
3. Murdoch J, Muller NL. Pulmonary sarcoidosis: changes on follow-up CT examination. AJR Am J Roentgenol. 1992;159:473–7.
4. Paslawski M, Krzyzanowski K, Zlomaniec J. Lymphangitis carcinomatosa in thin section computed tomography. Ann Univ Mariae Curie Sklodowska Med. 2004;59:1–5.
5. Stein MG, Mayo J, Muller N, Aberle DR, Webb WR, Gamsu G. Pulmonary lymphangitic spread of carcinoma: appearance on CT scans. Radiology. 1987;162:371–5.

# 5 Comet Tail Sign

## Definition

The sign has been originally described on chest radiographs. It is formed by distorted blood vessel(s) and a focal area of atelectatic lung adjacent to pleural thickening. The vessel(s) are seen as curvilinear soft tissue density or densities, extending from the medial margin of the atelectatic lung to the pulmonary hilum. When the vessels are multiple thus there are multiple tails, the vessels are more likely parachute; then, parachute sign may be used (Fig. 5.1). The sign is due to contracted fibrous scarring and shrinking pleural disease with rounded atelectasis. Likewise, on CT, swirling of bronchi and vessels extending from the hilum and converging on the atelectatic lung help produce comet tail appearance [1] (Figs. 5.1 and 5.2).

## Diseases Causing the Sign

The CT comet tail sign is specifically observed in *rounded atelectasis*.

## Distribution

The comet tail sign, which is identified in rounded atelectasis, is usually seen in the posterior aspect of the lower lung zones.

## Clinical Considerations

Rounded atelectasis is seen in patients with asbestos exposure [2].

## Rounded Atelectasis

### Pathology and Pathogenesis

Rounded atelectasis (RA) is a focal, pleural-based lesion resulting from pleural and subpleural scarring and atelectasis of the adjacent lung tissue. In cases reported in literatures, 60–70 % of patients with RA had been exposed to asbestos [3].

### Symptoms and Signs

Most patients with RA are asymptomatic and the lesions are incidentally founded on chest radiographs, simulating a lung mass. Respiratory symptoms include dyspnea, cough, and chest pain in the order of frequency [4].

### CT Findings

CT findings of RA are of a round or oval mass abutting a pleural surface, with swirling of the bronchi and vessels extending from the hilum and converging on the mass, producing a comet tail appearance, and with adjacent pleural thickening [5, 6] (Figs. 5.1 and 5.2). The central aspect of the mass usually has indistinct margins as a result of blurring by the entering vessels. Volume loss of the affected lobe is usually present. Air bronchograms are seen within the mass in about 60 % of cases. The atelectatic lung typically enhances significantly after injection of contrast material (Figs. 5.1 and 5.2). Synonyms include folded lung syndrome, helical atelectasis, Blesovsky syndrome, pleural pseudotumor, and pleuroma [7].

K.S. Lee et al., *Radiology Illustrated: Chest Radiology*, Radiology Illustrated,
DOI 10.1007/978-3-642-37096-0_5, © Springer-Verlag Berlin Heidelberg 2014

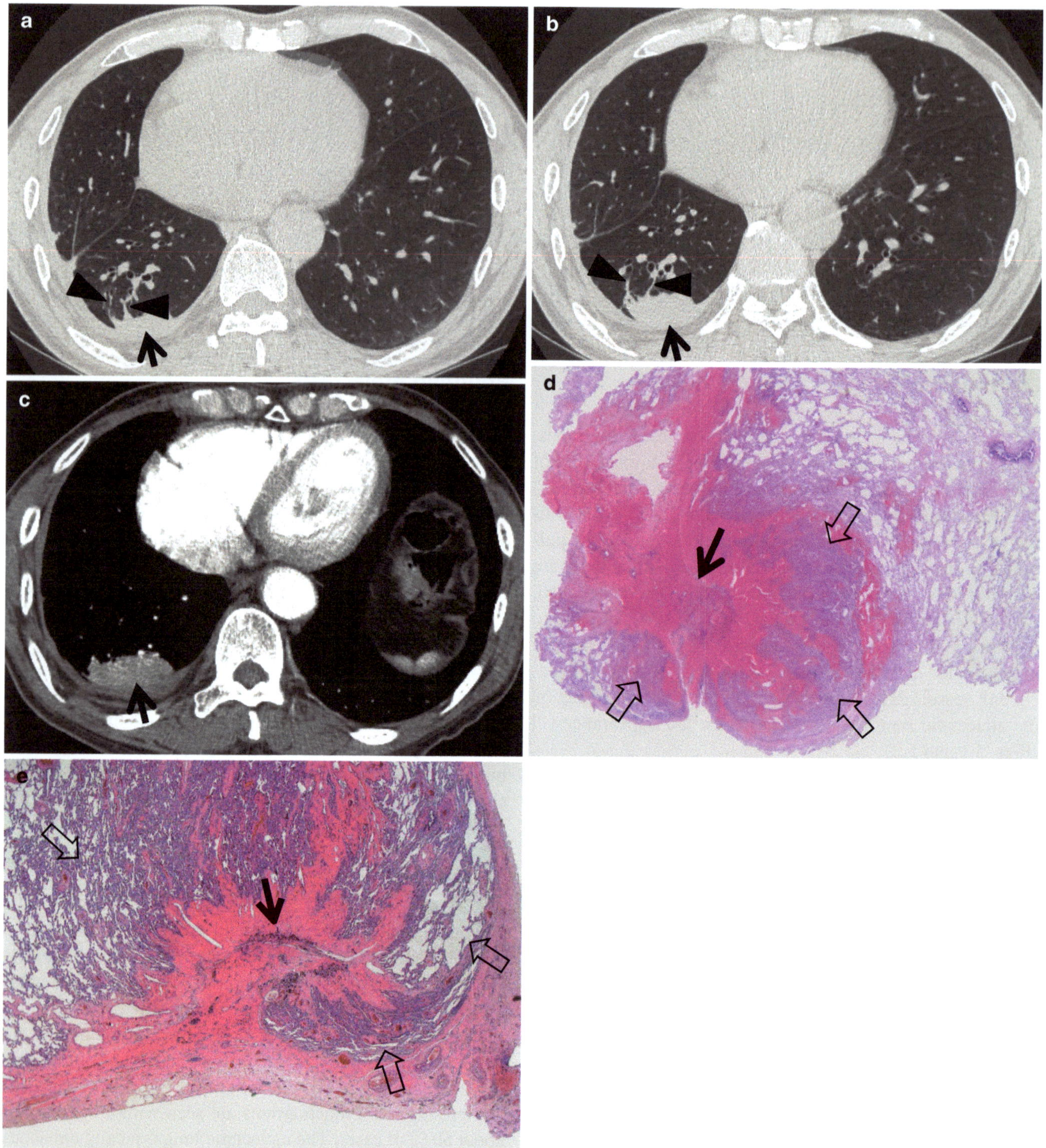


**Fig. 5.1** Rounded atelectasis in a 66-year-old man complaining of shortness of breath and cough. (**a, b**) Consecutive thin-section (1.5-mm section thickness) CT scans obtained at ventricular level show the atelectatic right lower lobe (*arrows*) abutting pleura. Also note two vascular curvilinear soft tissue attenuations (*arrowheads*), extending from anterior margin of the atelectatic lung to pulmonary hilum; these two structures may help explain parachute sign (please refer to definition of comet tail sign) on chest radiograph in this particular condition (rounded atelectasis). Also note right pleural effusion and thickening, posterior to the atelectatic lung, and extrapleural subcostal fat accumulation. (**c**) Mediastinal window image demonstrates the enhancing atelectatic lung (*arrow*) abutting pleura. (**d**) Low-magnification (×10) photomicrograph of pathologic specimen obtained from a different patient with rounded atelectasis depicts enfolded visceral pleura (*arrow*) curving into a rounded atelectatic lung that gestures wings (*open arrows*) of a vane. (**e**) High-magnification (×100) photomicrograph discloses more clearly enfolded visceral pleura (*arrow*) and rounded atelectatic lung (*open arrows*)

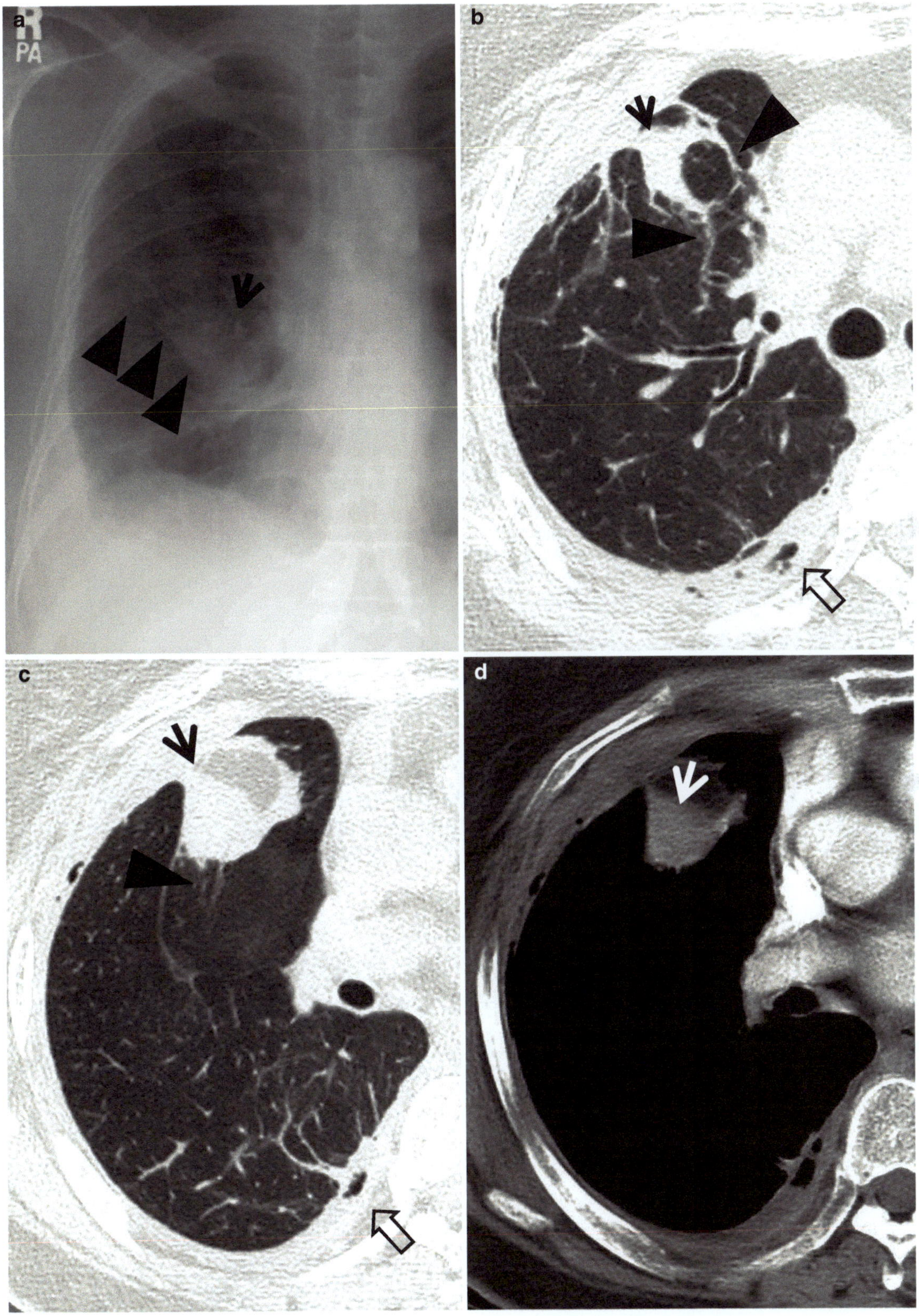


**Fig. 5.2** Rounded atelectasis simulating a lung mass in a 63-year-old man complaining of mild dyspnea and cough. (**a**) Chest radiograph shows right pleural effusion and a mass (*arrow*) in right middle lung zone superior to right minor fissure (*arrowheads*). (**b**, **c**) Thin-section (1.5-mm section thickness) CT scans obtained at levels of the right main bronchus (**b**) and bronchus intermedius (**c**), respectively, show the atelectatic right upper lobe (*arrows*) abutting anterior pleura. Also note vascular curvilinear soft tissue attenuations (*arrowheads*), extending from posterior margin of the atelectatic lung to pulmonary hilum. Also note right pleural effusion and thickening in posterior pleura (*open arrows*). (**d**) Mediastinal window of CT scan obtained at same level to (c) demonstrates the atelectatic right upper lobe (*arrow*). Also note right pleural effusion and thickening

## CT–Pathology Comparisons

Because of the pathogenetic association with pleural fibrosis, RA usually occurs in the peripheral lung adjacent to the visceral pleura. Pathologic examination shows pleural fibrosis overlying the abnormal lung parenchyma as well as invaginations of fibrotic pleura into the region of collapse. The appearance suggests that retraction of collagen in the pleura as it matures is the cause of the collapse [8].

## Patient Prognosis

RA usually remains stable over time; however, slow growth as well as diminution in size has been described [9].

## References

1. Lynch DA, Gamsu G, Ray CS, Aberle DR. Asbestos-related focal lung masses: manifestations on conventional and high-resolution CT scans. Radiology. 1988;169:603–7.
2. Chong S, Lee KS, Chung MJ, Han J, Kwon OJ, Kim TS. Pneumoconiosis: comparison of imaging and pathologic findings. Radiographics. 2006;26:59–77.
3. Kim GY, Park JY, Han JH, Kim TS, Kim JG. Rounded atelectasis: a brief case report. Korean J Pathol. 2003;37:279–81.
4. Cavazza A, Roggeri A, Rossi G, et al. Round atelectasis of the lung: clinicopathological study of 6 cases and review of the literature. Pathologica. 2003;95:50–6.
5. McHugh K, Blaquiere RM. CT features of rounded atelectasis. AJR Am J Roentgenol. 1989;153:257–60.
6. O'Donovan PB, Schenk M, Lim K, Obuchowski N, Stoller JK. Evaluation of the reliability of computed tomographic criteria used in the diagnosis of round atelectasis. J Thorac Imaging. 1997;12:54–8.
7. Hansell DM, Bankier AA, MacMahon H, McLoud TC, Muller NL, Remy J. Fleischner Society: glossary of terms for thoracic imaging. Radiology. 2008;246:697–722.
8. Peacock C, Copley SJ, Hansell DM. Asbestos-related benign pleural disease. Clin Radiol. 2000;55:422–32.
9. Szydlowski GW, Cohn HE, Steiner RM, Edie RN. Rounded atelectasis: a pulmonary pseudotumor. Ann Thorac Surg. 1992;53:817–21.

# CT Halo Sign

# 6

## Definition

CT halo sign is a CT finding of ground-glass opacity surrounding a nodule or mass. It was first described as a sign of hemorrhage around foci of invasive pulmonary aspergillosis [1] (Fig. 6.1).

## Diseases Causing the Sign

The halo sign is nonspecific and may be caused by several pathologic processes: hemorrhagic pulmonary nodules [2], tumor cell infiltration, and non-hemorrhagic inflammatory lesions. Hemorrhagic pulmonary nodules may occur in infectious diseases including *angioinvasive pulmonary aspergillosis* (Fig. 6.2), mucormycosis, and candidiasis and noninfectious diseases including antineutrophil cytoplasmic antibody (ANCA)-associated granulomatous vasculitis and primary and *metastatic hemorrhagic tumors* (Figs. 6.3 and 6.4). The hemorrhagic nodule can also be found in a patient with *pulmonary endometriosis with catamenial hemorrhage* [3, 4] (Fig. 6.5). Tumor cell infiltrations in lung adenocarcinomas, bronchus-associated lymphoid tissue (BALT) lymphoma, and pulmonary metastatic neoplasm may appear with the halo sign. *Eosinophilic lung disease* [5] (Fig. 6.1) and organizing pneumonia are representative of inflammatory lesions showing the halo sign (Table 6.1) [4].

## Distribution

The nodule and halo sign usually show random distribution without specific zonal, central–peripheral, or bronchovascular distribution. The nodule and halo sign may show subpleural distribution in angioinvasive pulmonary aspergillosis, metastatic hemorrhagic tumors, and non-hemorrhagic pulmonary metastatic neoplasms.

## Clinical Considerations

Angioinvasive pulmonary aspergillosis is seen in neutropenic subjects with immunosuppression (absolute neutrophil count, <500/L). ANCA-associated granulomatous vasculitis is usually associated with clinical presentation that included acute glomerulonephritis, chronic refractory sinusitis, or rhinorrhea. Serologic test including cytoplasmic ANCA is performed for the diagnosis of the disease. Catamenial hemorrhage occurs at the time of patient menstruation. Eosinophilic lung disease is usually seen in patients who have intake history of freshwater crabs [6] or raw cow liver [7].

**Key Points for Differential Diagnosis**

1. On CT scans, segmental areas of consolidation and surrounding ground-glass opacity or at least one nodule with the halo sign are seen in patients with angioinvasive pulmonary aspergillosis. However, the findings are nonspecific and can be seen in neutropenic patients with mucormycosis, organizing pneumonia, or pulmonary hemorrhage [8].
2. Patients with ANCA-associated granulomatous vasculitis may have localized areas of hemorrhage related to pulmonary nodules or may develop diffuse alveolar hemorrhage [4].
3. A single persistent nodule and surrounding halo sign may suggest the presence of invasive adenocarcinoma, BALT lymphoma, or organizing pneumonia [4].
4. Nodule(s) and halo sign in eosinophilic lung disease are usually multiple, migratory, and transient [5].

K.S. Lee et al., *Radiology Illustrated: Chest Radiology*, Radiology Illustrated,
DOI 10.1007/978-3-642-37096-0_6, © Springer-Verlag Berlin Heidelberg 2014

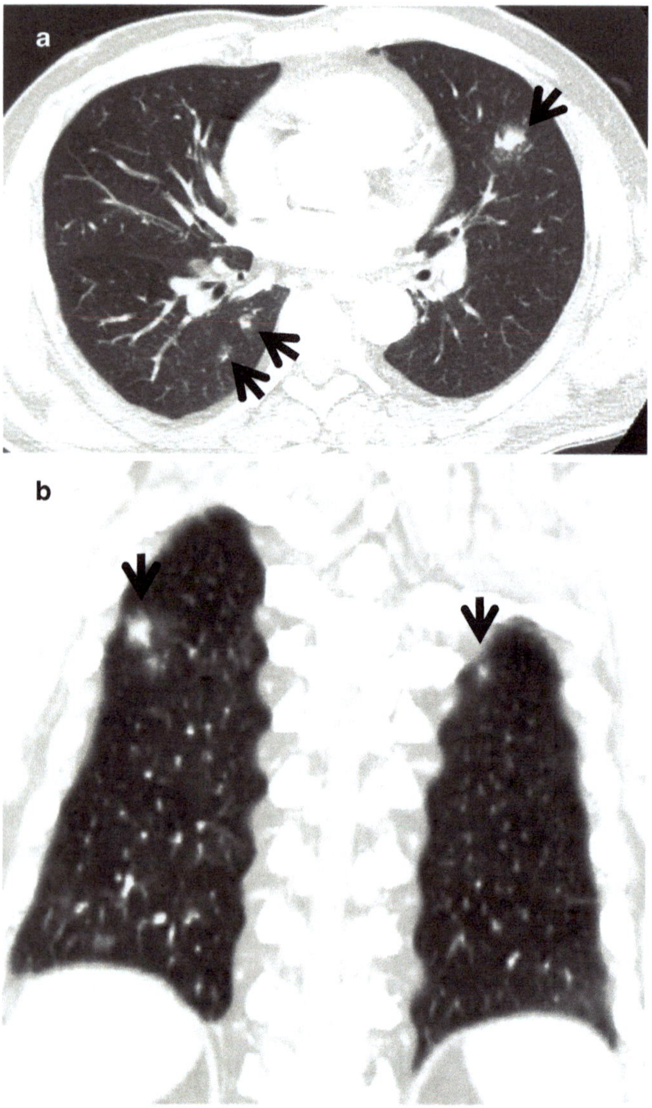


**Fig. 6.1** Toxocara canis and its larva migration in a 66-year-old man with colon cancer who had a history of raw cow liver intake. (**a**) Lung window of CT scan (2.5-mm section thickness) obtained at lower lobar bronchia level shows nodules (*arrows*) with surrounding halo sign in both lungs. (**b**) Coronal reformatted (2.0-mm section thickness) CT scan also demonstrates nodules (*arrows*) with halo sign

## Angioinvasive Pulmonary Aspergillosis

### Pathology and Pathogenesis

Central portion of the lesion is typically pale and shows a relatively intact underlying structure in a gross pathologic specimen. The peripheral portion demonstrates a rim of hemorrhage or consolidation. Histologically, coagulative necrosis and its permeation by numerous fungal hyphae are seen (Fig. 6.2). Invasion into small- to medium-sized pulmonary arteries within the necrotic portion is common. Depending on patient immune capability (with recovery of absolute neutrophil count), the junction between the necrosis and viable parenchyma shows a variably severe neutrophilic infiltrate. Release of enzymes from the neutrophils may result in the separation of a portion of the necrotic tissue from the adjacent lung, resulting in an intracavitary sequestrum (the so-called lung ball).

### Symptoms and Signs

Prolonged neutropenia, hematopoietic stem cell transplantation (HSCT), solid organ transplantation, high-dose corticosteroid therapy, and AIDS are the risk factors for developing invasive pulmonary aspergillosis. Clinical presentation often mimics that of acute bacterial pneumonia. High fever, nonproductive cough, hemoptysis, pleuritic chest pain, and dyspnea are the most frequent symptoms.

### CT Findings

The characteristic HRCT findings consist of nodules surrounded by a halo of ground-glass opacity and wedge-shaped pleural-based areas of consolidation (Fig. 6.2). In approximately 50 % of cases, the nodules undergo cavitation, manifested as an air crescent surrounding a round, eccentric opacity [1]. The air-crescent sign in angioinvasive aspergillosis is usually seen during convalescence.

### CT–Pathology Comparisons

Nodules with ground-glass halo on CT correspond pathologically to the foci of the necrotic lung surrounded by viable but hemorrhagic lung parenchyma [9]. Wedge-shaped pleural-based consolidation areas are related to more extensive intralobular hemorrhage or true parenchymal infarction.

### Patient Prognosis

The rate of successful outcomes is increasing with newer antifungal agents. Voriconazole was more effective than amphotericin B as initial therapy for invasive pulmonary aspergillosis and was associated with significantly improved survival (71 vs. 58 %, respectively). Higher mortality occurred in the patients with extrapulmonary aspergillosis and allogeneic HSCT recipients. Combination antifungal therapy can be given as salvage therapy. The value of aggressive surgical resection for localized form of invasive pulmonary aspergillosis is unclear [10, 11].

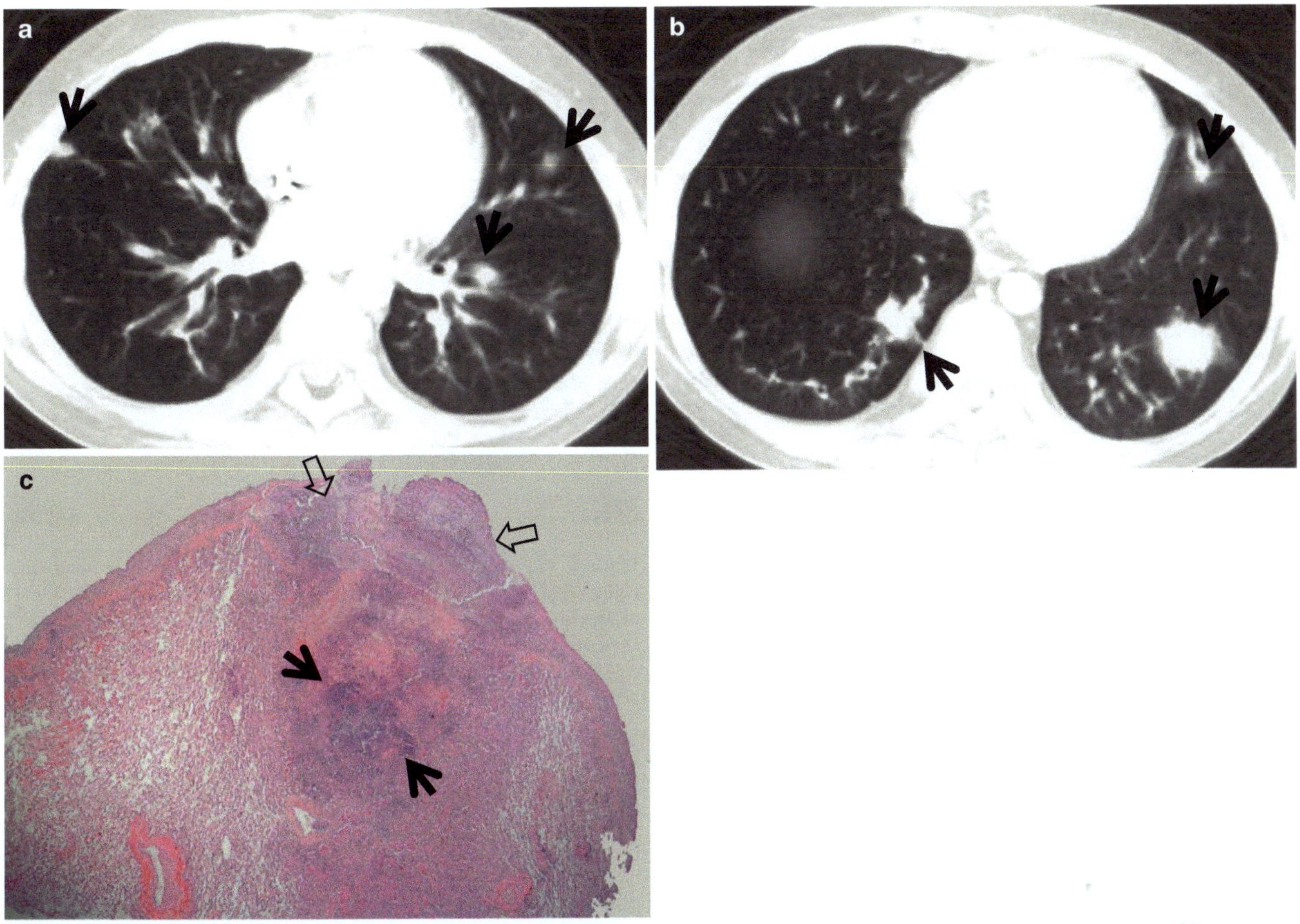


**Fig. 6.2** Invasive pulmonary aspergillosis in an 11-year-old boy with acute lymphocytic leukemia and neutropenia. (**a, b**) Lung window of CT (5.0-mm section thickness) scans obtained at levels of the inferior pulmonary vein (**a**) and liver dome (**b**), respectively, shows nodules (*arrows*) with halo sign in both lungs. Also note ground-glass opacity along bronchovascular bundles. (**c**) High-magnification photomicrograph of pathologic specimen obtained from the left lower lobe with wedge resection by using video-assisted thoracoscopic surgery discloses necrotic abscess containing blue area of fungal colonization (*arrows*) in central portion of lesion. Fungal organisms extend to pleural space (*open arrows*)

## Metastatic Hemorrhagic Tumors

### Pathology and Pathogenesis

The capillary bed of the lung is an effective filter of tumor emboli, and secondary tumors in the lung are therefore the usual immediate source of metastases in other organs. The terminal bronchopneumonia with abscess or hemorrhage adjacent to the tumor may also follow airway obstruction.

### Symptoms and Signs

Due to peritumoral hemorrhage secondary to the fragility of neovascular tissue, cough, blood-tinged sputum, and dyspnea can occur in the patients with lung metastases from hypervascular tumors. Symptoms and signs related to the primary site of malignancy usually exist.

### CT Findings

On CT, hematogenous metastatic nodules range from a few millimeters to several centimeters in diameter, and when multiple they are usually of varying in size. The nodules tend to be most numerous in the outer third of the lungs, particularly the subpleural regions of the lower zones, and have a random distribution within the secondary pulmonary lobules. Metastases most commonly are round and have smooth margins. Metastatic hemorrhagic tumors such as angiosarcoma, Kaposi sarcoma, choriocarcinoma, and melanoma have a halo of ground-glass opacity surrounding nodules (Figs. 6.3 and 6.4) [2, 4].

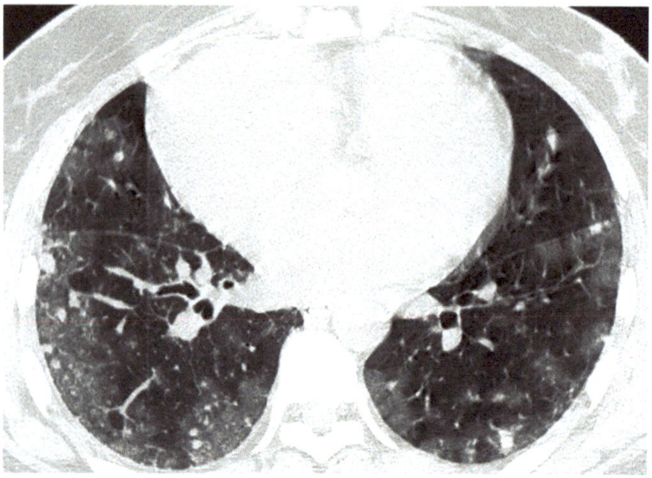

**Fig. 6.3** Hemorrhagic metastasis in a 52-year-old woman with renal cell carcinoma. Lung window of CT (5.0-mm section thickness) scan obtained at level of the interior pulmonary vein shows multiple solid nodules surrounded by ground-glass opacity, suggesting hemorrhagic metastasis

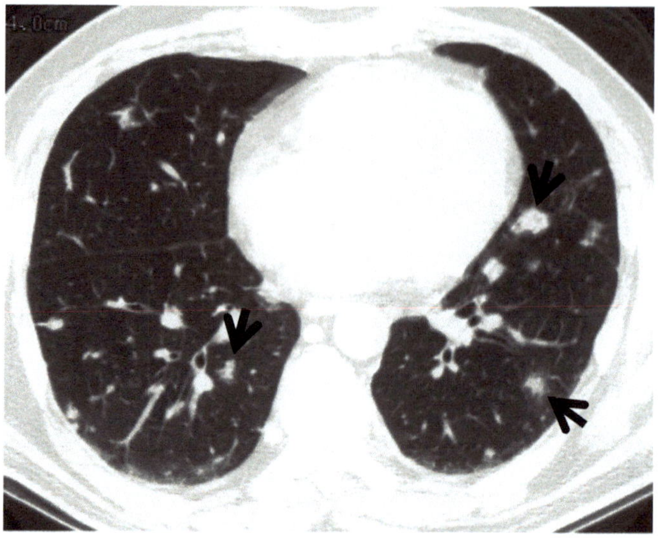

**Fig. 6.4** Nodules with halo sign in a 28-year-old man with melanoma. Lung window of CT (5.0-mm section thickness) scan obtained at level of the interior pulmonary vein shows multiple variable-sized nodules (*arrows*) having surrounding halo (hemorrhagic metastases)

### CT–Pathology Comparisons

A halo of ground-glass opacity surrounding metastatic nodules corresponds to extensive hemorrhage in the nodule and adjacent lung parenchyma. In these conditions, hemorrhage is regarded to be present owing to the fragility of the neovascular tissue with resultant thrombosis and rupture [4].

### Patient Prognosis

Advanced stage of the malignancy makes the prognosis very grave.

## Pulmonary Endometriosis with Catamenial Hemorrhage

### Pathology and Pathogenesis

The heterotopic tissue consists of both stroma and glands and reproduces the appearances of normal endometrium in every way (Fig. 6.5). Decidual change takes place in pregnancy, and cyclic hemorrhagic disruption, with consequent hemosiderosis, may obscure the nature of the tissue, in which case immunocytochemistry may be used to demonstrate estrogen and progesterone receptors and in the stromal component CD10 [12].

### Symptoms and Signs

Pulmonary endometriosis with catamenial hemorrhage is characterized by recurrent hemoptysis occurring within 24–48 h after the start of each menstruation cycle in female patients in the reproductive age. Hemoptysis is usually small in amount and lasts a few days. It is frequently accompanied by cough and chest discomfort. The history of the obstetric procedure, especially induced abortion, is common [13].

### CT Findings

During menstruation, focal consolidation with a relatively well-defined margin and ground-glass opacity are common CT findings of pulmonary parenchymal endometriosis (Fig. 6.5) [3, 4]. However, CT scans obtained after menstruation demonstrate marked improvement of pulmonary consolidation and nodules. Other findings of thoracic endometriosis include thin-walled cavities or bullous formation and catamenial hemothorax or pneumothorax.

### CT–Pathology Comparisons

CT findings of consolidation, nodules, and ground-glass opacity in pulmonary endometriosis can be presumed to represent pulmonary hemorrhage. Hemorrhage could result from the rupture of the capillaries in the endometrial tissue particles trapped within pulmonary vascular network [3, 4].

## Patient Prognosis

When the site of pulmonary endometriosis is confirmed by chest CT to be localized and fixed, surgical resection can be tried. Medical treatment with progestational agents or gonadotropin-releasing hormones may be applied if hemoptysis continues with conservative therapy. Variable results in terms of short- and long-term outcome have been reported [14].

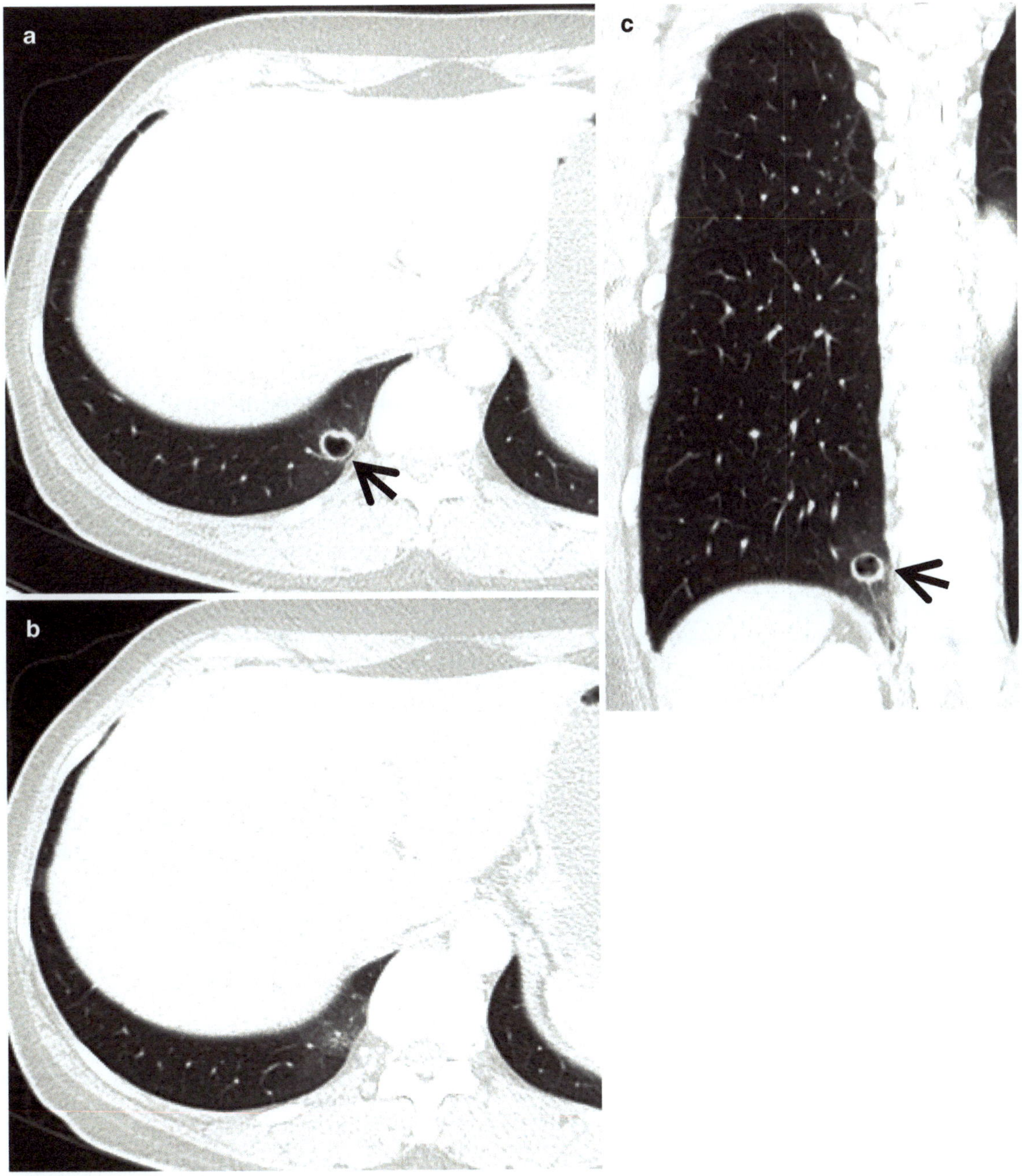


**Fig. 6.5** Pulmonary endometriosis showing halo sign in a 46-year-old woman. (**a, b**) Lung window of consecutive CT scans (2.5-mm section thickness) obtained at levels of liver dome shows a cystic lesion (*arrow*) of eccentric wall thickness depicting surrounding ground-glass opacity halo in the right lung base. (**c**) Coronal reformatted (2.0-mm section thickness) image demonstrates cystic lesion with halo sign (*arrow*). (**d**) High-magnification (×100) photomicrograph of pathologic specimen obtained from the right lower lobe with wedge resection by using video-assisted thoracoscopic surgery discloses a nodule composed of many well-formed endometrial glands and admixed stroma. Also note a large dilated gland-forming cyst within central portion of nodule. *Inset*: stroma is pale pink and is composed of bland-looking oval or spindle cells (×200)

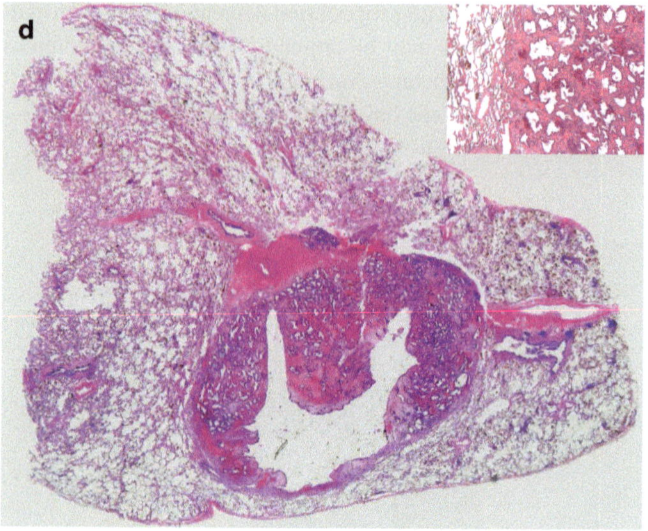


Fig. 6.5 (continued)

Table 6.1 Common diseases manifesting as CT halo sign

| Disease | Key points for differential diagnosis |
|---|---|
| Infectious disease | |
| Angioinvasive pulmonary aspergillosis | Nodules with a GGO, wedge-shaped pleural-based areas of consolidation |
| Mucormycosis | Nodules and masses with CT and reversed halo |
| Candidiasis | |
| ANCA-associated granulomatous vasculitis | Multiple, bilateral, subpleural nodules or masses |
| Hemorrhagic metastasis | Multiple nodules with GGO halo, varying in size |
| Pulmonary endometriosis | Focal consolidation and GGO during menstruation |
| Eosinophilic lung disease | Migrating multifocal subpleural nodules with GGO halo |

*Note*: *GGO* ground-glass opacity, *ANCA* antineutrophil cytoplasmic antibody

## Eosinophilic Lung Disease (Parasitic Infestation)

### Pathology and Pathogenesis

Secondary eosinophilic lung disease caused by parasites can manifest as simple, acute, chronic, or incidental eosinophilic pneumonia [15].

### Symptoms and Signs

The most common parasitic infections for pulmonary eosinophilia are caused by *Strongyloides*, *Ascaris*, *Toxocara*, *Paragonimus*, and *Ancylostoma* species [16]. Symptoms are usually minimal but could be severe, including low-grade fever, dry cough, substernal chest discomfort, dyspnea, wheezing, and blood-tinged sputum to frank hemoptysis. Blood and sputum eosinophilia is the most common laboratory abnormality.

### CT Findings

Parasitic infestation most commonly results in findings similar to Loeffler's syndrome. Pulmonary visceral larva migrans such as *Ascaris suum or Toxocara canis* appears on CT as migrating multifocal subpleural nodules with halo of ground-glass opacity and ill-defined margin (Fig. 6.1) [17]. Pleuropulmonary paragonimiasis usually manifests as a necrotic subpleural nodule with focal pleural thickening and subpleural streaky opacity connecting the pleura and the nodule. More than half of cases, this nodule has adjacent areas of ground-glass opacity [6].

### CT–Pathology Comparisons

In cases of pulmonary visceral larva migrans, mutifocal subpleural nodules with a halo of ground-glass opacity are related to patchy interstitial thickening, an inflammatory exudate composed largely of eosinophils, and alveolar hemorrhage and edema [18]. In cases of pleuropulmonary paragonimiasis, subpleural nodule with a necrotic low attenuation is related to necrotic granuloma and organizing pneumonia [6].

### Patient Prognosis

Antihelminthic therapy is necessary to eradicate the infection caused by *Strongyloides*, *Ascaris*, and *Paragonimus*. The role of antihelminthic agents in the treatment of *Toxocara* is not established.

## References

1. Kuhlman JE, Fishman EK, Siegelman SS. Invasive pulmonary aspergillosis in acute leukemia: characteristic findings on CT, the CT halo sign, and the role of CT in early diagnosis. Radiology. 1985;157:611–4.
2. Primack SL, Hartman TE, Lee KS, Muller NL. Pulmonary nodules and the CT halo sign. Radiology. 1994;190:513–5.
3. Chung SY, Kim SJ, Kim TH, et al. Computed tomography findings of pathologically confirmed pulmonary parenchymal endometriosis. J Comput Assist Tomogr. 2005;29:815–8.
4. Kim Y, Lee KS, Jung KJ, Han J, Kim JS, Suh JS. Halo sign on high resolution CT: findings in spectrum of pulmonary diseases with pathologic correlation. J Comput Assist Tomogr. 1999;23:622–6.
5. Jeong YJ, Kim KI, Seo IJ, et al. Eosinophilic lung diseases: a clinical, radiologic, and pathologic overview. Radiographics. 2007;27:617–37. discussion 637–619.

6. Kim TS, Han J, Shim SS, et al. Pleuropulmonary paragonimiasis: CT findings in 31 patients. AJR Am J Roentgenol. 2005;185:616–21.
7. Choi D, Lim JH, Choi DC, et al. Transmission of Toxocara canis via ingestion of raw cow liver: a cross-sectional study in healthy adults. Korean J Parasitol. 2012;50:23–7.
8. Won HJ, Lee KS, Cheon JE, et al. Invasive pulmonary aspergillosis: prediction at thin-section CT in patients with neutropenia–a prospective study. Radiology. 1998;208:777–82.
9. Hruban RH, Meziane MA, Zerhouni EA, Wheeler PS, Dumler JS, Hutchins GM. Radiologic-pathologic correlation of the CT halo sign in invasive pulmonary aspergillosis. J Comput Assist Tomogr. 1987;11:534–6.
10. Segal BH, Walsh TJ. Current approaches to diagnosis and treatment of invasive aspergillosis. Am J Respir Crit Care Med. 2006;173:707–17.
11. Limper AH, Knox KS, Sarosi GA, et al. An official American Thoracic Society statement: treatment of fungal infections in adult pulmonary and critical care patients. Am J Respir Crit Care Med. 2011;183:96–128.
12. Flieder DB, Moran CA, Travis WD, Koss MN, Mark EJ. Pleuro-pulmonary endometriosis and pulmonary ectopic deciduosis: a clinicopathologic and immunohistochemical study of 10 cases with emphasis on diagnostic pitfalls. Hum Pathol. 1998;29:1495–503.
13. Kim CJ, Nam HS, Lee CY, et al. Catamenial hemoptysis: a nation-wide analysis in Korea. Respiration. 2010;79:296–301.
14. Channabasavaiah AD, Joseph JV. Thoracic endometriosis: revisiting the association between clinical presentation and thoracic pathology based on thoracoscopic findings in 110 patients. Medicine (Baltimore). 2010;89:183–8.
15. Kuzucu A. Parasitic diseases of the respiratory tract. Curr Opin Pulm Med. 2006;12:212–21.
16. Chitkara RK, Krishna G. Parasitic pulmonary eosinophilia. Semin Respir Crit Care Med. 2006;27:171–84.
17. Sakai S, Shida Y, Takahashi N, et al. Pulmonary lesions associated with visceral larva migrans due to Ascaris suum or Toxocara canis: imaging of six cases. AJR Am J Roentgenol. 2006;186:1697–702.
18. Martinez S, Restrepo CS, Carrillo JA, et al. Thoracic manifestations of tropical parasitic infections: a pictorial review. Radiographics. 2005;25:135–55.

# 7 Galaxy Sign

## Definition

A large pulmonary nodule composed of multiple small nodules and surrounded by many very smaller satellite nodules is called a galaxy sign [1] (Fig. 7.1).

## Diseases Causing the Sign

The nodule(s) with CT galaxy sign is (are) observed in patients with pulmonary sarcoidosis and *active pulmonary tuberculosis* [2] (Table 7.1) (Figs. 7.2 and 7.3).

## Distribution

The CT galaxy sign in pulmonary sarcoidosis, as in the cases of other pulmonary sarcoidosis, is usually located in the upper and middle lung zones but can also be seen in the lower lung zones. In tuberculosis, the galaxy sign is noticed specifically in the upper lobes or the superior segments of the lower lobes.

## Clinical Considerations

Tuberculous galaxy sign indicates active disease, thus reversible to antituberculous chemotherapy [2]. Also the galaxy sign in sarcoidosis is reversible. According to a report of Heo and his colleagues, a single galaxy sign is far more frequent in patients with tuberculosis than in those with sarcoidosis [2].

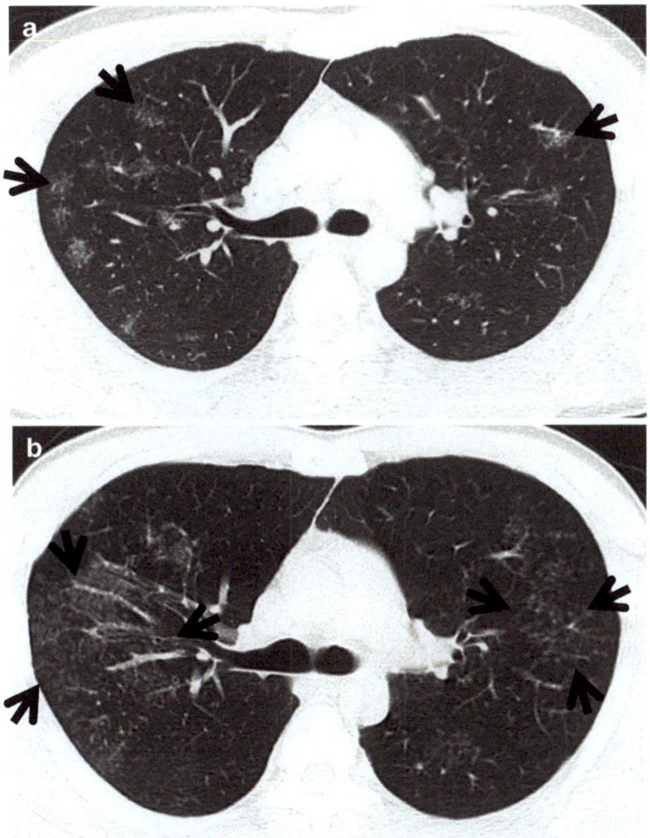


**Fig. 7.1** CT galaxy sign in a 23-year-old man with pulmonary sarcoidosis. (**a**, **b**) Consecutive thin-section (2.5-mm section thickness) CT scans obtained at levels of the right upper lobar bronchi show multifocal areas of CT galaxy sign (*arrows*) that are comprised of multiple small nodules and surrounded by many very small satellite nodules, particularly in the right upper lobe. Mediastinal window images (not shown here) demonstrated enlarged lymph nodes in the mediastinum and hilum, bilaterally

K.S. Lee et al., *Radiology Illustrated: Chest Radiology*, Radiology Illustrated,
DOI 10.1007/978-3-642-37096-0_7, © Springer-Verlag Berlin Heidelberg 2014

**Table 7.1** Common diseases manifesting as galaxy sign

| Disease | Key points for differential diagnosis |
|---|---|
| Sarcoidosis | Associated with lymphadenopathy |
| Pulmonary tuberculosis | Associated with tree-in-bud pattern, upper lung predominance |

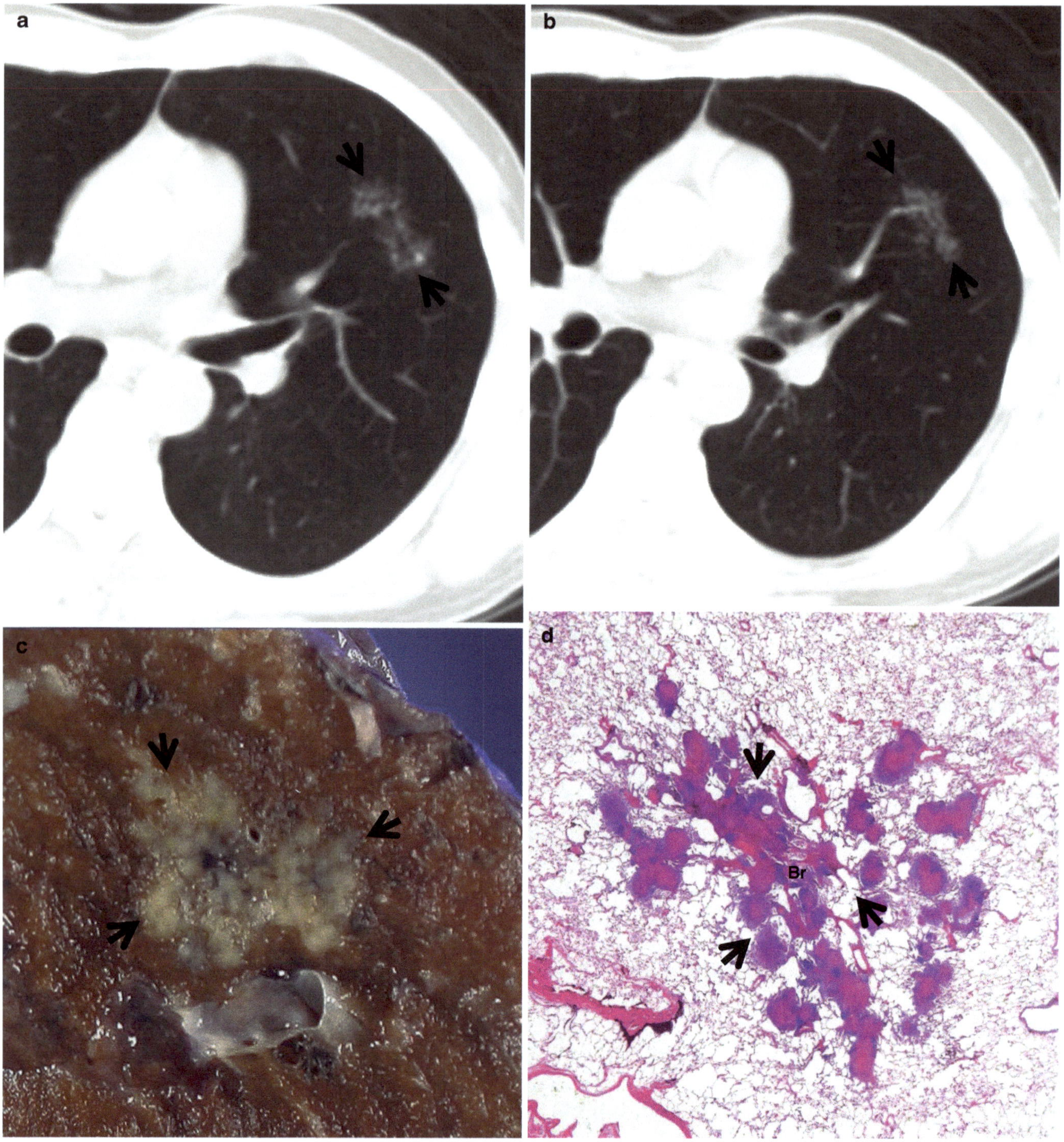


**Fig. 7.2** CT galaxy sign in a 44-year-old man with active pulmonary tuberculosis. (**a**, **b**) Consecutive (5.0-mm section thickness, low-dose technique) CT scans obtained at level of the right bronchus intermedius show CT galaxy sign (*arrows*) in superior lingular segment of the left upper lobe. On these relatively thick-section CT images, caution should be given not to interpret this galaxy sign as ground-glass opacity lesion, thus invasive lung adenocarcinoma. (**c**) Gross pathology specimen obtained from the left upper lobe with surgical lung biopsy demonstrates nodular aggregation (*arrows*) of small granulomas. (**d**) Low-magnification (×4) photomicrograph discloses nodular aggregation of granulomas having central necrosis in the peribronchiolar interstitium. Granulomas are concentrated toward the center of nodular cluster (*arrows*) than in its periphery. *Br* bronchiole

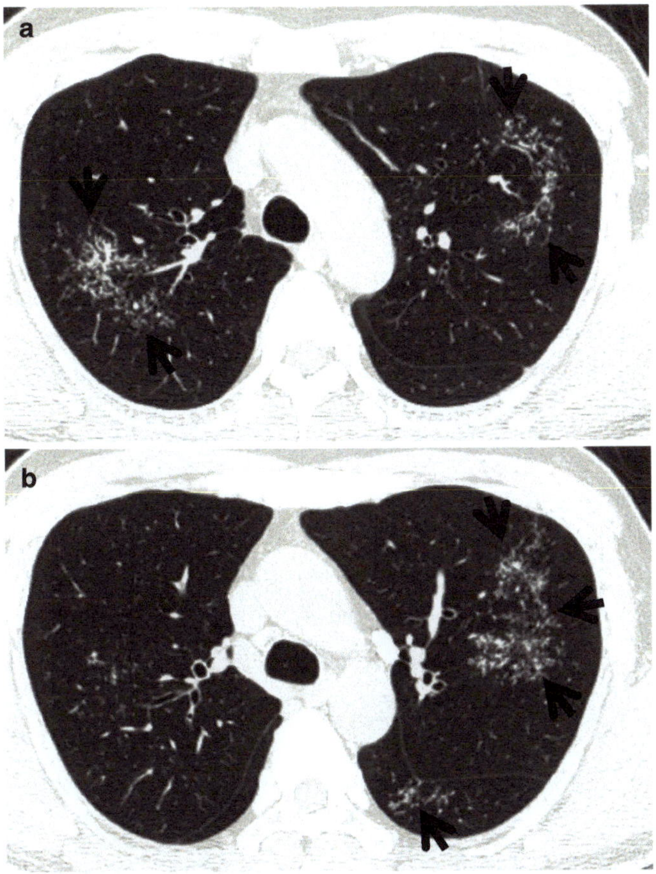


Fig. 7.3 CT galaxy sign in a 53-year-old man with active pulmonary tuberculosis. (**a**, **b**) Lung window of thin-section (2.5-mm section thickness) CT scans obtained at levels of the aortic arch (**a**) and azygos arch (**b**), respectively, shows CT galaxy sign (*arrows*) in both upper lobes and superior segment of the left lower lobe

**Key Points for Differential Diagnosis**

1. The presence of single rather than multiple CT galaxy sign favors the diagnosis of pulmonary tuberculosis.
2. Zonal predominance is more prominent in tuberculous galaxy sign with specific involvement of the upper lobes (upper zone) and the superior segments (middle lung zone) of the lower lobes.
3. In tuberculous galaxy sign, it is accompanied by tree-in-bud sign, whereas enlarged hilar or mediastinal lymph node enlargement is much more frequent in sarcoidosis [2].

## Galaxy Sign in Pulmonary Tuberculosis

### Pathology and Pathogenesis

The histologic reaction of tuberculosis is primarily granulomatous and necrotizing with cavitation; lesions may progress to fibrosis and calcification [3]. Coalescence of multiple granulomas may form galaxy sign (clustered tuberculous granulomas) (Figs. 7.2 and 7.3).

### Symptoms and Signs

Cough is the most common symptom of active pulmonary tuberculosis. It may be nonproductive but sputum is usually present as the disease progresses. Hemoptysis and pleuritic chest discomfort can occur. Constitutional symptoms, including fever, malaise, fatigue, weight loss, night sweating, and anorexia are often accompanied. Patients may asymptomatic [4].

### CT Findings

CT findings of a single clustered nodule with CT galaxy sign, clustered nodules with CT galaxy sign in the upper lobe and superior segment of the lower lobe, or CT galaxy sign not associated with lymphadenopathy or associated with tree-in-bud patterns favor the diagnosis of pulmonary tuberculosis rather than sarcoidosis [2] (Figs. 7.2 and 7.3).

### CT–Pathology Comparisons

CT galaxy sign on HRCT reflects a coalescence of multiple granulomas. Granulomas are much more concentrated toward the center of the cluster than in its periphery, and individual macroscopic granulomas can be identified when granulomas are not so densely assembled [1] (Fig. 7.2).

### Patient Prognosis

Cure rate for drug-sensitive tuberculosis is more than 95 % with the current standard four-drug treatment regimen of first-line drugs (isoniazid, rifampicin, pyrazinamide, and ethambutol) for 6 months [4]. Prolonged medication for at least 20 months with second-line drugs is necessary for multidrug-resistant (MDR) tuberculosis. Extensively drug-resistant (XDR) tuberculosis is extremely difficult to treat. When the disease of MDR or XDR tuberculosis is localized, surgical resection of the lung lesion can be done with medical therapy.

## References

1. Nakatsu M, Hatabu H, Morikawa K, et al. Large coalescent parenchymal nodules in pulmonary sarcoidosis: "sarcoid galaxy" sign. AJR Am J Roentgenol. 2002;178:1389–93.
2. Heo JN, Choi YW, Jeon SC, Park CK. Pulmonary tuberculosis: another disease showing clusters of small nodules. AJR Am J Roentgenol. 2005;184:639–42.
3. Leung AN. Pulmonary tuberculosis: the essentials. Radiology. 1999;210:307–22.
4. Zumla A, Raviglione M, Hafner R, von Reyn CF. Tuberculosis. N Engl J Med. 2013;368:745–55.

# 8 Reversed Halo Sign

## Definition

Reversed halo sign, which was named originally from the disease cryptogenic organizing pneumonia, refers to a focal, rounded area of ground-glass opacity surrounded by a more or less complete ring of consolidation [1, 2] (Fig. 8.1).

## Diseases Causing the Sign

The reversed halo sign was first described as being relatively specific for *cryptogenic organizing pneumonia* (*COP*) (Fig. 8.2) or COP-like reaction but was later observed in several other infectious and noninfectious diseases. *Pulmonary mucormycosis* (former pulmonary zygomycosis) (Fig. 8.3) and invasive pulmonary aspergillosis may manifest the reversed halo sign [3]. Other causes of the reversed halo sign include noninvasive fungal infections such as paracoccidioidomycosis, histoplasmosis, and *Pneumocystis jirovecii* pneumonia [4]. Furthermore, pulmonary infarction [5], antineutrophil cytoplasmic antibody-associated granulomatous vasculitis (former Wegener's granulomatosis), radiofrequency ablation, and *lymphomatoid granulomatosis* (Fig. 8.4) may also lead to this finding [6, 7] (Table 8.1).

## Distribution

The reversed halo sign in COP may have its distribution along the subpleural lungs or the bronchovascular bundles [1]. In invasive fungal infection in immunocompromised patients, the sign appears as a large single lesion. In noninvasive fungal infection, the reversed halo sign(s) is usually associated with ground-glass opacity, small centrilobular nodules, or areas of consolidation, and the lesions are usually bilateral and asymmetric [4]. The reversed halo sign in chronic eosinophilic pneumonia may show upper and mid lung zone predominance, whereas pulmonary infarction may show subpleural location in pulmonary infarction.

## Clinical Considerations

In neutropenic patients, the presence of reversed halo sign may suggest invasive fungal infection. Approximately 40 % of patients with chronic eosinophilic pneumonia have asthma; thus, reversed halo sign in asthmatics may imply chronic eosinophilic pneumonia [8]. In the situation of clinically pulmonary embolic disease, the presence of reversed halo sign hints the diagnosis of pulmonary infarction.

**Key Points for Differential Diagnosis**

1. On CT scans, the reversed halo sign is observed in approximately 20 % of COP patients [1].
2. The reversed halo sign, along with the halo sign, is highly suggestive of early infection by an angioinvasive fungus; the halo sign and reversed halo sign are most commonly associated with invasive pulmonary aspergillosis and pulmonary mucormycosis, respectively [3].
3. In paracoccidioidomycosis, the reversed halo sign is seen in 10 % of patients with active *Paracoccidioides brasiliensis* infection [4].
4. The reversed halo sign findings may be specifically useful for making a diagnosis of pulmonary infarction, when direct findings of thromboembolism are absent, especially when CT examination is delayed relative to symptom onset [5].

K.S. Lee et al., *Radiology Illustrated: Chest Radiology*, Radiology Illustrated,
DOI 10.1007/978-3-642-37096-0_8, © Springer-Verlag Berlin Heidelberg 2014

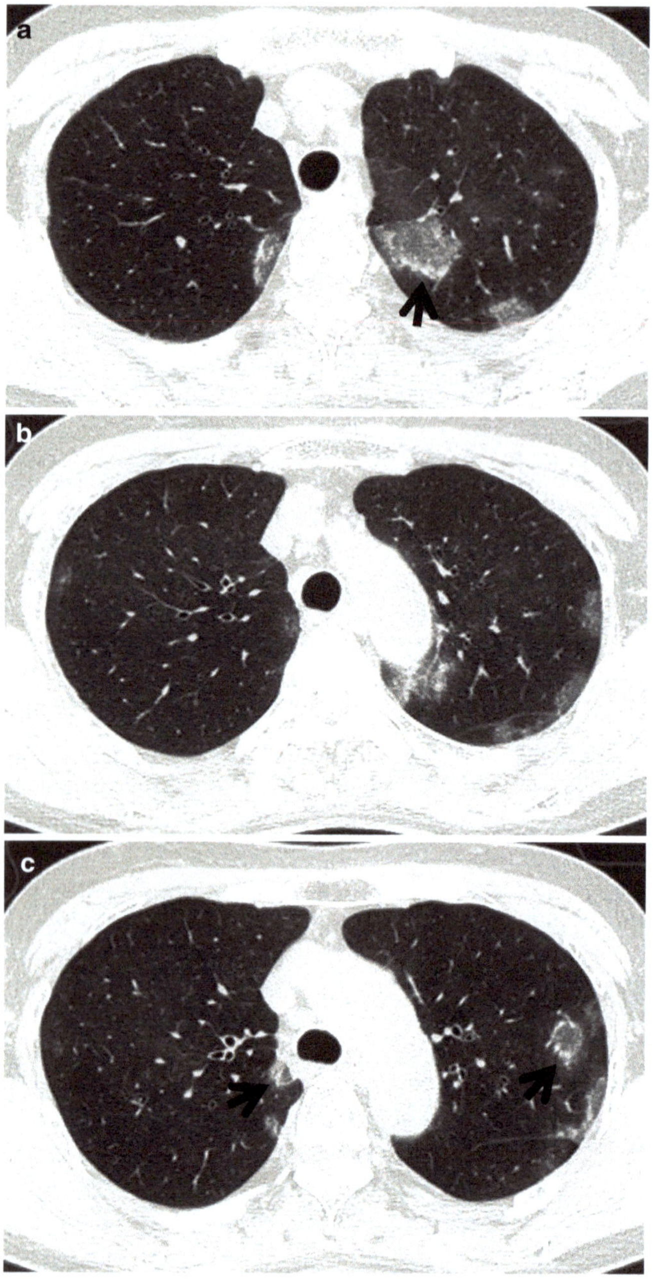


**Fig. 8.1** Reversed halo sign in a 55-year-old asthmatic woman and chronic eosinophilic pneumonia. (**a**–**c**) Lung window images of thin-section (1.5-mm section thickness) scans obtained at levels of the great vessels (**a**), aortic arch (**b**), and azygos arch (**c**), respectively, show multifocal areas of ground-glass opacity in both lungs. Please note reversed halo sign (ground-glass opacity surrounded by a more or less complete ring of consolidation) (*arrows*) in both upper lobes

## Cryptogenic Organizing Pneumonia and Reversed Halo Sign

### Pathology and Pathogenesis

COP is a predominantly airspace-filling, active fibrosing process that involves distal bronchioles, alveolar ducts, and peribronchiolar alveoli in varying proportions (Fig. 8.2). The fibrosis is easily recognized at low magnification because it stains lightly and assumes the round to oval, elongated, branching shapes in airspaces. The process is sharply demarcated from the adjacent areas of normal parenchyma [9].

### Symptoms and Signs

The mean age of COP at presentation is about 50–55 years (range 21–80 years). The duration of symptoms prior to diagnosis is usually less than 2 months [10]. In typical presentation, it begins with a flu-like illness characterized by fever, malaise, fatigue, weight loss, and cough, followed by the development of dyspnea. The clinical presentation of COP is often confused with that of community-acquired pneumonia. Hemoptysis and finger clubbing are rare. Chest auscultation reveals fine inspiratory crackles in both lower lungs.

### CT Findings

The typical CT findings also consist of unilateral or bilateral areas of airspace consolidation [11]. In approximately 60 % of cases, the consolidation involves mainly the subpleural or peribronchial lung regions or both [12]. Areas of ground-glass opacity are commonly present in association with the areas of consolidation. Small, ill-defined nodules, often in a centrilobular distribution, are seen in 30–50 % of cases [12]. An air bronchogram with traction bronchiectasis may be seen in patients who have extensive consolidation and are usually restricted to these areas. Occasionally, the disease is manifested as a large nodule or mass-like area of consolidation. On CT scans, the reversed halo sign is observed in approximately 20 % of COP patients [1] (Fig. 8.2).

### CT–Pathology Comparisons

The areas of consolidation correspond histologically to the regions of lung parenchyma that show airspace fibrosis [13]. The ground-glass opacities correlate with areas of alveolar septal inflammation and minimal airspace fibrosis. The small nodules are related to foci of organizing pneumonia limited to the peribronchiolar region and/or to fibroblastic tissue plugs within the bronchiolar lumen. The central ground-glass opacity of the reversed halo sign corresponds histopathologically to the area of alveolar septal inflammation and cellular debris, and the ring-shaped peripheral airspace consolidation of the reversed halo sign, to the area of organizing pneumonia within the alveolar ducts [1].

### Patient Prognosis

In general, COP improves rapidly with the administration of corticosteroid therapy. Complete recovery with physiologic

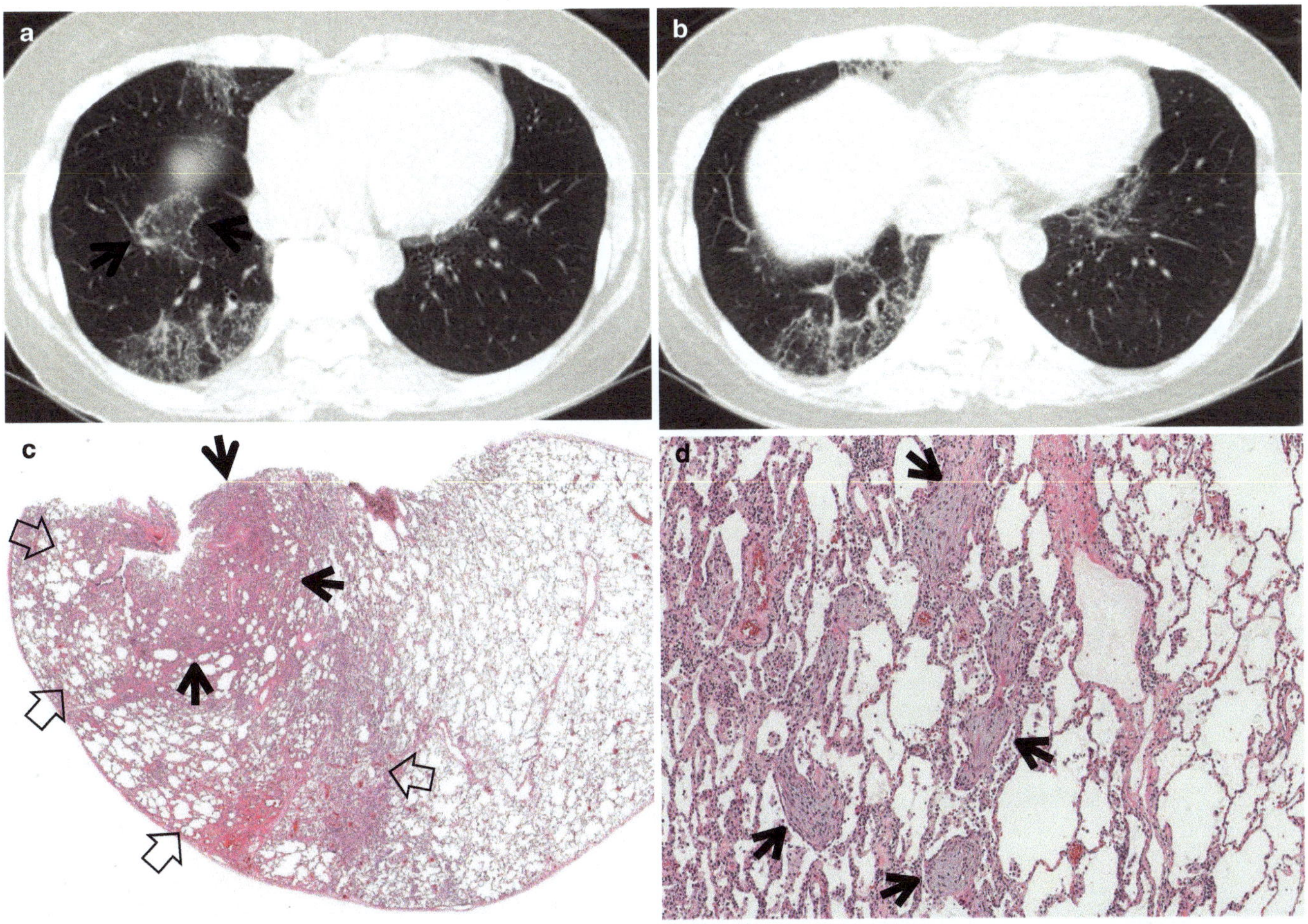


**Fig. 8.2** Cryptogenic organizing pneumonia showing reversed halo sign in a 58-year-old woman. (**a, b**) Lung window images of thin-section (2.5-mm section thickness) scans obtained at levels of the suprahepatic inferior vena cava (**a**) and liver dome (**b**), respectively, show multifocal areas of ground-glass opacity in both lungs. Also note reversed halo sign area (*arrows*). (**c**) Low-magnification (×8) photomicrograph demonstrates somewhat denser area of consolidative area (*arrows*) and less dense area (*open arrows*) of interstitial inflammatory cell infiltration areas. Combination of these denser and less dense areas helps form reversed halo sign. (**d**) High-magnification (×100) photomicrograph discloses polyps (*arrows*) of fibroblast tissue within lumens of respiratory bronchioles, alveolar ducts, and alveoli. The interstitium is moderately thickened by mononuclear inflammatory cell infiltrates

improvement and normalization of the chest lesion is observed in two-thirds of patients. Spontaneous improvement also has been reported. Relapse may occur when the corticosteroids are tapered. Rapidly progressive fatal form can have a clinical course of acute interstitial pneumonia, showing a high mortality [14].

## Pulmonary Mucormycosis

### Pathology and Pathogenesis

The characteristic pathology features of pulmonary mucormycosis are extensive parenchymal and vascular invasion by mycelia, with resultant hemorrhagic infarction. The organisms can be differentiated from *Aspergillus* because they are wider, nonseptate, fragmented, and having irregular branching points, often at 90° angles [15].

### Symptoms and Signs

Pulmonary mucormycosis is an important opportunistic mycosis in severely immunocompromised patients with hematologic malignancies and recipients of stem cell transplantation [15]. The clinical presentations of pulmonary mucormycosis are similar to those caused by *Aspergillus*. Concomitant sinus infection, oral necrotic lesions in the hard palate, and chest wall cellulitis are suggestive of pulmonary mucormycosis. Refractory fever despite broad spectrum antibiotics, nonproductive cough, progressive dyspnea, and pleuritic chest pain are common.

### CT Findings

The most common CT findings of pulmonary mucormycosis are nodules or consolidation [16]. Consolidations are most commonly posterior, abutting the pleura. They may be

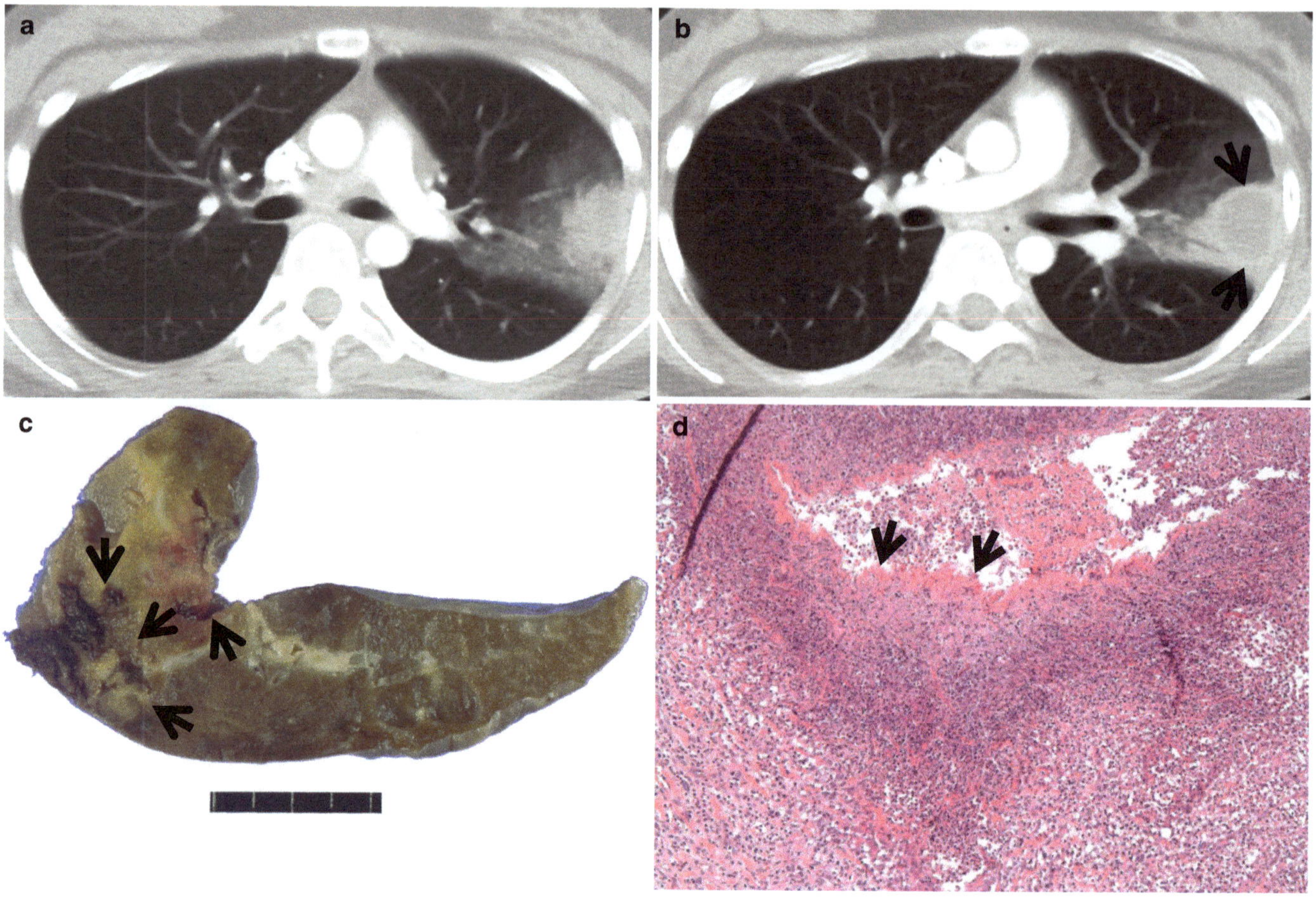

**Fig. 8.3** Pulmonary mucormycosis in a 17-year-old woman who had a history of anaplastic large cell lymphoma 5 years ago. (**a**, **b**) Lung window images of enhanced consecutive CT scans (5.0-mm section thickness) obtained at levels of the right bronchus intermedius show dense consolidation surrounded by ground-glass opacity (a kind of halo sign). Please note internal reversed halo sign (*arrows*) formed by central necrosis and peripheral enhancing ring of consolidation. (**c**) Cut surface of gross specimen obtained with wide wedge resection of the left upper lobe by using video-assisted thoracoscopic surgery demonstrates invasive fungal consolidative lesion harboring necrotic cavity (*arrows*). (**d**) High-magnification photomicrograph (×100) discloses necrotizing pneumonia. Please note fungal organisms that have broad hyphae (*arrows*), thin wall, and little (pauci) septa

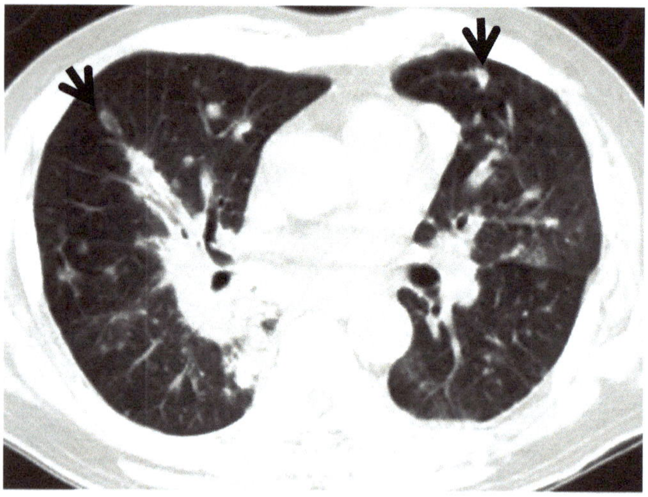

**Fig. 8.4** Lymphomatoid granulomatosis in a 70-year-old man showing reversed halo sign. Lung window image of CT scan (5.0-mm section thickness) obtained at level of the left lower lobar bronchus shows multiple variable-sized nodules in both lungs. Please also note bilaterally enlarged hilar lymph nodes. Some nodules show reversed halo sign (*arrows*)

**Table 8.1** Common diseases manifesting as reversed halo sign

| Disease | Key points for differential diagnosis |
|---|---|
| Cryptogenic organizing pneumonia | Reversed halo sign, unilateral and bilateral consolidation with peribronchovascular and subpleural distribution |
| Infectious disease | |
| Mucormycosis | Reversed and CT halo sign |
| Invasive pulmonary aspergillosis | Reversed and CT halo sign |
| Paracoccidioidomycosis, histoplasmosis | |
| Pulmonary infarction | Subpleural location |
| ANCA-associated granulomatous vasculitis | Multiple, bilateral, subpleural nodules or masses |
| Radiofrequency ablation | |
| Lymphomatoid granulomatosis | Nodules and masses with central low attenuation and peripheral rim enhancement, CT halo or reversed halo sign |

*Note*: *ANCA* antineutrophil cytoplasmic antibody

wedge-shaped and may have air bronchograms. Nodules and masses may have central low attenuation and may cavitate. CT halo sign and reversed halo sign are also seen (Fig. 8.3). Reversed halo sign is an early sign seen in 4 % of patients with pulmonary fungal infection and is significantly more common in pulmonary mucormycosis than in invasive pulmonary aspergillosis [17].

### CT–Pathology Comparisons

Reversed halo sign in invasive fungal infection are histopathologically associated with infarcted lung tissue, with a greater amount of hemorrhage at the periphery than in the center [17].

### Patient Prognosis

Timely diagnosis of pulmonary mucormycosis is critical in the outcome of this infection because it rapidly spreads to the contralateral lung and distal organs if not promptly treated. The first-line antifungal agents typically used for aspergillosis, such as voriconazole, lack activity against *Mucorales*. The overall mortality rate of pulmonary mucormycosis ranges from 50 to 70 % but increases up to 95 % with extrathoracic dissemination. To improve survival, surgical debridement of infected tissue as well as antifungal agents should be performed on an urgent basis.

## Lymphomatoid Granulomatosis

### Pathology and Pathogenesis

The lungs contain nodules of pinkish-gray tissue, the largest of which show central necrosis and cavitation. Alternatively, areas of confluent consolidation may be seen. Microscopically, most cases show broad tracts of necrosis separated by a mixed angiocentric infiltrate that includes usually scanty pleomorphic atypical lymphoid cells. While most of the lymphocytes stain for T-cell markers, the atypical lymphoid cells stain as B cells. The degree of cellular atypia varies considerably. The lesions are graded 1–3 on the degree of lymphocytic atypia, the presence of necrosis, and the polymorphic/monomorphic nature of the infiltrate, grade 3 lesions being synonymous with angiocentric lymphomas [18].

### Symptoms and Signs

The most common symptoms include fever, persistent productive cough, dyspnea, and chest tightness [19]. The presentation is typically insidious, and lung lesions may wax and wane. Constitutional symptoms such as weight loss, malaise, and fatigue may be present. Symptoms related to the other organ involvements of the skin, central nervous system, and kidney can occur.

### CT Findings

Characteristic CT findings are pulmonary nodules and masses with central low attenuation and peripheral rim enhancement, ground-glass halo, or reversed halo sign [6, 20] (Fig. 8.4). The nodules and masses are lower lobe predominant with a peribronchovascular and/or subpleural distribution [20]. Coarse irregular opacities and small thin-walled cysts are also seen [21].

### CT–Pathology Comparisons

Pulmonary nodules and masses are histologically caused by intravascular and perivascular infiltration of atypical lymphoid cells [21]. A low-attenuation center is corresponded to the histologic findings of central necrosis, and peripheral rim enhancement of the nodules is related to the angioinvasive and angio-destructive nature of lymphomatoid granulomatosis [20].

Reversed halo sign in lymphomatoid granulomatosis may be related to a central area of airspace filling with edema fluid and foamy histiocytes, surrounded by a denser rim of lymphocytic infiltration [6].

### Patient Prognosis

Lymphomatoid granulomatosis is usually an EBV-driven lymphoproliferative disease in immunocompromised patients; immunosuppressive agents should be discontinued if at all. Specific therapy with corticosteroids, anti-CD20 monoclonal antibodies such as rituximab, interferon-alpha-2b, and combination chemotherapy have showed a variable success rate [19].

## References

1. Kim SJ, Lee KS, Ryu YH, et al. Reversed halo sign on high-resolution CT of cryptogenic organizing pneumonia: diagnostic implications. AJR Am J Roentgenol. 2003;180:1251–4.
2. Hansell DM, Bankier AA, MacMahon H, McLoud TC, Muller NL, Remy J. Fleischner Society: glossary of terms for thoracic imaging. Radiology. 2008;246:697–722.
3. Georgiadou SP, Sipsas NV, Marom EM, Kontoyiannis DP. The diagnostic value of halo and reversed halo signs for invasive mold infections in compromised hosts. Clin Infect Dis. 2011;52:1144–55.
4. Gasparetto EL, Escuissato DL, Davaus T, et al. Reversed halo sign in pulmonary paracoccidioidomycosis. AJR Am J Roentgenol. 2005;184:1932–4.
5. Revel MP, Triki R, Chatellier G, et al. Is it possible to recognize pulmonary infarction on multisection CT images? Radiology. 2007;244:875–82.

6. Benamore RE, Weisbrod GL, Hwang DM, et al. Reversed halo sign in lymphomatoid granulomatosis. Br J Radiol. 2007;80: e162–6.
7. Marchiori E, Zanetti G, Hochhegger B, Irion KL, Carvalho AC, Godoy MC. Reversed halo sign on computed tomography: state-of-the-art review. Lung. 2012;190:389–94.
8. Kim Y, Lee KS, Choi DC, Primack SL, Im JG. The spectrum of eosinophilic lung disease: radiologic findings. J Comput Assist Tomogr. 1997;21:920–30.
9. Myers JL, Colby TV. Pathologic manifestations of bronchiolitis, constrictive bronchiolitis, cryptogenic organizing pneumonia, and diffuse panbronchiolitis. Clin Chest Med. 1993;14:611–22.
10. Cordier JF. Cryptogenic organising pneumonia. Eur Respir J. 2006;28:422–46.
11. Lee KS, Kullnig P, Hartman TE, Muller NL. Cryptogenic organizing pneumonia: CT findings in 43 patients. AJR Am J Roentgenol. 1994;162:543–6.
12. Muller NL, Staples CA, Miller RR. Bronchiolitis obliterans organizing pneumonia: CT features in 14 patients. AJR Am J Roentgenol. 1990;154:983–7.
13. Nishimura K, Itoh H. High-resolution computed tomographic features of bronchiolitis obliterans organizing pneumonia. Chest. 1992;102:26S–31.
14. Cohen AJ, King Jr TE, Downey GP. Rapidly progressive bronchiolitis obliterans with organizing pneumonia. Am J Respir Crit Care Med. 1994;149:1670–5.
15. Hamilos G, Samonis G, Kontoyiannis DP. Pulmonary mucormycosis. Semin Respir Crit Care Med. 2011;32:693–702.
16. Jamadar DA, Kazerooni EA, Daly BD, White CS, Gross BH. Pulmonary zygomycosis: CT appearance. J Comput Assist Tomogr. 1995;19:733–8.
17. Wahba H, Truong MT, Lei X, Kontoyiannis DP, Marom EM. Reversed halo sign in invasive pulmonary fungal infections. Clin Infect Dis. 2008;46:1733–7.
18. Guinee Jr DG, Perkins SL, Travis WD, Holden JA, Tripp SR, Koss MN. Proliferation and cellular phenotype in lymphomatoid granulomatosis: implications of a higher proliferation index in B cells. Am J Surg Pathol. 1998;22:1093–100.
19. Roschewski M, Wilson WH. Lymphomatoid granulomatosis. Cancer J. 2012;18:469–74.
20. Chung JH, Wu CC, Gilman MD, Palmer EL, Hasserjian RP, Shepard JA. Lymphomatoid granulomatosis: CT and FDG-PET findings. Korean J Radiol. 2011;12:671–8.
21. Lee JS, Tuder R, Lynch DA. Lymphomatoid granulomatosis: radiologic features and pathologic correlations. AJR Am J Roentgenol. 2000;175:1335–9.

# 9 Tree-in-Bud Sign

## Definition

Tree-in-bud sign refers to the condition in which small centrilobular nodules less than 10 mm in diameter are associated with centrilobular branching nodular structures [1] (Fig. 9.1). The small nodules represent lesions involving the small airways. However, vascular lesions involving the arterioles and capillaries may simulate the centrilobular small nodules and branching nodular structures (vascular tree-in-bud sign) [2–5] (Fig. 9.2).

## Diseases Causing the Sign

The localized tree-in-bud sign is typically seen in infectious bronchiolitis, *aspiration bronchiolitis*, and bronchopneumonia including tuberculosis and nontuberculous mycobacterial pulmonary disease. Vascular tree-in-bud sign can be observed in *foreign-body-induced necrotizing pulmonary vasculitis (cellulose and talc granulomatosis)* [2–4] and in localized pulmonary lymphatic metastasis [5] (Table 9.1). For diseases related to this chapter, please refer to section "Small Nodules with Centrilobular Distribution" in Chap. 18 and Chap. 26.

## Distribution

In infectious and aspiration bronchiolitis, the tree-in-bud sign shows middle and lower lung zone predominance. The upper lobes and the superior segment of the lower lobes are usually involved in tuberculosis, whereas the right middle lobe and lingular division of the left upper lobe are typical location of nodular bronchiectatic form of nontuberculous mycobacterial pulmonary disease.

In foreign-body-induced necrotizing vasculitis and in localized lymphatic metastasis, the vascular tree-in-bud sings demonstrate lower lung zone and subpleural predominance.

## Clinical Considerations

Tree-in-bud pattern with bronchial wall thickening is one (accounts for 31 % in one series) of the important CT findings of community-acquired respiratory viral infection in adults [6]. Predisposing factors for aspiration bronchiolitis include structural abnormalities of the pharynx, esophageal disorders, neurologic defects, and chronic illness [7]. Nontuberculous mycobacterial disease, nodular bronchiectatic form, is seen in an elderly lady who has lowered body mass index, and tuberculosis is a common infectious disease in immunocompromised hosts. Foreign-body-induced necrotizing vasculitis (cellulose and talc granulomatosis) is common among drug addicts who grind up and intravenously inject various drugs such as amphetamines, methylphenidate, or hydromorphone. These drugs are prepared as oral medication [3].

**Key Points for Differential Diagnosis**

1. Various diseases show this pattern of lung abnormality and thus distinction of one disease from others, the presence of associated imaging findings, along with patient history and clinical presentation, is often useful in suggesting the specific cause of this pattern (Table 9.1).

## Aspiration Bronchiolitis

### Pathology and Pathogenesis

Aspiration of gastric contents results in a chemical burn of the tracheobronchial tree and pulmonary parenchyma with an intense parenchymal inflammatory reaction. Once localized to the lung, neutrophils play a key role in the development of lung injury through the release of oxygen radicals and proteases. Acid aspiration pneumonitis reduces host

K.S. Lee et al., *Radiology Illustrated: Chest Radiology*, Radiology Illustrated,
DOI 10.1007/978-3-642-37096-0_9, 

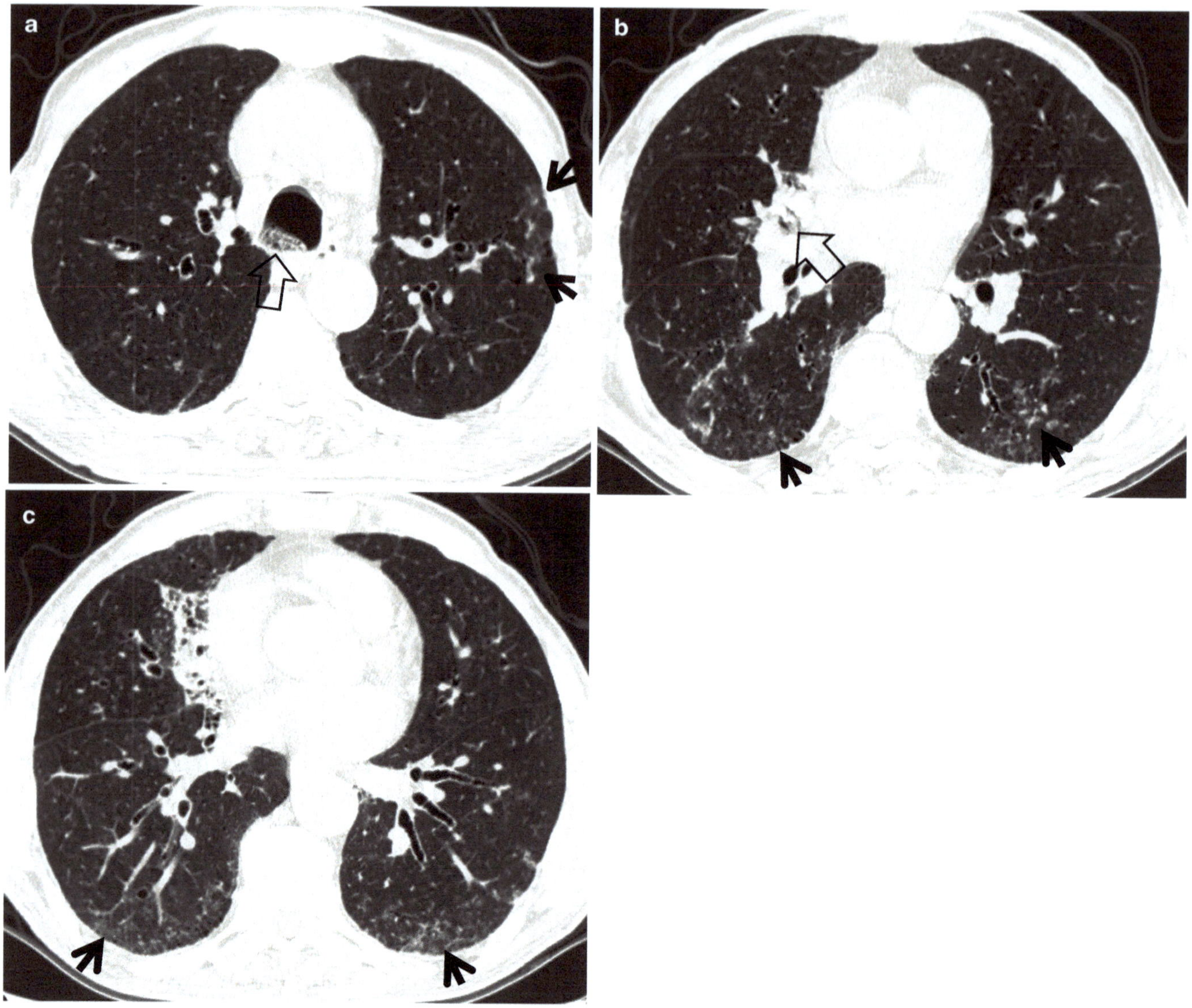


**Fig. 9.1** Aspiration pneumonia in a 66-year-old man with Parkinson's disease. (**a–c**) Lung window images of thin-section (1.0-mm section thickness) CT scans obtained at levels of the azygos arch (**a**), right middle lobar bronchus (**b**), and inferior pulmonary veins (**c**), respectively, show multifocal areas of tree-in-bud signs (*arrows*) in both lungs and parenchymal consolidation in the right middle lobe. Also note large amount of secretion (*open arrows*) in tracheobronchial trees.

defenses against infection, increasing the risk of superinfection. In these circumstances, the pulmonary inflammatory response is likely to result from both bacterial infection and the inflammatory response of the gastric particulate matter [8].

## Symptoms and Signs

Diffuse aspiration bronchiolitis is suspected in elderly patients with recurrent episodes of bronchorrhea, bronchospasm, and dyspnea [8]. It frequently presents with acute onset of symptoms while sleeping. Occult aspiration in the elderly is usually associated with neurologic impairment, esophageal dysmotility, and gastroesophageal reflux.

## CT Findings

HRCT manifestations include centrilobular nodules and uni- or bilateral foci of branching areas of increased attenuation with a tree-in-bud appearance in the dependent portions of both lungs [9] (Fig. 9.1).

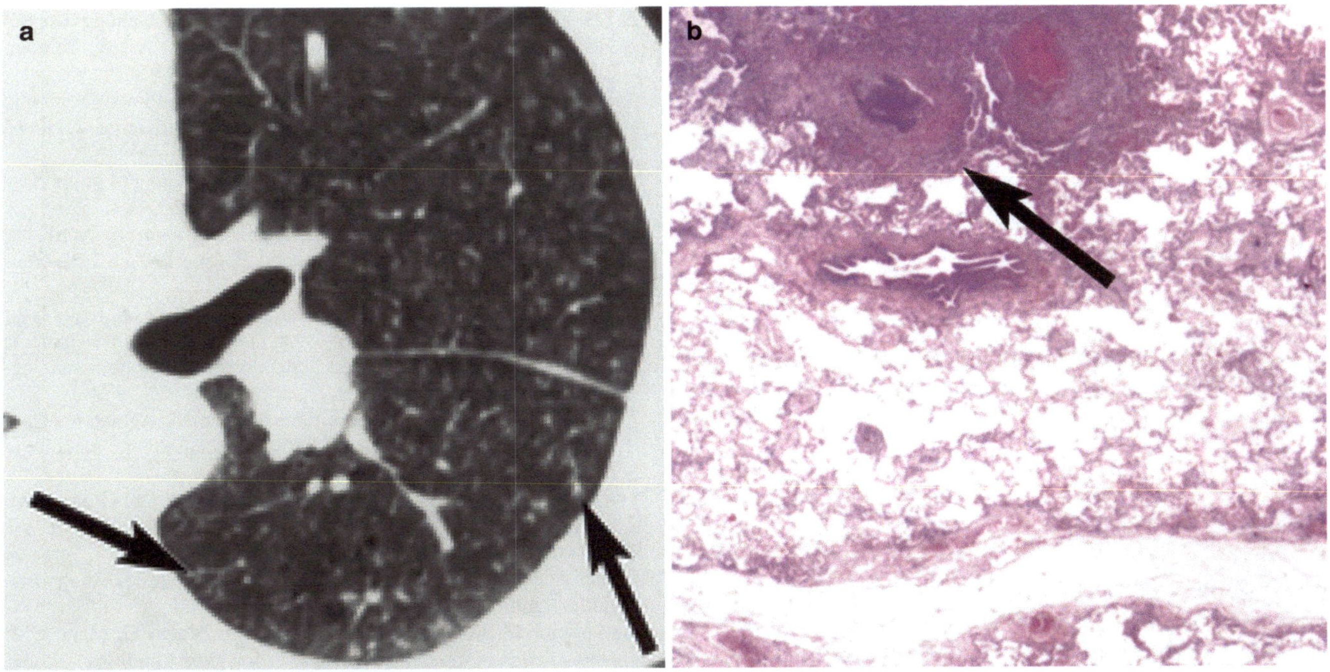


**Fig. 9.2** Cellulose granulomatosis (foreign-body-induced pulmonary vasculitis) in a 37-year-old man who is a drug abuser. (**a**) Thin-section (1.5-mm collimation) CT scan obtained at level of left interlobar pulmonary artery shows diffuse pulmonary involvement with ill-defined centrilobular small nodules (*arrows*). Note also nodular branching structures (tree-in-bud sign). (**b**) Low-magnification (×40) photomicrograph demonstrates necrotizing vasculitis at the central portion of secondary pulmonary lobule (*arrow*) (Reprinted from Han et al. [3] with permission)

**Table 9.1** Common diseases manifesting as tree-in-bud sign

| Disease | Key points for differential diagnosis |
|---|---|
| Infectious bronchiolitis | Tree-in-bud signs in mid and lower lung zone |
| Aspiration bronchiolitis | Tree-in-bud signs in the dependent portion |
| Tuberculosis | Tree-in-bud sign in the upper lobe and the superior segment of lower lobe |
| Nontuberculous mycobacterial disease | Tree-in-bud sign in the right middle lobe and lingular segment of the left upper lobe |
| Foreign-body-induced pulmonary vasculitis | Tree-in-bud sign with lower lung zone and subpleural predominance |
| Localized pulmonary lymphatic metastasis | Tree-in-bud sign with lower lung zone and subpleural predominance |

## CT–Pathology Comparisons

Centrilobular nodules and tree-in-bud patterns reflect the bronchiolar distribution of aspirated material.

## Patient Prognosis

Treatment consists of broad-spectrum antibiotics and management of the underlying dysphagia.

# Foreign-Body-Induced Pulmonary Vasculitis (Cellulose and Talc Granulomatosis)

## Pathology and Pathogenesis

Intravascular foreign materials and their associated granulomatous reaction in vessel walls cause tree-in-bud appearance at CT. Materials responsible for this disorder include insoluble particles such as microcrystalline cellulose, talc, and corn starch, which are used as fillers in tablets taken orally. These substances become trapped in the pulmonary vasculature, causing thrombosis, inflammation, and eventually giant cell reaction [3] (Fig. 9.2).

## Symptoms and Signs

Presentation of patients with talc granulomatosis can range from asymptomatic to fulminant disease [10]. It produces slowly progressive dyspnea on exertion (even after intravenous drug use has ceased), dry cough, nonspecific chest pain, and, occasionally, anorexia, weight loss, and mild fever. Lung sounds are usually normal. History of occupational exposure or of drug addiction is the major clue to the diagnosis.

## CT Findings

CT manifestations of cellulose granulomatosis consist of diffuse centrilobular small nodules and a tree-in-bud pattern [11] (Fig. 9.2).

## CT–Pathology Comparisons

Tree-in-bud pattern seen on HRCT in patients with cellulose granulomatosis represents intra-arteriolar accumulation of microcrystalline cellulose with associated adjacent granulomatous reaction (Fig. 9.2).

## Patient Prognosis

There are no established treatments for talc granulomatosis. Patients must stop the intravenous drug use. Success with steroids has been reported [12], but most believe that there is no benefit from corticosteroid therapy. Lung transplantation is considered a last option for patients with end-stage disease.

## References


1. Im JG, Itoh H, Shim YS, et al. Pulmonary tuberculosis: CT findings–early active disease and sequential change with antituberculous therapy. Radiology. 1993;186:653–60.
2. Lee KS, Kim TS, Han J, et al. Diffuse micronodular lung disease: HRCT and pathologic findings. J Comput Assist Tomogr. 1999;23:99–106.
3. Han D, Lee KS, Franquet T, et al. Thrombotic and nonthrombotic pulmonary arterial embolism: spectrum of imaging findings. Radiographics. 2003;23:1521–39.
4. Chung MP, Yi CA, Lee HY, Han J, Lee KS. Imaging of pulmonary vasculitis. Radiology. 2010;255:322–41.
5. Moon JW, Lee HY, Han J, Lee KS. Tree-in-bud sign as a manifestation of localized pulmonary lymphatic metastasis from a pancreas cancer. Intern Med. 2011;50:3027–9.
6. Shiley KT, Van Deerlin VM, Miller Jr WT. Chest CT features of community-acquired respiratory viral infections in adult in patients with lower respiratory tract infections. J Thorac Imaging. 2010;25:68–75.
7. Rossi SE, Franquet T, Volpacchio M, Gimenez A, Aguilar G. Tree-in-bud pattern at thin-section CT of the lungs: radiologic-pathologic overview. Radiographics. 2005;25:789–801.
8. Marik PE. Pulmonary aspiration syndromes. Curr Opin Pulm Med. 2011;17:148–54.
9. Franquet T, Gimenez A, Roson N, Torrubia S, Sabate JM, Perez C. Aspiration diseases: findings, pitfalls, and differential diagnosis. Radiographics. 2000;20:673–85.
10. Marchiori E, Lourenco S, Gasparetto TD, Zanetti G, Mano CM, Nobre LF. Pulmonary talcosis: imaging findings. Lung. 2010;188:165–71.
11. Bendeck SE, Leung AN, Berry GJ, Daniel D, Ruoss SJ. Cellulose granulomatosis presenting as centrilobular nodules: CT and histologic findings. AJR Am J Roentgenol. 2001;177:1151–3.
12. Chau CH, Yew WW, Lee J. Inhaled budesonide in the treatment of talc-induced pulmonary granulomatosis. Respiration. 2003;70:439.

# 10 Gloved Finger Sign or Toothpaste Sign

## Definition

Gloved finger sign is originally described on chest radiography and represents mucoid impaction of the branching bronchi [1]. The sign is formed by branching tubular, toothpaste, or fingerlike densities [2]. On CT, the dilated bronchi, filled and impacted with mucus (usually fluid attenuation but variable depending on the constituents of content in the dilated bronchi), generate a gloved finger appearance [3] (Fig. 10.1).

## Diseases Causing the Sign

Any airway obstructive lesions may result in gloved finger sign. Benign and malignant neoplasms (Fig. 10.2) causing airway obstruction can cause distal bronchiectasis and mucoid impaction. Developmental airway disease, *bronchial atresia* (Fig. 10.1), usually appears as gloved finger sign. Broncholithiasis, *bronchial tuberculosis and stricture* (Fig. 10.3), intralobar pulmonary sequestration, and *foreign-body aspiration* may also cause mucoid impaction and gloved finger sign. *Allergic bronchopulmonary aspergillosis* (ABPA) (Figs. 10.4 and 10.5) and cystic fibrosis with or without ABPA are the two most common nonobstructive diseases causing gloved finger sign on radiologic examinations [2] (Table 10.1).

## Distribution

Congenital bronchial atresia involves the parahilar airways [4]. Broncholithiasis is characterized and associated with peribronchial calcific nodal disease and thus involves usually the segmental bronchi [5]. Aneurysmal appearance of the medium-sized bronchi is seen on CT scans in bronchial tuberculosis [6]. ABPA characteristically involves central airways. Mucus plugging and bronchiectasis usually involve the airways of the upper and middle lung zones in cystic fibrosis.

## Clinical Considerations

Almost all patients with ABPA have asthma [7]. In approximately two-thirds of patients with bronchial atresia, the lesions are incidentally found. The remaining patients complain of cough, hemoptysis, fever, and shortness of breath [8]. Hemoptysis is a usual sign in broncholithiasis; it may be massive. Other parenchymal tuberculous lesions usually accompany gloved finger sign in bronchial tuberculosis. Cystic fibrosis is a disease of children, adolescence, and young adults, and most signs and symptoms affect the respiratory or the digestive system.

**Key Points for Differential Diagnosis**

1. Bronchiectasis with mucoid impaction is common in ABPA but occurs only occasionally in asthmatic patients with a positive skin test to *A. fumigatus* but without other features of the disease [9].
2. Gloved finger sign and bronchial obstruction are usually accompanied by mosaic perfusion area (hyperlucent lung) of the surrounding lung parenchyma [4].
3. CT helps localize correctly the endobronchial or peribronchial location of calcified lymph nodes in broncholithiasis [5].
4. Other parenchymal tuberculous lesions usually accompany gloved finger sign in bronchial tuberculosis [6].

## Bronchial Atresia

### Pathology and Pathogenesis

Atresia of a segmental or subsegmental bronchus classically results in a central mucus-filled cyst (mucocele) at the distal point of atresia, dilated distal airways with mucus, and

K.S. Lee et al., *Radiology Illustrated: Chest Radiology*, Radiology Illustrated,
DOI 10.1007/978-3-642-37096-0_10, © Springer-Verlag Berlin Heidelberg 2014

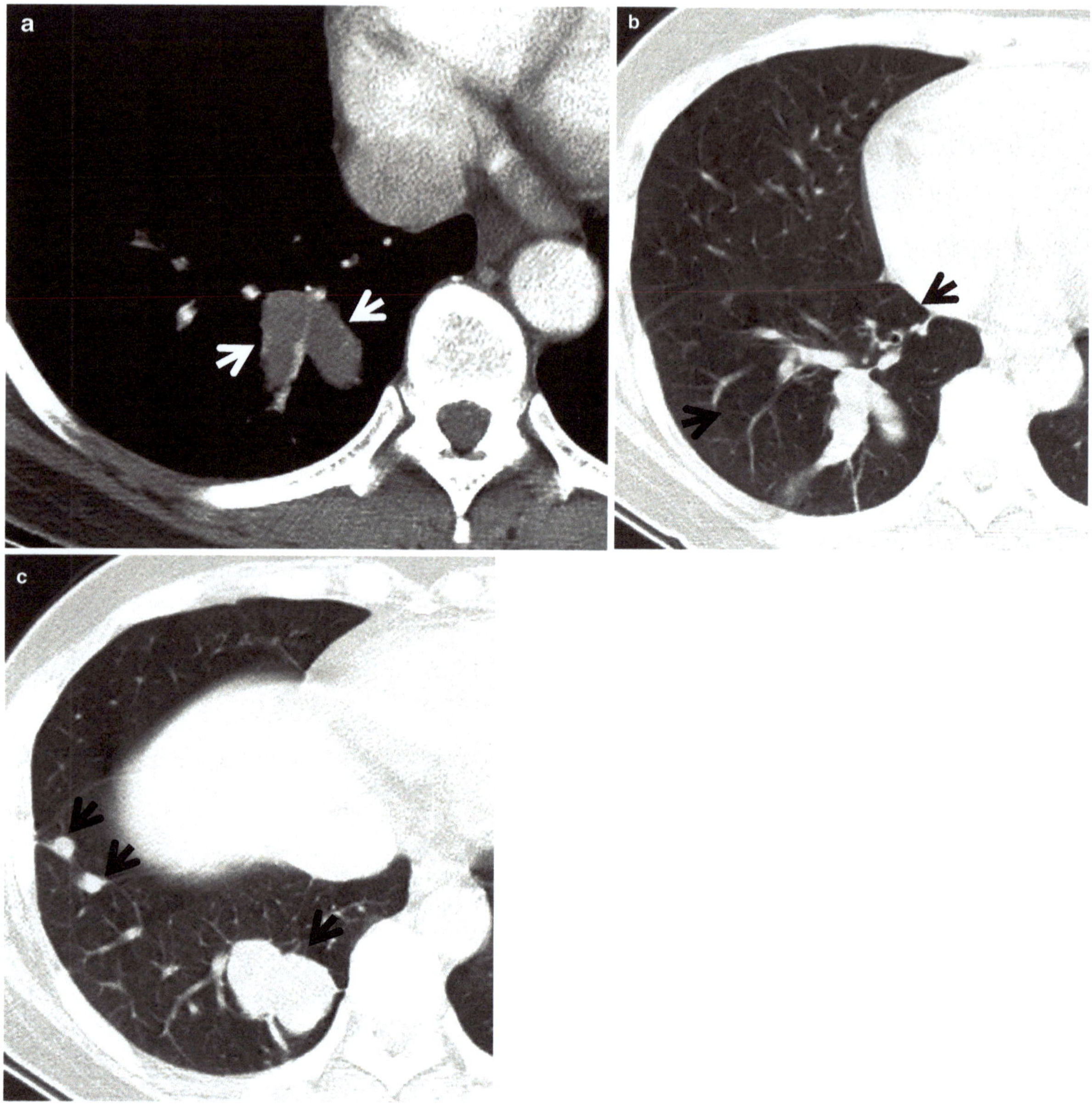


**Fig. 10.1** Bronchial atresia showing gloved finger appearance in a 43-year-old woman. (**a**) Mediastinal window image of enhanced CT scan (5.0-mm section thickness) obtained at level of the suprahepatic inferior vena cava shows V-shaped low-attenuation lesion (*arrows*) in the right lower lobe. (**b**) Lung window image of CT scan obtained at similar level to (a) demonstrates same branching lesion. Please note low-attenuation area (*arrows*) surrounding branching lesion. (**c**) CT scan obtained at level of liver dome displays branching nodular lesions (*arrows*) in the right lower lobe

hyperinflated microcystic distal parenchyma. Abundant inspissated mucus is typically noted within proximal airway lumens immediately distal to the focus of atresia and adjacent airspaces. Mucus-filled bronchus is continuous with the distal airways but has no connection with the more proximal airways. Infection may result in inflammation and fibrosis. The distal hyperinflation is due to collateral ventilation and air trapping [10].

## Symptoms and Signs

The left upper lobe is most commonly involved (two-thirds of patients), particularly the apicoposterior segmental bronchus. Most patients with bronchial atresia are asymptomatic, but dyspnea, chest pain, recurrent pneumonia up to 20 % of patients, pneumothorax, hemoptysis, and asthma have been reported [11].

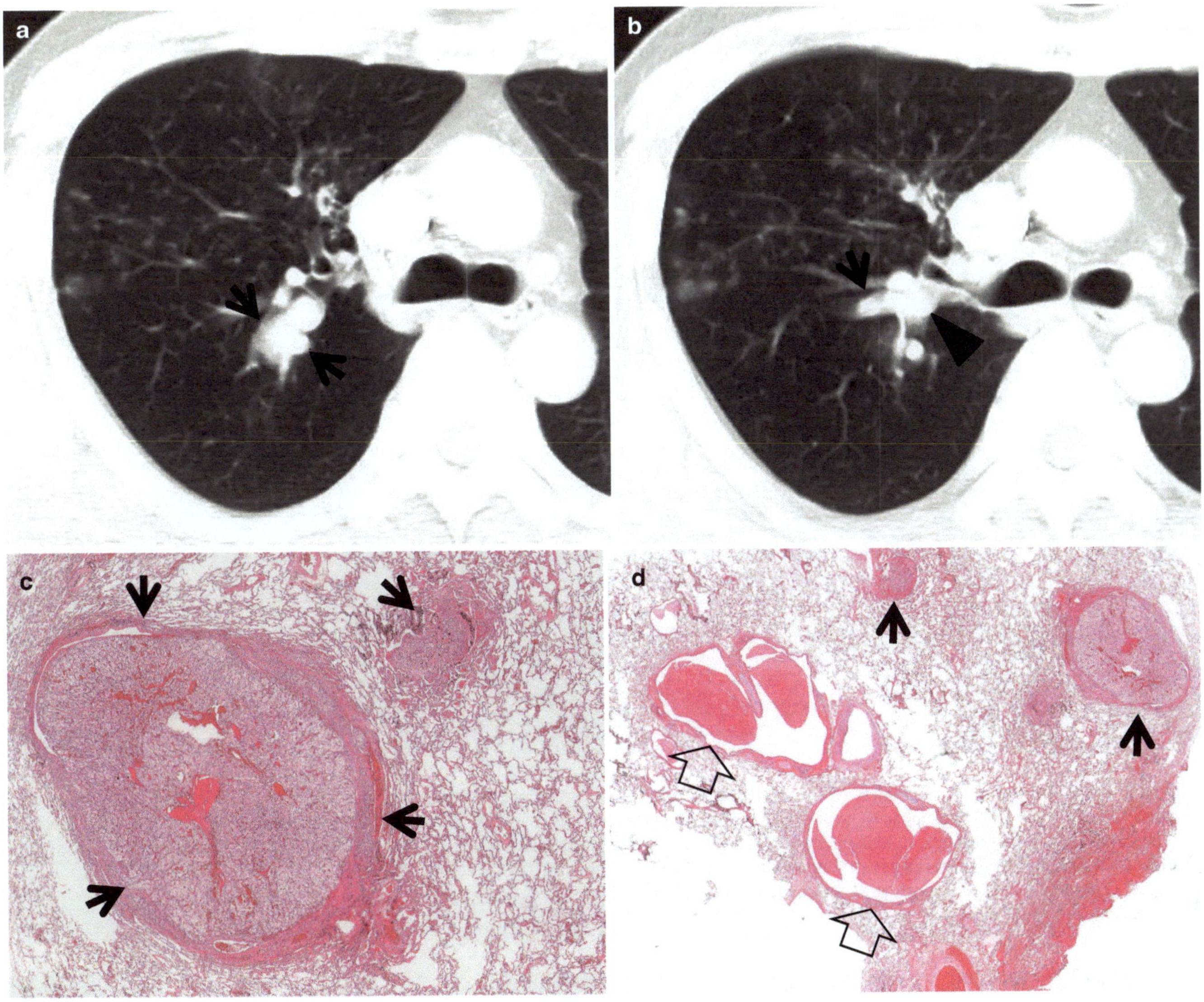


**Fig. 10.2** Gloved finger sign associated with mucus retention in airways distal to endobronchial metastasis in a 54-year-old man with renal cell carcinoma. (**a**, **b**) Lung window images of CT scans (5.0-mm section thickness) obtained at levels of the azygos arch (**a**) and main bronchi (**b**), respectively, show branching tubular lesions (*arrows*) in posterior segment of the right upper lobe, representing mucus plugging. Also note endobronchial tumor (*arrowhead*) in the posterior segmental bronchus of the right upper lobe. Bronchoscopic biopsy disclosed endobronchial metastatic renal cell carcinoma nodule (not shown here). Small centrilobular nodules and branching nodular structures in anterior segment of the right upper lobe are due to concurrent nontuberculous mycobacterial pulmonary disease. (**c**) High-magnification photomicrograph (×200) of pathologic specimen obtained from the right upper lobe with right upper lobectomy (from a different patient but with same disease) displays endobronchial tumor nodules (*arrows*). (**d**) High-magnification photomicrograph (×100) discloses endobronchial tumor nodules (*arrows*) and distal mucus plugging (*open arrows*) within the dilated bronchi

## CT Findings

Characteristic CT findings of bronchial atresia include bronchial occlusion, mucoid impaction with bronchial dilatation (bronchocele) immediately distal to the atretic bronchus, and decreased vascularity and attenuation and increased volume of the affected segment [12, 13] (Fig. 10.1). It most commonly affects the apicoposterior segmental bronchus of the left upper lobe, followed by segmental bronchi of the right upper lobe, the right middle lobe, and rarely the right lower lobe [14].

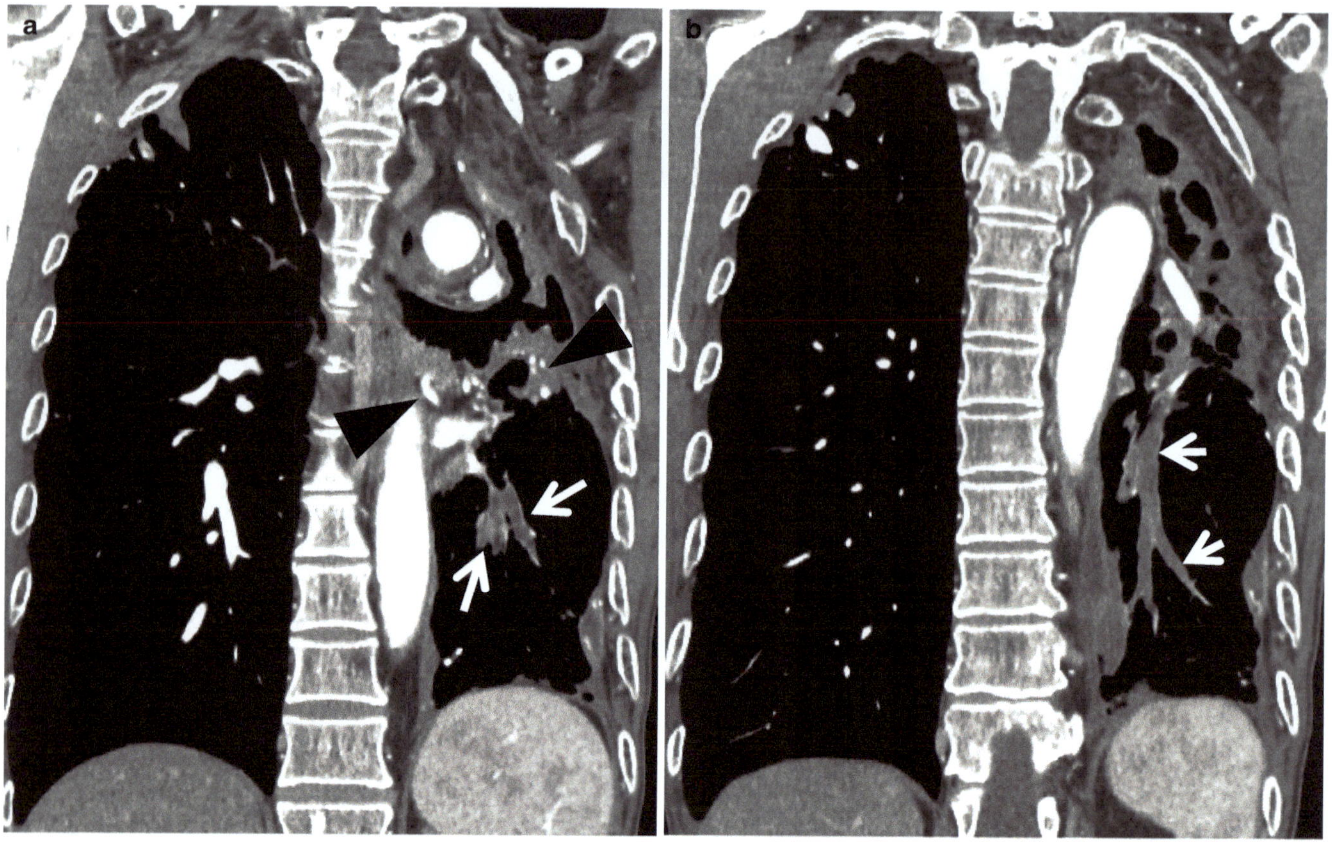


**Fig. 10.3** Gloved finger sign associated with tuberculous bronchial stricture involving the left lower lobar bronchus in a 67-year-old man who had a history of previous tuberculous infection. (**a, b**) Mediastinal window and coronal reformatted images (2.0-mm section thickness) of enhanced CT scans obtained at levels of the descending thoracic aorta show branching tubular lesions (*arrows*) in the left lower lobe, representing mucus plugging. Also note the hypertrophied left bronchial artery and its branches (*arrowheads*) and destroyed left upper lobe owing to tuberculous infection

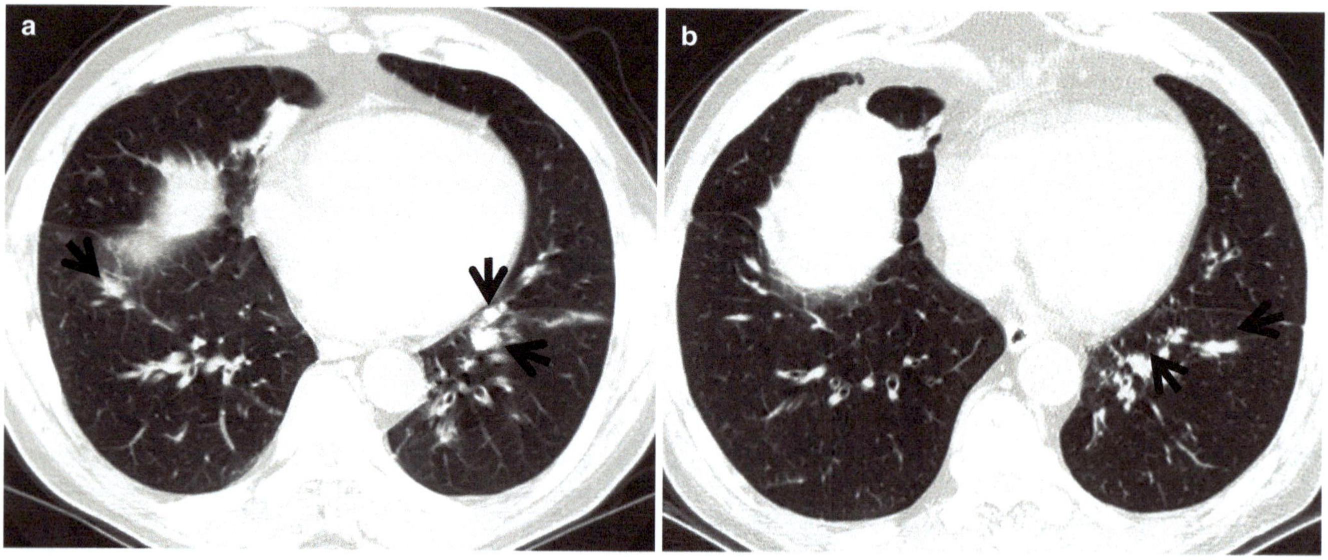


**Fig. 10.4** Allergic bronchopulmonary aspergillosis in a 64-year-old asthmatic man. (**a, b**) Lung window images of consecutive CT scans (2.5-mm section thickness) obtained at levels of liver dome show mucus plugging (*arrows*) in the dilated bronchi in both lower lobes. Also note the dilated bronchi (bronchiectasis) without mucus filling

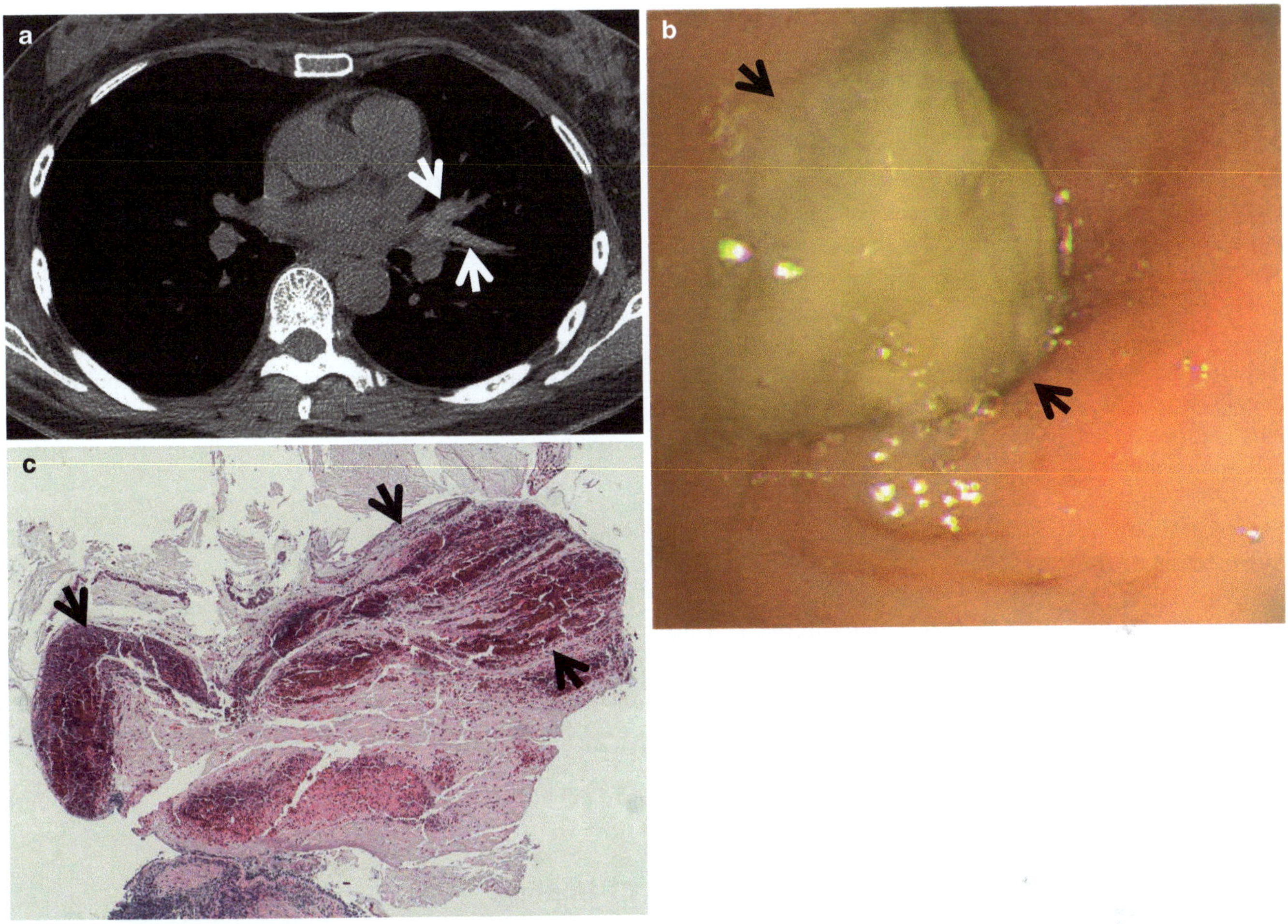


**Fig. 10.5** Allergic bronchopulmonary aspergillosis in a 56-year-old asthmatic woman. (**a**) Mediastinal window of unenhanced CT scan (2.5-mm section thickness) obtained at level of the right middle lobar bronchus shows high-attenuation V-shaped branching structures (*arrows*) in lingular division of the left upper lobe. (**b**) Bronchoscopy depicts yellow mucus (*arrows*) obstructing lingular divisional bronchus. (**c**) Low magnification (×8) photomicrograph obtained with bronchoscopic biopsy discloses allergic mucin (mucus plus eosinophils) (*arrows*) containing calcifications

**Table 10.1** Common diseases manifesting as gloved finger sign

| Disease | Key points for differential diagnosis |
|---|---|
| Benign and malignant neoplasms causing airway obstruction | |
| Bronchial atresia | Bronchocele in the apicoposterior segment of the left upper lobe |
| Broncholithiasis | Endobronchial or peribronchial location of calcified lymph nodes |
| Bronchial tuberculosis | Aneurysmal appearance of medium-sized bronchi |
| Foreign-body aspiration | Intrabronchial foreign body with gloved finger sign |
| ABPA | Central bronchiectasis with high-attenuation mucus plugging |

*Note*: *ABPA* allergic bronchopulmonary aspergillosis

## CT–Pathology Comparisons

Pathologically, the bronchial tree peripheral to the point of obliteration is patent and has a normal number of airways and airspaces. This results in the accumulation of mucus and an attendant mucocele immediately distal to the atresia. The alveoli in the lung supplied by the atretic bronchus are ventilated by collateral pathways and show features of air trapping with hyperinflation.

## Patient Prognosis

Treatment is usually conservative. Surgery is only indicated when major clinical symptoms are present.

## Bronchial Tuberculosis and Mucoid Impaction

### Pathology and Pathogenesis

Airway tuberculosis in its proximal form may mimic a neoplasm and is noteworthy for extensive necrosis and often large numbers of bacilli. The characteristic granulomatous morphology may not be visible around the necrotic material. The distal airway involved with mucoid impaction is dilated, and its wall shows nonspecific chronic inflammatory changes varying from a mild infiltrate to a severe reaction that includes many eosinophils. The affected airway may be merely distended and therefore returns to normal after the plug is expectorated, or its wall may be largely destroyed by the inflammation.

### Symptoms and Signs

Clinical manifestations of bronchial tuberculosis may be acute, insidious, or delayed. It is frequently misdiagnosed as bronchial asthma. Common symptoms include cough, shortness of breath, wheezing and fever, and hemoptysis [15]. On chest auscultation, diminished breath sound, rhonchus, and fixed wheezing can be heard.

### CT Findings

The principal CT findings of bronchial tuberculosis are circumferential wall thickening and luminal narrowing, with the involvement of a long segment of the bronchi. However, aneurysmal appearance of medium-sized bronchi with abrupt ending of the air column and without narrowing of proximal airway is another CT feature of bronchial tuberculosis (Fig. 10.3) [6].

### CT–Pathology Comparisons

Aneurysmal appearances of the medium-sized bronchi represent large caseating granulomas filling the lumen of the medium-sized bronchi [6].

### Patient Prognosis

The eradication of *Mycobacterium tuberculosis* and the prevention of bronchial stenosis are the main goals for the treatment of bronchial tuberculosis. Delayed diagnosis results in the permanent fibrotic stricture of the involved bronchial trees. Standard treatment with antituberculosis drugs should be given promptly once it is diagnosed. Symptomatic bronchial stenosis even after the antituberculosis chemotherapy can be relieved by bronchoscopic intervention therapy (balloon dilation, laser therapy, or stent insertion) or reconstructional bronchial surgery.

## Foreign-Body Aspiration

### Pathology and Pathogenesis

The inhalation of a foreign body is especially common in children, while the narrow, pliable bronchi of infants are particularly liable to be compressed by distended pulmonary arteries at points where they are in close anatomic proximity.

### Symptoms and Signs

Symptoms of foreign-body aspiration can vary from life-threatening airway obstruction or death to nonspecific symptoms. Sudden onset of choking sensation and intractable cough is the most common. Other symptoms include cough, fever, breathlessness, and wheezing [16]. Older patients are more likely to be mistakenly diagnosed as chronic obstructive pulmonary disease or pneumonia.

### CT Findings

Although foreign bodies may become lodged in any location of the tracheobronchial tree, the most common sites are the right lower lobe, intermediate bronchus, and left main bronchus [17]. Chest CT images often show the intrabronchial foreign body and associated features such as atelectasis, hyperlucency, bronchiectasis, lobar consolidation, mucoid impaction with gloved finger sign, a tree-in-bud pattern, and a thickened bronchial wall adjacent to the foreign body [18].

### CT–Pathology Comparisons

CT findings of bronchiectasis and mucoid impaction with gloved finger sign and air trapping with a resultant decrease in perfusion of the compromised segment or lobe result from the remnants of aspirated foreign bodies for long periods of time [17].

### Patient Prognosis

After initial airway support, prompt removal of foreign body is necessary to avoid complications. Both rigid and flexible bronchoscopies can be utilized to remove the foreign bodies in the airway.

## Allergic Bronchopulmonary Aspergillosis

### Pathology and Pathogenesis

The hallmark of allergic bronchopulmonary aspergillosis (ABPA) is "allergic mucin" which is composed of abundant eosinophilic mucin, mixed with eosinophils, eosinophil cytoplasmic debris, occasional Charcot–Leyden crystals, as well as calcium oxalate crystals (Fig. 10.5). There are rare fungal hyphae in the mucin. Various combinations of asthmatic changes, bronchocentric granulomatosis, and eosinophilic pneumonia are commonly seen [19].

### Symptoms and Signs

Clinically, the patients with ABPA present with chronic asthma, recurrent pulmonary infiltrates, and bronchiectasis. Most complain of low-grade fever, wheezing, bronchial hyperreactivity, hemoptysis, or productive cough. Expectoration of brownish mucus plugs is seen in 31–69 % of patients [19]. Patients may be minimally symptomatic or asymptomatic.

### CT Findings

CT findings of ABPA consist primarily of mucoid impaction and bronchiectasis involving predominantly the segmental and subsegmental bronchi of the upper lobes, along with centrilobular small nodules or branching linear structures [20] (Figs. 10.4 and 10.5). Bronchiectasis with mucoid impaction generates a gloved finger sign. In approximately 30 % of patients, the impacted mucus is highly opaque or demonstrates frank calcification at CT [21] (Fig. 10.5).

### CT–Pathology Comparisons

Airway colonization by *Aspergillus* causes persistent inflammation and fibrosis, leading to segmental and subsegmental bronchiectasis and mucoid impaction [22]. High-attenuation mucus plugging is related to the presence of calcium salts [23]. Centrilobular small nodules on CT reflect the presence of dilated bronchioles filled with mucus or necrotic debris.

### Patient Prognosis

Institution of glucocorticoids to control the immunologic activity and close monitoring for detection of relapses are the two important aspects of the management of ABPA. Because of frequent relapses (up to 45 %) with the lower doses of glucocorticoids, a higher dose and prolonged duration of corticosteroid therapy are necessary. Antifungal therapy with itraconazole can be given with corticosteroid therapy in the relapsed patients.

## References


1. Mintzer RA, Neiman HL, Reeder MM. Mucoid impaction of a bronchus. JAMA. 1978;240:1397–8.
2. Nguyen ET. The gloved finger sign. Radiology. 2003;227:453–4.
3. Collins J. CT signs and patterns of lung disease. Radiol Clin North Am. 2001;39:1115–35.
4. Matsushima H, Takayanagi N, Satoh M, et al. Congenital bronchial atresia: radiologic findings in nine patients. J Comput Assist Tomogr. 2002;26:860–4.
5. Conces Jr DJ, Tarver RD, Vix VA. Broncholithiasis: CT features in 15 patients. AJR Am J Roentgenol. 1991;157:249–53.
6. Cha JH, Han J, Park HJ, et al. Aneurysmal appearance of medium-sized bronchi: a peripheral manifestation of endobronchial tuberculosis. AJR Am J Roentgenol. 2009;193:W95–9.
7. Kim Y, Lee KS, Choi DC, Primack SL, Im JG. The spectrum of eosinophilic lung disease: radiologic findings. J Comput Assist Tomogr. 1997;21:920–30.
8. Wang Y, Dai W, Sun Y, Chu X, Yang B, Zhao M. Congenital bronchial atresia: diagnosis and treatment. Int J Med Sci. 2012;9:207–12.
9. Angus RM, Davies ML, Cowan MD, McSharry C, Thomson NC. Computed tomographic scanning of the lung in patients with allergic bronchopulmonary aspergillosis and in asthmatic patients with a positive skin test to Aspergillus fumigatus. Thorax. 1994;49:586–9.
10. Kunisaki SM, Fauza DO, Nemes LP, et al. Bronchial atresia: the hidden pathology within a spectrum of prenatally diagnosed lung masses. J Pediatr Surg. 2006;41:61–5; discussion 61–5.
11. Desir A, Ghaye B. Congenital abnormalities of intrathoracic airways. Radiol Clin North Am. 2009;47:203–25.
12. Kinsella D, Sissons G, Williams MP. The radiological imaging of bronchial atresia. Br J Radiol. 1992;65:681–5.
13. Beigelman C, Howarth NR, Chartrand-Lefebvre C, Grenier P. Congenital anomalies of tracheobronchial branching patterns: spiral CT aspects in adults. Eur Radiol. 1998;8:79–85.
14. Jederlinic PJ, Sicilian LS, Baigelman W, Gaensler EA. Congenital bronchial atresia. A report of 4 cases and a review of the literature. Medicine (Baltimore). 1987;66:73–83.
15. Xue Q, Wang N, Xue X, Wang J. Endobronchial tuberculosis: an overview. Eur J Clin Microbiol Infect Dis. 2011;30:1039–44.
16. Boyd M, Chatterjee A, Chiles C, Chin Jr R. Tracheobronchial foreign body aspiration in adults. South Med J. 2009;102:171–4.
17. Limper AH, Prakash UB. Tracheobronchial foreign bodies in adults. Ann Intern Med. 1990;112:604–9.
18. Zissin R, Shapiro-Feinberg M, Rozenman J, Apter S, Smorjik J, Hertz M. CT findings of the chest in adults with aspirated foreign bodies. Eur Radiol. 2001;11:606–11.
19. Agarwal R. Allergic bronchopulmonary aspergillosis. Chest. 2009;135:805–26.
20. Neeld DA, Goodman LR, Gurney JW, Greenberger PA, Fink JN. Computerized tomography in the evaluation of allergic bronchopulmonary aspergillosis. Am Rev Respir Dis. 1990;142:1200–5.
21. Franquet T, Muller NL, Gimenez A, Guembe P, de La Torre J, Bague S. Spectrum of pulmonary aspergillosis: histologic, clinical, and radiologic findings. Radiographics. 2001;21:825–37.
22. Zander DS. Allergic bronchopulmonary aspergillosis: an overview. Arch Pathol Lab Med. 2005;129:924–8.
23. Logan PM, Muller NL. High-attenuation mucous plugging in allergic bronchopulmonary aspergillosis. Can Assoc Radiol J. 1996;47:374–7.

# 11 Lobar Atelectasis Sign

## Definition

Atelectasis is derived from the Greek words *ateles* and *ektasis* meaning "incomplete expansion or stretching" [1]. The terms "atelectasis," "collapse," and "loss of lung volume" are used synonymously implying reduced inflation of the lung. In broad sense, atelectasis denotes diminished air within the lung associated with volume decrease, and generally, it manifests as increased density. Atelectasis can be differentiated by its volume decrease from consolidation in which volume is maintained because air is replaced by liquid or cells of approximately equal volume (Figs. 11.1, 11.2, 11.3, 11.4, 11.5, 11.6, and 11.7).

## Disease Causing the Sign

Various causes of lobar atelectasis are enlisted in Table 11.1.

## Distribution

All five lobes of both lungs can be involved with lobar atelectasis process. Because the right lung has three lobes, three kinds (middle and lower lobes, upper and middle lobes, and upper and lower lobes) of combined lobar atelectasis may occur in the right lung [2].

## Clinical Considerations

According to its pathophysiologic mechanisms, atelectasis is classified as follows:

(1) resorption (obstructive) atelectasis by central obstruction; (2) adhesive atelectasis from surfactant deficiency, as in hyaline membrane disease of newborn; (3) passive atelectasis associated with pneumothorax and pleural effusion; (4) compressive atelectasis by adjacent masses or elevated diaphragm; (5) cicatrization atelectasis by pulmonary fibrosis; and (6) gravity-dependent atelectasis [3, 4] (Table 11.1). Atelectasis is one of the most important radiologic findings, which should not be missed on chest radiograph, because it may suggest a hidden central malignancy. There are other peculiar entities of atelectasis, which are peripheral lobar atelectasis, migrating lobar atelectasis, platelike atelectasis, and rounded atelectasis.

**Key Points for Differential Diagnosis**

1. As a cause of resorption (obstructive) atelectasis, bronchogenic carcinoma is the most important one (Figs. 11.1, 11.2, 11.3, and 11.5). In a middle-aged or elderly smoker with unexplained lobar atelectasis or recurrent pneumonia, the diagnosis of bronchogenic carcinoma should be strongly suggested. The other various kinds of malignant endobronchial tumors can also obstruct the bronchi, resulting in resorption (obstructive) atelectasis, and these are bronchial carcinoid, adenoid cystic carcinoma, mucoepidermoid carcinoma, and endobronchial metastasis (breast cancer, renal cell carcinoma, melanoma, colon cancer). Rarely, benign endobronchial tumors (hamartoma, lipoma, leiomyoma, papilloma, neurogenic tumor, fibroma) can also be found as an obstructing mass.
2. Resorption (obstructive) atelectasis takes place also from obstruction of the peripheral small airways by mucus plugging. For example, postoperative patients with thoracic or abdominal trauma receiving intensive care frequently develop left lower lobe atelectasis. This results partly from impaired mucociliary clearance of secretions, which are retained in the peripheral airways with distal resorption (obstructive) atelectasis [5].

K.S. Lee et al., *Radiology Illustrated: Chest Radiology*, Radiology Illustrated,
DOI 10.1007/978-3-642-37096-0_11, 

3. Although bronchial neoplasm, mucus plug, and occasionally inflammatory bronchostenosis are the most frequent causes of lobar atelectasis in adults, bronchial tumors are uncommon in children. Instead, pneumonia is the most common cause of atelectasis, in which the inflammatory exudate and secretion obstruct the airways which are smaller and more vulnerable to mucus obstruction than in adults (Figs. 11.4 and 11.6). Mucus plugging can also develop in other conditions such as bronchial asthma or cystic fibrosis. Aspirated foreign body (such as peanut) is another important cause of lobar atelectasis in children (Fig. 11.6).

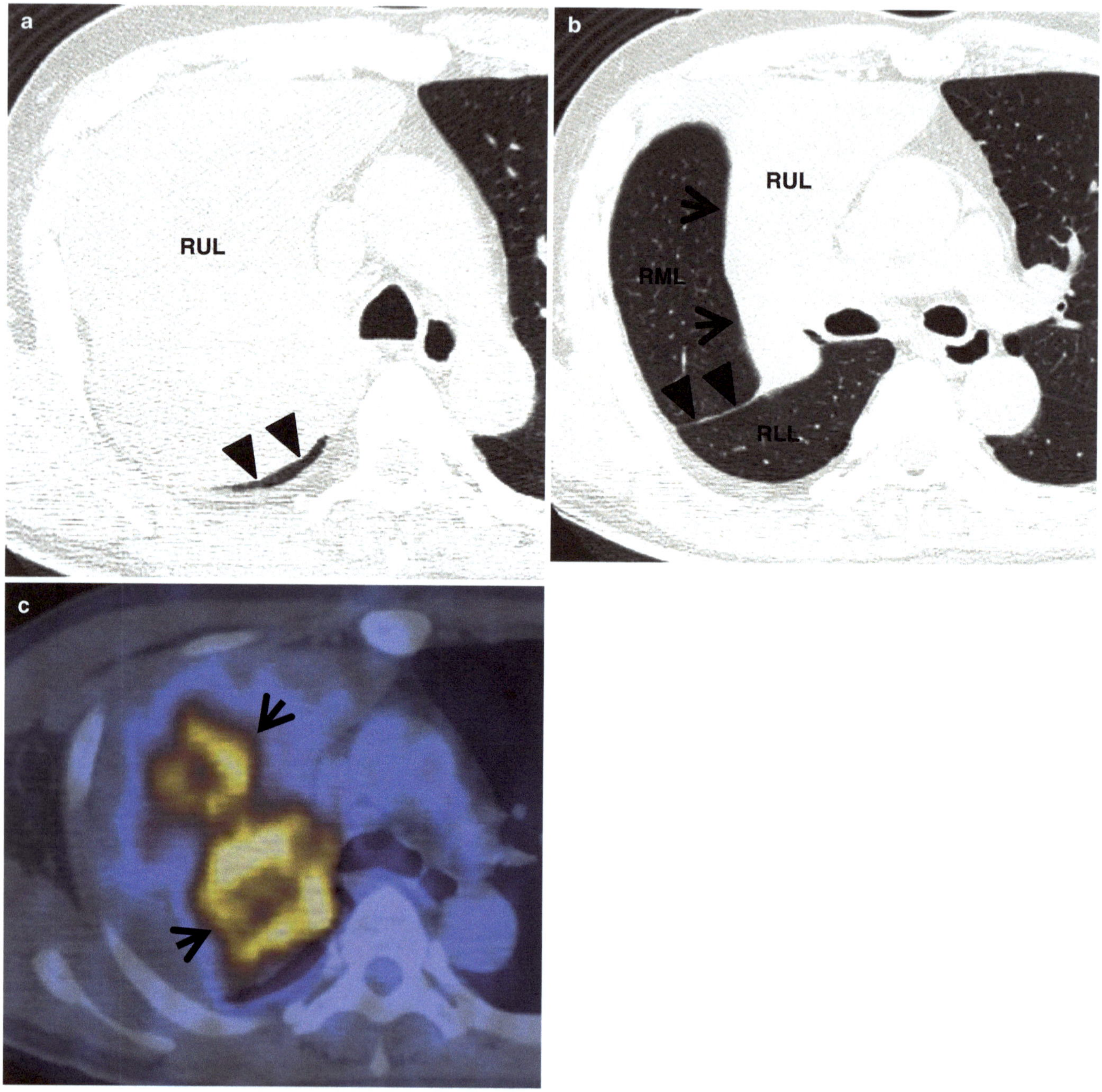


**Fig. 11.1** Right upper lobar atelectasis associated central squamous cell carcinoma in a 53-year-old man. (**a**, **b**) Lung window images of CT scans (5.0-mm section thickness) obtained at levels of the aortic (**a**) and azygos (**b**) arches, respectively, show the atelectatic right upper lobe. Also note the atelectatic right upper lobe marginated posteriorly by the right major fissure (*arrowheads*) and superiorly elevated right middle lobe marginated by right minor fissure (*arrows*). *RUL* right upper lobe, *RML* right middle lobe, *RLL* right lower lobe. (**c**) $^{18}$Fluorine fluorodeoxyglucose (FDG) PET demonstrates increased FDG uptake (*arrows*) within central bronchogenic carcinoma. The atelectatic right upper lobe surrounds the tumor

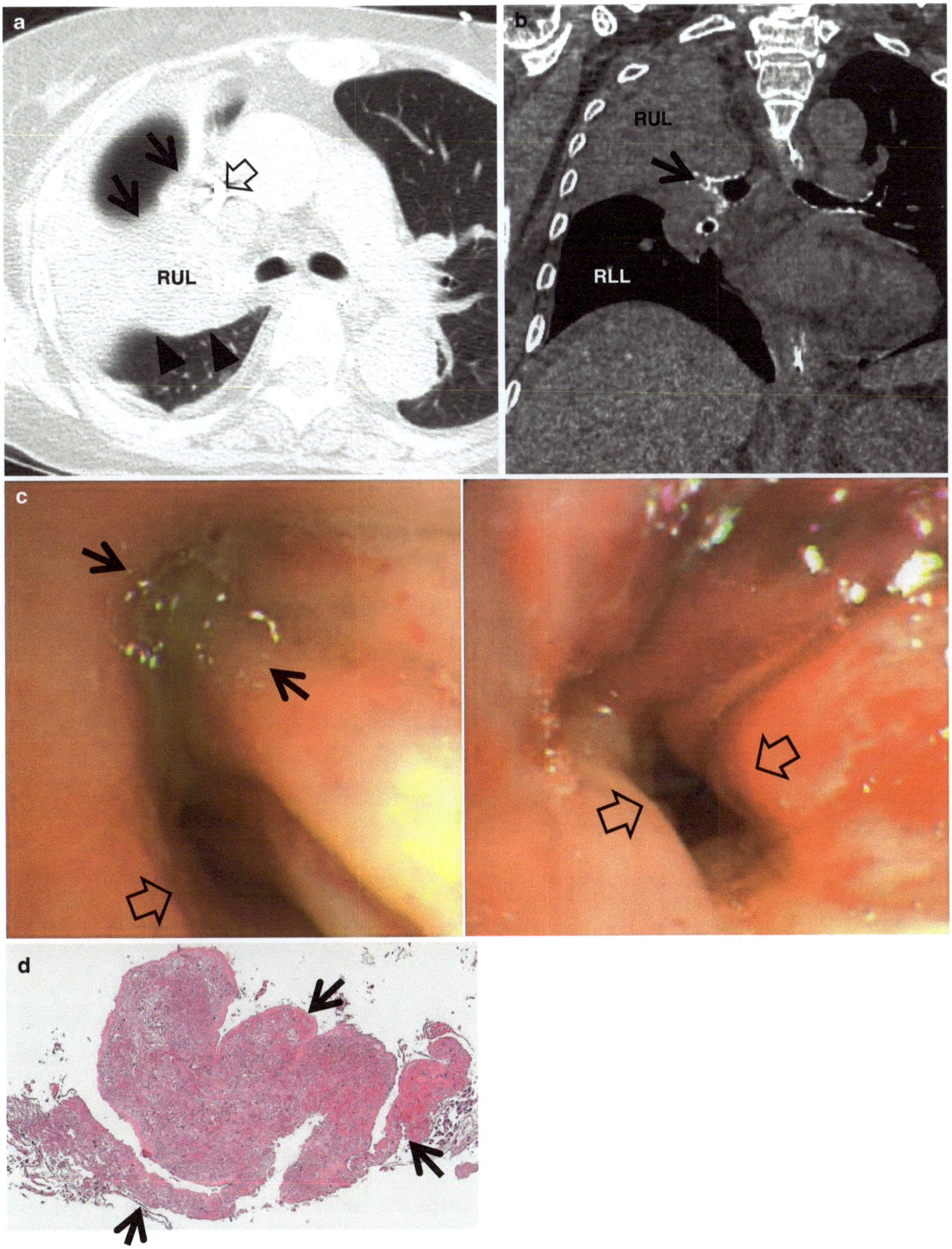


**Fig. 11.2** Right upper lobe atelectasis due to bronchial aspergillosis in a 62-year-old woman who has diffuse large B-cell lymphoma. (**a**) Lung window image of CT scan (2.5-mm section thickness) obtained at level of the main bronchi shows the atelectatic right upper lobe bounded anteriorly by right minor fissure (*arrows*) and posteriorly by right major fissure (*arrowheads*). A central venous line (*open arrow*) is inserted for chemotherapy. *RUL* right upper lobe. (**b**) Coronal reformatted image (2.0-mm section thickness) demonstrates the obliterated right upper lobar bronchus (*arrow*) with intraluminal soft tissue, causing right upper lobar atelectasis. Also note diffuse calcification in airway walls. *RUL* right upper lobe, *RLL* right lower lobe. (**c**) Bronchoscopy displays obliterated the right upper lobar bronchus (*arrows*) with white necrotic tissue and surrounding mucosal inflammation and edema. The right bronchus intermedius also demonstrates 50 % luminal narrowing (*open arrows*) with edema and inflammation. (**d**) High-magnification (×200) photomicrograph of pathologic specimen obtained with bronchoscopic biopsy discloses numerous fungal hyphae (*arrows*) infiltrating bronchial wall

4. The essential signs of lobar atelectasis are increased opacity of the involved lobe and the evidences of volume decrease. The signs can be divided into (1) direct signs, displacement of interlobar fissures and crowding of pulmonary blood vessels and major bronchi, and (2) indirect signs, pulmonary opacification; elevation of the diaphragm; shift of the trachea, heart, mediastinum, and hilum; compensatory hyperexpansion of the adjacent lung; approximation of the ribs; and juxtaphrenic peak.

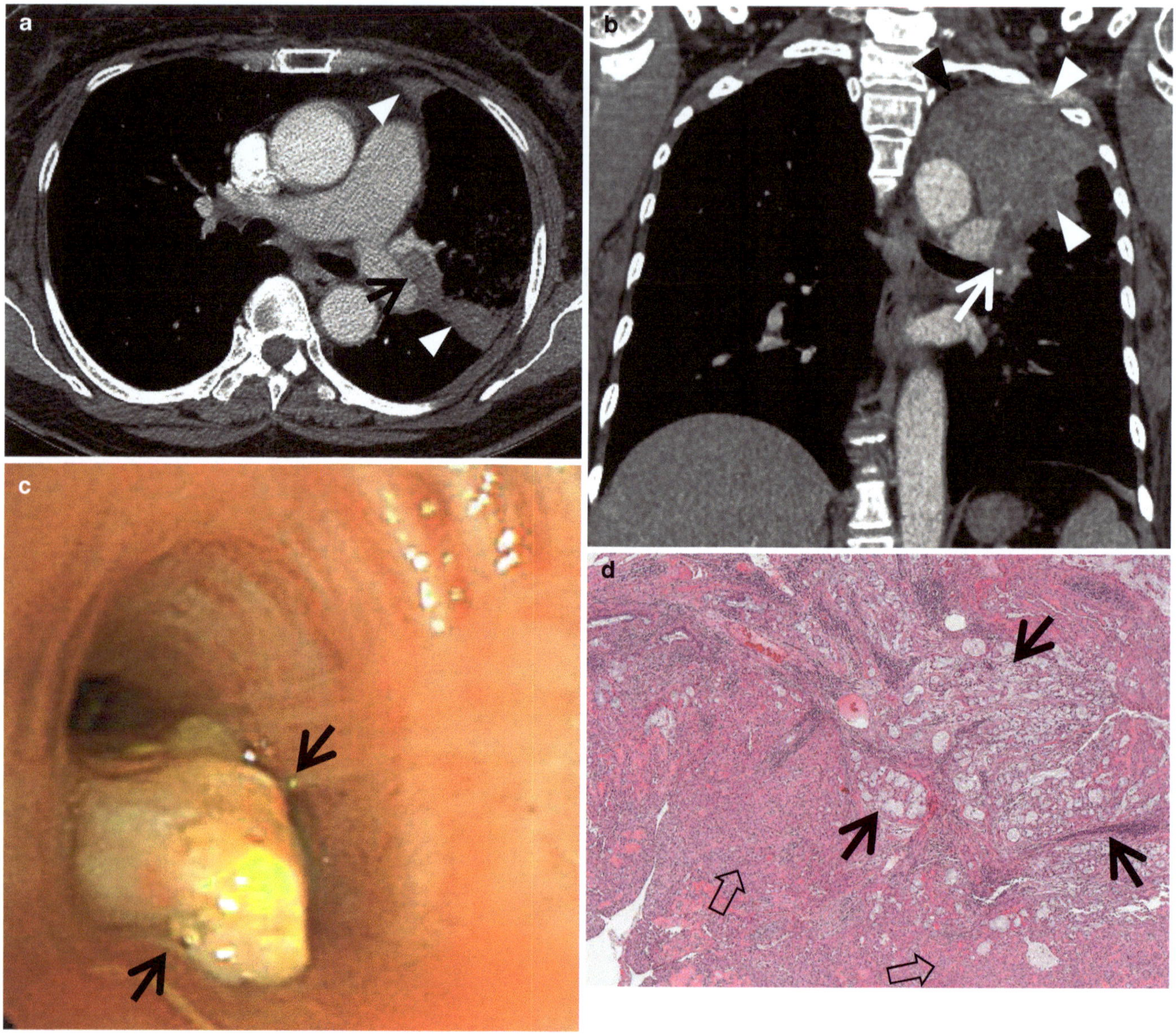


**Fig. 11.3** Left upper lobar atelectasis owing to mucoepidermoid carcinoma arising from the left upper lobar bronchus in a 69-year-old woman. (**a**) Enhanced CT scan (2.5-mm section thickness) obtained at level of the distal left main bronchus shows an endobronchial nodule (*arrow*) obstructing the left upper lobar bronchus. Also note the atelectatic left upper lobe (*arrowheads*). (**b**) Coronal reformatted (2.0-mm section thickness) CT scan demonstrates endobronchial nodule (*arrow*) and the atelectatic left upper lobe (*arrowheads*). (**c**) Bronchoscopy displays whitish-yellow nodule (*arrows*) obstructing the left upper lobar bronchus. (**d**) High-magnification (×100) photomicrograph of pathologic specimen obtained with left upper lobectomy discloses glandular spaces containing mucus (*arrows*) admixed with sheets of epidermoid cells (*open arrows*), diagnostic of mucoepidermoid carcinoma

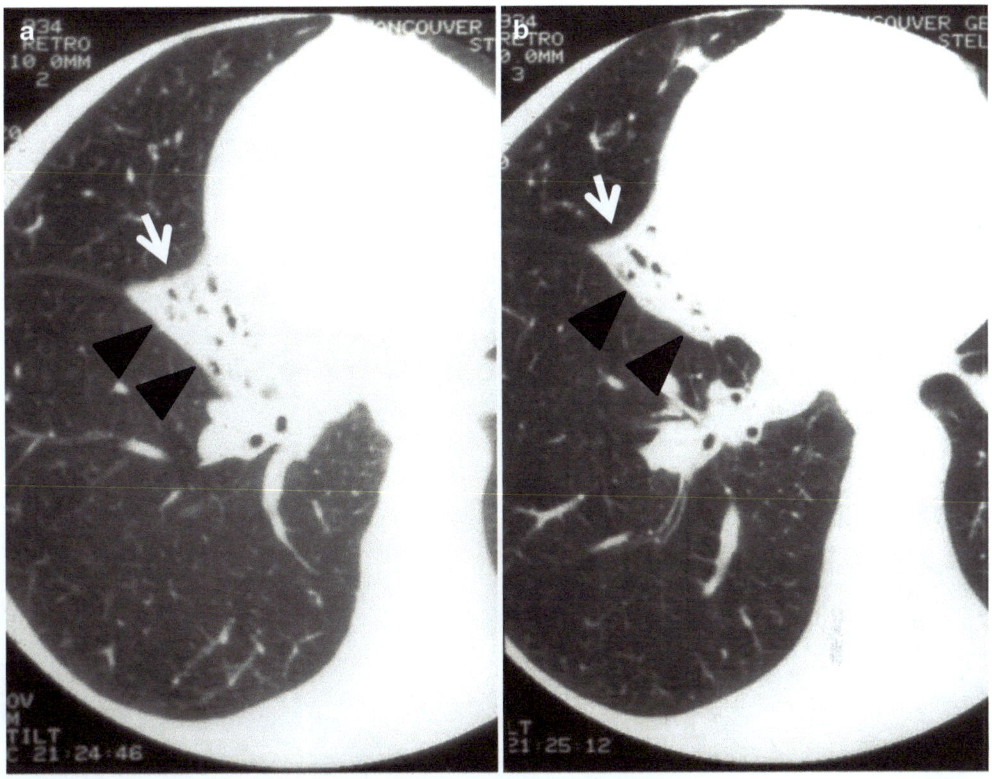


**Fig. 11.4** Right middle lobar atelectasis (right middle lobe syndrome) in a 72-year-old man. (**a**, **b**) Consecutive CT scans (1.5-mm section thickness) obtained at level of the right inferior pulmonary vein show the atelectatic right middle lobe marginated by right minor (*arrows*) and major (*arrowheads*) fissures. Anterior margin (right minor fissure) of the atelectatic right middle lobe is somewhat wavy, whereas posterior margin (right major fissure) of the lobe is sharp

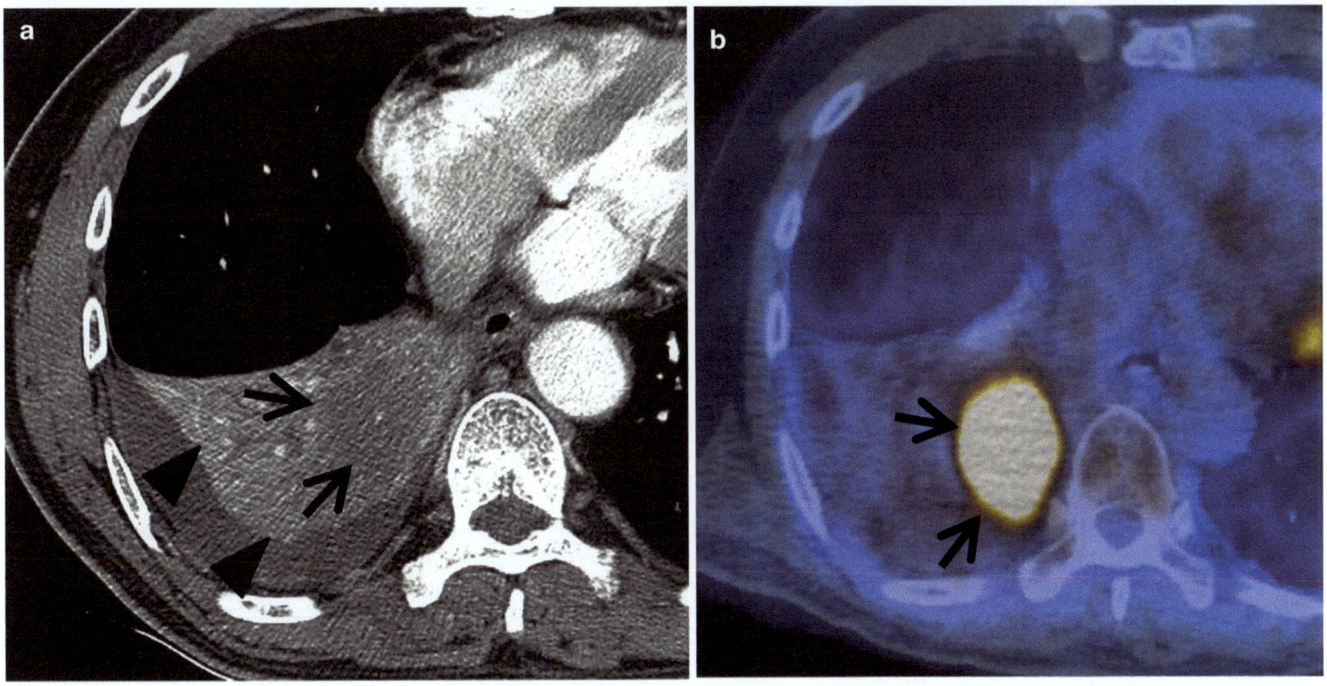


**Fig. 11.5** Right lower lobar atelectasis in a 61-year-old man who has squamous cell carcinoma involving the right lower lobe. (**a**) Mediastinal window image of enhanced CT scan (2.5-mm section thickness) obtained at ventricular level shows low-attenuation mass (*arrows*) and associated right lower lobar atelectasis (enhancing area, *arrowheads*). Also note right pleural effusion. (**b**) $^{18}$Fluorine fluorodeoxyglucose (FDG) PET demonstrates increased FDG uptake (*arrows*) within central bronchogenic carcinoma. The atelectatic right lower lobe surrounds the tumor

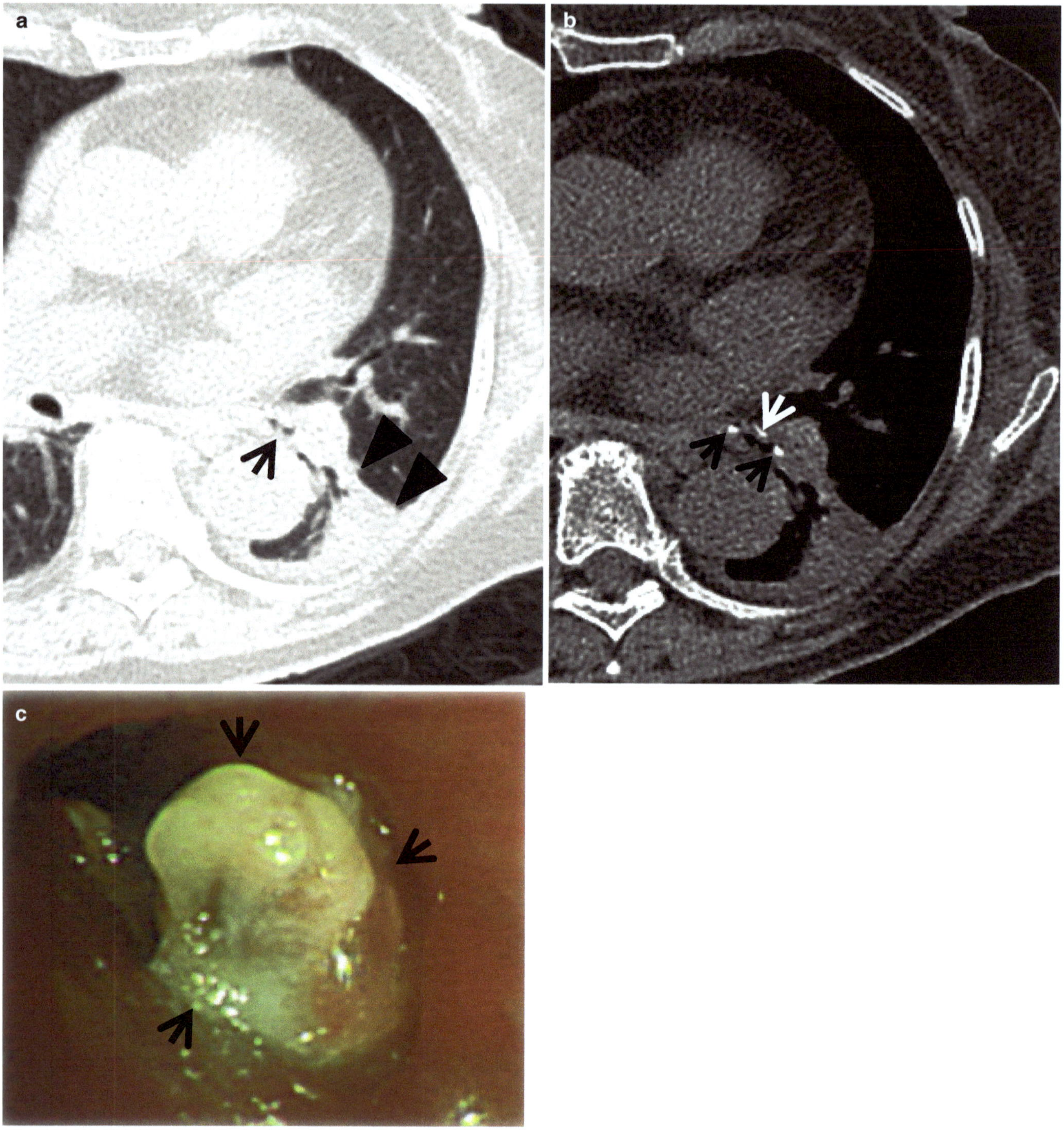


**Fig. 11.6** Left lower lobar atelectasis related to aspirated foreign body in an 82-year-old woman. (**a**) Lung window of CT scan (2.5-mm section thickness) obtained at the left lower lobar bronchus level shows the narrowed left lower lobar bronchus (*arrow*) and volume decrease of left lower lobe bounded laterally by left major fissure (*arrowheads*). (**b**) Mediastinal window image demonstrates peribronchial calcific attenuations (*arrows*) that are associated with left lower lobar bronchial narrowing. (**c**) Bronchoscopy displays inflamed granulation tissue (*arrows*) obstructing the left lower lobar bronchus. (**d**) Low-magnification (×4) of pathologic specimen obtained with rigid bronchoscopy discloses combination of cartilage (*arrows*), bone fragment (*arrowhead*), and necrotic tissue with bacteria (*Actinomyces*) (*open arrows*) that has caused granulation tissue obstructing left lower lobar bronchus

Fig. 11.6 (continued)

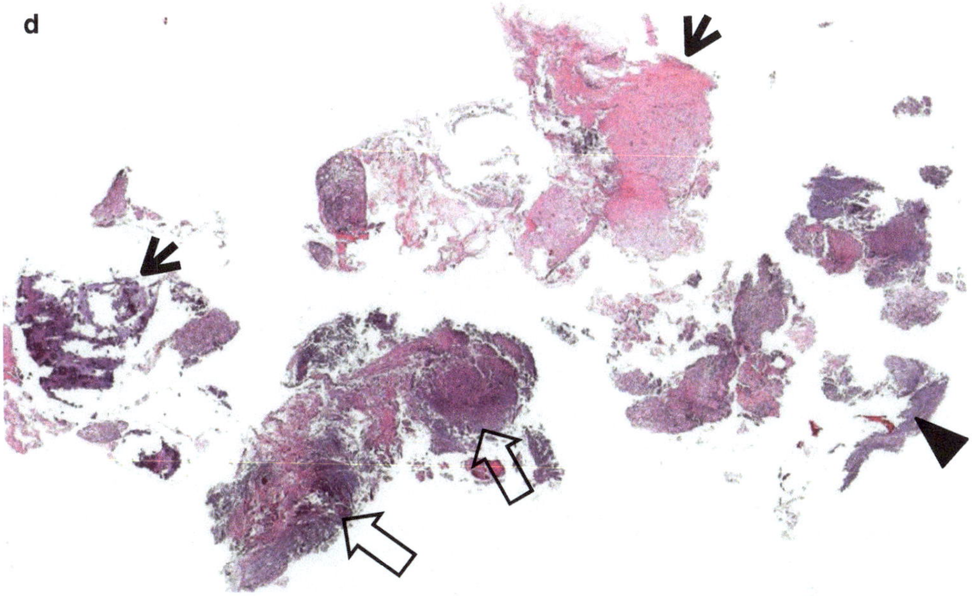


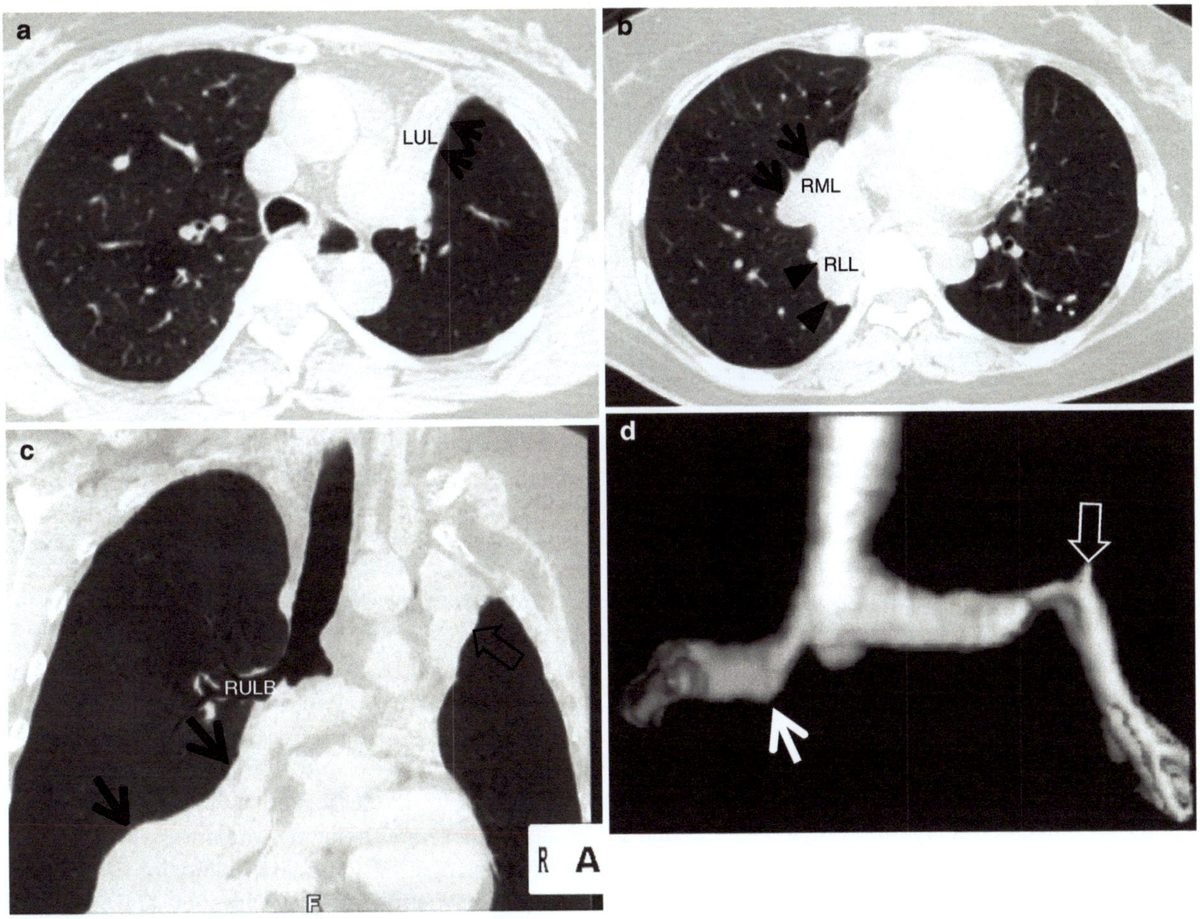


Fig. 11.7 Trilobar atelectasis involving the right middle and lower lobar bronchi and left upper lobar bronchus in a 34-year-old woman with bronchial tuberculosis, fibrotic stage. (**a**) Lung window of CT scan (5.0-mm section thickness) obtained at carinal level shows the atelectatic left upper lobe (*arrows*) marginated laterally by the elevated left lower lobe. *LUL* left upper lobe. (**b**) CT scan obtained at level of the segmental bronchi of the left lower lobe demonstrates the atelectatic right middle lobe (*RML*) and right lower lobe (*RLL*) bounded laterally by right minor (*arrows*) and major (*arrowheads*) fissures, respectively. (**c**) Minimum-intensity projection (MIP) image clearly depicts the atelectatic right middle and lower lobes (*arrows*) and left upper lobe (*open arrow*). Please note the patent right upper lobar bronchus (*RULB*) and aerated right upper lobe filling entire right hemothorax. (**d**) Three-dimensional image made with shaded-surface display (SSD) technique discloses clearly obliterated bronchus intermedius (*arrow*) and left upper lobar bronchus (*open arrow*). Also note irregular narrowing of both main bronchi

**Table 11.1** The etiology of atelectasis

| |
|---|
| I. Resorption atelectasis (obstructive atelectasis) |
| A. Tumor |
| 1. Bronchogenic carcinoma |
| 2. Malignant endobronchial tumors (carcinoid, adenoid cystic carcinoma, mucoepidermoid carcinoma) |
| 3. Endobronchial metastasis (breast cancer, renal cell carcinoma, melanoma, colon cancer) |
| 4. Benign endobronchial tumors (hamartoma, lipoma, papilloma, neurogenic tumor, fibroma) |
| B. Inflammatory |
| 1. Endobronchial tuberculosis (endobronchial granuloma, fibrotic bronchial stricture, broncholithiasis) |
| 2. Fungal infection |
| C. Miscellaneous |
| 1. Mucus plugging (thoracic or abdominal pain, trauma, postoperative status, general anesthesia, endotracheal intubation) |
| 2. Foreign-body aspiration |
| 3. Diffuse bronchostenosis (amyloidosis, ANCA-associated granulomatous vasculitis) |
| 4. Extrinsic bronchial compression (metastatic hilar lymph nodes, large left atrium, aortic aneurysm) |
| II. Adhesive atelectasis |
| A. Respiratory distress syndrome of the newborn |
| B. Pulmonary embolism |
| C. Acute radiation pneumonitis |
| D. Viral pneumonia |
| III. Passive atelectasis |
| A. Simple pneumothorax |
| B. Pleural effusion, hemothorax |
| C. Diaphragmatic eventration or paralysis |
| IV. Compressive atelectasis |
| A. Large intrathoracic tumor |
| B. Large emphysematous bulla |
| C. Tension pneumothorax |
| D. Increased intra-abdominal pressure (massive ascites, pregnancy, intestinal obstruction) |
| V. Cicatrization atelectasis |
| A. Chronic destructive tuberculosis |
| B. Chronic fungal infection |
| C. Radiation fibrosis |
| D. Idiopathic pulmonary fibrosis |
| E. Other pulmonary fibrosis (scleroderma, pneumoconiosis, asbestosis, sarcoidosis) |

*Note*: *ANCA* antineutrophil cytoplasmic antibody

## Right Upper Lobar Atelectasis

Golden's S sign denotes a centrally located mass with associated lobar atelectasis. In general, the atelectatic lobe shows a concave border pushed by the hyperexpanding adjacent lobe. In the presence of a central obstructing mass, the focal convex bulge by the mass coupled with the concave border of an atelectatic lobe makes a wavy interface, termed Golden's S sign.

On CT scan the atelectatic right upper lobe (RUL) manifests as a triangular or trapezoid soft tissue attenuation abutting the anterior chest wall and the upper mediastinum [6, 7]. It is bordered laterally by the elevated minor fissure and posteriorly by the major fissure. The major fissure maintains its original contour, whether straight, concave, or convex (Figs. 11.1 and 11.2).

## Left Upper Lobar Atelectasis

On CT scans, the atelectatic left upper lobe (LUL) forms a homogeneous opacity based on the anterior chest wall and the mediastinum (Fig. 11.3). Typically, the posterior margin has a V-shaped contour from the lung apex to the hilum, where the apex of the V merges with the hilar vessels and bronchi. These are the hilar structures, which are relatively fixed in position, thus tethering the major fissure into the V shape. The superior segment of the left lower lobe (LLL) is pulled forward along both the medial and lateral limbs of the V. The part of the superior segment that follows the medial limb forms a tongue of the lung between the mediastinum and the atelectatic LUL. This tongue is visible on PA radiographs making the aortic arch clearly discernible and has been called the Luftsichel (air-crescent) or periaortic lucency.

Less commonly, the major fissure may have a straight border rather than a V-shaped contour.

## Right Middle Lobar Atelectasis

On CT scans, the atelectatic right middle lobe (RML) is triangular or trapezoidal in shape. Its posterior border, demarcated by the major fissure, is usually well defined because the major fissure crosses the axial scan plane almost perpendicularly. On the other hand, the interface between RML and RUL is often less distinct because of dome-shaped contour of the minor fissure (Fig. 11.4). However, as the minor fissure is pushed down by the overexpanding RUL and getting a more oblique orientation, the anterior margin of the RML becomes more distinct.

## Lower Lobar Atelectasis

On CT scans, the lower lobes lose volume in a posteromedial direction, pulling down the major fissure in the axial plane. The lateral portion of this fissure demonstrates a greater degree of mobility because the medial portion is fixed to the mediastinum by the hilar structures and the inferior pulmonary ligament. The resultant appearance of the atelectatic lower lobe is a triangular opacity which lies posteromedially in the lower thoracic cavity abutting the spine (Figs. 11.5 and 11.6).

## Combined Atelectasis of the Right Middle and Lower Lobes

Because the bronchus intermedius is the common pathway to the RML and RLL, a single localized lesion involving the bronchus intermedius gives rise to combined atelectasis of these lobes. The bronchial obstruction can be caused by a tumor, a foreign body, a mucous plug, or an inflammatory stricture.

On CT scans, the atelectatic RML and RLL occupy the lower hemithorax and abut the right cardiac border medially and the right hemidiaphragm inferiorly (Fig. 11.7).

## Combined Atelectasis of the Right Upper and Middle Lobes

For combined atelectasis of the RUL and RML to occur, the bronchi of both lobes must be narrowed or occluded by a single or two separate lesions while the bronchus intermedius remains patent, thus allowing the RLL to remain expanded. Combined atelectasis of the RUL and RML can occur with bronchogenic carcinoma, metastatic tumor, carcinoid tumor, mucous plug, and bronchial inflammation. In bronchogenic carcinoma, the primary tumor can obstruct one bronchus and cause the other bronchus to be obstructed by direct extension through the lung parenchyma or peribronchial sheath or by lymphadenopathy [2].

On CT scan, the atelectatic RUL and RML cause a wedge-shaped area of soft tissue attenuation abutting the chest wall anteriorly and the ascending aorta and right cardiac border medially. This wedge-shaped opacification extends inferiorly to the level of the right atrium. The major fissure is displaced anteriorly, and the hyperexpanded lower lobe fills most of the right hemithorax.

## Combined Atelectasis of the Right Upper and Lower Lobes

Combined atelectasis of the RUL and RLL is rare. It may be due to mucous plugs occurring simultaneously in the bronchi of the RUL and RLL. On CT scans, the minor fissure is higher than normal because of the RUL atelectasis, and the major fissure is more posterior than normal because of the RLL atelectasis. The RML is overinflated filling the right hemithorax.

## References


1. Woodring JH, Reed JC. Types and mechanisms of pulmonary atelectasis. J Thorac Imaging. 1996;11:92–108.
2. Lee KS, Logan PM, Primack SL, Muller NL. Combined lobar atelectasis of the right lung: imaging findings. AJR Am J Roentgenol. 1994;163:43–7.
3. Proto AV, Tocino I. Radiographic manifestations of lobar collapse. Semin Roentgenol. 1980;15:117–73.
4. Lansing AM. Radiological Changes in Pulmonary Atelectasis. Arch Surg. 1965;90:52–6.
5. Gamsu G, Singer MM, Vincent HH, Berry S, Nadel JA. Postoperative impairment of mucous transport in the lung. Am Rev Respir Dis. 1976;114:673–9.
6. Raasch BN, Heitzman ER, Carsky EW, Lane EJ, Berlow ME, Witwer G. A computed tomographic study of bronchopulmonary collapse. Radiographics. 1984;4:195–232.
7. Naidich DP, McCauley DI, Khouri NF, Leitman BS, Hulnick DH, Siegelman SS. Computed tomography of lobar collapse: 1. Endobronchial obstruction. J Comput Assist Tomogr. 1983;7:745–57.

# 12 Decreased Opacity with Cystic Airspace

## Cavity

### Definition

A cavity is a gas-filled space, shown as a lucency or low-attenuation area, with identifiable wall (usually >4 mm in thickness) (Fig. 12.1). It can be seen within pulmonary consolidation, a mass, or a nodule. A cavity is usually produced by the expulsion or drainage of a necrotic portion of the lesion via the airways. It may contain a fluid level [1, 2].

### Diseases Causing the Cavity

Cavities are present in a wide variety of infectious and noninfectious processes. Malignancies are the most frequent noninfectious process causing lung cavitary lesion(s) and include primary lung cancer (*squamous cell carcinoma*) (Fig. 12.1), lymphoma, and Kaposi sarcoma particularly in HIV-infected patients, lymphomatoid granulomatosis, and metastasis from an extrathoracic malignancy. Other noninfectious causes are antineutrophil cystoplasmic antibody (ANCA)-associated granulomatous vasculitis (former Wegener's granulomatosis), pulmonary embolism and infarction and necrosis, and *Langerhans cell histiocytosis* (eosinophilic granuloma) (Fig. 12.2). Infectious conditions comprise bacterial infection (necrotizing pneumonia and lung abscess, *septic pulmonary embolism* (Fig. 12.3), and nocardiosis), mycobacterial infection (*Mycobacterium tuberculosis* (Fig. 12.4) and nontuberculous mycobacterial [NTM] pulmonary disease (Fig. 12.5)), fungal infection (aspergillosis (Figs. 12.6 and 12.7), zygomycosis, coccidioidomycosis, and cryptococcosis), and parasitic infection (*paragonimiasis*) [1] (Table 12.1) (Fig. 12.8).

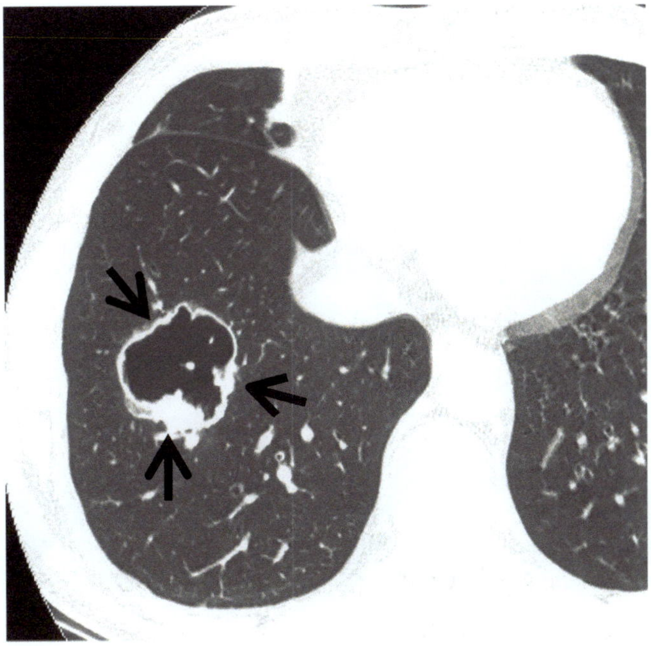

**Fig. 12.1** Squamous cell carcinoma in a 69-year-old smoker man. Lung window image of thin-section (1.5-mm section thickness) CT scan obtained at level of suprahepatic inferior vena cava shows a cavitary lesion (*arrows*) having irregular and variable wall thickness in right lower lobe

### Distribution

In Langerhans cell histiocytosis, the cavitating nodules are associated with noncavitating nodules and are distributed mainly in the upper and middle lung zones, sparing the lower lung zones. The presence of a single or multiple large cavitary lesions in the upper lobes suggests the diagnosis of mycobacterial disease [3]. In NTM disease, cavitation is common in the upper lobes and frequently associated with apical pleural thickening and pulmonary emphysema (upper lobe fibrocavitary form) [4]. In pleuropulmonary paragonimiasis, necrotic or cavitary nodules or masses are usually located in the subpleural or subfissural areas [5].

### Clinical Considerations

Cigarette smoking is highly related to pulmonary Langerhans cell histiocytosis, and the cavitating nodules in the disease

K.S. Lee et al., *Radiology Illustrated: Chest Radiology*, Radiology Illustrated,
DOI 10.1007/978-3-642-37096-0_12, © Springer-Verlag Berlin Heidelberg 2014

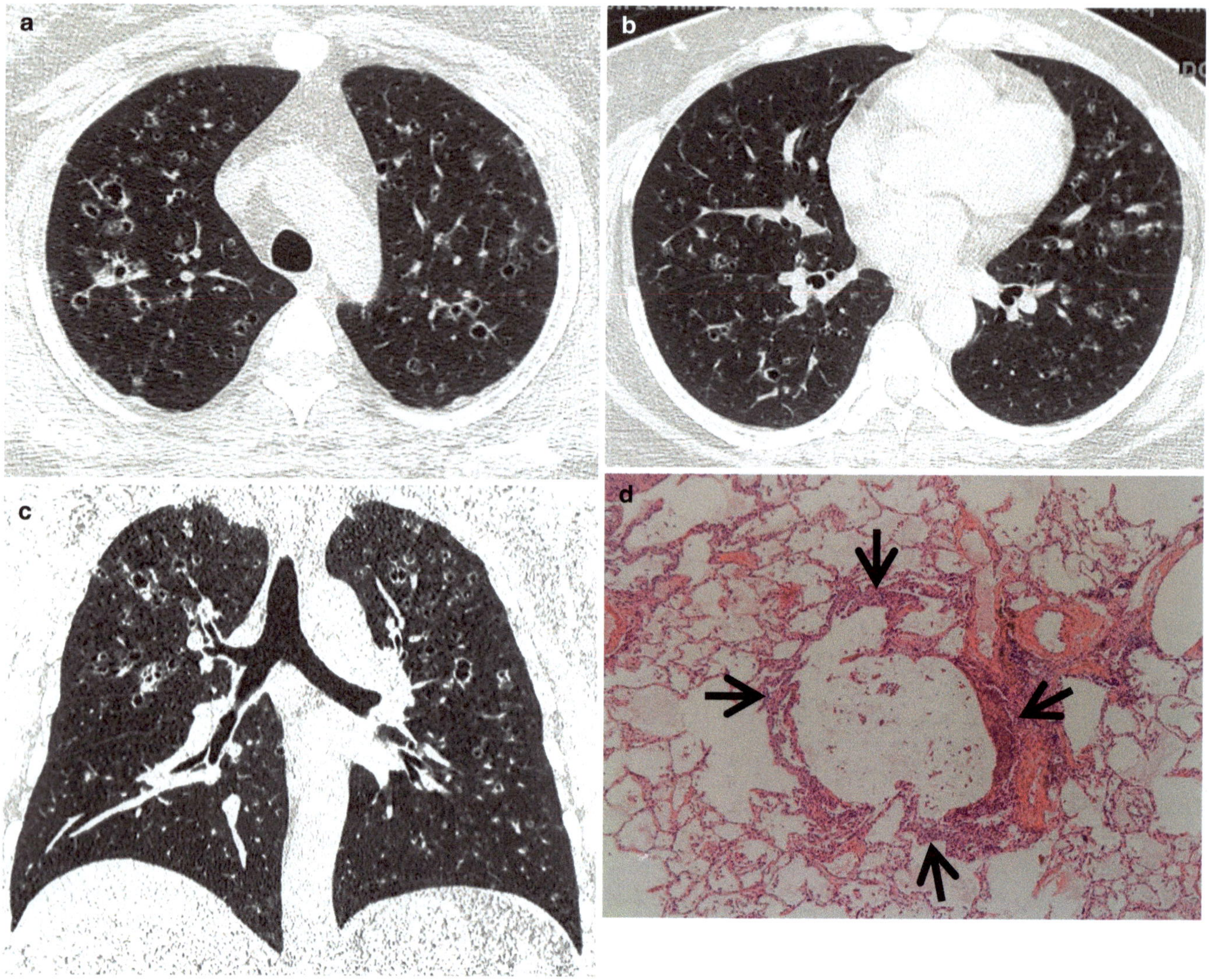


**Fig. 12.2** Pulmonary Langerhans cell histiocytosis in a 47-year-old smoker woman (20-pack-year smoking history). (**a**, **b**) Lung window images of thin-section (1.5-mm section thickness) CT scans obtained at levels of aortic arch (**a**) and inferior pulmonary veins (**b**), respectively, show cavitating and noncavitating nodules in both lungs. Also note variable wall thickness of cavitating nodular lesions. (**c**) Coronal reformatted image (2.0-mm section thickness) demonstrates nodular lesions with upper and middle lung zone predominance. (**d**) High-magnification (×100) photomicrograph of surgical biopsy specimen obtained from left upper lobe discloses a cystic lesion (*arrows*) having relatively thick wall which is composed of numerous Langerhans cells and other inflammatory cells. Also note mild inflammatory cell infiltration in pericystic interstitium (alveolar walls)

are reversible with corticosteroid or cytotoxic drug therapy [6]. In tuberculous infection, imaging findings have implications as for host immune status (e.g., lymph node enlargement and lower lung zone parenchymal opacity in HIV-infected patients) of patients, but whether a patient's disease is due to recently transmitted (epidemiologically primary infection) or remotely acquired infection (reactivation tuberculosis) cannot be determined from the radiographic findings [7]. The most common risk factor for pulmonary nocardiosis is underlying lung disease such as asthma, bronchiectasis, or chronic obstructive pulmonary disease. People with systemic immunodeficiency associated with cancer chemotherapy, HIV infection, organ transplantation, or long-term corticosteroid use are also at increased risk for pulmonary *Nocardia* infection [1]. Cryptococcal infections are mostly common in immunocompromised patients such as those with AIDS, who underwent organ transplantation, or who have a hematologic malignancy. These infections are relatively rare in immunocompetent patients [8]. Paragonimiasis infection occurs when humans eat infected crabs or crayfish containing metacercaria of *Paragonimus*.

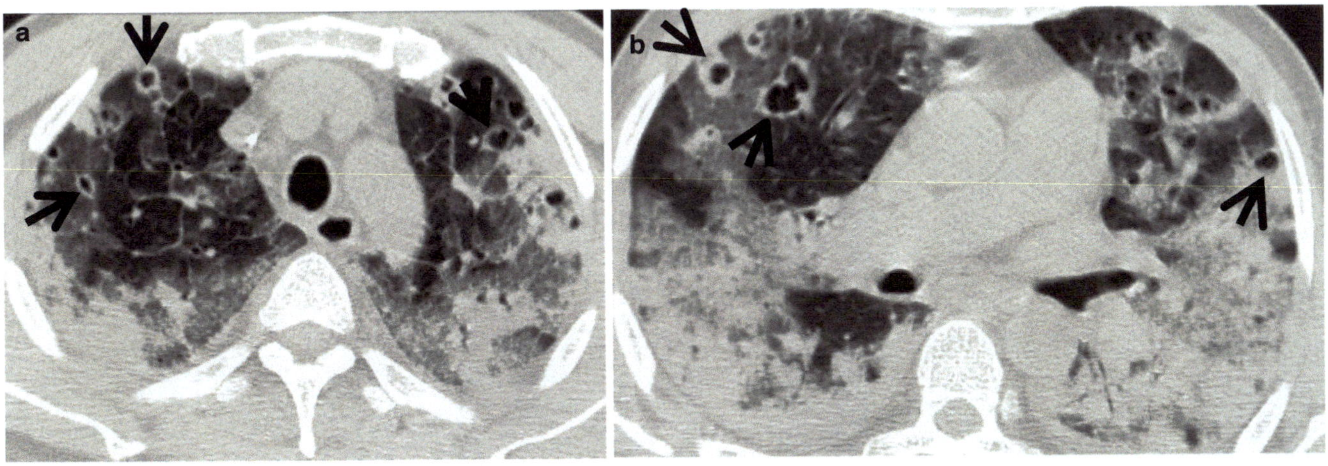


**Fig. 12.3** Septic lung in a 58-year-old man with methicillin-sensitive *Staphylococcus aureus* who has a history of electric burn on his left thigh. (**a**, **b**) Lung window images of CT (2.5-mm section thickness) scans obtained at levels of aortic arch (**a**) and right bronchus intermedius (**b**), respectively, show bilateral extensive areas of ground-glass opacity and consolidation. Also note variable-sized cavitary lesions (*arrows*) in both lungs. Pleural effusions are also seen, bilaterally

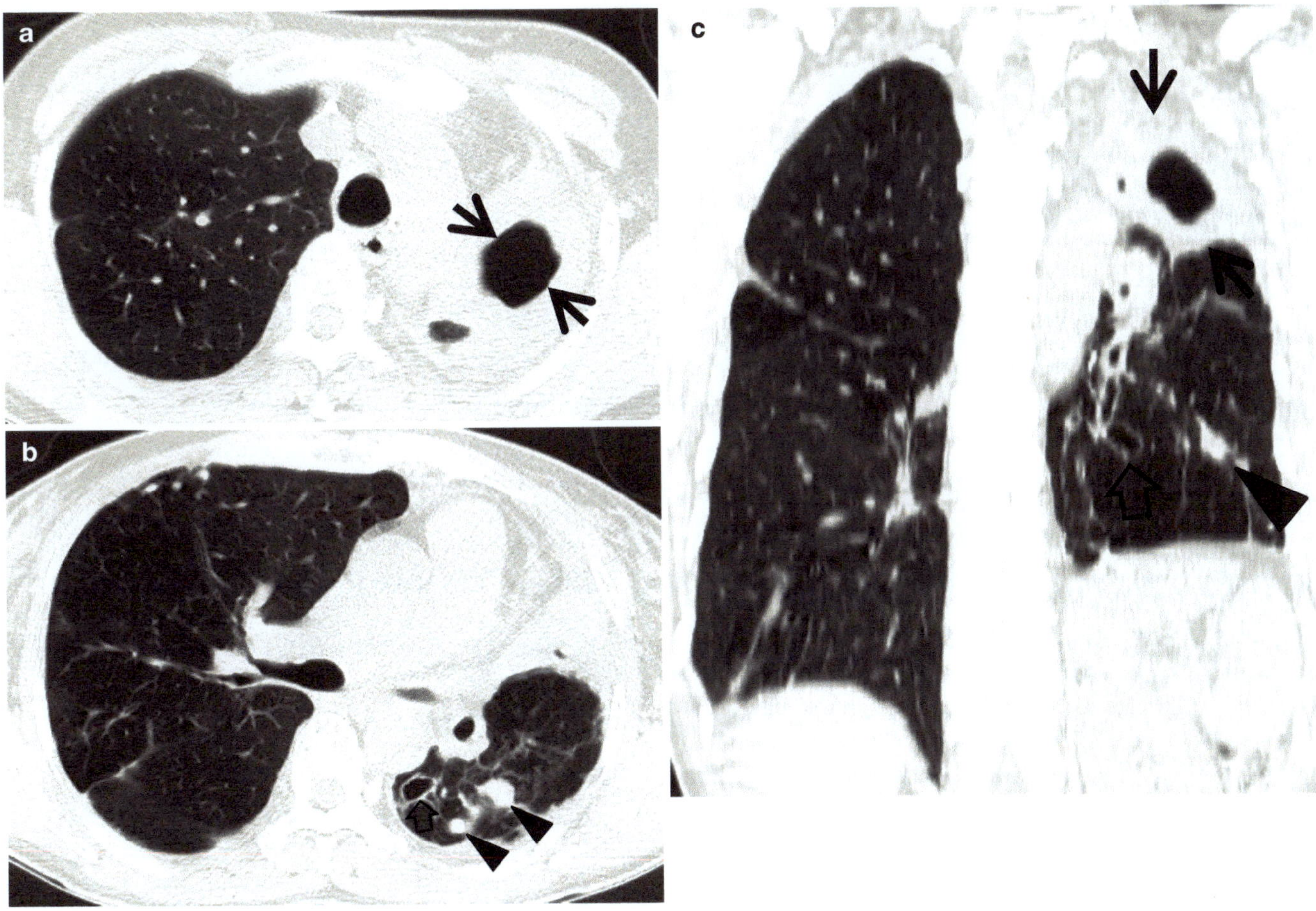


**Fig. 12.4** Multidrug-resistant pulmonary tuberculosis in a 49-year-old woman. (**a**, **b**) Lung window images of CT (2.5-mm section thickness) scans obtained at levels of aortic arch (**a**) and right upper lobar bronchus (**b**), respectively, show a large thick-walled cavitary lesion (*arrows* in **a**) in volume decreased left upper lobe and another smaller cavity (*open arrow*) and nodular lesions (*arrowheads*) in left lower lobe. Also note left pleural effusion and subcentimeter nodules in right upper lobe. (**c**) Coronal reformatted (2.0-mm section thickness) CT image demonstrates left upper lobe cavity (*arrows*) and thin-walled cavity (*open arrow*) and nodular lesion (*arrowhead*) in left lower lobe. Please note left pleural effusion. (**d**) Gross pathologic specimen obtained with left pneumonectomy displays a large cavity (*arrows*) in the left upper lobe, thin-walled cavity (*open arrow*) in the left lower lobe, multiple nodules containing caseation necrosis (*arrowheads*), and marked bronchial thickening due to inflammatory and fibrotic changes. (**e**) High-magnification (×100) photomicrograph of pathologic specimen discloses a necrotizing granuloma having palisading epithelioid histiocytes and eosinophilic materials (*arrows*) on its periphery and central caseating necrotic materials (*C*). *Inset*: small necrotizing granuloma

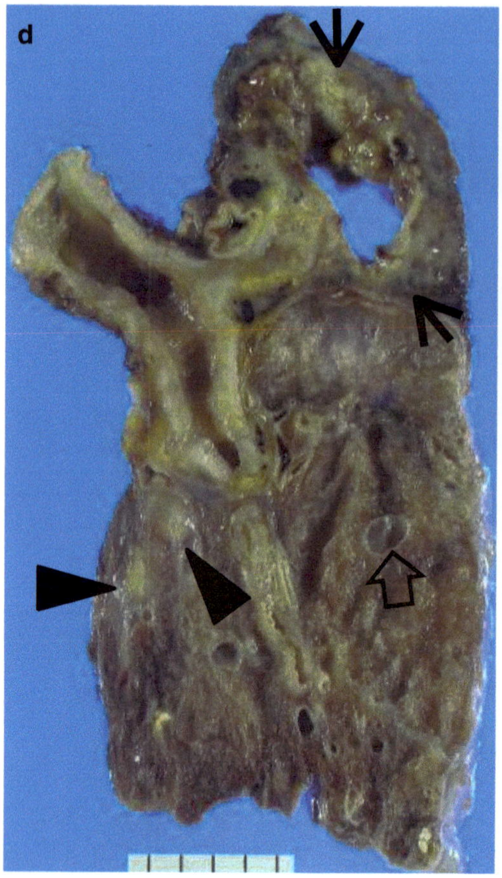


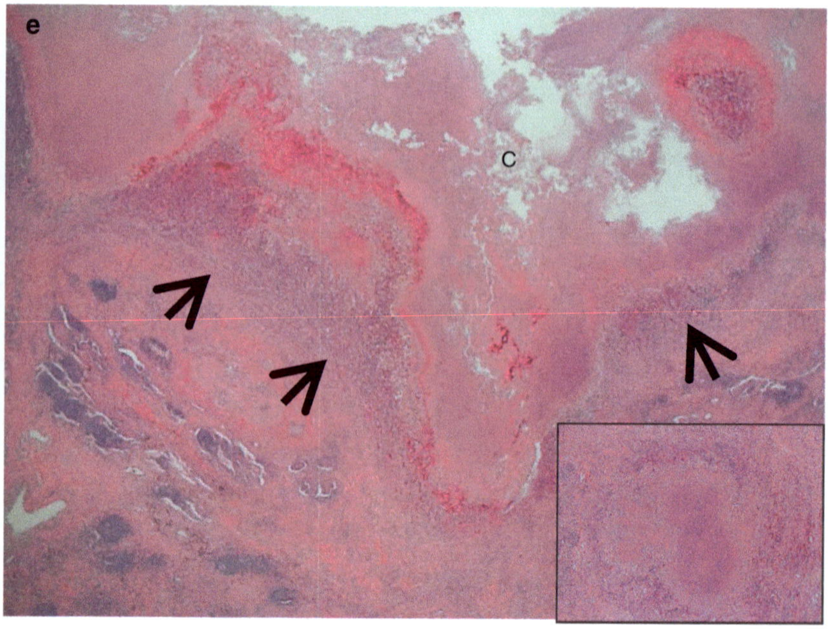


Fig. 12.4 (continued)

**Key Points for Differential Diagnosis**

1. In cavitary squamous cell carcinoma, the borders of tumor are often irregular or lobulated. The cavities are usually thick walled and have a nodular inner surface. Discordance between the inner and outer walls of a cavitary lesion (e.g., smooth inner walls and uneven outer walls or uneven outer and inner walls and discordant uneven sectors) is more common in peripheral lung cancer cavity, and concordance between the walls (e.g., smooth inner and outer walls or uneven outer and inner walls and concordant uneven sectors) is more common in single pulmonary tuberculous cavity. Thus, analyzing the characteristics of cavitary internal and external walls on CT is valuable in differentiating between peripheral lung cancer cavity and single pulmonary tuberculous thick-walled cavity [9].
2. In pulmonary tuberculosis, satellite centrilobular nodules or tree-in-bud patterns suggesting bronchogenic spread usually seen around the cavities. The presence of multiple cavities and young patient age (20s or 30s) suggest multidrug-resistant (MDR) tuberculosis [10].
3. The presence of a cavity on CT of the lung may help exclude the diagnosis of viral infection in immunocompromised patients and lung infection [11].
4. The air-crescent sign in invasive pulmonary aspergillosis, defined as crescents of air surrounding nodular lesions, is observed in up to 63 % of patients. The sign, occurring in about half of the patients with recovery from neutropenia, is caused by tissue ischemia and subsequent necrosis due to fungal angioinvasion [12]. Whether a mural nodule within a cavitary lesion is contrast-enhanced or not is one of the most important features in making a

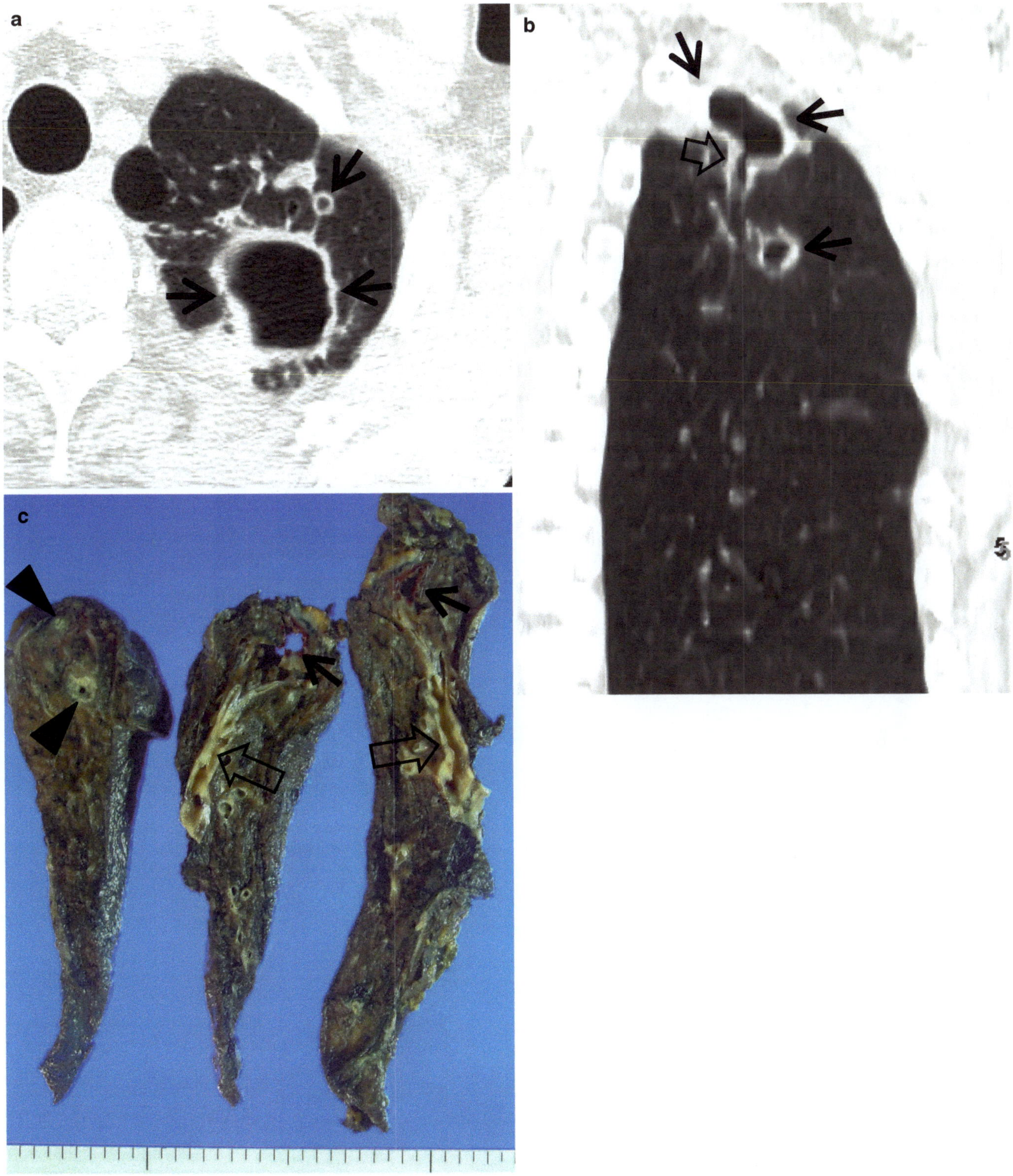


Fig. 12.5 Nontuberculous mycobacterial pulmonary disease of upper lobe fibrocavitary form (*M. intracellulare*) in a 64-year-old man. (**a**) Lung window image of CT scan (2.5-mm section thickness) obtained at level of great vessels shows relatively even cavity wall thickness (*arrows*) in left apical area. Also note variable-sized nodules. (**b**) Coronal reformatted image (2.0-mm section thickness) demonstrates two cavitary lesions (*arrows*) in left upper lobe. Also note wall thickening (*open arrow*) of bronchus draining larger cavity. (**c**) Gross pathologic specimen obtained with left upper lobectomy discloses several thin-walled cavities (*arrows*), variable-sized granulomas (*arrowheads*), and bronchiectasis (*open arrows*)

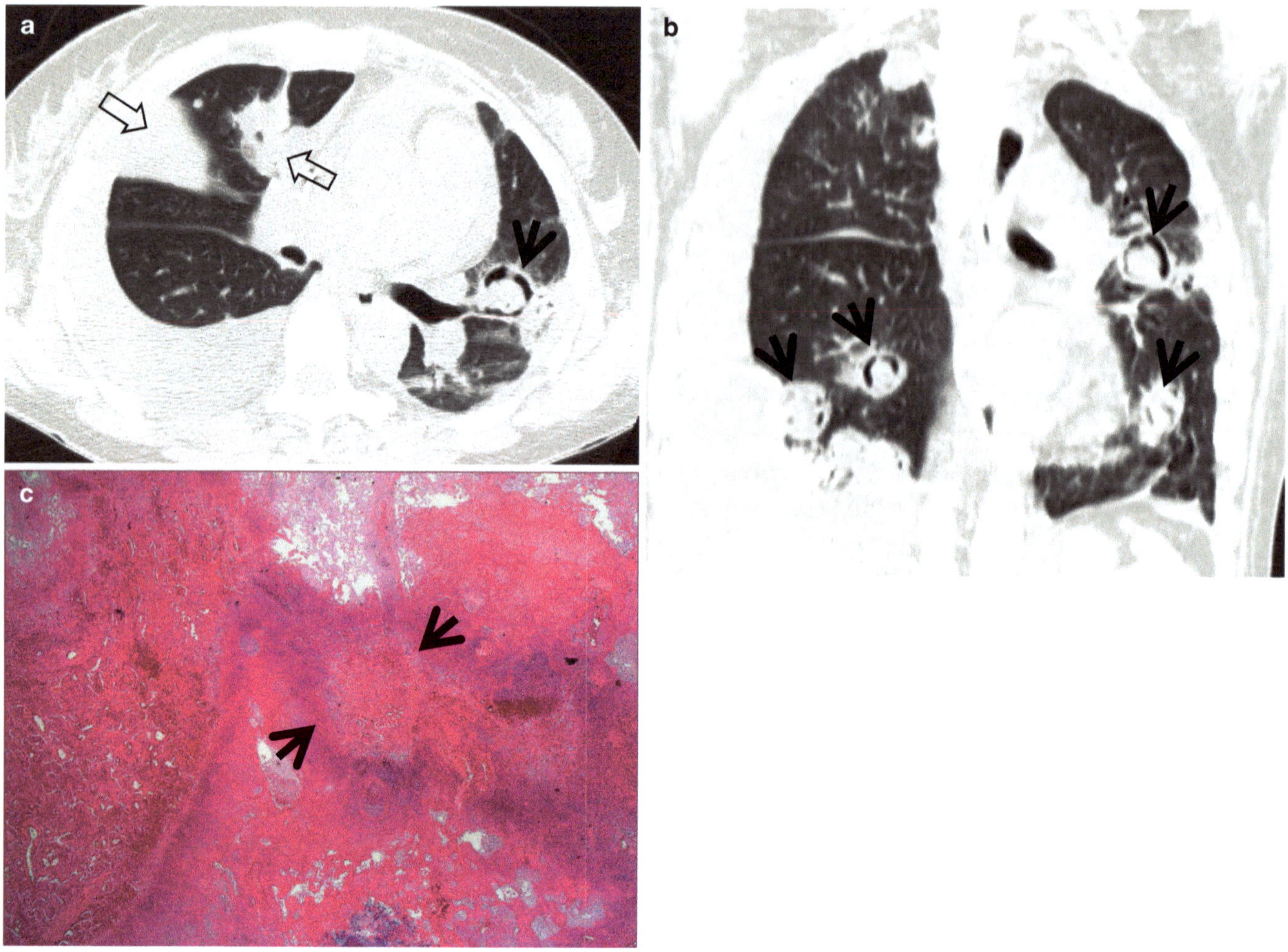


**Fig. 12.6** Invasive pulmonary aspergillosis in a 27-year-old woman with acute myeloid leukemia. (**a**) Lung window image of CT scan (2.5-mm section thickness) obtained at level of right bronchus intermedius shows a cavitating nodule (crescent sign) (*arrow*) in lingular division of left upper lobe and cavitating and noncavitating areas (*open arrows*) of consolidation in right upper lobe. Also note bilateral pleural effusions. (**b**) Coronal reformatted image (2.0-mm section thickness) demonstrates multiple cavitating nodules (*arrows*) showing crescent sign. (**c**) High-magnification (×100) photomicrograph of surgical biopsy specimen disclosed fungal organisms (*arrows*) within cavitated infarction area

differential diagnosis between an intracavitary aspergilloma and a cavitary lung cancer [13].

5. The presence of a "feeding vessel" sign, in which a distinct vessel is seen leading to the center of a pulmonary nodule, may suggest the diagnosis of septic embolism, but the sign is nonspecific (may be seen in pulmonary metastatic nodules) [14].
6. According to one CT report [8], cavitation within lung lesions in pulmonary cryptococcosis was noted in only four (17 %) of 23 patients. The lung lesions of cryptococcosis in non-AIDS patients show an indolent course, slowly progressive even without adequate treatment and does not show a rapid resolution even with antifungal treatment [8].
7. Subpleural or subfissural necrotic nodule with adjacent pleural thickening and subpleural linear opacities (worm migration track) leading to a necrotic nodule can be an important clue in the diagnosis of pleuropulmonary paragonimiasis on CT [5].

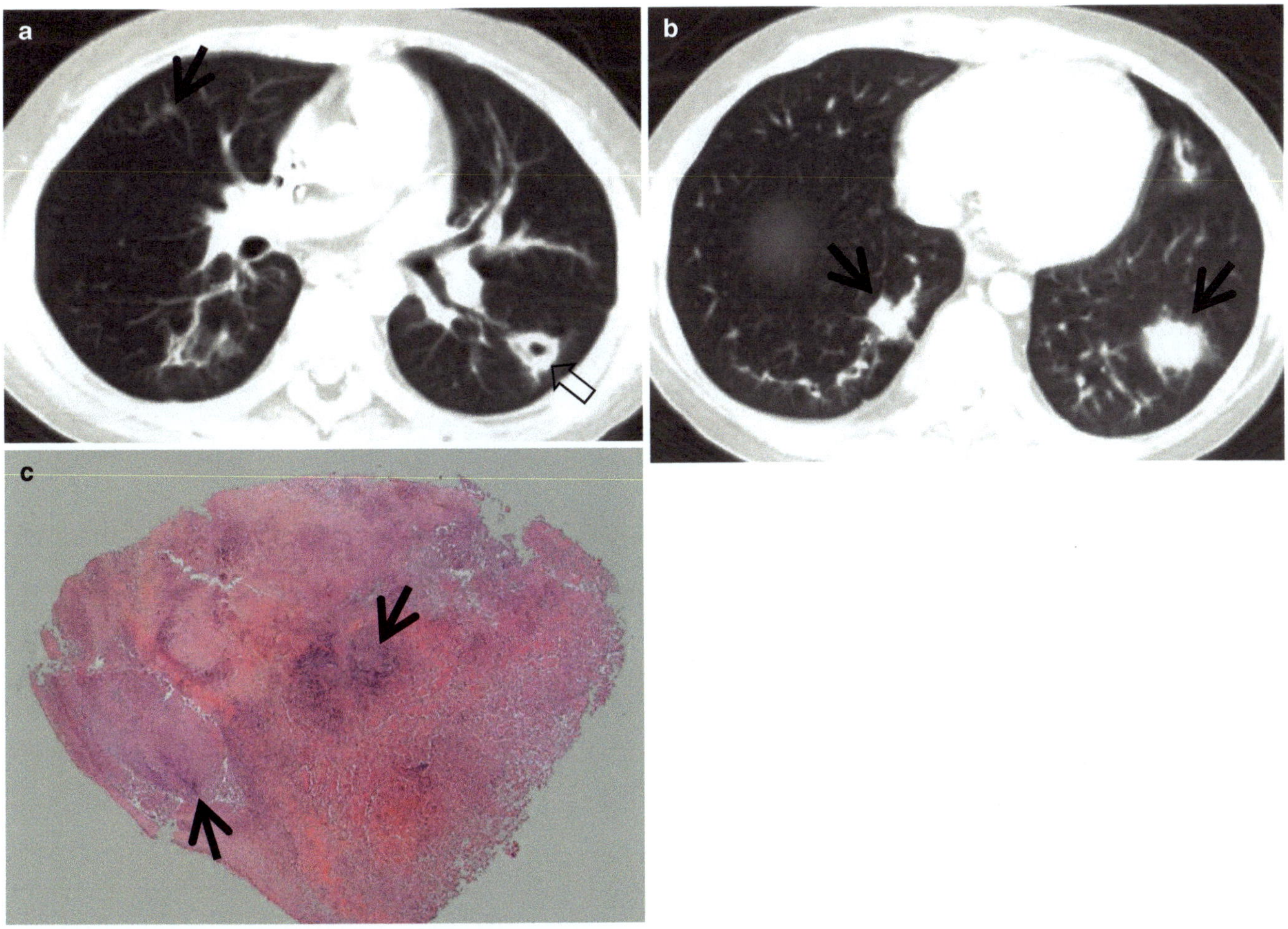

**Fig. 12.7** Invasive pulmonary aspergillosis in an 11-year-old boy with acute lymphoblastic leukemia. (**a**, **b**) Lung window images of CT (5.0-mm section thickness) scans obtained at levels of right bronchus intermedius (**a**) and liver dome (**b**), respectively, show multiple nodules (*arrows*) showing halo sign. Also note a cavitating nodule (*open arrow*) in superior segment of left lower lobe. (**c**) High-magnification (×100) photomicrograph of surgical lung biopsy specimen discloses necrotizing fungal pneumonia with abscess formation. Please note blue fungal hyphae (*arrows*) in necrotic spaces

**Table 12.1** Common diseases manifesting as cavity

| Disease | Key points for differential diagnosis |
|---|---|
| Primary lung cancer (squamous cell carcinoma) | Thick-walled cavity with a nodular inner surface |
| ANCA-associated granulomatous vasculitis | Multiple, bilateral, subpleural nodules, or masses |
| Lymphomatoid granulomatosis | Pulmonary nodules and masses with central low attenuation and peripheral rim enhancement, and ground-glass opacity halo |
| Pulmonary infarction | Peripheral wedge-shaped consolidation with central lucencies |
| Langerhans cell histiocytosis | Cavitating and noncavitating nodules in upper and middle lung zones |
| Lung abscess | |
| Septic pulmonary embolism | Multiple, peripheral nodules with a feeding vessel sign |
| Mycobacterial infection | Single or multiple large cavitary lesion in the upper lobes, satellite centrilobular nodules |
| Fungal infection | Cavity with an air-crescent sign |
| Parasitic infection (PW) | Cavitary nodules or masses in the subpleural or subfissural areas |

*Note*: *ANCA* antineutrophil cytoplasmic antibody, *PW Paragonimus westermani*

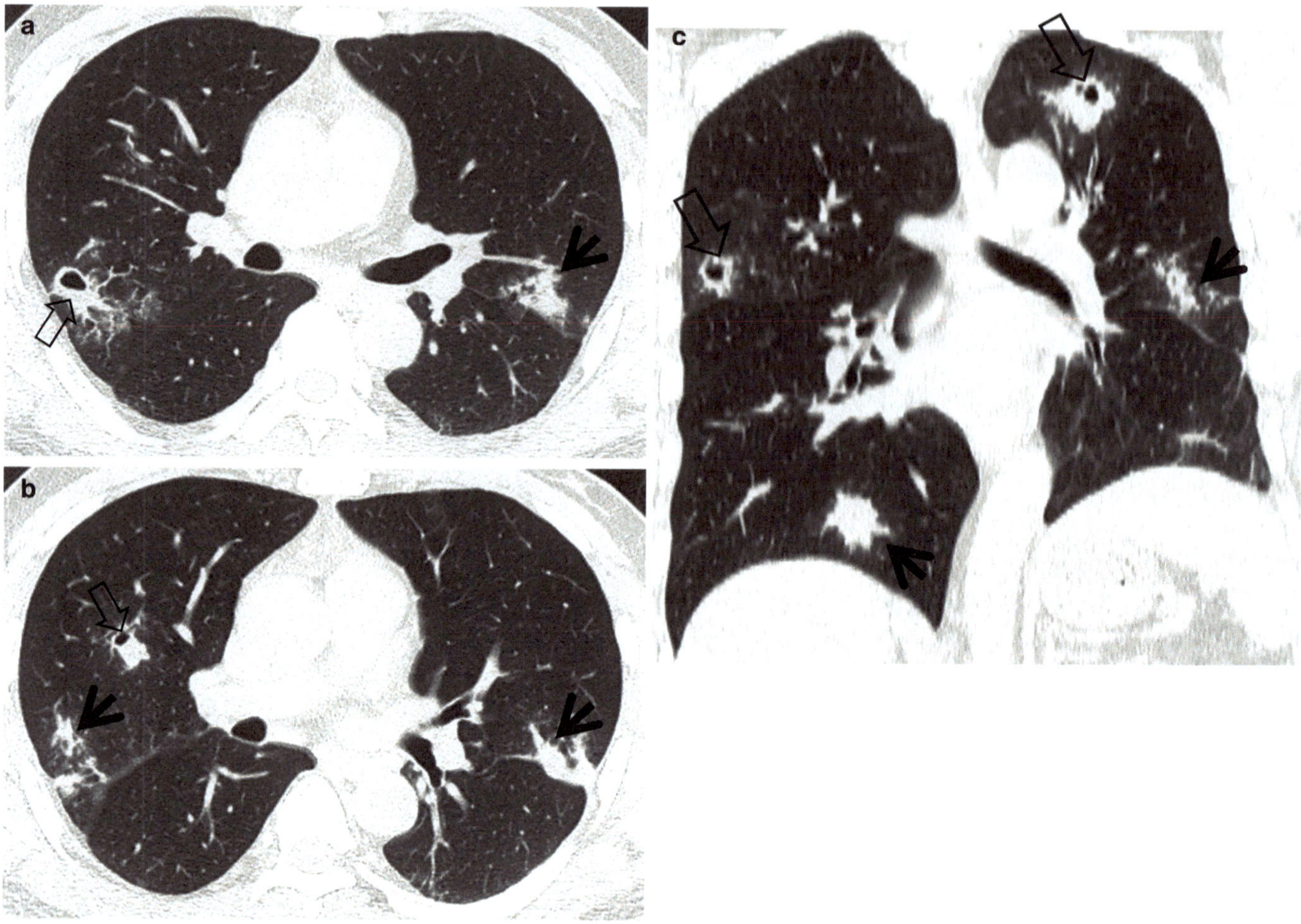


**Fig. 12.8** Pulmonary *Paragonimus westermani* (PW) infestation in a 46-year-old man proved by sputum smear showing parasitic eggs and positive ELISA test for PW. (**a**, **b**) Lung window images of consecutive CT (2.5-mm section thickness) scans obtained at levels of right bronchus intermedius show multiple nodules with (*open arrows*) or without (*arrows*) internal cavity. (**c**) Coronal reformatted image (2.0-mm section thickness) demonstrates multiple cavitating (*open arrows*) and noncavitating (*arrows*) nodules in both lungs

## Lung Squamous Cell Carcinoma as a Cavitary Lesion

### Pathology and Pathogenesis

Squamous cell carcinoma (SCC) is a malignant epithelial tumor showing keratinization or intercellular bridges that arise from bronchial epithelium. Two-thirds of SCCs are centrally located, arising from proximal bronchi, and one-third of cases are peripherally located (Fig. 12.1). Tumors are firm gray-white masses with areas of necrosis and cavitation, and central lesions often have endobronchial growth, which may occlude the lumen of airways and cause obstructive changes. Tumor cells are polygonal and hyperchromatic and have irregular nuclei and prominent nucleoli; the amount of cytoplasm is variable from abundant to scanty. There are several histologic variants as follows: papillary variant, clear-cell variant, small-cell variant, basaloid variant, and alveolar space-filling type of peripheral SCC [15].

### Symptoms and Signs

Hemoptysis is an important feature of SCC of the lung that can be related both to central airway location of the tumor and to an increased propensity to cavitation [16]. Shortness of breath and fever occur due to atelectasis and postobstructive pneumonia. In general, it tends to be locally aggressive with less frequent metastasis to distant organ than adenocarcinoma of the lung. Chest wall invasion causes chest pain. Hypercalcemia may be present as a paraneoplastic syndrome secondary to secretion of parathyroid hormone-related protein.

### CT Findings

The most common radiologic abnormality of SCC is a large central mass and atelectasis secondary to the airway obstruction [17]. One-third of SCCs present as intraparenchymal nodules or masses that lack apparent connection to a bronchus (Fig. 12.1). There has been a more recent shift, however, to a greater percentage of tumors occurring in the periphery of the lung with 53 % in one study [18]. The borders of the nodule are often irregular or lobulated. Approximately 10 % of SCCs show cavitation. The cavities are usually thick walled and have a nodular inner surface. Discordance between the inner and outer walls of a cavitary lesion (e.g., smooth inner walls and uneven outer walls or uneven outer and inner walls and discordant uneven sectors) is more common in peripheral lung cancer cavity and concordance between the walls (e.g., smooth inner and outer walls or uneven outer and inner walls and concordant uneven sectors) is more common in single pulmonary tuberculous cavity. Thus, the characterization of a cavitary lesion according to its cavitary internal and external walls on CT is valuable in differentiating between peripheral lung cancer cavity and single pulmonary tuberculous thick-walled cavity [9].

### CT-Pathology Comparisons

In SCC, necrosis of the central portion of the tumor is common, especially in larger ones. Possibly because of their intimate association with proximal airways, the necrotic material can drain relatively easily and cavity formation is common. Occasionally, a cavity results from infection and abscess formation in an area of obstructive pneumonitis. Nodular inner surface of cavity is probably related to local differences in necrosis and growth rate within the tumor.

### Patient Prognosis

Surgical resection is a potentially curative treatment of the early stage of SCC of the lung, with a 5-year survival rate up to 70 %. Combined modality therapy with surgery, radiotherapy, and chemotherapy can improve the survival in the patients with stages II and III. Clinical trials with novel targeted agents for advanced stage lung cancer are ongoing. Prognosis is poor (5-year survival 1 %) in the stage IV group.

## Langerhans Cell Histiocytosis

### Pathology and Pathogenesis

Langerhans cell histiocytosis (LCH) is a rare interstitial lung disease caused by proliferation of Langerhans cells. It can either be limited to the lung (pulmonary LCH) or be part of a systemic LCH. Langerhans cells are characterized by large, folded nuclei, vesicular chromatin, and abundantly pale to eosinophilic cytoplasm. LCH can be divided into two phases: early cellular (proliferative) and late fibrotic phases. Early cellular phase is characterized by nodular proliferation of Langerhans cells centered on small airways, such as terminal bronchioles, and cystic dilatation of involved airways and eosinophils is commonly seen (Fig. 12.2). In late fibrotic phase, Langerhans cells are diminished and replaced by fibrous tissue [6].

### Symptoms and Signs

Clinical presentation of pulmonary LCH is variable [19]. Despite diffuse lung involvement, symptoms can be minor or absent. Initially patients often attribute their symptoms to smoking. Dry cough and dyspnea on exertion are present in approximately two-thirds of the patients. Spontaneous pneumothorax responsible for chest pain occurs in up to 20 %. Bone lesions (<20 %), diabetes insipidus with polyuria and polydipsia (5 %), and skin lesions are the most common extrapulmonary manifestations.

### CT Findings

The incidence of these findings depends on the stage of disease. The most common thin-section CT findings of early LCH are multiple poorly defined small nodules with a centrilobular distribution [20, 21] (Fig. 12.2). Nodules measure 1–5 mm in diameter, although larger nodules are seen in approximately 30 % of cases. Their margins may be smooth or irregular. Larger nodules may show lucent centers. As the disease progresses, the nodules tend to cavitate, and a combination of cysts and nodules is characteristic (Fig. 12.2). Cysts are often seen in association with nodules but may be the only HRCT finding. They range from a few millimeters to several centimeters in diameter and may be round or irregular in shape. Regardless of the stage, the abnormalities are most severe in the upper and mid-lung zones; the lung bases are relatively spared (Fig. 12.2). Less common findings include reticular pattern, interlobular septal thickening, large bullae, and ground-glass opacity. The radiologic abnormalities may regress, resolve completely, become stable, or progress to advanced cystic changes. According to a study, more than half of patients show improvement on follow-up CT scans because even thin-walled cysts harbor active inflammatory cells in their walls and show improvement with treatment [6]. Spontaneous pneumothorax is seen in approximately 10 % of patients.

### CT-Pathology Comparisons

LCH is histopathologically characterized by peribronchiolar proliferation and infiltration of Langerhans cells that form stellate nodules. With progression, cellular nodules are transformed into cavitary nodules or thin-walled cysts (Fig. 12.2). In advanced stages, fibrotic scars are surrounded by enlarged and distorted air spaces. Centrilobular nodules seen on HRCT correspond histopathologically to the area of peribronchiolar granulomas composed of Langerhans cell, eosinophils, lymphocytes, and macrophages [6]. Lucent centers seen in large nodules correspond to a dilated bronchiole surrounded by thickened peribronchiolar interstitium. Thick- and thin-walled cystic lesions seen on CT consist of a central cavity surrounded by a thick and thin wall composed of Langerhans cell sheets and eosinophils. In thin-walled cysts, inflammatory cell infiltrations along the alveolar walls as well as pericystic emphysema are seen. Bizarre cysts seen on CT have irregular and wavy wall on pathology, and the walls of cystic lesions are composed of numerous Langerhans and other inflammatory cells or fibrotic changes. Several cysts coalesce with surrounding cysts via the destruction of their walls.

### Patient Prognosis

The natural history of the disease is widely variable and unpredictable [19]. Approximately 50 % of patients experience a favorable outcome, with after the cessation of smoking or with glucocorticoid therapy. Approximately 10–20 % of patients have early severe manifestations, consisting of recurrent pneumothorax or progressive respiratory failure. Finally, 30–40 % of patients show persistent symptoms of variable severity that remain stable over time.

## Septic Pulmonary Embolism

### Pathology and Pathogenesis

Septic pulmonary embolism causes lung abscess and septic infarction. Localized suppurative necrosis of lung tissue and cavitation containing necrotic fluid or debris are observed.

### Symptoms and Signs

Septic pulmonary embolism is an uncommon disorder presenting with fever; respiratory symptoms such as cough, sputum, hemoptysis, chest pain, and dyspnea; and lung infiltrates in the presence of an extrapulmonary source of infection [22]. Since infected thrombus can cause lung abscess, septic infarction, empyema, bronchopleural fistula, shock, and death; respiratory symptoms are variable and often nonspecific. Historically, septic pulmonary embolism has been associated with intravenous drug use, pelvic thrombophlebitis, and suppurative processes in the head and neck. However, increasing use of indwelling catheters and devices as well as increasing numbers of immunocompromised patients has changed the epidemiology and clinical manifestations of septic pulmonary embolism.

### CT Findings

Septic pulmonary embolism is characterized by the presence of multiple nodules that usually measure 1–3 cm in diameter and that frequently cavitate [23] (Fig. 12.3). The nodules often have ill-defined margins and have a feeding vessel sign [14]. The subpleural wedge-shaped areas of consolidation often with central areas of necrosis or cavitation are also seen. According to a study, cavitation within the nodules is more common in pulmonary septic embolism caused by gram-positive microorganisms, whereas ill-defined margins are more common in pulmonary septic embolism caused by gram-negative microorganisms [24].

### CT-Pathology Comparisons

Nodules seen on CT correspond to areas of infarction and hemorrhage caused by ischemia and neutrophilic exudates and necrosis of lung parenchyma caused by toxins from organisms. The subpleural wedge-shaped areas of consolidation correspond to areas of hemorrhage or infarction caused by occlusion of pulmonary arteries by septic emboli.

### Patient Prognosis

Early diagnosis is the most important to improve the prognosis. With appropriate antimicrobial therapy and control of the infectious source, resolution of the illness and avoidance of potential complications can be expected.

## Cavitary Pulmonary Tuberculosis

### Pathology and Pathogenesis

Pulmonary tuberculosis (TB) is usually seen as a necrotizing consolidative process predominantly in lung apices. Pulmonary TB may be seen as a Ghon lesion (1–2 cm, round, white-gray pulmonary nodule with central necrosis), a Ghon complex (Ghon lesion plus hilar lymphadenopathy), or a Ranke complex (fibrosis and calcification of the Ghon complex via cell-mediated immunity). Histologically, both necrotizing (caseating) and nonnecrotizing granulomas can be seen in lung parenchyma or lymph nodes. Organisms (4-μm beaded rods) can be demonstrated using acid-fast stains (Ziehl–Neelsen), although a negative acid-fast stain does not rule out tuberculosis. Langerhans-type multinucleated giant cells are frequently seen [25] (Fig. 12.4).

### Symptoms and Signs

Cough is the most common symptom of pulmonary TB. Cavitary pulmonary TB is often accompanied by hemoptysis. Constitutional symptoms, including fever, malaise, fatigue, weight loss, night seating, and anorexia, are often present [26].

## CT Findings

The CT findings of active cavitary pulmonary TB include cavities, centrilobular small nodules, and branching linear structures, giving a tree-in-bud appearance, lobular consolidation, and bronchial wall thickening [25, 27]. Cavitation in single or multiple sites is evident in 40–45 % of active pulmonary TB [28] (Fig. 12.4). Walls of cavities may range from thin and smooth to thick and nodular; air–fluid levels have been reported to occur in 9–21 % of tuberculous cavities. Bronchogenic spread of disease occurs when an area of caseous necrosis liquefies and communicates with the bronchial tree. Bronchogenic spread manifests as centrilobular small nodules and tree-in-bud patterns around or distant site from the cavities.

## CT-Pathology Comparisons

The CT findings of active cavitary pulmonary TB include cavities, centrilobular small nodules and branching linear structures, lobular consolidation, and bronchial wall thickening [25, 27]. Cavitation is centrilobular in location, and several centrilobular cavities progressively coalesce into a larger cavity (Fig. 12.4). The wall of the cavity consists of caseous materials, epithelioid cells with multinucleated giant cells, granulation tissue, and a fibrous capsule. Histopathologic analysis indicates that centrilobular small nodules occur as a result of impaction of caseous material within or around the terminal or respiratory bronchioles and sometimes within the alveolar ducts. The airways show a yellowish thickening of the wall with caseation necrosis. Centrilobular nodules grow and coalesce into lobular consolidation, consisting of centrally located granulomas that contain caseation necrosis and marginal nonspecific inflammation.

## Patient Prognosis

Cure rate for drug-sensitive TB is more than 95 % with the current standard four-drug treatment regimen of first-line drugs (isoniazid, rifampicin, pyrazinamide, and ethambutol) for 6 months [26]. Prolonged medication for at least 20 months with second-line drugs is necessary for multidrug-resistant TB. Extensively drug-resistant TB is extremely difficult to treat. When the disease of drug-resistant cavitary TB is localized, surgical resection of the lung lesion can be done with medical therapy.

# Paragonimiasis

## Pathology and Pathogenesis

Paragonimiasis is infection by trematodes of the genus *Paragonimus*, with most infections of humans with flukes of this genus attributed to *P. westermani*. It is an important human disease in Far East Asia and parts of Latin America and Africa. The use of raw or incompletely cooked crabs or crayfish and their juices for food or medicine is the most important method of transmission. The worm evokes a cystic necrotizing granulomatous and fibrotic response with tissue eosinophilia. The ova of *Paragonimus* are approximately 80 µm in size and show a flattened operculum [5].

## Symptoms and Signs

Initially, pulmonary paragonimiasis manifests as chronic cough and hemoptysis. Chest pain and dyspnea can occur when pneumothorax or hydropneumothorax develops. Subcutaneous nodules can be found in the advanced case.

## CT Findings

Typical CT findings of pleuropulmonary paragonimiasis are a poorly marginated subpleural or subfissural nodule that frequently contains a low-opacity necrotic area or cavity (Fig. 12.8), focal pleural thickening, and subpleural linear attenuation lesions leading to a necrotic peripheral nodule, thin-walled cyst, pneumothorax, or hydropneumothorax [5, 29]. These imaging findings correlate well with the stage of the disease [29]. Early findings are caused by the migration of juvenile worms and include pneumothorax or hydropneumothorax, airspace consolidation, and linear opacities. Later findings resulting from worm cysts include subpleural nodules or masses, thin-walled cysts, and bronchiectasis.

## CT-Pathology Comparisons

In a study of the correlation between CT and histologic findings in pleuropulmonary paragonimiasis, the subpleural nodule is a necrotic granuloma containing multiple eggs and organizing pneumonia with granulation tissue. Adjacent pleural thickening is composed of fibrotic thickening with some areas of lymphocytic infiltration [5].

## Patient Prognosis

Praziquantel (75 mg/kg/day for 3 days) is the drug of choice for pulmonary paragonimiasis. With this regimen, relapse occurred in about 2 % of the cases [30].

# Cyst

## Definition

A cyst is a round parenchymal lucency or low-attenuating area with a well-defined interface with normal lung. Cysts have variable wall thickness but are usually thin-walled (<2 mm) (Fig. 12.9). The cysts usually contain air but occasionally contain fluid or solid material [2]. Cysts may be located in the subpleural region or within the lung.

A bleb is a small gas-containing space within the visceral pleural or in the subpleural lung, not larger than 10 mm in diameter. It appears as a thin-walled cystic air space contiguous to the pleura (Fig. 12.10). A bulla is an airspace measuring more than 10 mm in diameter, sharply demarcated by a thin wall that is no greater than 1 mm in thickness (Fig. 12.11). Bullae can be seen in a subpleural location or within the lung parenchyma. A bulla is usually accompanied by emphysematous changes in the adjacent lung.

Pneumatocele is a thin-walled, gas-filled space in the lung. It appears as a round, thin-walled airspace. Once believed to be a combination of parenchymal necrosis and check-valve airway obstruction, the mechanism of pneumatocele formation

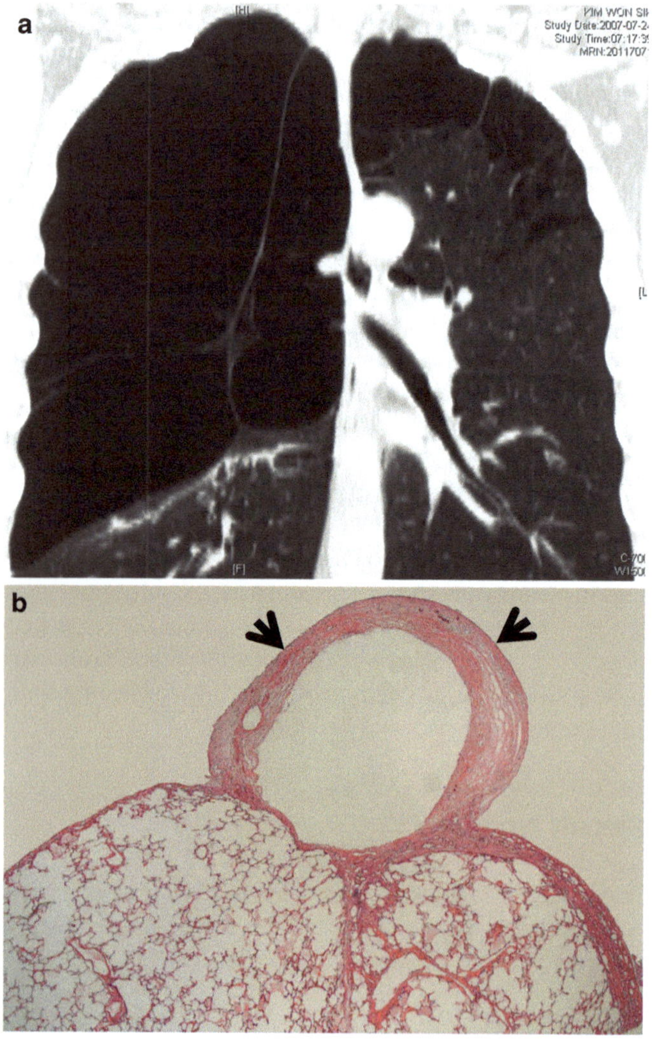


**Fig. 12.9** Vanishing lung syndrome in a 51-year-old male smoker. (**a**) Coronal reformatted (2.0-mm-section thickness) CT image shows multiple variable-sized air-filled cystic lesions in bilateral upper and right middle lung zones. (**b**) High-magnification (×100) photomicrograph of pathologic specimen obtained from lung apex in a different patient demonstrates an air-filled bulla (*arrows*) attached to underlying lung

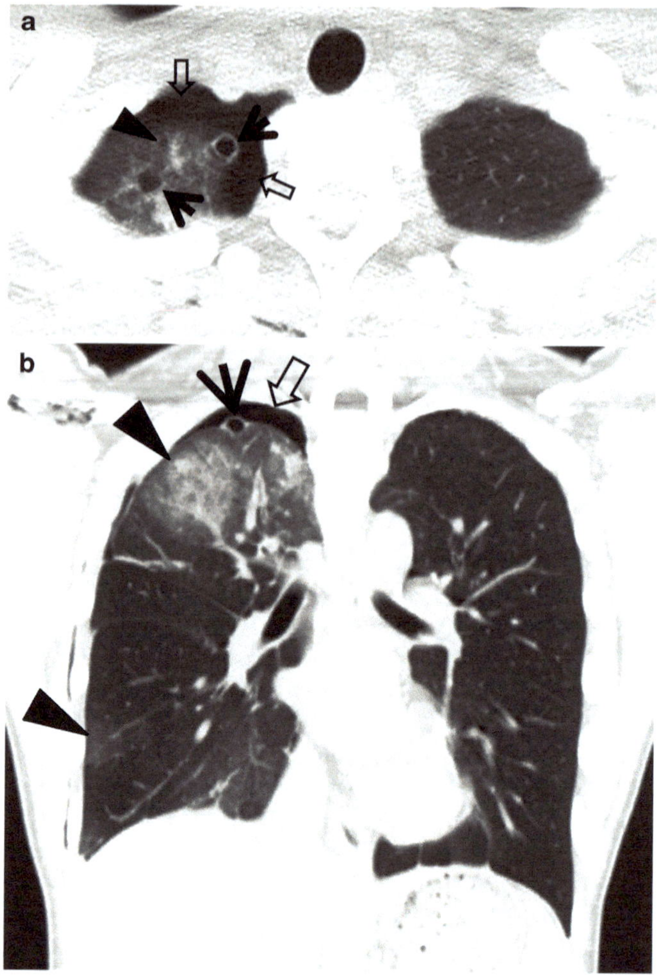


**Fig. 12.10** Pneumothorax due to ruptured blebs in an 18-year-old boy. (**a**) Lung window image of CT scan (2.5-mm-section thickness) obtained at levels of great vessels shows small multiple air-filled cysts (blebs, *arrows*) in right apex. Also note pneumothorax (*open arrows*), which was caused by ruptured bleb (*arrowhead*). (**b**) Coronal reformatted image (2.0-mm-section thickness) demonstrates bleb (*arrow*), pneumothorax (*open arrow*), and re-expansion pulmonary edema (*arrowheads*) in right lung

is suggested newly by Boisset [31] and is as follows: bronchial inflammation ruptures the bronchiolar walls and causes the formation of "air corridors" in the interstitium of the bronchiolar wall. Air dissects down these corridors to the pleura and forms pneumatoceles, a form of subpleural emphysema.

## Diseases Causing the Cyst

The differential diagnosis for lung cysts is broad and encompasses multisystem diseases in addition to cystic diseases isolated to the chest [32]. *Blebs, bullae, and pneumatoceles*, as a localized lesion or an extensive disease, are most frequently encountered cystic lung lesions. Interstitial lung diseases that may cause scattered or isolated pulmonary cysts include early form of Langerhans cell histiocytosis (LCH), lymphangioleiomyomatosis, lymphocytic interstitial pneumonia, desquamative interstitial pneumonia, and subacute hypersensitivity

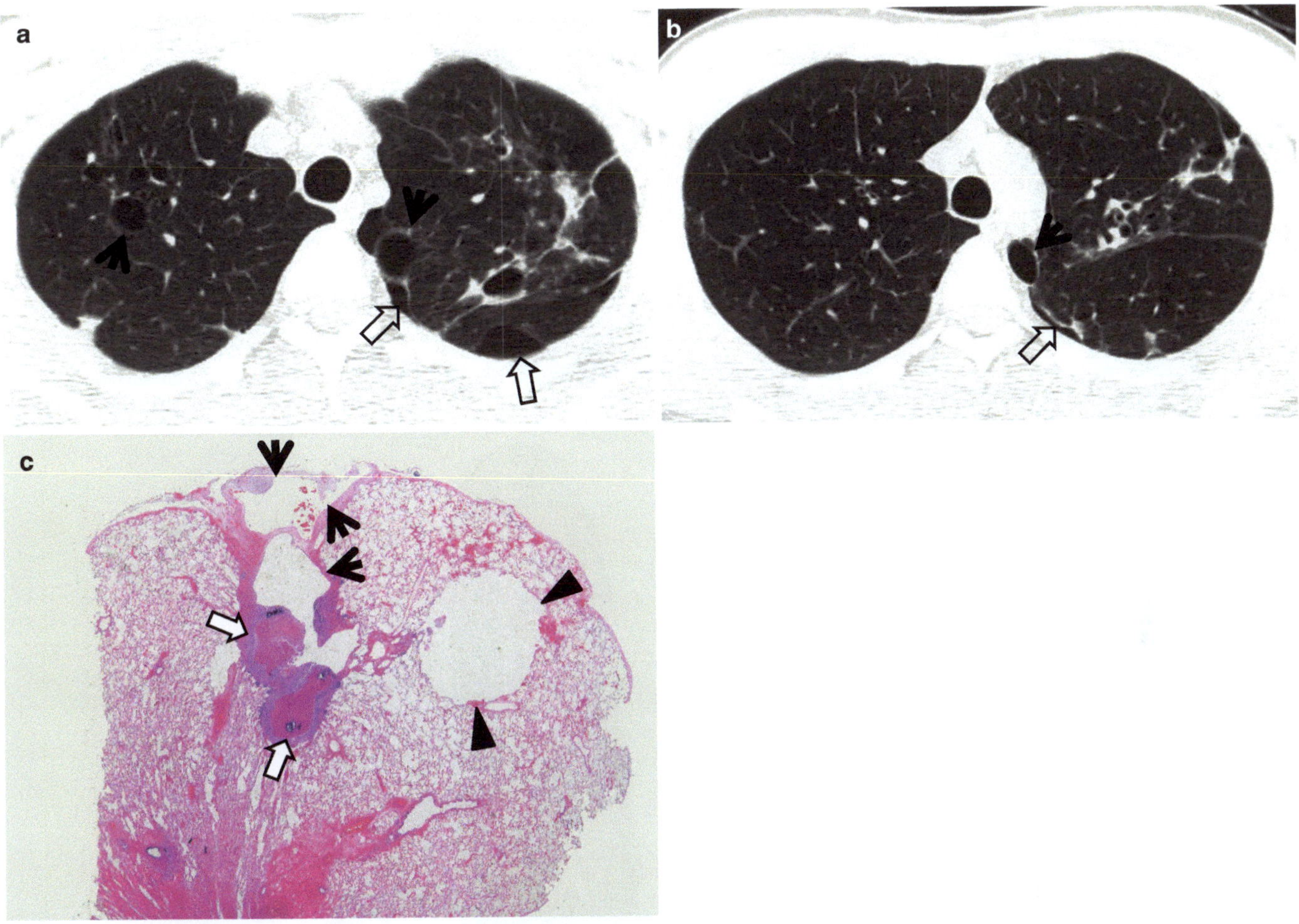


**Fig. 12.11** Bullae and tuberculous granulomas in a 56-year-old man. (**a**, **b**) Lung window images of CT scans (2.5-mm-section thickness) obtained at levels of great vessels (**a**) and aortic arch (**b**), respectively, show multiple small air-filled cysts (bullae) (*arrows*), variable-sized nodular lesions of tuberculosis, and pneumothorax (*open arrows*) in left pleural space due to ruptured bulla. Also note bronchiectasis in left upper lobe. (**c**) High-magnification (×100) photomicrograph obtained from left lung apex demonstrates an air-filled bullae (*arrows*) attached to underlying lung. Also note multiple tuberculous granulomas (*open arrows*) adjacent to bullae. Pulmonary emphysema (*arrowheads*) is also seen

pneumonitis. Developmental lesions such as *pulmonary sequestration* (Fig. 12.12), *congenital cystic adenomatoid malformation* (*CCAM*) (Fig. 12.13), *and pulmonary bronchogenic cyst* (Fig. 12.14) may present with localized air-filled or fluid-filled cystic lesions or their aggregation [34]. Malignant causes include cystic pulmonary metastasis, cystic fibrohistiocytic tumor, and cystic mesenchymomas. Infectious diseases (*Staphylococcal pneumonia* (Fig. 12.15), *Pneumocystis jirovecii pneumonia* (Fig. 12.16), pleuropulmonary paragonimiasis), *trauma/barotrauma* (Fig. 12.17), and Birt–Hogg–Dube syndrome also cause pulmonary cysts (Table 12.2).

## Distribution

In LCH, the cysts are typically diffusely distributed, with predominance in the lung apices and relative sparing of the lung bases [35]. Unlike in LCH, cysts may involve the juxtaphrenic recesses and spare the extreme apices in lymphangioleiomyomatosis [36]. In lymphocytic interstitial pneumonia, cysts are distributed in a scattered, random distribution [37]. Identification of small cysts admixed within the ground glass opacity is a unique feature to desquamative interstitial pneumonia [38]. Developmental lung anomalies usually involve lower lobes [34]. Although upper lobe predominance has been reported, cysts may involve any portion of the lungs in *Pneumocystis jirovecii* pneumonia [39]. Cysts in Birt–Hogg–Dube syndrome have lower lung zone predominance [40].

## Clinical Considerations

Cigarette smoking is highly related to pulmonary LCH and desquamative interstitial pneumonia. Lymphangioleiomyomatosis is almost exclusive to women of childbearing age. Lymphocytic interstitial pneumonia is often associated with collagen vascular disorders, in particular Sjogren's syndrome, but is also seen in patients with HIV infection. Pulmonary sequestration and CCAM should be suspected in young adults with nonresolving or recurrent lower

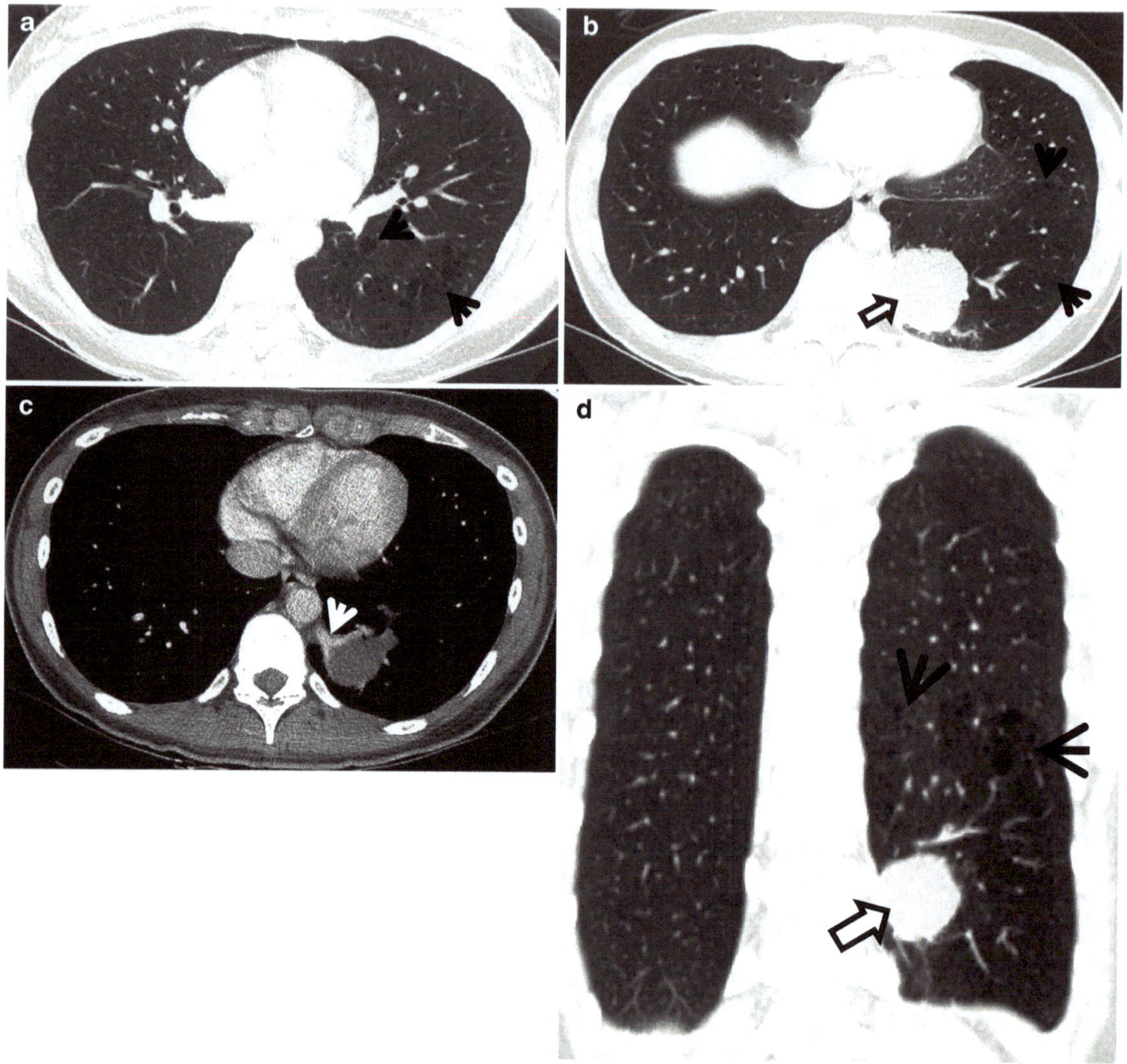


**Fig. 12.12** Pulmonary sequestration in a 24-year-old woman. (**a**, **b**) Lung window images of CT scans (2.5-mm-section thickness) obtained at levels of inferior pulmonary veins (**a**) and liver dome (**b**), respectively, show unusual air-filled cystic aggregation (*arrows*) and a round soft-tissue mass (*open arrows*) in left lower lobe. (**c**) Mediastinal window image obtained at level of suprahepatic inferior vena cava demonstrates a low-attenuation soft-tissue mass that is being supplied by a systemic artery (*arrow*) arising from descending thoracic aorta. (**d**) Coronal reformatted CT image (2.0-mm-section thickness) exhibits a soft tissue mass (*open arrow*) and cystic lesion aggregation (*arrows*) in left lower lobe

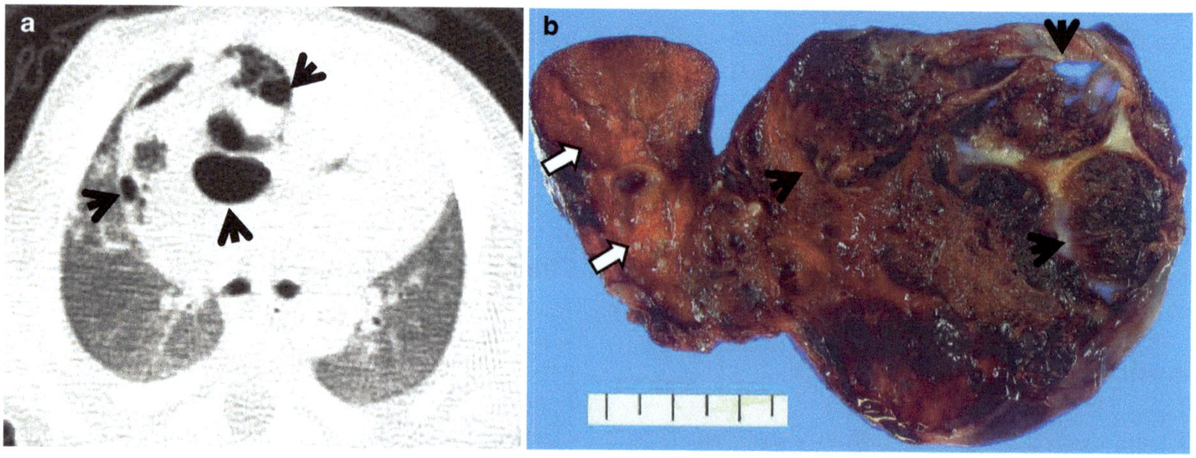


**Fig. 12.13** Congenital cystic adenomatoid malformation in a 7-month-old boy. (**a**) Lung window image of CT scan (5.0-mm-section thickness) obtained at level of main bronchi shows a round soft-tissue lesion harboring multiple air-filled cystic lesions (*arrows*) in right upper lobe. (**b**) Cut surface of gross pathologic specimen obtained with right upper lobectomy demonstrates multilocular cystic changes (*arrows*), some of which contain blood. Residual resected lung exhibits consolidation (*open arrows*). (**c**) Low-magnification (×40) photomicrograph of pathologic specimen discloses variable-sized thin-walled cysts lined by thin-layer of respiratory epithelium. Several cysts contain blood and are interconnected (*arrows*)

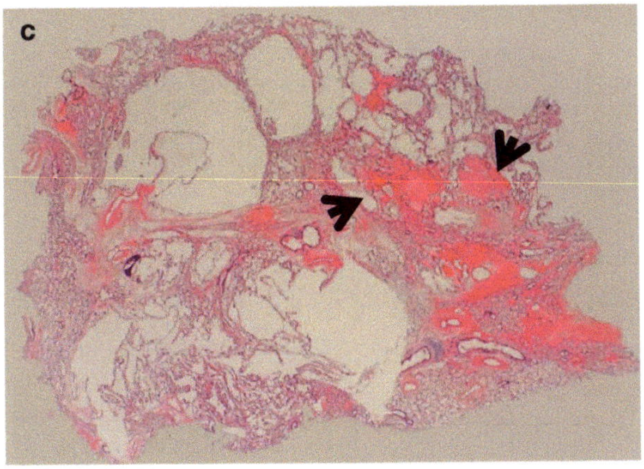


Fig. 12.13 (continued)

lobe pneumonia. *Pneumocystis jirovecii* pneumonia usually occurs in immunocompromised hosts, particularly those with deficiency in cell-mediated immunity (patients with HIV infection, organ transplantation, hematologic malignancy, patients undergoing chemotherapy, or long-term corticosteroid therapy). The incidence of cysts has been reported to be lower in patients without HIV infection than in HIV-infected patients [41] and cysts may resolve after treatment and clearing of infection [42]. Pneumatocele in Staphylococcal pneumonia is seen more often in children than in adults and increases in size over several days to weeks. Blunt thoracic trauma may result in pulmonary laceration (traumatic pseudocyst) when there is a disruption of the lung parenchyma. It is usually encountered in young patients, whose compliant chest wall permits the transmission of great compressive

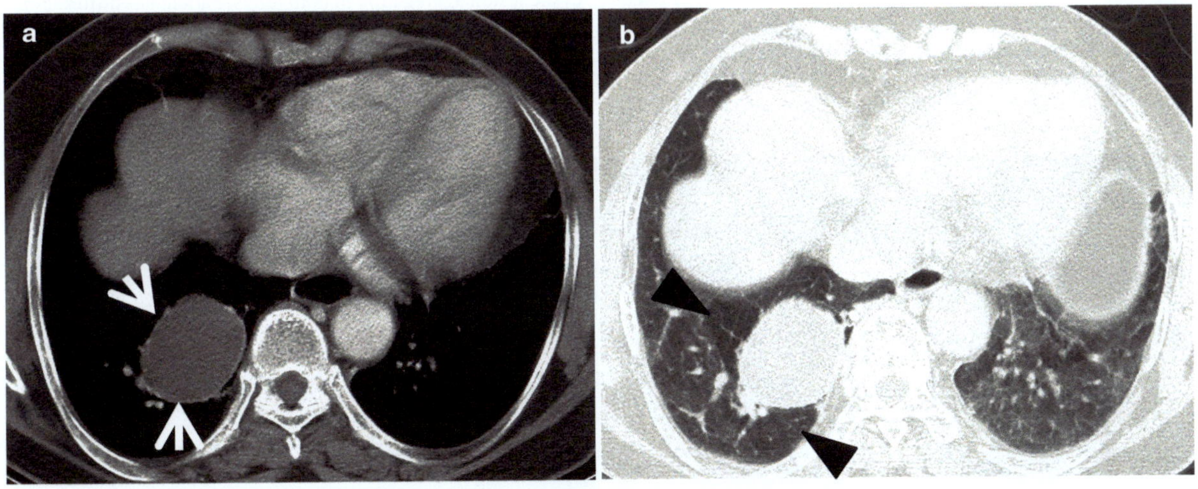


Fig. 12.14 Intrapulmonary bronchogenic cyst in a 61-year-old woman. (**a**) Mediastinal window image of enhanced CT scan (5.0-mm-section thickness) obtained at level of liver some shows a 45-mm-sized well-defined homogeneous low-attenuation (9 HU) lesion (*arrows*) in right lower lobe. (**b**) Lung window image demonstrate cystic lesion and surrounding low-attenuation mosaic perfusion (*arrowheads*) (Reprinted from Ref. [33] with permission)

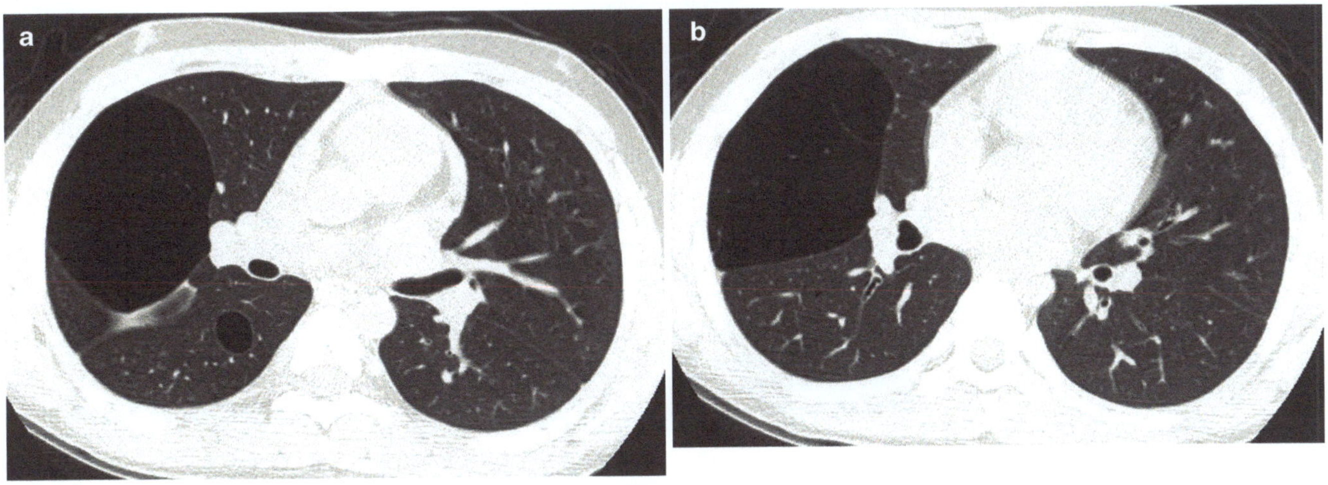


Fig. 12.15 Pneumatoceles as sequelae of *Staphylococcus* pneumonia in a 47-year-old man. (**a, b**) Lung window images of CT scans (2.5-mm-section thickness) obtained at levels of proximal (**a**) and distal (**b**) bronchus intermedius, respectively, show two air-filled cystic lesions of different size in right upper lobe and right lower lobe. Patient suffered from pneumonia for 3 weeks

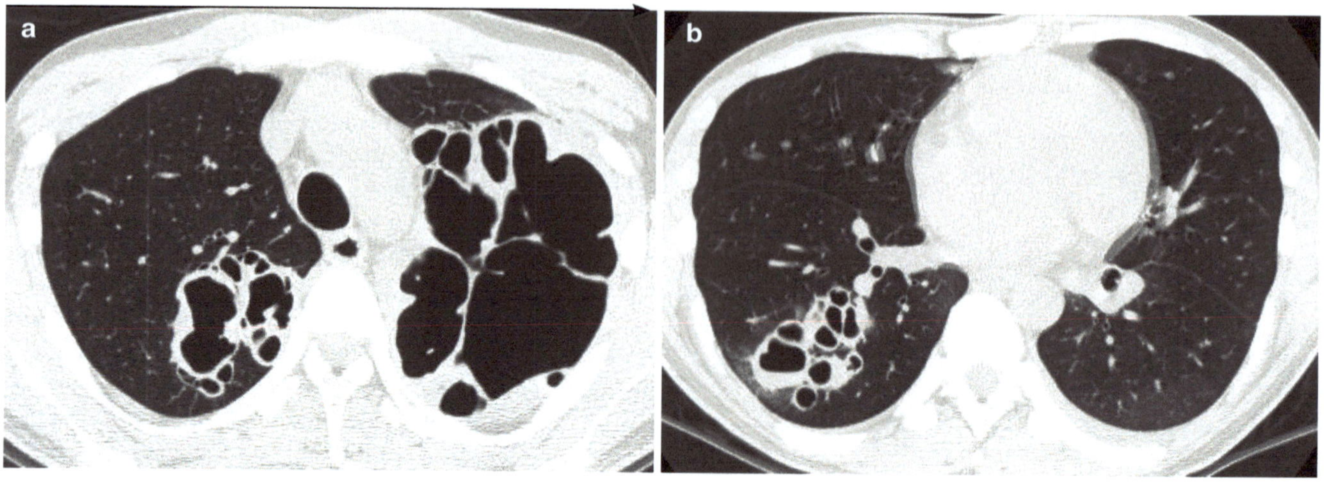

**Fig. 12.16** Multiseptated air-filled cystic lesions in both lungs in a 27-year-old man with HIV infection and *Pneumocystis jirovecii* pneumonia. (**a**, **b**) Lung window images of CT scans (2.5-mm-section thickness) obtained at levels of aortic arch (**a**) and right inferior pulmonary vein (**b**), respectively, show multifocal areas of air-filled multiseptated cystic lesion aggregation in both lungs. Patient has diffuse ground-glass opacity lesions on CT scans obtained 2 weeks prior

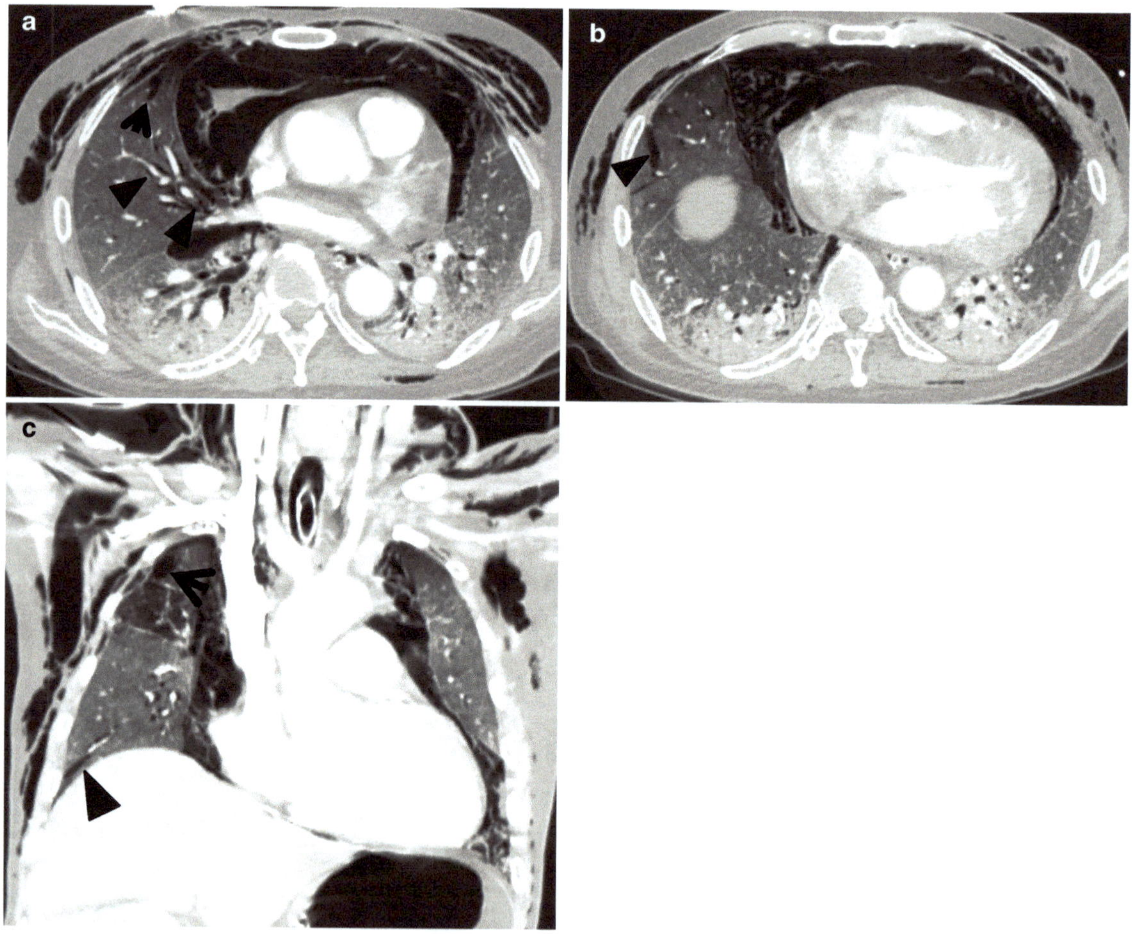

**Fig. 12.17** Traumatic pneumatocele in a 31-year-old man with traffic accident. (**a**, **b**) Lung window images of CT scans (5.0-mm-section thickness) obtained at levels of right inferior pulmonary vein (**a**) and liver dome (**b**), respectively, show an air-filled traumatic cyst (*arrow* in **a**) in right middle lobe. Also note interstitial emphysema tracking pulmonary arteries (*arrowheads*), traumatic lung contusion (increased lung attenuation in both lungs), pneumomediastinum and subcutaneous emphysema in both lungs and bilateral chest walls. (**c**) Coronal reformatted image (2.5-mm-section thickness) demonstrates pneumatocele (*arrow*) in right upper lobe, interstitial emphysema (*arrowhead*) in right lower lobe, and pneumomediastinum and subcutaneous emphysema in both hemithoraces

**Table 12.2** Common diseases manifesting as cyst

| Disease | Key points for differential diagnosis |
|---|---|
| Bullae, blebs, pneumatoceles | Usually associated with centrilobular or paraseptal emphysema |
| Langerhans cell histiocytosis | Nodules, cavitary nodules, and bizarre shaped, uneven-sized cysts with upper and middle lung zone predominance in a smoker |
| Lymphangioleiomyomatosis | Multiple or a few scattered cysts in a woman who presents with a pneumothorax |
| Lymphocytic interstitial pneumonia | Associated with GGO and poorly defined centrilobular nodules |
| Desquamative interstitial pneumonia | Lack of a perceptible cyst wall and areas of GGO around the cysts in smoker |
| Congenital cystic adenomatoid malformation, Pulmonary sequestration | Multiple, thin walled complex cysts |
| Bronchogenic cyst | Areas of mosaic low attenuation and band-like linear attenuation adjacent to the cyst |
| Burt–Hogg–Dube syndrome | Lung cysts found at the lung bases in patients with a solid renal mass |
| Trauma/barotrauma | Cysts are usually surrounded by contusion |
| Parasitic infection (PW) | Associated with cavitary nodules or masses in the subpleural or subfissural areas |
| *Pneumocystis jirovecii* pneumonia | Cysts are accompanied by various degree of GGO |
| Staphylococcal pneumonia | Associated with bronchopneumonia pattern |
| Malignant cystic tumor | |

*Note*: *GGO* ground glass opacity, *PW Paragonimus Westermani*

forces to the lung parenchyma and the laceration of the lung parenchyma. If a family history of recurrent pneumothoraces is elicited, a diagnosis of Birt–Hogg–Dube syndrome may be suggested [43]. This condition is associated with pneumothoraces, renal cell carcinomas, and skin fibrofolliculomas.

**Key Points for Differential Diagnosis**

1. When assessing pulmonary cysts on HRCT, the most important feature that allows differentiation among diseases is their distribution. After then, careful observation of cyst shape and size, as well as for the presence of any ancillary findings are needed to refine the differential diagnosis.
2. Although it is not always possible to distinguish a bulla from a lung cyst or a pneumatocele, bullae are uncommon as isolated findings, except in the lung apices, and are usually associated with evidence of extensive centrilobular or paraseptal emphysema. The distinction between bleb and bulla is difficult on HRCT, but is of little practical significance.
3. The combination of nodules, cavitary nodules, and bizarre shaped, uneven-sized cysts with upper and middle lung zone predominance in a smoker allows a confident diagnosis of LCH [35].
4. Although diffusely distributed multiple lung cysts are the characteristic features of lymphangioleiomyomatosis, a few scattered cysts in a woman who presents with a pneumothorax may signify an early form of lymphangioleiomyomatosis.
5. Predominant CT findings of lymphocytic interstitial pneumonia (ground-glass opacity and poorly defined centrilobular nodules) and combinations of interlobular septal thickening, thickening of bronchovascular bundles, and scattered distribution of cysts may be helpful in differentiating lymphocytic interstitial pneumonia from other cystic diseases [35].
6. A combination of lack of a perceptible cyst wall and areas of ground-glass opacity around the cysts in individuals exposed to cigarette smoking is a characteristic feature of desquamative interstitial pneumonia [35].
7. The presence of multiple thin-walled, complex cystic masses usually allows the diagnosis of CCAM or pulmonary sequestration. The essential feature in the diagnosis of pulmonary sequestration is demonstration of the systemic arterial supply to the abnormal lung [44].
8. The identification of cystic lesions in an HIV-positive patient is highly suggestive of *Pneumocystis jirovecii* pneumonia. *Pneumocystis* pneumonia cysts are usually accompanied by various degrees of ground-glass opacity.
9. Birt–Hogg–Dube syndrome may manifest as a spontaneous pneumothorax or as lung cysts found at the lung bases in patients with a solid renal mass. The cysts are usually randomly scattered and have lower lung zone predominance. The large dominant cysts tend to be located in the lung bases and may be multiseptated [45].

## Blebs and Bullae

### Pathology and Pathogenesis

Bulla is a pathological entity caused by the confluence of two or more of the terminal elements of the bronchial tree. They may be found subsequent to any condition that interferes with normal respiratory mechanism that produces increased intra-alveolar pressure. A single bulla is a rarity;

they vary in size from that of a large vesicle to that of a large grape fruit. Bullae are formed in the lungs of patients afflicted with vesicular emphysema; blebs are present in cases of interstitial emphysema. A bleb is formed by the rupture of the alveolar wall; the air escaping through the tear separates the pleura from the alveolar wall lying underneath it, much like a dissecting aneurysm [46] (Figs. 12.9 and 12.10).

### Symptoms and Signs

Blebs and bullae rarely cause respiratory symptoms until pneumothorax or giant bullae develop. Many patients are clinically silent. Shortness of breath and nonspecific chest discomfort due to compression of surrounding lung tissue can occur in giant bullae.

### CT Findings

See the definition of bulla and bleb (Figs. 12.9, 12.10, and 12.11).

### CT-Pathology Comparisons

Also see the definition of bulla and bleb.

### Patient Prognosis

No therapy is necessary for asymptomatic patients. Patients with large bullae should receive surgical bulla resection. If resection is not possible, they should have regular follow-up to prevent potential acute complications such as pneumothorax and to exclude the development of lung cancer associated with pulmonary bullae. With smoking cessation and optimization of bronchodilator therapy, resolution of giant bullae has been reported [47].

## Pulmonary Sequestration

### Pathology and Pathogenesis

Pulmonary sequestration is a malformation in which a portion of lung is detached from the remaining normal lung and receives its blood supply from a systemic artery. The anomaly may be intralobar or extralobar. Pathologically, intralobar sequestrations are located within normal lung but are generally well demarcated from the surrounding parenchyma and do not communicate with the normal bronchi [48]. Venous drainage is almost always via the pulmonary venous system. Extralobar sequestrations are completely enclosed by a pleural membrane [49]. Venous drainage of extralobar sequestrations is via systemic veins.

### Symptoms and Signs

Pulmonary sequestrations in adults are usually asymptomatic and the abnormality is found incidentally on a chest radiograph or CT. The most common clinical manifestations are related to superimposed infection, in which cases the signs and symptoms are those of acute pneumonia.

### CT Findings

The most common CT findings of intralobar pulmonary sequestration consist of focal areas of lucency or irregular cystic spaces with or without fluid [50]. Extralobar sequestration is visualized as a homogeneous opacity or well-circumscribed mass or occasionally cystic areas on CT [50]. The vast majority are situated in the posterior basal segment of a lower lobe. Demonstration of the systemic arterial supply is essential for the diagnosis and this anomalous vessel is typically seen coursing from the lower thoracic or upper abdominal aorta through the inferior pulmonary ligament into the sequestered lung [44] (Fig. 12.12).

### CT-Pathology Comparisons

Pathologically, intralobar sequestrations usually consist of one or more cystic spaces resembling dilated bronchi with a variable amount of intervening solid tissue. Therefore, they appear as cystic spaces with or without fluid on CT. Extralobar sequestration usually contain immature lung tissue and few airways and are completely enclosed by a pleural membrane, so they appear as a well-circumscribed mass on CT.

### Patient Prognosis

Surgical resection is the treatment of choice for patients with infection or symptoms resulting from compression of normal lung tissue [51]. Reported postoperative complications are uncommon and the prognosis following surgical excision is excellent [52].

## Congenital Cystic Adenomatoid Malformation

### Pathology and Pathogenesis

CCAM is characterized by a multicystic mass, a pulmonary tissue with an abnormal proliferation of bronchial structures [53]. Three main morphologic subtypes (type I, large, multiloculated cysts greater than 2 cm in diameter; type II, uniform small cysts less than 2 cm in diameter; type III, solid appearing lesions that microscopically demonstrate tiny cysts) have been described (Fig. 12.13).

### Symptoms and Signs

In adults, CCAM may be an incidental finding or may be accompanied by symptoms related to recurrent respiratory infections. Less common complications include pneumothorax and the development of carcinoma [54].

### CT Findings

The characteristic CT findings of CCAM typically consist of a unilocular or multiloculated cyst or a complex soft tissue and cystic mass ranging from 4 to 12 cm in diameter [55]. They are usually located in the lower lobes. Type I lesions have at least one cyst greater than 2 cm in diameter, and type II lesions area characterized by multiple thin-walled cysts ranging from 2 to 20 mm in diameter (Fig. 12.12).

### CT-Pathology Comparisons

On CT-pathology correlation, areas of consolidation correspond histologically to areas of glandular or bronchiolar structures with or without areas of endogenous lipid or organizing pneumonia or mucus plugs. Low attenuation areas at CT correspond to areas of air-filled microcysts blended with normal lung parenchyma [56].

### Patient Prognosis

Because the majority of cases are associated with recurrent infection and risk for the development of carcinoma, the treatment of choice is surgical resection.

## Intrapulmonary Bronchogenic Cyst

### Pathology and Pathogenesis

Bronchogenic cyst results from abnormal separation of localized portions of the tracheobronchial tree from the adjacent airways between the 3rd and 24th weeks of gestation [53].

### Symptoms and Signs

The majority of bronchogenic cysts is asymptomatic and found incidentally on a chest radiograph or CT.

### CT Findings

Most bronchogenic cysts are located in the mediastinum, but 10–30 % in the lung [57]. CT demonstrates a homogeneous cystic mass with a thin smooth wall. In about half of cases, the cyst shows homogeneous attenuation at water density, whereas the attenuation of the others is higher than water density [58]. Occasionally, bronchogenic cysts are air filled and multilocular. The lung adjacent to bronchogenic cysts shows areas of mosaic low attenuation and band-like linear attenuation [59] (Fig. 12.14).

### CT-Pathology Comparisons

Pathologically, bronchogenic cysts are thin-walled, unilocular, and spherical in shape. They are filled with either mucoid or serous fluid. Therefore, they appear as a homogeneous cystic mass with water attenuation. In about half of cases, the cysts have a higher attenuation, which results from the presence of protein or, less commonly, hemorrhage or calcium oxalate within the mucoid cyst [58]. Areas of mosaic attenuation and band-like linear attenuation adjacent to bronchogenic cysts histologically correspond to emphysema and bronchiolization or fibrotic changes [59].

### Patient Prognosis

The majority of bronchogenic cysts in adults are removed surgically.

## Pneumatoceles in Staphylococcal Pneumonia

### Pathology and Pathogenesis

Pulmonary pneumatoceles are areas of regional obstructive emphysema usually developing as a complication (inflammatory narrowing of a bronchus) of staphylococcal pneumonia. They are thin-walled, air-containing, cyst-like structures which may occur at any age but are most frequently seen in infancy [33].

### Symptoms and Signs

Staphylococcal pneumonia typically occurs in cases of influenza (airborne transmission) or nosocomial pneumonia, particularly ventilator-associated pneumonia. The clinical presentation of pneumonia caused by *Staphylococcus aureus* is usually similar to those by other etiological agents. However, rapid progression of pulmonary lesions, frequent complications such as pleural effusion, empyema and septic shock, and high mortality are not uncommon.

### CT Findings

The typical pattern of *Staphylococcal* pneumonia at presentation is bronchopneumonia manifested as centrilobular nodules, tree-in-bud pattern, and lobular, subsegmental or segmental areas of consolidation [60]. The areas of consolidation may be patchy or confluent, unilateral or bilateral but usually involve two or more lobes. Segmental atelectasis is common but air bronchograms are infrequent. Common complications are formations of abscess and pneumatoceles (Fig. 12.15). Abscess formation can be identified in about 15–30 % of patients [61]. Pneumatocele characteristically increases in size over several days to weeks and is seen more often in children (40–75 %) than in adults (15 %) [60, 62].

### CT-Pathology Comparisons

The typical histologic pattern of *Staphylococcal* pneumonia is bronchopneumonia. Because proximal airways are usually filled with inflammatory exudates, segmental atelectasis is common, and air bronchograms are infrequent. *Staphylococcal* pneumonia begins as a focus of consolidation followed by abscess formation, cavitation and pneumatocele formation. Pneumatocele presumably results from drainage of a focus of necrotic lung parenchyma followed by check-valve obstruction of the airway subtending it, enabling air to enter the parenchymal space during inspiration, but preventing its egress during expiration [63].

### Patient Prognosis

Early diagnosis and appropriate administration of appropriate antimicrobial therapy are the most important for the treatment of Staphylococcal pneumonia. Methicillin resistance is increasingly frequent (more than 60 % of strains from intensive care units in the USA) in this organism [64]. Vancomycin, linezolid, and teicoplanin are antibiotics approved for the treatment of nosocomial pneumonia due to methicillin-resistant *Staphylococcus aureus*.

## Cystic Lesions in *Pneumocystis jirovecii* Pneumonia

### Pathology and Pathogenesis

*Pneumocystis* pneumonia in humans is an opportunistic infection caused by *Pneumocystis jirovecii* (former *P. carinii*) (PJP), an ascomycetous fungus, in patients with impaired immunity. The classic findings of PJP in sections of lung stained with Hematoxylin and Eosin (H & E) are widening of the alveolar septa with an infiltrate of mononuclear cells and foamy honeycombed acellular exudates within the alveolar spaces. This exudate consists of aggregated cysts and trophozoites that are not visualized on H & E staining [65].

### Symptoms and Signs

PJP can occur in immunocompromised individuals, especially hematopoietic stem and solid organ transplants, those receiving high-dose corticosteroid therapy and persons with advanced HIV infection [65]. A slow indolent time course with symptoms of pneumonia progressing over weeks to months is characteristic in HIV-infected patients. Fulminant respiratory failure associated with fever and dry cough is typical in non-HIV-infected patients.

### CT Findings

On CT of patients with PJP, the prevalence of cysts ranges from approximately 10–34 % [42] (Fig. 12.16). Cysts may vary in appearance, with differing shapes and sizes and various degrees of wall thickness. Cysts are usually multiple and bilateral, and they may be found in either a subpleural or an intraparenchymal location. Although upper lobe predominance has been reported, cysts may involve any portion of the lungs. PJP cysts are usually accompanied by various degrees of ground-glass opacity. Cystic *pneumocystis* pneumonia is associated with an increased incidence of spontaneous pneumothorax, which is believed to occur in association with rupture of subpleural cysts.

### CT-Pathology Comparisons

Cystic formation in PJP is probably related to infiltration of organisms into the parenchymal interstitium with subsequent necrosis and cavitation [66].

### Patient Prognosis

The first-line drug for treatment and prevention is trimethoprim-sulfamethoxazole. To reduce the incidence of respiratory failure due to a severe inflammation caused by microbial degradation after antimicrobial therapy, the addition of corticosteroids is indicated for all patients with HIV infection and confirmed cases [65].

## Traumatic Lung Cysts

### Pathology and Pathogenesis

Injury to the lung parenchyma caused by nonpenetrating chest trauma is frequently accompanied by pulmonary contusion and intrapulmonary hemorrhage, but the development of a traumatic lung pseudocyst is a rare occurrence. Pseudocysts are considered to be due to tearing or laceration of the lung parenchyma [67].

## Symptoms and Signs

Traumatic lung cyst is a very rare manifestation of blunt chest injury. It develops early after trauma, requires no specific treatment, and resolves spontaneously after a period of up to a few months [68]. Its main significance lies in that it has to be differentially diagnosed from cavitary lung lesions of other origin. Symptoms are nonspecific and include chest pain, hemoptysis, and shortness of breath. The majority of the reported cases had concomitant injuries, such as pneumothorax, hemopneumothorax, or pulmonary hematoma.

## CT Findings

Pulmonary laceration (traumatic lung cyst) occurs when there is a disruption of the lung parenchyma, resulting in a cavity in the lung. It appears as a round or oval cavity or cyst on CT [69, 70] (Fig. 12.17). Traumatic cysts may be filled with air, blood, or both air and blood. Over time, they become increasingly filled with blood and then regress. They may be single or multiple and unilocular or multilocular in appearance. In acute setting, traumatic cysts are usually surrounded by contusion. Traumatic cysts heal more slowly than contusion and may last up to several months.

## CT-Pathology Comparisons

Because of the normal pulmonary elastic recoil, lung tissues surrounding a laceration pull back from the laceration itself. This results in the laceration manifesting at CT as a round or oval cavity or cyst, instead of having the linear appearance typically seen in other solid organ. Traumatic pulmonary pseudocysts develop through a mechanism that allows the transmission of great compressive forces to the lung parenchyma. The latter undergoes a rapid compression and decompression that causes the formation of small parenchymal lacerations, affecting both the alveoli and the interstitium. Around these lacerations, the elastic lung tissue retracts, thus leaving small cavities or cysts that are filled with air or fluid [71].

## Patient Prognosis

Traumatic lung cysts typically change in shape and size, and may become larger during the first 2 weeks of observation [68]. After that time, they start to get smaller until eventual resolution. It requires no specific treatment and resolves spontaneously after a period of up to a few months.

## References


1. Gadkowski LB, Stout JE. Cavitary pulmonary disease. Clin Microbiol Rev. 2008;21:305–33, table of contents.
2. Hansell DM, Bankier AA, MacMahon H, McLoud TC, Muller NL, Remy J. Fleischner Society: glossary of terms for thoracic imaging. Radiology. 2008;246:697–722.
3. Yang YW, Kang YA, Lee SH, et al. Aetiologies and predictors of pulmonary cavities in South Korea. Int J Tuberc Lung Dis. 2007;11:457–62.
4. Koh WJ, Kwon OJ, Lee KS. Nontuberculous mycobacterial pulmonary diseases in immunocompetent patients. Korean J Radiol. 2002;3:145–57.
5. Kim TS, Han J, Shim SS, et al. Pleuropulmonary paragonimiasis: CT findings in 31 patients. AJR Am J Roentgenol. 2005;185: 616–21.
6. Kim HJ, Lee KS, Johkoh T, et al. Pulmonary Langerhans cell histiocytosis in adults: high-resolution CT-pathology comparisons and evolutional changes at CT. Eur Radiol. 2011;21:1406–15.
7. Geng E, Kreiswirth B, Burzynski J, Schluger NW. Clinical and radiographic correlates of primary and reactivation tuberculosis: a molecular epidemiology study. JAMA. 2005;293:2740–5.
8. Song KD, Lee KS, Chung MP, et al. Pulmonary cryptococcosis: imaging findings in 23 non-AIDS patients. Korean J Radiol. 2010;11:407–16.
9. Li BG, Ma DQ, Xian ZY, et al. The value of multislice spiral CT features of cavitary walls in differentiating between peripheral lung cancer cavities and single pulmonary tuberculous thick-walled cavities. Br J Radiol. 2012;85:147–52.
10. Cha J, Lee HY, Lee KS, et al. Radiological findings of extensively drug-resistant pulmonary tuberculosis in non-AIDS adults: comparisons with findings of multidrug-resistant and drug-sensitive tuberculosis. Korean J Radiol. 2009;10:207–16.
11. Franquet T, Muller NL, Gimenez A, Martinez S, Madrid M, Domingo P. Infectious pulmonary nodules in immunocompromised patients: usefulness of computed tomography in predicting their etiology. J Comput Assist Tomogr. 2003;27:461–8.
12. Kim MJ, Lee KS, Kim J, Jung KJ, Lee HG, Kim TS. Crescent sign in invasive pulmonary aspergillosis: frequency and related CT and clinical factors. J Comput Assist Tomogr. 2001;25:305–10.
13. Park Y, Kim TS, Yi CA, Cho EY, Kim H, Choi YS. Pulmonary cavitary mass containing a mural nodule: differential diagnosis between intracavitary aspergilloma and cavitating lung cancer on contrast-enhanced computed tomography. Clin Radiol. 2007;62:227–32.
14. Dodd JD, Souza CA, Muller NL. High-resolution MDCT of pulmonary septic embolism: evaluation of the feeding vessel sign. AJR Am J Roentgenol. 2006;187:623–9.
15. Travis WD, Brambilla E, Muller-Hermelink HK, Harris CC, editors. Pathology and genetics of tumours of the lung pleura, World Health Organization classification of tumours. Lyon: IARC Press; 2004.
16. Drilon A, Rekhtman N, Ladanyi M, Paik P. Squamous-cell carcinomas of the lung: emerging biology, controversies, and the promise of targeted therapy. Lancet Oncol. 2012;13:e418–26.
17. Rosado-de-Christenson ML, Templeton PA, Moran CA. Bronchogenic carcinoma: radiologic-pathologic correlation. Radiographics. 1994; 14:429–46; quiz 447–8.
18. Funai K, Yokose T, Ishii G, et al. Clinicopathologic characteristics of peripheral squamous cell carcinoma of the lung. Am J Surg Pathol. 2003;27:978–84.
19. Tazi A. Adult pulmonary Langerhans' cell histiocytosis. Eur Respir J. 2006;27:1272–85.
20. Kulwiec EL, Lynch DA, Aguayo SM, Schwarz MI, King Jr TE. Imaging of pulmonary histiocytosis X. Radiographics. 1992;12: 515–26.

21. Abbott GF, Rosado-de-Christenson ML, Franks TJ, Frazier AA, Galvin JR. From the archives of the AFIP: pulmonary Langerhans cell histiocytosis. Radiographics. 2004;24:821–41.
22. Cook RJ, Ashton RW, Aughenbaugh GL, Ryu JH. Septic pulmonary embolism: presenting features and clinical course of 14 patients. Chest. 2005;128:162–6.
23. Kuhlman JE, Fishman EK, Teigen C. Pulmonary septic emboli: diagnosis with CT. Radiology. 1990;174:211–3.
24. Kwon WJ, Jeong YJ, Kim KI, et al. Computed tomographic features of pulmonary septic emboli: comparison of causative microorganisms. J Comput Assist Tomogr. 2007;31:390–4.
25. Lee JY, Lee KS, Jung KJ, et al. Pulmonary tuberculosis: CT and pathologic correlation. J Comput Assist Tomogr. 2000;24:691–8.
26. Zumla A, Raviglione M, Hafner R, von Reyn CF. Tuberculosis. N Engl J Med. 2013;368:745–55.
27. Jeong YJ, Lee KS. Pulmonary tuberculosis: up-to-date imaging and management. AJR Am J Roentgenol. 2008;191:834–44.
28. Miller WT, Miller Jr WT. Tuberculosis in the normal host: radiological findings. Semin Roentgenol. 1993;28:109–18.
29. Im JG, Whang HY, Kim WS, Han MC, Shim YS, Cho SY. Pleuropulmonary paragonimiasis: radiologic findings in 71 patients. AJR Am J Roentgenol. 1992;159:39–43.
30. Singh TS, Sugiyama H, Rangsiruji A. Paragonimus & paragonimiasis in India. Indian J Med Res. 2012;136:192–204.
31. Boisset GF. Subpleural emphysema complicating staphylococcal and other pneumonias. J Pediatr. 1972;81:259–66.
32. Beddy P, Babar J, Devaraj A. A practical approach to cystic lung disease on HRCT. Insights Imaging. 2011;2:1–7.
33. Flaherty RA, Keegan JM, Sturtevant HN. Post-pneumonic pulmonary pneumatoceles. Radiology. 1960;74:50–3.
34. Zylak CJ, Eyler WR, Spizarny DL, Stone CH. Developmental lung anomalies in the adult: radiologic-pathologic correlation. Radiographics. 2002;22(Spec No):S25–43.
35. Koyama M, Johkoh T, Honda O, et al. Chronic cystic lung disease: diagnostic accuracy of high-resolution CT in 92 patients. AJR Am J Roentgenol. 2003;180:827–35.
36. Rappaport DC, Weisbrod GL, Herman SJ, Chamberlain DW. Pulmonary lymphangioleiomyomatosis: high-resolution CT findings in four cases. AJR Am J Roentgenol. 1989;152:961–4.
37. Silva CI, Flint JD, Levy RD, Muller NL. Diffuse lung cysts in lymphoid interstitial pneumonia: high-resolution CT and pathologic findings. J Thorac Imaging. 2006;21:241–4.
38. Lynch DA, Travis WD, Muller NL, et al. Idiopathic interstitial pneumonias: CT features. Radiology. 2005;236:10–21.
39. Chow C, Templeton PA, White CS. Lung cysts associated with Pneumocystis carinii pneumonia: radiographic characteristics, natural history, and complications. AJR Am J Roentgenol. 1993;161:527–31.
40. Ayo DS, Aughenbaugh GL, Yi ES, Hand JL, Ryu JH. Cystic lung disease in Birt-Hogg-Dube syndrome. Chest. 2007;132:679–84.
41. Hardak E, Brook O, Yigla M. Radiological features of Pneumocystis jirovecii pneumonia in immunocompromised patients with and without AIDS. Lung. 2010;188:159–63.
42. Boiselle PM, Crans Jr CA, Kaplan MA. The changing face of Pneumocystis carinii pneumonia in AIDS patients. AJR Am J Roentgenol. 1999;172:1301–9.
43. Menko FH, van Steensel MA, Giraud S, et al. Birt-Hogg-Dube syndrome: diagnosis and management. Lancet Oncol. 2009;10:1199–206.
44. Ahmed M, Jacobi V, Vogl TJ. Multislice CT and CT angiography for non-invasive evaluation of bronchopulmonary sequestration. Eur Radiol. 2004;14:2141–3.
45. Agarwal PP, Gross BH, Holloway BJ, Seely J, Stark P, Kazerooni EA. Thoracic CT findings in Birt-Hogg-Dube syndrome. AJR Am J Roentgenol. 2011;196:349–52.
46. Wiese ER. Bulla of the lung. Dis Chest. 1946;12:238–41.
47. Byrd Jr RP, Roy TM. Spontaneous resolution of a giant pulmonary bulla: what is the role of bronchodilator and anti-inflammatory therapy? Tenn Med. 2013;106:39–42.
48. Frazier AA, Rosado de Christenson ML, Stocker JT, Templeton PA. Intralobar sequestration: radiologic-pathologic correlation. Radiographics. 1997;17:725–45.
49. Rosado-de-Christenson ML, Frazier AA, Stocker JT, Templeton PA. From the archives of the AFIP. Extralobar sequestration: radiologic-pathologic correlation. Radiographics. 1993;13:425–41.
50. Ikezoe J, Murayama S, Godwin JD, Done SL, Verschakelen JA. Bronchopulmonary sequestration: CT assessment. Radiology. 1990;176:375–9.
51. Shanmugam G, MacArthur K, Pollock JC. Congenital lung malformations – antenatal and postnatal evaluation and management. Eur J Cardiothorac Surg. 2005;27:45–52.
52. DeParedes CG, Pierce WS, Johnson DG, Waldhausen JA. Pulmonary sequestration in infants and children: a 20-year experience and review of the literature. J Pediatr Surg. 1970;5:136–47.
53. Berrocal T, Madrid C, Novo S, Gutierrez J, Arjonilla A, Gomez-Leon N. Congenital anomalies of the tracheobronchial tree, lung, and mediastinum: embryology, radiology, and pathology. Radiographics. 2004;24:e17.
54. Ioachimescu OC, Mehta AC. From cystic pulmonary airway malformation, to bronchioloalveolar carcinoma and adenocarcinoma of the lung. Eur Respir J. 2005;26:1181–7.
55. Patz Jr EF, Muller NL, Swensen SJ, Dodd LG. Congenital cystic adenomatoid malformation in adults: CT findings. J Comput Assist Tomogr. 1995;19:361–4.
56. Kim WS, Lee KS, Kim IO, et al. Congenital cystic adenomatoid malformation of the lung: CT-pathologic correlation. AJR Am J Roentgenol. 1997;168:47–53.
57. St-Georges R, Deslauriers J, Duranceau A, et al. Clinical spectrum of bronchogenic cysts of the mediastinum and lung in the adult. Ann Thorac Surg. 1991;52:6–13.
58. Mendelson DS, Rose JS, Efremidis SC, Kirschner PA, Cohen BA. Bronchogenic cysts with high CT numbers. AJR Am J Roentgenol. 1983;140:463–5.
59. Yoon YC, Lee KS, Kim TS, Kim J, Shim YM, Han J. Intrapulmonary bronchogenic cyst: CT and pathologic findings in five adult patients. AJR Am J Roentgenol. 2002;179:167–70.
60. Macfarlane J, Rose D. Radiographic features of staphylococcal pneumonia in adults and children. Thorax. 1996;51:539–40.
61. Chartrand SA, McCracken Jr GH. Staphylococcal pneumonia in infants and children. Pediatr Infect Dis. 1982;1:19–23.
62. Dines DE. Diagnostic significance of pneumatocele of the lung. JAMA. 1968;204:1169–72.
63. Quigley MJ, Fraser RS. Pulmonary pneumatocele: pathology and pathogenesis. AJR Am J Roentgenol. 1988;150:1275–7.
64. Ramirez P, Fernandez-Barat L, Torres A. New therapy options for MRSA with respiratory infection/pneumonia. Curr Opin Infect Dis. 2012;25:159–65.
65. Gilroy SA, Bennett NJ. Pneumocystis pneumonia. Semin Respir Crit Care Med. 2011;32:775–82.
66. Gurney JW, Bates FT. Pulmonary cystic disease: comparison of Pneumocystis carinii pneumatoceles and bullous emphysema due to intravenous drug abuse. Radiology. 1989;173:27–31.
67. Shirakusa T, Araki Y, Tsutsui M, et al. Traumatic lung pseudocyst. Thorax. 1987;42:516–9.
68. Stathopoulos G, Chrysikopoulou E, Kalogeromitros A, et al. Bilateral traumatic pulmonary pseudocysts: case report and literature review. J Trauma. 2002;53:993–6.
69. Kaewlai R, Avery LL, Asrani AV, Novelline RA. Multidetector CT of blunt thoracic trauma. Radiographics. 2008;28:1555–70.
70. Tsitouridis I, Tsinoglou K, Tsandiridis C, Papastergiou C, Bintoudi A. Traumatic pulmonary pseudocysts: CT findings. J Thorac Imaging. 2007;22:247–51.
71. Fagan CJ, Swischuk LE. Traumatic lung and paramediastinal pneumatoceles. Radiology. 1976;120:11–8.

# 13 Decreased Opacity without Cystic Airspace

## Mosaic Attenuation

### Definition

Mosaic attenuation pattern appears as patchwork of regions of differing attenuation that may represent (a) patchy interstitial disease, (b) obliterative small airway disease, or (c) occlusive vascular disease [1, 2]. Mosaic attenuation pattern caused by the latter two disease categories is called mosaic perfusion (Figs. 13.1 and 13.2). The combination of mixed lung attenuations (combination of ground-glass opacity, normal lung, and reduced lung attenuation as a result of mosaic perfusion) often gives the lung a geographic appearance and has been termed the *head-cheese sign*.

### Diseases Causing the Mosaic Attenuation Pattern

Causes of mosaic attenuation pattern include infiltrative lung disease, airway disease, and vascular disease. Mosaic attenuation can be seen in a variety of airway diseases including bronchiectasis, *cystic fibrosis* (Fig. 13.2), allergic bronchopulmonary aspergillosis (ABPA), asthma, and *constrictive bronchiolitis* (Fig. 13.1). Vascular causes of mosaic perfusion include *chronic pulmonary thromboembolism* (Fig. 13.3) and *pulmonary arterial hypertension* (Fig. 13.4) (Table 13.1). Various interstitial lung diseases characterized by patchy areas of ground-glass opacity (GGO) are also the causes of mosaic attenuation pattern. Please note Chaps. 20 and 21 areas of GGO with or without reticulation. Mixed infiltrative and obstructive diseases (hypersensitive pneumonitis, sarcoidosis, atypical infection with associated bronchiolitis) also cause mosaic attenuation pattern.

### Distribution

In cystic fibrosis, proximal or perihilar bronchi are always involved when bronchiectasis is present. All lobes are typically involved, although early in the disease, abnormalities show often predominantly upper lobe predominance in their distribution [3]. Although there are some overlaps, areas of mosaic perfusion in cystic fibrosis correspond to pulmonary lobules or subsegments [4], whereas those in chronic thromboembolism are typically segmental or subsegmental in distribution [5]. In subacute hypersensitivity pneumonitis, areas of GGO are usually diffuse, bilateral, and symmetric. However, areas of mosaic perfusion are multifocal and usually have a configuration consistent with involvement of single or multiple adjacent pulmonary lobules [6].

### Clinical Considerations

Cystic fibrosis results from an autosomal-recessive genetic defect in the structure of the cystic fibrosis transmembrane regulator protein, which leads to abnormal chloride transport across epithelial membranes [7]. ABPA results from both type I and type III hypersensitivity reactions to the endobronchial growth of Aspergillus species and is characteristically associated with eosinophilia, symptoms of asthma, and typical imaging findings [8]. Conditions associated with constrictive bronchiolitis include heart–lung or lung transplantation, chronic allograft rejection, allogeneic bone marrow transplantation with chronic graft-versus-host disease, and collagen vascular disease, especially rheumatoid arthritis [9]. Pulmonary arterial hypertension may be idiopathic or arise in association with chronic pulmonary thromboembolism; pulmonary embolism caused by tumor cells, parasitic material, or foreign material; parenchymal lung disease; liver disease; vasculitis; human immunodeficiency virus infection; or a left-to-right cardiac shunt [5]. Most cases of hypersensitivity pneumonitis develop only after many years of inhaling allergens, which include microbes, animal or plant proteins, and certain chemicals [10].

K.S. Lee et al., *Radiology Illustrated: Chest Radiology*, Radiology Illustrated,
DOI 10.1007/978-3-642-37096-0_13, © Springer-Verlag Berlin Heidelberg 2014

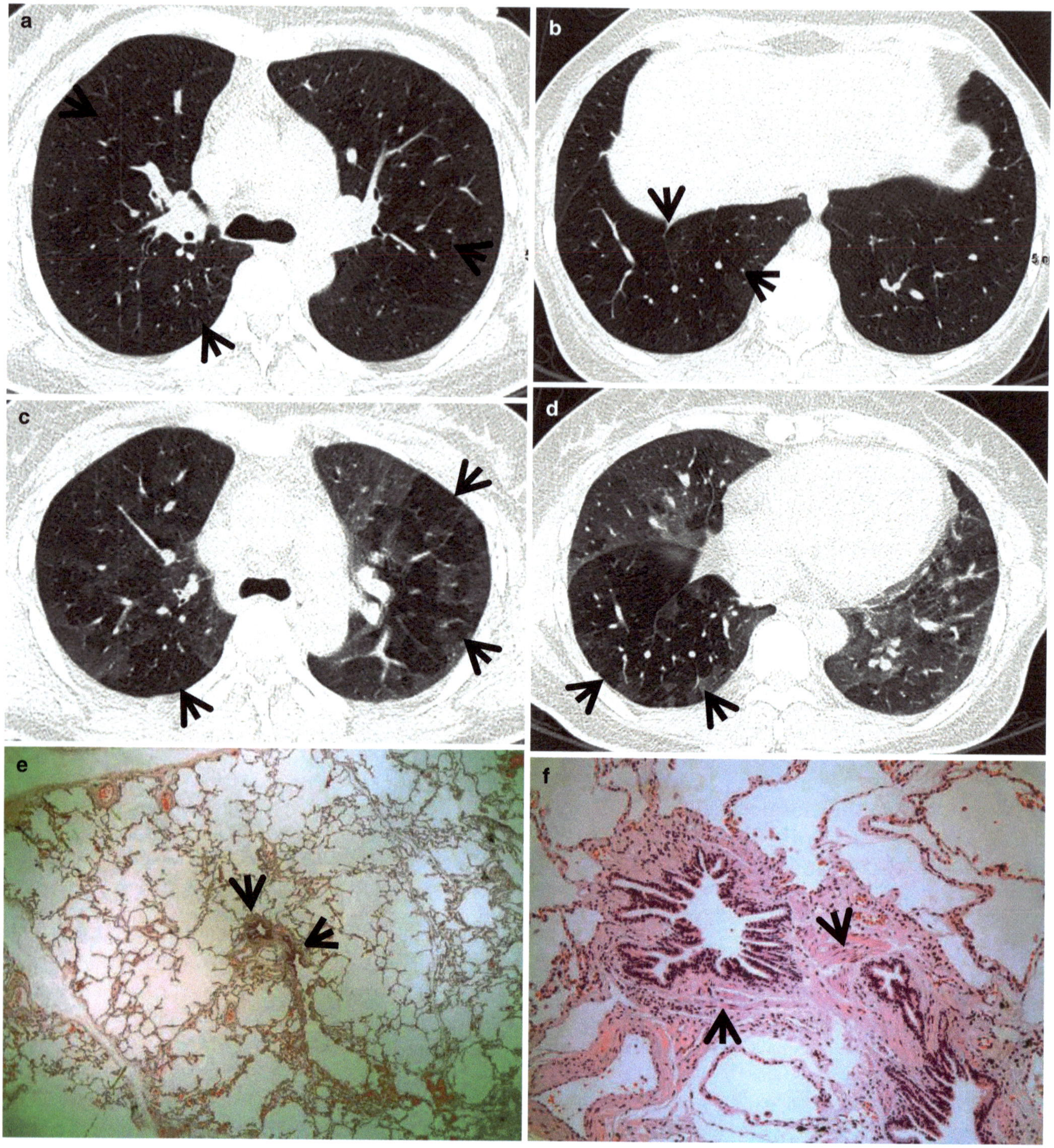


**Fig. 13.1** Constrictive bronchiolitis in a 45-year-old woman. (**a**, **b**) Lung window images of thin-section (1.5-mm section thickness) CT scans obtained at levels of main bronchi (**a**) and liver dome (**b**), respectively, show patchy areas of mosaic perfusion (*arrows*) in both lungs. (**c**, **d**) Expiratory CT scans obtained at similar levels to (**a**, **c**) and (**b**, **d**), respectively, demonstrate air trapping (*arrows*) more clearly in both lungs. (**e**) Low-magnification (×40) photomicrograph of pathologic specimen obtained with surgical lung biopsy displays bronchiolar collagen-type fibrosis inducing luminal narrowing (*arrows*) of a membranous bronchiole. (**f**) High-magnification photomicrograph (×200) discloses fibrous thickening of lamina propria between epithelium and muscularis mucosa (*arrows*)

**Key Points for Differential Diagnosis**

1. Regardless of its cause, when mosaic perfusion is present, pulmonary vessels in the areas of decreased opacity often appear smaller than vessels in relatively dense areas of the lung [11, 12]. This discrepancy can be quite helpful in distinguishing mosaic perfusion from patchy appearance of GGO. In patients with GGO, vessels usually appear equal in size throughout the lungs.
2. In patients with mosaic perfusion resulting from airway diseases, abnormally dilated or thick-walled airways may be visible in the relatively lucent lung regions [2], and lobular areas of low attenuation are common [13]. Air trapping on expiratory scans is often helpful in confirming the diagnosis. Attenuation differences are accentuated scans obtained on expiration [14].
3. In patients with mosaic perfusion resulting from vascular diseases, areas of low attenuation are usually larger than lobules. In patients with mosaic perfusion occurring in association with chronic pulmonary embolism or pulmonary arterial hypertension, enlargement of the main pulmonary arteries may be visible.

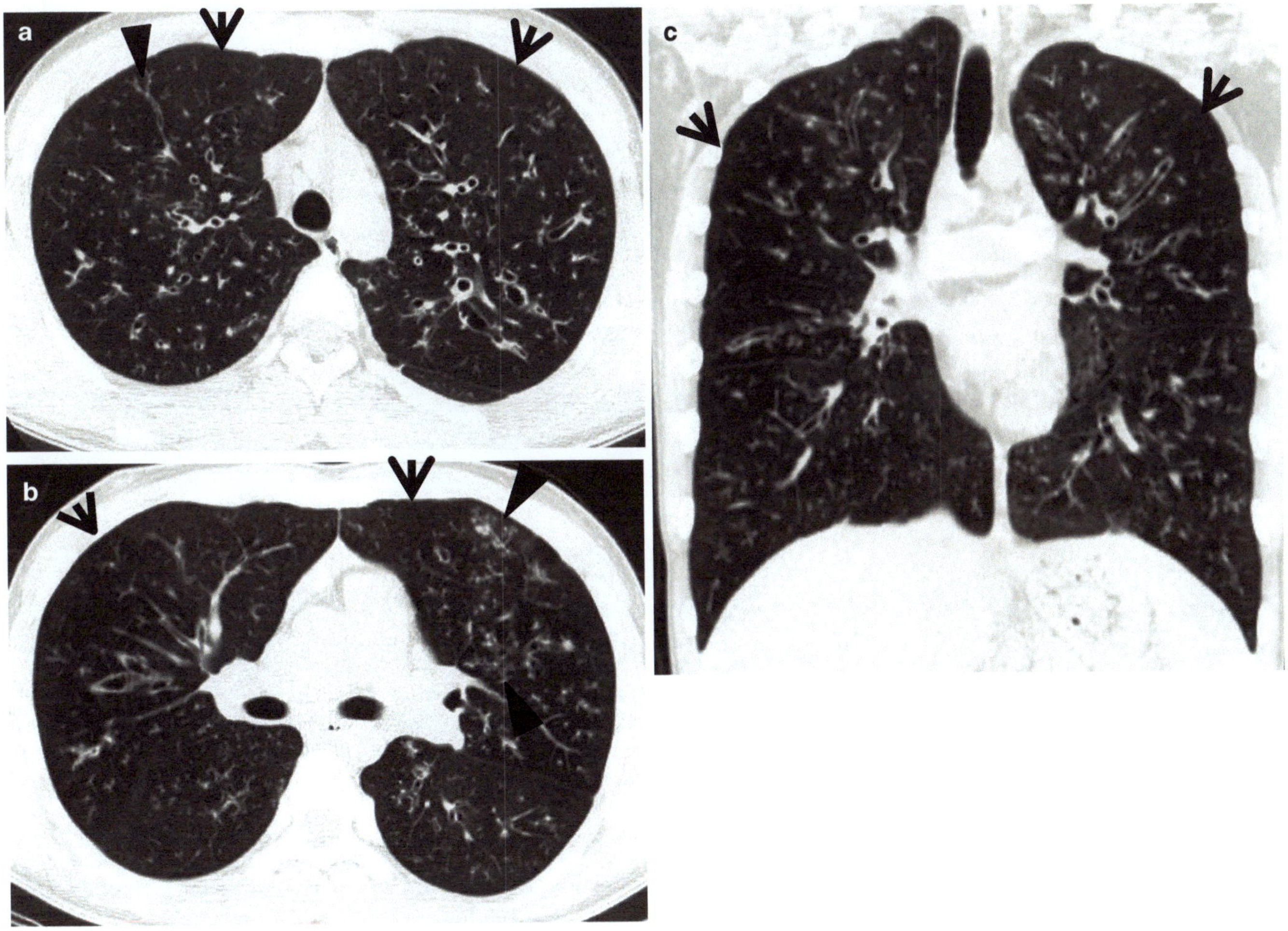


**Fig. 13.2** Cystic fibrosis in a 24-year-old man who underwent lung transplantation. (**a**, **b**) Lung window images of thin-section (2.5-mm section thickness) CT scans obtained at levels of aortic arch (**a**) and main bronchi (**b**), respectively, show extensive areas of bronchiectasis and cellular bronchiolitis (*arrowheads*) in both lungs. Also note bilateral patchy areas of mosaic attenuation (*arrows*). (**c**) Coronal reformatted CT image (2.0-mm section thickness) demonstrates bronchiectasis and cellular bronchiolitis in both lungs. Also note patchy areas of mosaic attenuation (*arrows*), in which oligemia (decreased caliber of vessels) findings are clearly visualized. (**d**) Gross pathology and photomicrographs at corresponding area indicated by bars of explanted lungs disclose pus in bronchiectatic or bronchiolectatic airways. In a portion of right lung, airway wall fibrosis and resultant postobstructive airway dilatation are seen (*open arrows*)

d

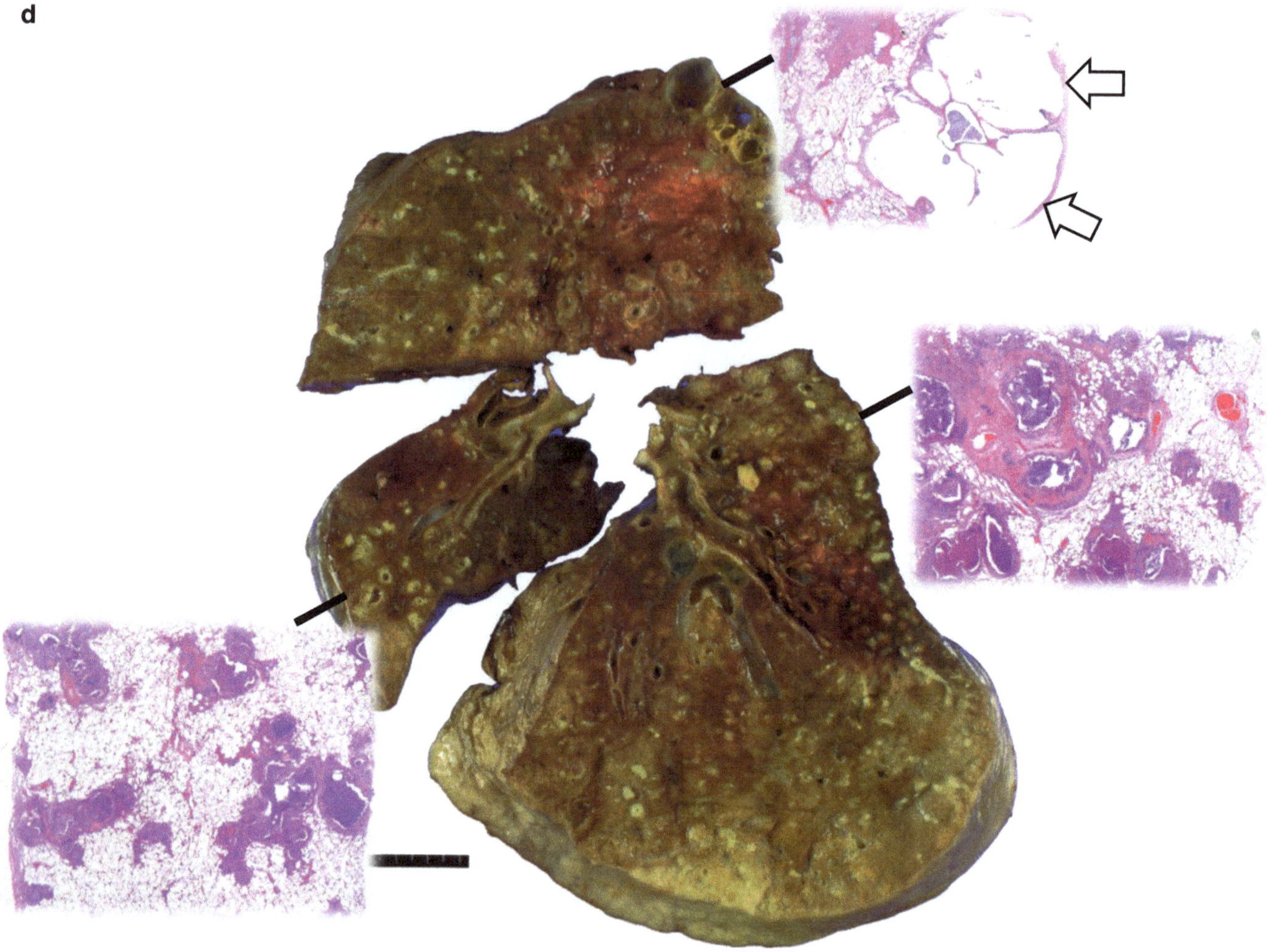

Fig. 13.2 (continued)

4. Characteristic CT vascular signs including webs or bands, intimal irregularities, abrupt narrowing, or complete obstruction of the pulmonary arteries with enlarged main pulmonary arteries enable the diagnosis of chronic pulmonary thromboembolism in patients with mosaic perfusion [15].
5. Data from electrocardiographically (ECG)-gated multidetector CT studies show that functional parameters such as right pulmonary artery distensibility, systolic–diastolic right ventricular outflow tract dimensions, and diastolic wall thickness can be measured with good interobserver agreement and used as reliable criteria for a diagnosis of pulmonary hypertension [16]. Mosaic lung perfusion is found significantly more often among those with pulmonary arterial hypertension due to vascular disease than among those with pulmonary arterial hypertension due to cardiac or lung disease (74 % [17 of 23] vs. 8 % [3 of 38] of the patients in one series) [17].
6. The head-cheese sign is usually indicative of mixed infiltrative and obstructive disease, usually associated with bronchiolitis. In patients with this appearance, the presence of GGO is caused by lung infiltration, whereas the presence of mosaic perfusion with decreased vessels sign is usually caused by small airway disease. The combination of GGO on inspiratory scans and air trapping on expiratory scans is considered indicative of a mixed infiltrative and obstructive disease such as hypersensitivity pneumonitis [14].

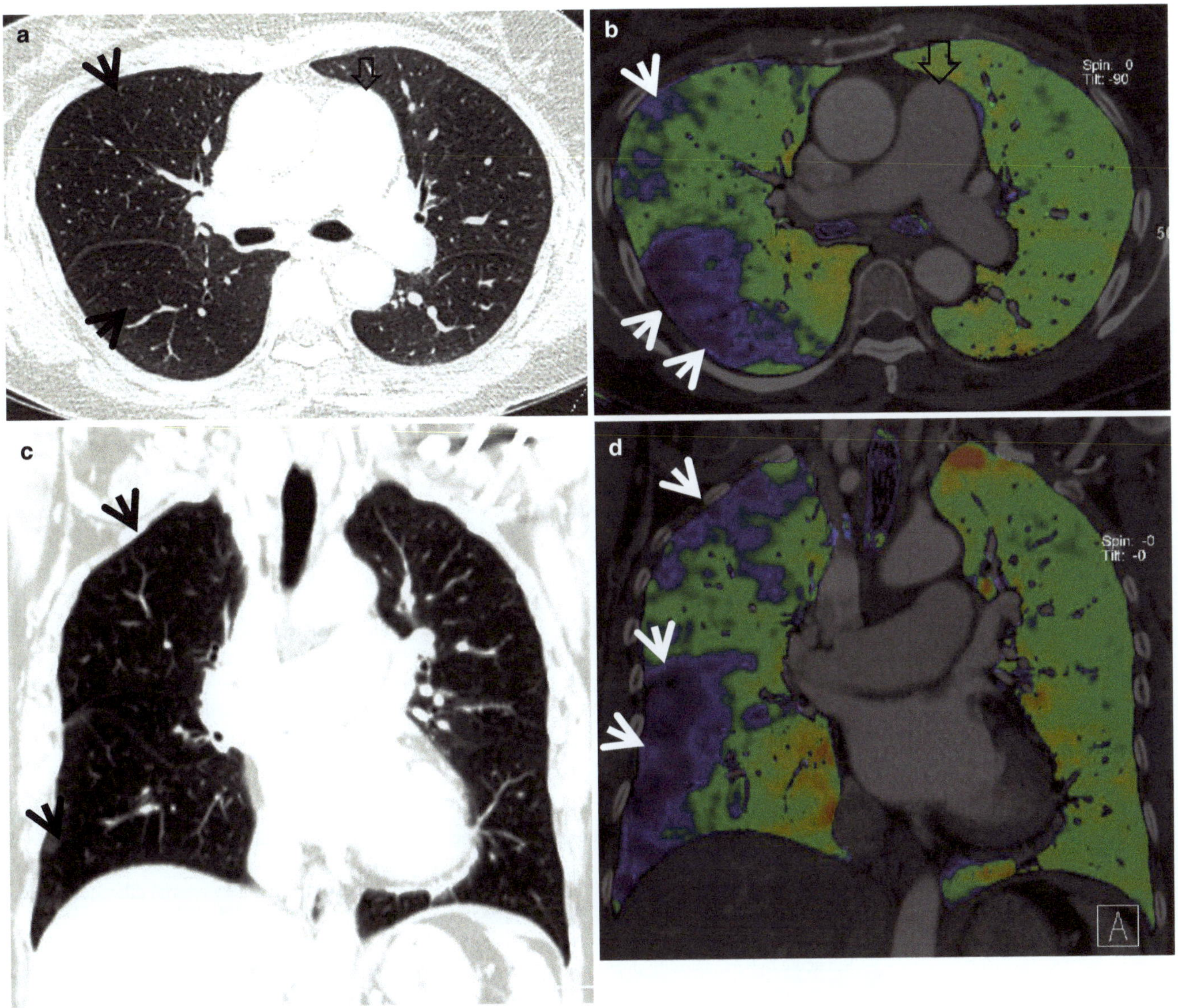


**Fig. 13.3** Mosaic perfusion in a 58-year-old woman with chronic thromboembolism and pulmonary arterial hypertension. (**a**) Lung window image of CT scan (1.0-mm section thickness) obtained at level of main bronchi shows mosaic attenuation areas (*arrows*) in right lung. Also note markedly enlarged main pulmonary artery. (**b**) Iodine perfusion map obtained with dual-source dual-energy CT clearly demonstrates areas of mosaic perfusion (*arrows*, *blue-colored areas*). (**c**) Coronal reformatted image (2.0-mm section thickness) shows multifocal areas (*arrows*) of mosaic attenuation. (**d**) Iodine perfusion map depicts more clearly mosaic perfusion areas (*arrows*)

## Cystic Fibrosis

### Pathology and Pathogenesis

Cystic fibrosis is an autosomal-recessive disease with a mutation of cystic fibrosis transmembrane conductance regulator (CFTR) gene and multisystem involvement. Patients have abnormal transport of chloride and sodium across the respiratory epithelium, resulting in thickened airway secretions and susceptibility to recurrent infections. Grossly, widespread bronchiectasis (more severe in upper lobe) with thick mucus plugs, pleural fibrosis or adhesions, pneumonic consolidation, and lobar atelectasis are seen in an end-stage disease (Fig. 13.2). Microscopically, acute and chronic inflammations involving the large and small airways associated with bronchial gland and goblet cell hyperplasia, squamous metaplasia, and mucostasis are frequently seen (Fig. 13.2).

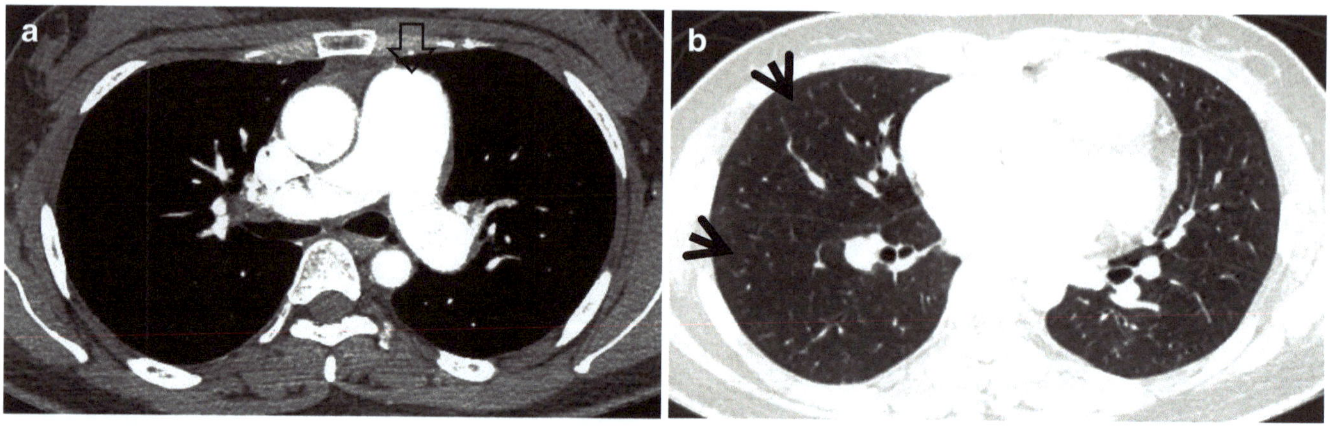


Fig. 13.4 Mosaic perfusion in a 28-year-old woman with idiopathic pulmonary arterial hypertension. (**a**) Mediastinal window image of enhanced CT (1.0-mm section thickness) scan obtained at level of main bronchi shows markedly enlarged main pulmonary artery (*open arrow*). (**b**) Lung window image obtained at level of right inferior pulmonary vein demonstrates suspicious areas of mosaic attenuation (*arrows*)

Table 13.1 Common diseases manifesting as mosaic attenuation

| Disease | Key points for differential diagnosis |
|---|---|
| Airway disease | |
| Bronchiectasis | Bronchial dilatation with peribronchial thickening, signet ring sign |
| Cystic fibrosis | Mosaic perfusion, bronchiectasis involving upper lobes |
| ABPA | Central bronchiectasis with high-attenuation mucus plugging, mosaic perfusion |
| Asthma | Thickening and narrowing of the medium-sized and small bronchi, cylindrical bronchiectasis, centrilobular nodules, multifocal and patchy areas of mosaic perfusion |
| Constrictive bronchiolitis | Mosaic perfusion, air trapping on expiratory scans |
| Vascular disease | |
| Chronic pulmonary thromboembolism | Mosaic perfusion, ipsilateral airway dilatation, vascular findings of chronic embolism |
| Pulmonary arterial hypertension | Mosaic perfusion, central pulmonary arterial dilatation in the absence of detectable intraluminal thrombi |
| Mixed infiltrative and obstructive disease | |
| Subacute hypersensitivity pneumonitis | Combination of GGO on inspiratory scan and air trapping on expiratory scan |
| Sarcoidosis | Associated with perilymphatic micronodules |
| Atypical pneumonia with bronchiolitis | Patchy areas of GGO and centrilobular nodules, mosaic perfusion |

*Note*: *ABPA* allergic bronchopulmonary aspergillosis, *GGO* ground-glass opacity

## Symptoms and Signs

Since cystic fibrosis is a genetic disease resulting in complications in multiple organs, especially involving the lungs and pancreas, it mimics a number of other diseases. Usual respiratory presentations in adults include cough, sputum, wheezing, dyspnea, recurrent respiratory tract infection, and cor pulmonale if advanced. Usual gastrointestinal presentations in adults are recurrent abdominal pain, biliary cirrhosis with portal hypertension, and recurrent pancreatitis. Infertility may occur.

## CT Findings

The predominant HRCT finding in early stage of cystic fibrosis is a mosaic perfusion due to air trapping related to small airway disease. Other typical CT features include bronchiectasis and peribronchial thickening, mainly involving the upper lobes, and centrilobular nodules or a tree-in-bud pattern and atelectasis or consolidation secondary to mucous plugging [3, 18] (Fig. 13.2). Bronchiectasis is most often cylindrical, but varicose and cystic bronchiectasis can be seen in advanced cases.

## CT–Pathology Comparisons

Cystic fibrosis causes abnormal mucous gland secretions and the subsequent effect of inflammation and infection on airways [3]. The earliest and most universal pathologic lesion of cystic fibrosis is mucous obstruction of bronchioles and small bronchi (Fig. 13.2). A mosaic perfusion, which is the predominant early HRCT findings of cystic fibrosis, is caused by air trapping related to mucous obstruction and inflammation of bronchioles and small bronchi (Fig. 13.2). The elicited inflammatory response damages the normal structure of the airways, and bronchiectasis develops. Upper lobe predominance of bronchiectasis and peribronchial thickening may reflect an effect of gravity on the elastin-damaged parenchymal tissue. Obstruction of airways by mucous plugs results in centrilobular small nodules or a tree-in-bud pattern and atelectasis or consolidation on HRCT.

## Patient Prognosis

Treatment consists of control of mucus retention and chronic infection in the lungs, replacement of pancreatic enzymes, and nutritional therapy. New therapeutic approaches, including pharmacologic interventions and gene transfer, offer hope for further advances [19]. Lung transplantation has become an accepted therapy for respiratory failure secondary to cystic fibrosis. The outcome is highly variable, but 50 % of patients can now be expected to survive beyond 37 years.

# Constrictive Bronchiolitis

## Pathology and Pathogenesis

Constrictive bronchiolitis is a small airway disease in which variable narrowing or obliteration of airway lumens occurs. Histologically, the disease shows submucosal scarring, concentric luminal narrowing, adventitial scarring, and chronic inflammation. In the late stage, the lumen is completely occluded by the fibrosis (Fig. 13.1).

## Symptoms and Signs

Clinically, constrictive bronchiolitis is characterized by progressive airflow obstruction with poor responsiveness to medical therapy and high mortality rates [20]. Patients complain of cough and dyspnea, which progress relentlessly over weeks to months. Physical examination reveals inspiratory squeaks in 40–60 % of patients.

## CT Findings

The main HRCT findings usually consist of areas of mosaic perfusion associated with vessels of decreased caliber on inspiratory scans and air trapping on expiratory scans [21]. Air trapping on expiratory HRCT is the most sensitive sign to detect constrictive bronchiolitis on HRCT [22] (Fig. 13.1). Central and peripheral bronchiectasis is also commonly present. Other findings include centrilobular small nodules and tree-in-bud patterns.

## CT–Pathology Comparisons

Mosaic perfusion on HRCT is presumably caused by hypoventilation of the alveoli distal to the bronchial obstruction, which leads to secondary vasoconstriction. This vasoconstriction can be seen on CT scans as areas of decreased attenuation [23] (Fig. 13.1). Bronchiectasis may be secondary to the constrictive bronchiolitis itself or to a prior insult to the bronchial wall. Centrilobular small nodules and tree-in-bud patterns on HRCT are caused by peribronchiolar thickening and bronchiolectasis with secretions [24].

## Patient Prognosis

Prognosis of constrictive bronchiolitis, irrespective of etiology, is poor. Most patients progressively deteriorate and are ultimately fatal due to respiratory failure within months to years. Macrolide antibiotics exhibit immunomodulatory effects and have been used.

# Chronic Pulmonary Thromboembolism

## Pathology and Pathogenesis

Chronic pulmonary thromboembolism (PE) causes pulmonary hypertension secondary to obstruction of arteries due to organized thrombi. In the lung of chronic PE, distended capillaries, multifocal microscopic foci of alveolar wall necrosis with focal inflammation, small amount of fibrinous exudate, and edema fluid can be seen. Variable amount of bronchopneumonia may be accompanied.

## Symptoms and Signs

Patients with chronic PE typically present with nonspecific symptoms occurring in those with other causes of pulmonary hypertension [25]. The symptoms include progressive dyspnea on exertion, chronic fatigue, chest discomfort, palpitations, or syncope. Cardiac murmur may be heard. Lower extremity edema, ascites, hepatomegaly, and cyanosis can be found.

### CT Findings

The most common pulmonary parenchymal finding of chronic PE is a mosaic perfusion pattern (combination of areas of decreased attenuation and perfusion adjacent to areas of increased attenuation and perfusion) [15] (Fig. 13.3). Mosaic perfusion patterns are typically distributed in segmental and subsegmental patterns [26]. Chronic PE may also be associated with ipsilateral airway dilatation [27]. Vascular findings of chronic PE include webs or bands, intimal irregularities, abrupt narrowing or complete obstruction of pulmonary arteries, and enlargement of main pulmonary artery [15].

### CT–Pathology Comparisons

The areas of decreased attenuation and vascularity on HRCT correspond to the lung distal to partially or completely occluded vessels, whereas the areas of increased attenuation and vascularity are the result of blood flow redistribution to the normal lung. It has been postulated that airway dilatation is secondary to retraction of fibrous tissue within the vascular lumen [27].

### Patient Prognosis

Historical data indicate that chronic PE, if left untreated, is associated with a poor 5-year survival, ranging from 10 to 40 % [25]. Patients should receive lifelong anticoagulation therapy. Pulmonary thromboendarterectomy is the procedure of choice in symptomatic patients with chronic PE. The overall perioperative mortality rates at experienced centers range from 4 to 7 %. Pulmonary thromboendarterectomy has improved the 6-year survival rate up to 75 %.

## Idiopathic Pulmonary Arterial Hypertension

### Pathology and Pathogenesis

Medial hypertrophy and concentric or eccentric intimal fibrosis of the pulmonary arteries (muscular arteries) are seen in all forms of pulmonary hypertension [28].

### Symptoms and Signs

The most common presenting symptom in patients with pulmonary arterial hypertension is dyspnea on exertion [29]. Other common complaints include fatigue, lack of energy, chest pain, syncope, palpitations, and lower extremity edema. On auscultation, an accentuated pulmonic component of S2 is present in most patients with pulmonary arterial hypertension.

### CT Findings

Characteristic vascular features of idiopathic pulmonary arterial hypertension on CT are central pulmonary artery dilatation, usually in the absence of detectable intraluminal thrombi, small tortuous peripheral vessels representing plexogenic arteriopathy, and an abrupt decrease in the caliber of segmental and subsegmental arteries [5]. Additional CT findings include right heart enlargement, pericardial effusion, and mosaic perfusion pattern in lung parenchyma (Fig. 13.4). Mosaic perfusion pattern in idiopathic pulmonary arterial hypertension is characterized by focal perivascular hyper-attenuating areas in a peripheral or perihilar distribution or small, scattered, well-defined areas of low attenuation corresponding to the anatomic unit of a secondary pulmonary lobule with adjacent areas of increased attenuation in a patchy and diffuse distribution [30]. Dilatation of bronchial and nonbronchial systemic arteries is less commonly seen than in pulmonary hypertension due to chronic PE.

### CT–Pathology Comparisons

Central pulmonary artery enlargement on CT is associated with wall thickening of elastic and large muscular arteries along with their luminal dilatation. Thickening is predominantly the result of intimal fibrosis in the larger vessels and a combination of intimal fibrosis and medial muscle hypertrophy and hyperplasia in the smaller muscular branches. In large dilated vessels, atherosclerotic plaques, sometimes complicated by calcification, also may be seen.

The plexogenic pulmonary arteriopathy is seen in the muscular pulmonary arteries, most characteristic of which is a plexiform lesion referring to localized focus of vascular dilatation associated with an intraluminal plexus of slit-like vascular channels separated by a variable number of fibroblast-like cells. The lesion is noted in a short distance beyond the origin of a small supernumerary branch (usually 100–200 um in diameter). Additional pathology in plexogenic arteriopathy is the presence of arterial intimal fibrous tissue with a solid appearance and being distributed in a more or less concentric fashion in the vessel lumen. Occasionally, the intimal fibrosis is eccentric in location or traverses the lumen. The plexogenic arteriopathy is thought to be related to the vascular pruning (central arterial enlargement, peripheral vascular obliteration, and mosaic perfusion).

## Patient Prognosis

With advances in knowledge of the disease and the availability of newer therapeutic agents, such as endothelin receptor antagonists, phosphodiesterase inhibitors, and prostanoids, survival of patients with idiopathic pulmonary arterial hypertension has improved but still remains suboptimal. The French Registry demonstrated that 1-, 2-, and 3-year survivals of pulmonary arterial hypertension are 85.7, 69.5, and 54.9 % for incident cases, respectively [31].

# Airway Disease (Bronchiectasis and Bronchiolectasis)

## Definition

Bronchiectasis is irreversible localized or diffuse bronchial dilatation, usually resulting from chronic infection, proximal airway obstruction, or congenital bronchial abnormality [1, 32] (Fig. 13.5). Morphologic criteria on thin-section CT scans include bronchial dilatation with respect to the accompanying pulmonary artery (signet ring sign), lack of tapering of bronchi, and identification of bronchi within 1 cm of the pleural surface [33] (Fig. 13.5). Bronchiectasis may be classified as cylindric, varicose, or cystic, depending on the appearance of the affected bronchi. It is often accompanied by bronchial wall thickening, mucoid impaction (please note Chap. 10), and small airway abnormalities [33].

Bronchiolectasis is defined as dilatation of bronchioles. When dilated bronchioles are filled with exudates and are thick walled, they are visible as a tree-in-bud pattern or as centrilobular nodules on CT [34].

Traction bronchiectasis and bronchiolectasis, respectively, represent irregular bronchial and bronchiolar dilatation caused by surrounding retractile pulmonary fibrosis [35].

## Diseases Causing the Bronchiectasis and Bronchiolectasis

Bronchiectasis can result from chronic or severe bacterial infection (*Staphylococcus*, *Klebsiella*, *Mycobacterium tuberculosis*, nontuberculous mycobacterial disease), fungal (histoplasmosis) infection, and viral (Swyer-James-MacLeod syndrome, HIV infection) infection (Fig. 13.6). Bronchiectasis may occur in association with a variety of genetic abnormalities, especially those with abnormal mucociliary clearance, immune deficiency, or structural abnormalities of the bronchus or bronchial wall (cystic fibrosis, alpha-1-antitrypsin deficiency, *dyskinetic cilia syndrome* (Fig. 13.7), Williams–Campbell syndrome, Mounier–Kuhn syndrome, immunodeficiency syndromes). Noninfectious causes of bronchiectasis include allergic bronchopulmonary aspergillosis (ABPA); asthma, bronchial obstruction by tumor, foreign body, or congenital abnormalities; and systemic diseases (collagen vascular disease and inflammatory bowel disease). Bronchiectasis may also occur in patients with constrictive bronchiolitis including chronic graft-versus-host disease (Table 13.2). Bronchiolectasis is usually associated with bronchiolitis (please refer to section "Small Nodules with Centrilobular Distribution" in Chap. 18). In patients with lung fibrosis (usual interstitial pneumonia, nonspecific interstitial pneumonia) and distortion of lung architecture (pulmonary tuberculosis), traction bronchiectasis and bronchiolectasis are commonly present.

## Distribution

Bronchiectasis as sequelae of pulmonary tuberculosis typically involves upper lobes [36]. In nodular bronchiectatic form of nontuberculous mycobacterial disease, bronchiectasis usually involves the right middle lobe, lingular division of the left upper lobe, and both lower lobes. In cystic fibrosis, proximal or perihilar bronchia are always involved when bronchiectasis is present. All lobes are typically involved, although early in the disease, abnormalities show often predominantly upper lobe predominance in their distribution [3]. Although central or diffuse bilateral bronchiectasis is common in patients with dyskinetic cilia syndrome, bronchiectasis involves predominantly or exclusively the lower lobes [37]. In Williams–Campbell syndrome, varicose and cystic bronchiectases are limited to the fourth-, fifth-, and sixth-generation bronchi [38]. ABPA typically involves segmental and subsegmental bronchi of the upper lobes.

## Clinical Considerations

Cystic fibrosis results from an autosomal-recessive genetic defect in the structure of the cystic fibrosis transmembrane regulator protein, which leads to abnormal chloride transport across epithelial membranes [7]. The major clinical manifestations of cystic fibrosis are obstructive pulmonary disease and pancreatic insufficiency. Dyskinetic cilia syndrome is a group of autosomal-recessive disorders associated with defective ciliary structure and function and

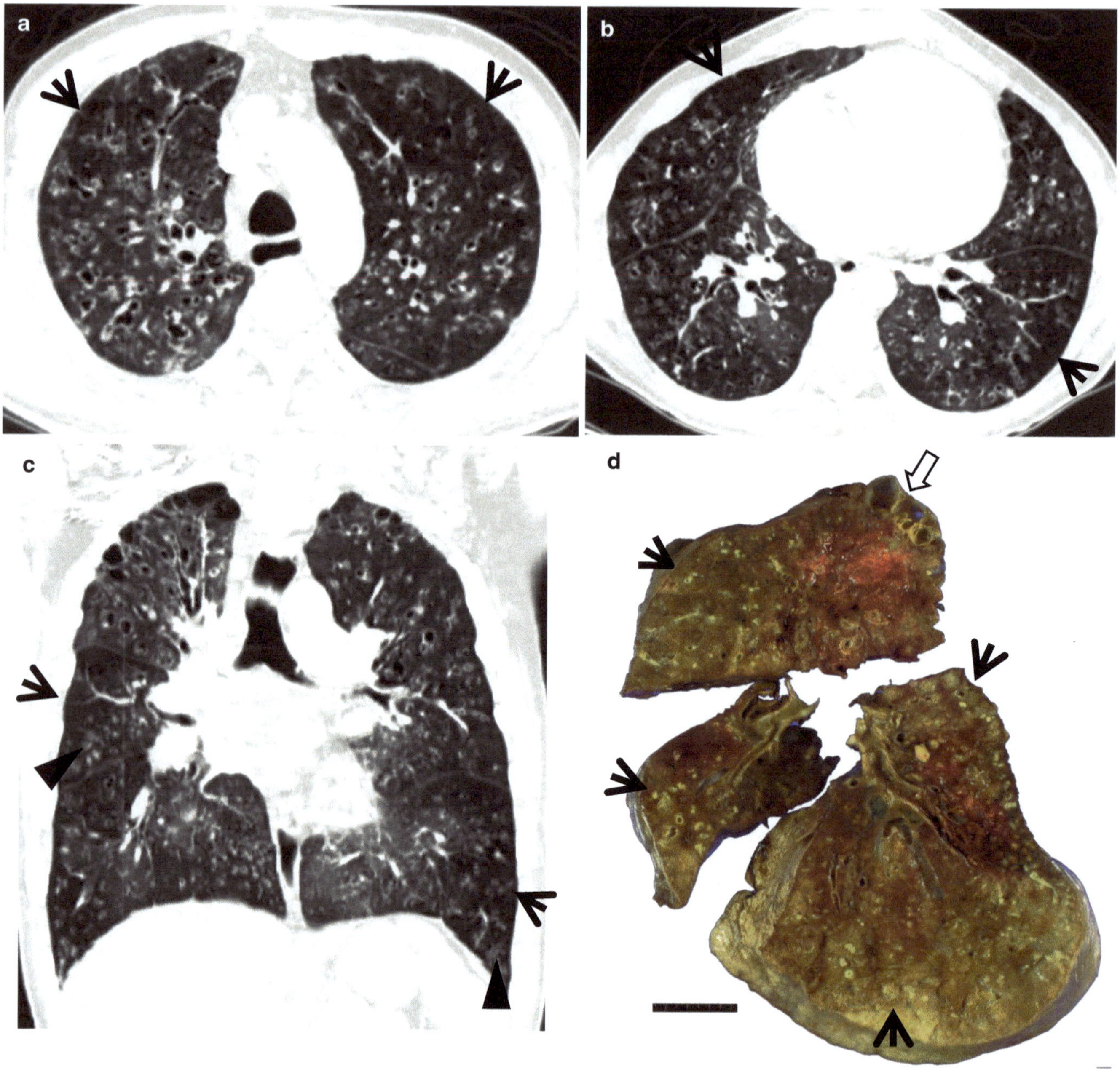


**Fig. 13.5** Extensive bronchiectasis in both lungs in a 44-year-old man in whom specific causes for bronchiectasis could not be elucidated. Patient received bilateral lung transplantation. (**a**, **b**) Lung window images of CT scans (2.5-mm section thickness) obtained at levels of aortic arch (**a**) and basal segmental bronchi (**b**), respectively, show extensive bronchiectasis in both lungs. Also note patchy areas (*arrows*) of mosaic attenuation. (**c**) Coronal reformatted CT image (2.0-mm section thickness) demonstrates extensive bronchiectasis and cellular bronchiolitis of tree-in-bud signs (*arrowheads*) in both lungs. Also note patchy areas (*arrows*) of mosaic attenuation. (**d**) Gross pathologic specimen of explanted right lung discloses bronchiectatic and bronchiolectatic airways filled with abscess (numerous yellow necrotic nodules, *arrows*) down to membranous bronchiolar level. Also note bullae (*open arrow*) in right upper lobe

predispose to sinusitis, recurrent pulmonary infections, and bronchiectasis [39]. Situs inversus totalis or heterotaxy is seen in approximately 50 % of patients. Williams–Campbell syndrome is a congenital form of bronchiectasis usually identified in infancy. It shows familial clustering and may be associated with other congenital abnormalities [40]. ABPA results from both type I and type III hypersensitivity reactions to the endobronchial growth of *Aspergillus* species and is characteristically associated with eosinophilia, symptoms of asthma, and typical imaging findings [8]. It is seen almost exclusively in patients with asthma or cystic fibrosis.

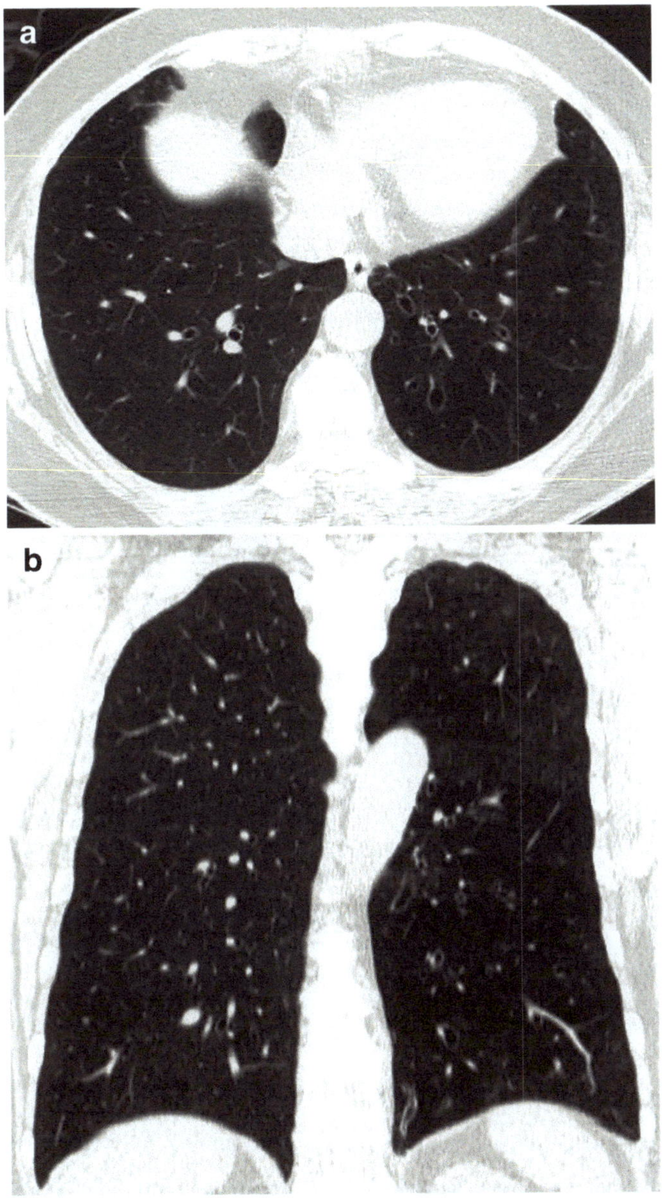

Fig. 13.6 Swyer-James-MacLeod syndrome in a 71-year-old woman. (a) Lung window images of CT scans (2.5-mm section thickness) obtained at level of liver dome show bronchiectasis in left lower lobe. Also note mosaic attenuation in bronchiectatic left lower lobe. (b) Coronal reformatted image (2.0-mm section thickness) demonstrates bronchiectasis exclusively in left lung. Also note decreased lung attenuation in left lung

**Key Points for Differential Diagnosis**

1. Reported diagnostic accuracy of HRCT in predicting specific etiologies of bronchiectasis range from 35 to 61 % [41, 42]. In a study, correct diagnosis was reached in 68 % of cases in cystic fibrosis, 67 % of cases in tuberculosis, and 56 % of cases in ABPA [42]. In this study, a bilateral upper lobe distribution was most commonly seen in patients with cystic fibrosis (76 %) and ABPA (56 %), whereas unilateral upper lobe distribution was most common in patients with tuberculosis, and a lower lobe distribution was most often seen in patients after childhood viral infections.
2. HRCT findings of bronchiectasis and bronchiolitis involving more than five lobes, especially when associated with lobular consolidation or a cavity, are highly suggestive of nontuberculous mycobacterial pulmonary disease [43].
3. In addition to bronchiectasis, Swyer-James-MacLeod syndrome is characterized by a hyperlucent lung or lobe, decreased vascularity, and normal or decreased size of the involved lung or lobe on inspiratory images and air trapping on expiratory images [44].
4. Except for Kartagener's syndrome (situs inversus, sinusitis, bronchiectasis), the imaging findings of dyskinetic cilia syndrome are nonspecific.
5. The characteristic HRCT findings of ABPA consist of bronchiectasis and mucoid impaction involving mainly the segmental and subsegmental bronchi of the upper lobes. Although these findings are characteristic features of ABPA, the sensitivity of central bronchiectasis proved to be only 37 % in diagnosing ABPA [37]. In 30 % of patients, the mucoid impaction has high attenuation on CT [45].
6. Characteristic features of traction bronchiectasis are dilatation and beading of the bronchi within areas of fibrosis. In patients with honeycombing, traction bronchiolectasis appears as a cyst on HRCT [46].

## Swyer-James-MacLeod Syndrome

### Pathology and Pathogenesis

Swyer-James-MacLeod syndrome is a peculiar postinfectious constrictive bronchiolitis that usually affects the lung asymmetrically [47].

### Symptoms and Signs

Patients with Swyer-James-MacLeod syndrome frequently have a history of recurrent pulmonary infection and present with nonspecific respiratory symptoms, such as dyspnea on exertion, productive cough, and shortness of breath.

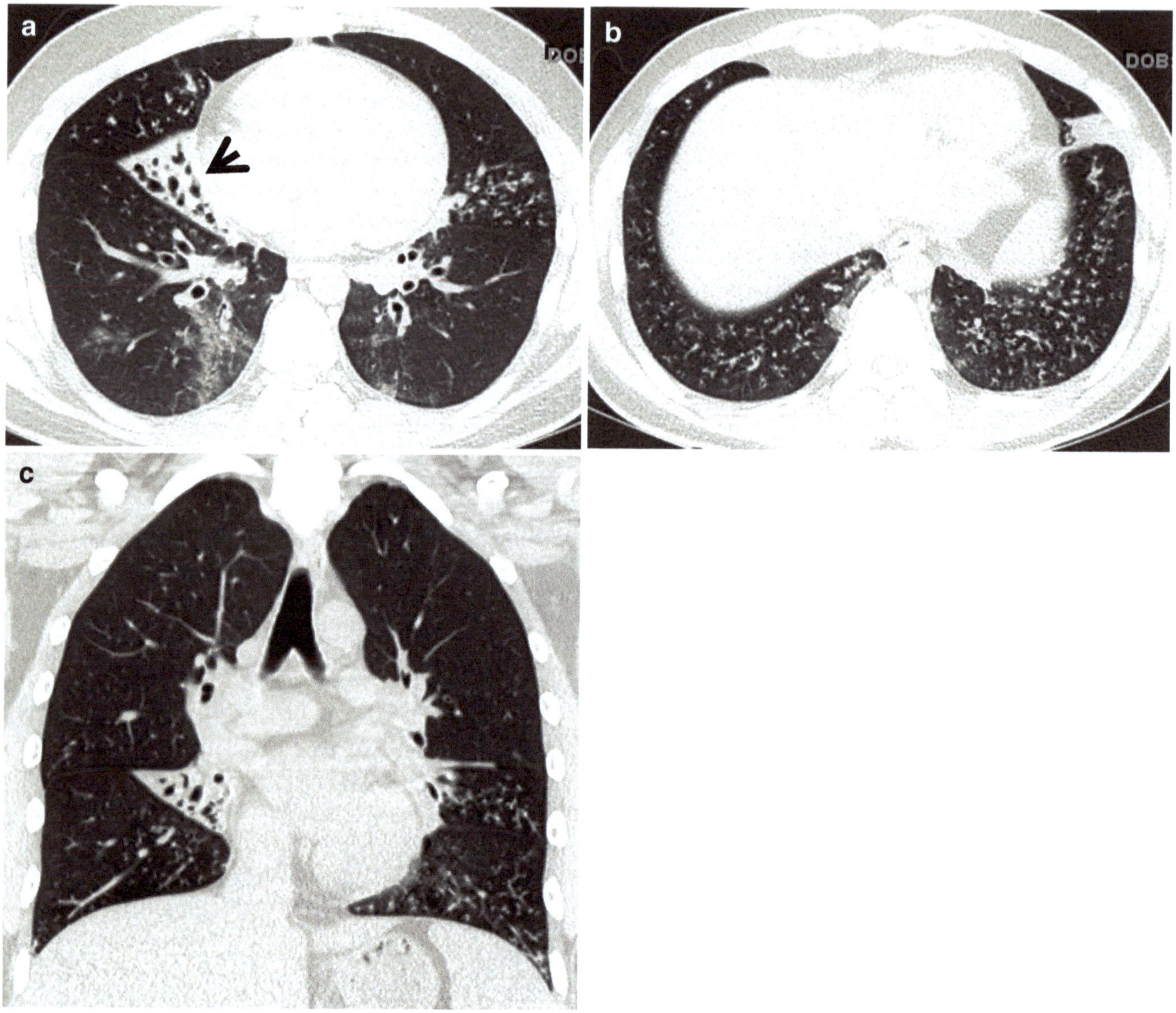


**Fig. 13.7** Ciliary dyskinesia syndrome in a 20-year-old man. (**a**, **b**) Lung window images of CT scans (2.5-mm section thickness) obtained at levels of basal segmental bronchi (**a**) and liver dome (**b**), respectively, show extensive bronchiectasis in right middle lobe (*arrow* in **a**), cellular bronchiolitis of tree-in-bud signs in both lungs, and patchy parenchymal opacity areas in both lower lobes. (**c**) Coronal reformatted image (2.0-mm section thickness) demonstrates bronchiectasis exclusively in right middle lobe and cellular bronchiolitis of tree-in-bud pattern in lower lung zones, bilaterally. Abnormal cilia were seen in nasal mucosal examination on electron microscopy (not shown here)

## CT Findings

The universal chest CT findings of Swyer-James-MacLeod syndrome are unilateral pulmonary hyperlucency and expiratory air trapping [48]. Bronchiectasis is seen in 60 % of cases (Fig. 13.6) and clinical features and prognosis of patients with Swyer-James-MacLeod syndrome will depend mainly on the presence or absence of saccular bronchiectasis [48]. Other findings include normal- or small-sized lung, lobar collapse, and bronchiectasis. Patchy areas of air trapping in the contralateral lung are also seen.

## CT–Pathology Comparisons

In Swyer-James-MacLeod syndrome, unilateral hyperlucency of lung results from decreased pulmonary blood flow secondary to obliterative bronchiolitis.

## Patient Prognosis

Unless severe pneumonia is complicated, clinical course of Swyer-James-MacLeod syndrome is relatively good.

**Table 13.2** Common diseases manifesting as bronchiectasis or bronchiolectasis

| Disease | Key points for differential diagnosis |
|---|---|
| Bacterial infection | |
| *Staphylococcus, Klebsiella* | |
| *Mycobacterium tuberculosis* | Bronchiectasis usually involves upper lobes |
| Nontuberculous mycobacterial disease | Bronchiectasis and bronchiolitis involving more than five lobes, especially when associated with lobular consolidation or a cavity |
| Viral infection | |
| Swyer-James-MacLeod syndrome | Unilateral pulmonary hyperlucency and expiratory air trapping |
| HIV infection | |
| Fungal (histoplasmosis) infection | |
| Genetic abnormalities | |
| Cystic fibrosis | Mosaic perfusion, bronchiectasis involving upper lobes |
| Alpha-1-antitrypsin deficiency | Associated with panacinar emphysema |
| Dyskinetic cilia syndrome | Central and diffuse bilateral bronchiectasis |
| Williams–Campbell syndrome | Varicose and cystic bronchiectasis are limited to the fourth-, fifth-, and sixth-generation bronchi |
| Mounier–Kuhn syndrome | |
| Immunodeficiency syndromes | |
| Noninfectious causes | |
| ABPA | Bronchiectasis involving segmental and subsegmental bronchi of the upper lobes. |
| Asthma | Thickening and narrowing of the medium-sized and small bronchi, cylindrical bronchiectasis, centrilobular nodules, multifocal and patchy areas of mosaic perfusion |
| Bronchial obstruction by tumor, foreign body, or congenital abnormalities | |
| Systemic diseases (collagen vascular disease and inflammatory bowel disease) | |

*Note*: *ABPA* allergic bronchopulmonary aspergillosis

## Dyskinetic Cilia Syndrome

### Pathology and Pathogenesis

The syndrome has been given its firm pathogenetic basis, when it was recognized that in many cases, the respiratory infections were the consequence of a developmental anomaly consisting of a reduced number of ciliary dynein arms. The term "immotile cilia syndrome" is introduced to encompass all patients with a developmental ciliary defect, regardless of their visceral anatomy, but later the term "primary ciliary dyskinesia" is substituted because the cilia show some movement although they do not beat effectively. The condition is inherited as an autosomal recessive with variable penetrance [49].

### Symptoms and Signs

Recurrent upper respiratory tract infection is the main clinical manifestation of early stage of dyskinetic cilia syndrome [50]. When chronic sinusitis and bronchiectasis eventually develop, patients complain of nasal obstruction and chronic production of purulent sputum, with episodes of pneumonia or hemoptysis. Sterility is present in most males due to loss of spermatozoal motility.

### CT Findings

The most common CT findings of dyskinetic cilia syndrome include peribronchial thickening, mucus plugging, bronchiectasis, air trapping, ground-glass opacity, or consolidation [51, 52]. Tree-in-bud patterns also may be seen. Pulmonary lesions in patients with dyskinetic cilia syndrome mainly affect the right middle lobe, the lingula, and the lower lobes. Situs inversus (Kartagener's syndrome) is seen in 50 % of patients (Fig. 13.7). Polysplenia and pectus excavatum are associated findings in approximately 8 % of cases.

### CT–Pathology Comparisons

The structurally abnormal cilia in dyskinetic cilia syndrome move ineffective and offer a condition predisposing to recurrent pulmonary infection and bronchiectasis.

## Patient Prognosis

Although dyskinetic cilia syndrome is not a curable disease, patients with this disorder often have a relatively long life span. Removal of infected secretions from the sinus and bronchial trees and appropriate use of antibiotics is the main therapy for this disorder.

## References

1. Hansell DM, Bankier AA, MacMahon H, McLoud TC, Muller NL, Remy J. Fleischner Society: glossary of terms for thoracic imaging. Radiology. 2008;246:697–722.
2. Worthy SA, Muller NL, Hartman TE, Swensen SJ, Padley SP, Hansell DM. Mosaic attenuation pattern on thin-section CT scans of the lung: differentiation among infiltrative lung, airway, and vascular diseases as a cause. Radiology. 1997;205:465–70.
3. Wood BP. Cystic fibrosis: 1997. Radiology. 1997;204:1–10.
4. Lynch DA, Brasch RC, Hardy KA, Webb WR. Pediatric pulmonary disease: assessment with high-resolution ultrafast CT. Radiology. 1990;176:243–8.
5. Grosse C, Grosse A. CT findings in diseases associated with pulmonary hypertension: a current review. Radiographics. 2010;30:1753–77.
6. Small JH, Flower CD, Traill ZC, Gleeson FV. Air-trapping in extrinsic allergic alveolitis on computed tomography. Clin Radiol. 1996;51:684–8.
7. Stern RC. The diagnosis of cystic fibrosis. N Engl J Med. 1997;336:487–91.
8. Jeong YJ, Kim KI, Seo IJ, et al. Eosinophilic lung diseases: a clinical, radiologic, and pathologic overview. Radiographics. 2007;27:617–37; discussion 637–9.
9. King Jr TE. Overview of bronchiolitis. Clin Chest Med. 1993;14:607–10.
10. Hirschmann JV, Pipavath SN, Godwin JD. Hypersensitivity pneumonitis: a historical, clinical, and radiologic review. Radiographics. 2009;29:1921–38.
11. Webb WR. High-resolution computed tomography of obstructive lung disease. Radiol Clin North Am. 1994;32:745–57.
12. Schwickert HC, Schweden F, Schild HH, et al. Pulmonary arteries and lung parenchyma in chronic pulmonary embolism: preoperative and postoperative CT findings. Radiology. 1994;191:351–7.
13. Im JG, Kim SH, Chung MJ, Koo JM, Han MC. Lobular low attenuation of the lung parenchyma on CT: evaluation of forty-eight patients. J Comput Assist Tomogr. 1996;20:756–62.
14. Arakawa H, Webb WR, McCowin M, Katsou G, Lee KN, Seitz RF. Inhomogeneous lung attenuation at thin-section CT: diagnostic value of expiratory scans. Radiology. 1998;206:89–94.
15. Han D, Lee KS, Franquet T, et al. Thrombotic and nonthrombotic pulmonary arterial embolism: spectrum of imaging findings. Radiographics. 2003;23:1521–39.
16. Revel MP, Faivre JB, Remy-Jardin M, Delannoy-Deken V, Duhamel A, Remy J. Pulmonary hypertension: ECG-gated 64-section CT angiographic evaluation of new functional parameters as diagnostic criteria. Radiology. 2009;250:558–66.
17. Sherrick AD, Swensen SJ, Hartman TE. Mosaic pattern of lung attenuation on CT scans: frequency among patients with pulmonary artery hypertension of different causes. AJR Am J Roentgenol. 1997;169:79–82.
18. Brody AS, Klein JS, Molina PL, Quan J, Bean JA, Wilmott RW. High-resolution computed tomography in young patients with cystic fibrosis: distribution of abnormalities and correlation with pulmonary function tests. J Pediatr. 2004;145:32–8.
19. Mogayzel Jr PJ, Naureckas ET, Robinson KA, et al. Cystic fibrosis pulmonary guidelines. Am J Respir Crit Care Med. 2013;187:680–9.
20. Lynch 3rd JP, Weigt SS, DerHovanessian A, Fishbein MC, Gutierrez A, Belperio JA. Obliterative (constrictive) bronchiolitis. Semin Respir Crit Care Med. 2012;33:509–32.
21. Worthy SA, Park CS, Kim JS, Muller NL. Bronchiolitis obliterans after lung transplantation: high-resolution CT findings in 15 patients. AJR Am J Roentgenol. 1997;169:673–7.
22. Leung AN, Fisher K, Valentine V, et al. Bronchiolitis obliterans after lung transplantation: detection using expiratory HRCT. Chest. 1998;113:365–70.
23. Hartman TE, Primack SL, Lee KS, Swensen SJ, Muller NL. CT of bronchial and bronchiolar diseases. Radiographics. 1994;14:991–1003.
24. Padley SP, Adler BD, Hansell DM, Muller NL. Bronchiolitis obliterans: high resolution CT findings and correlation with pulmonary function tests. Clin Radiol. 1993;47:236–40.
25. Klok FA, Mos IC, van Kralingen KW, Vahl JE, Huisman MV. Chronic pulmonary embolism and pulmonary hypertension. Semin Respir Crit Care Med. 2012;33:199–204.
26. Bergin CJ, Rios G, King MA, Belezzuoli E, Luna J, Auger WR. Accuracy of high-resolution CT in identifying chronic pulmonary thromboembolic disease. AJR Am J Roentgenol. 1996;166:1371–7.
27. Remy-Jardin M, Remy J, Louvegny S, Artaud D, Deschildre F, Duhamel A. Airway changes in chronic pulmonary embolism: CT findings in 33 patients. Radiology. 1997;203:355–60.
28. Price LC, Wort SJ, Perros F, et al. Inflammation in pulmonary arterial hypertension. Chest. 2012;141:210–21.
29. McLaughlin VV, Davis M, Cornwell W. Pulmonary arterial hypertension. Curr Probl Cardiol. 2011;36:461–517.
30. Moser KM, Fedullo PF, Finkbeiner WE, Golden J. Do patients with primary pulmonary hypertension develop extensive central thrombi? Circulation. 1995;91:741–5.
31. Humbert M, Sitbon O, Chaouat A, et al. Survival in patients with idiopathic, familial, and anorexigen-associated pulmonary arterial hypertension in the modern management era. Circulation. 2010;122:156–63.
32. Kang EY, Miller RR, Muller NL. Bronchiectasis: comparison of preoperative thin-section CT and pathologic findings in resected specimens. Radiology. 1995;195:649–54.
33. Naidich DP, McCauley DI, Khouri NF, Stitik FP, Siegelman SS. Computed tomography of bronchiectasis. J Comput Assist Tomogr. 1982;6:437–44.
34. Hansell DM. Small airways diseases: detection and insights with computed tomography. Eur Respir J. 2001;17:1294–313.
35. Hogg JC, Macklem PT, Thurlbeck WM. Site and nature of airway obstruction in chronic obstructive lung disease. N Engl J Med. 1968;278:1355–60.
36. Lee KS, Hwang JW, Chung MP, Kim H, Kwon OJ. Utility of CT in the evaluation of pulmonary tuberculosis in patients without AIDS. Chest. 1996;110:977–84.
37. Reiff DB, Wells AU, Carr DH, Cole PJ, Hansell DM. CT findings in bronchiectasis: limited value in distinguishing between idiopathic and specific types. AJR Am J Roentgenol. 1995;165:261–7.
38. Kaneko K, Kudo S, Tashiro M, Kishikawa T, Nakanishi Y, Yamada H. Case report: computed tomography findings in Williams-Campbell syndrome. J Thorac Imaging. 1991;6:11–3.
39. Rosen MJ. Chronic cough due to bronchiectasis: ACCP evidence-based clinical practice guidelines. Chest. 2006;129:122S–31.
40. Lee P, Bush A, Warner JO. Left bronchial isomerism associated with bronchomalacia, presenting with intractable wheeze. Thorax. 1991;46:459–61.

41. Lee PH, Carr DH, Rubens MB, Cole P, Hansell DM. Accuracy of CT in predicting the cause of bronchiectasis. Clin Radiol. 1995;50:839–41.
42. Cartier Y, Kavanagh PV, Johkoh T, Mason AC, Muller NL. Bronchiectasis: accuracy of high-resolution CT in the differentiation of specific diseases. AJR Am J Roentgenol. 1999;173:47–52.
43. Koh WJ, Lee KS, Kwon OJ, Jeong YJ, Kwak SH, Kim TS. Bilateral bronchiectasis and bronchiolitis at thin-section CT: diagnostic implications in nontuberculous mycobacterial pulmonary infection. Radiology. 2005;235:282–8.
44. Moore AD, Godwin JD, Dietrich PA, Verschakelen JA, Henderson Jr WR. Swyer-James syndrome: CT findings in eight patients. AJR Am J Roentgenol. 1992;158:1211–5.
45. Logan PM, Muller NL. High-attenuation mucous plugging in allergic bronchopulmonary aspergillosis. Can Assoc Radiol J. 1996;47:374–7.
46. Nishimura K, Kitaichi M, Izumi T, Nagai S, Kanaoka M, Itoh H. Usual interstitial pneumonia: histologic correlation with high-resolution CT. Radiology. 1992;182:337–42.
47. Kang EY, Woo OH, Shin BK, Yong HS, Oh YW, Kim HK. Bronchiolitis: classification, computed tomographic and histopathologic features, and radiologic approach. J Comput Assist Tomogr. 2009;33:32–41.
48. Lucaya J, Gartner S, Garcia-Pena P, Cobos N, Roca I, Linan S. Spectrum of manifestations of Swyer-James-MacLeod syndrome. J Comput Assist Tomogr. 1998;22:592–7.
49. Storm van's Gravesande K, Omran H. Primary ciliary dyskinesia: clinical presentation, diagnosis and genetics. Ann Med. 2005;37:439–49.
50. Lillington GA. Dyskinetic cilia and Kartagener's syndrome. Bronchiectasis with a twist. Clin Rev Allergy Immunol. 2001;21:65–9.
51. Kennedy MP, Noone PG, Leigh MW, et al. High-resolution CT of patients with primary ciliary dyskinesia. AJR Am J Roentgenol. 2007;188:1232–8.
52. Garcia-Pena P, Boixadera H, Barber I, Toran N, Lucaya J, Enriquez G. Thoracic findings of systemic diseases at high-resolution CT in children. Radiographics. 2011;31:465–82.

# 14 Air-Crescent Sign

## Definition

An air crescent is a collection of air in a crescentic shape that separates the wall of a cavity from an inner mass [1, 2] (Fig. 14.1).

## Diseases Causing the Sign

The air-crescent sign is often considered characteristic of either *Aspergillus colonization of preexisting cavities* (*aspergilloma*) (Figs. 14.1 and 14.2) or retraction of infracted lung in angioinvasive pulmonary aspergillosis. Other less common causes include tuberculosis, *Rasmussen's aneurysm* (Fig. 14.3), ANCA-associated granulomatous vasculitis (former Wegner's granulomatosis), complicated hydatid disease, hematoma, lung abscess, and necrotic lung cancer (Table 14.1).

## Distribution

Air-crescent sign in aspergilloma and tuberculosis usually occurs in the upper lobe. Rasmussen's aneurysms are usually distributed peripherally and beyond the branches of main pulmonary arteries [3]. Lung abscesses occur most commonly in the posterior segment of an upper lobe or the superior segment of a lower lobe. Hydatid cysts are usually located in the lower lobes.

## Clinical Considerations

Normal host immunity and the long period, often years, required for the formation of aspergilloma, can aid in distinguishing this condition from invasive aspergillosis. The most common underlying causes of aspergilloma are tuberculosis and sarcoidosis. Other conditions that occasionally may be associated with aspergilloma include bronchogenic cyst, pulmonary sequestration, and pneumatoceles secondary to *Pneumocystis jirovecii* infection. The air-crescent sign in invasive pulmonary aspergillosis is observed in up to 63 % of patients. The sign, occurring in about half of the patients with recovery from neutropenia, is caused by tissue ischemia and subsequent necrosis due to fungal angioinvasion [4].

Rasmussen's aneurysm occurs in chronic cavitary tuberculosis with 5 % of prevalence. Hemoptysis is the usual presenting symptom, which may be massive and life-threatening. Generalized symptoms and signs, such as diffuse alveolar hemorrhage, acute glomerulonephritis, chronic refractory sinusitis or rhinorrhea, imaging findings of nodules or cavities, and multisystemic disease, precede typical imaging findings in pulmonary vasculitis [5]. Lung abscess may result from aspiration or systemic spread of infection (septic embolism). Common causes of lung abscess include anaerobic bacteria, *Staphylococcus aureus, Pseudomonas aeruginosa, and Klebsiella pneumoniae.*

**Key Points for Differential Diagnosis**

1. Whether a mural nodule within a cavitary lesion is contrast enhanced or not is one of the most important features in making a differential diagnosis between an intracavitary aspergilloma and a cavitary lung cancer [6]. The aspergilloma usually moves when the patient change position.
2. Air-crescent sign in hydatid disease occurs when there is communication between the cyst and the airways. Air may enter the space between the pericyst and exocyst and produce a thin crescent of air around the periphery of the cyst. When cyst has ruptured into the bronchial tree, the collapsed endocyst–exocyst may be contrasted with surrounding air, resulting in the water-lily sign [7]. The cysts have homogeneous water density on CT [8].
3. A focal dilatation of one of the pulmonary segmental arteries present in the vicinity of a tuberculous cavity is almost a pathognomonic finding of Rasmussen's aneurysm.

K.S. Lee et al., *Radiology Illustrated: Chest Radiology*, Radiology Illustrated,
DOI 10.1007/978-3-642-37096-0_14, © Springer-Verlag Berlin Heidelberg 2014

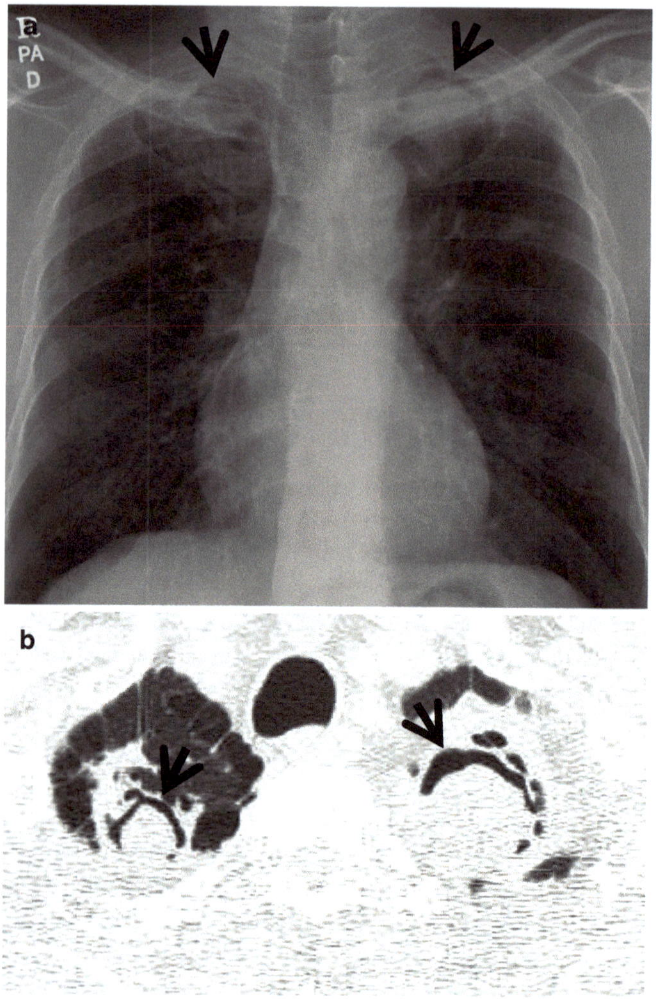


**Fig. 14.1** Air-crescent sign in aspergillomas growing within chronic tuberculous cavities in a 76-year-old man. (**a**) Chest radiograph shows air-crescent signs (*arrows*) in both apices. Also note small nodules in the bilateral upper lung zones. (**b**) Lung window image of thin-section (1.5-mm section thickness) CT scan obtained at level of great vessels demonstrates aspergillomas within cavities disclosing so-called air-crescent signs (*arrows*) in both lung apices. Also note parenchymal band in the right apex and bullae in both apices

## Aspergilloma

### Pathology and Pathogenesis

Aspergilloma is the fungus growth in the lumen of a cavity in the lung without invading the tissues (Fig. 14.2). The ball usually forms in an existing cavity, particularly an old tuberculous cavity (Fig. 14.1), bronchiectasis (Fig. 14.2), abscess, or emphysema, or in a congenital cyst. Aspergilloma formation has been observed both in the bronchiectatic lung distal to an obstructing carcinoma and within the cavity resulting from necrosis at the center of a peripheral carcinoma. Microscopically, an aspergilloma consists of a dense network of hyphae (Fig. 14.2), most of which are dead. Only the hyphae at the surface are well preserved.

### Symptoms and Signs

An aspergilloma may exist for years without causing symptoms [9]. Most patients experience mild hemoptysis, but severe hemoptysis may occur, particularly in patients with underlying tuberculosis. Hemoptysis is reported in 69–83 % of cases. Other symptoms include chronic cough and dyspnea that are probably more related to the underlying lung disease. Fever is rare.

### CT Findings

Characteristic CT findings of aspergilloma are intracavitary non-enhancing soft tissue mass with air-crescent sign [10] (Figs. 14.1 and 14.2). The aspergilloma usually moves when the patient changes position. It is often associated with thickening of the cavity wall and adjacent pleura [11, 12].

### CT–Pathology Comparisons

Conglomeration of intertwined fungal hyphae admixed with mucus and cellular debris appear as non-enhancing soft tissue mass on CT [13] (Fig. 14.2). The mass is separated from the wall of cavity by airspace, resulting in the air-crescent sign, and usually moves with position changes. Thickening of the cavity wall and pleura is due to a hypersensitivity reaction [11].

### Patient Prognosis

The natural history of aspergilloma is variable. In majority of cases, the lesion remains stable. The mortality rate from hemoptysis ranges from 2 to 14 %. In asymptomatic patients, no therapy is warranted. There is no consistent evidence that aspergilloma responds to antifungal agents. Bronchial artery embolization should be considered as a temporary measure to control bleeding in patients with life-threatening hemoptysis. The surgical resection is associated with relatively high morbidity and mortality that ranges between 1 and 23 %, although this seems to have improved over time.

## Rasmussen's Aneurysm

### Pathology and Pathogenesis

The involvement of blood vessels in pulmonary tuberculosis inducing obliterative endarteritis leads to the closure of the lumen of the pulmonary and bronchial arteries before their walls have been penetrated. However, caseation sometimes advances too quickly for the artery to become completely blocked, and an aneurysm may form where the

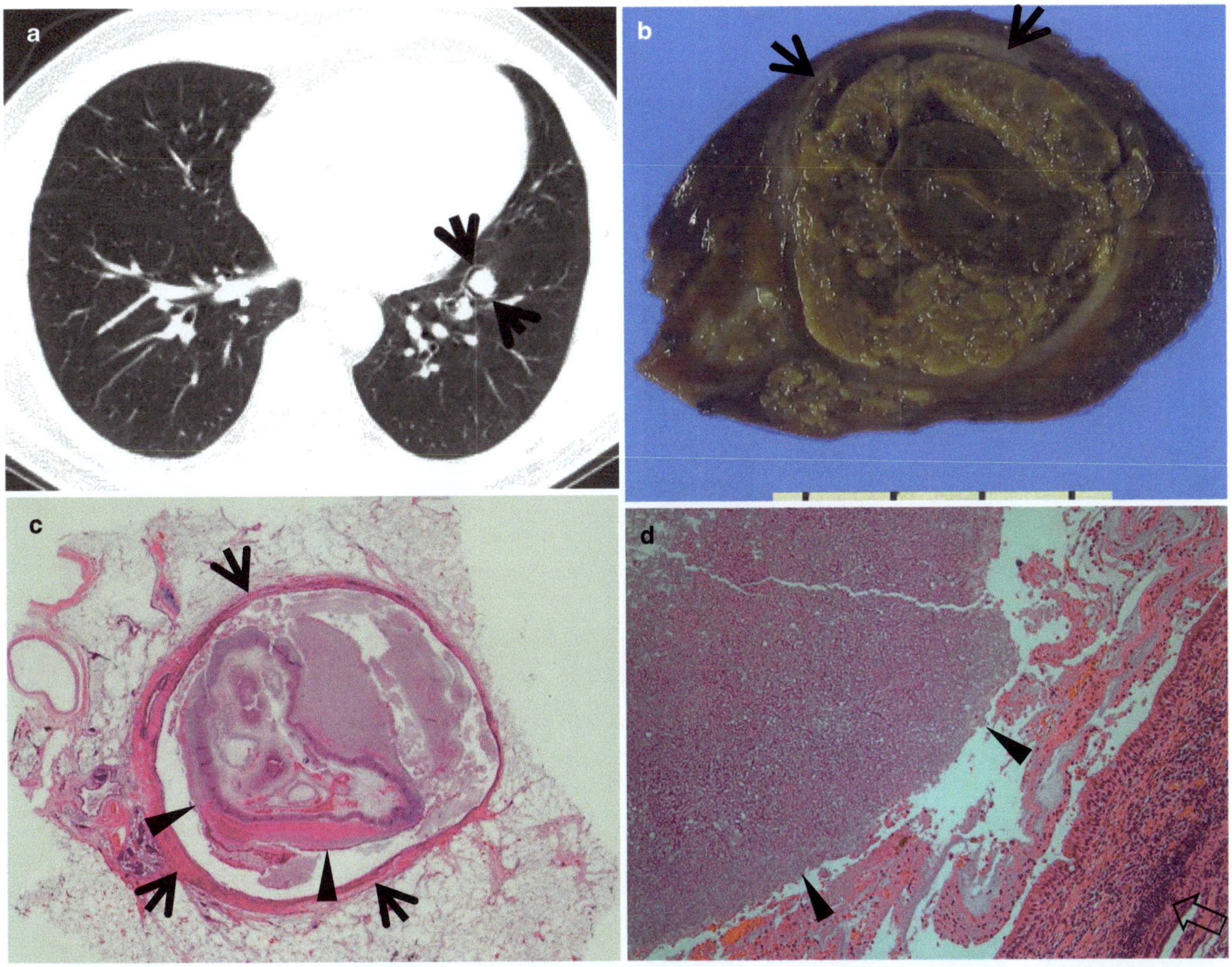


**Fig. 14.2** Air-crescent sign in an aspergilloma growing within a dilated bronchus in a 53-year-old man. (**a**) Lung window image of thin-section (1.5-mm section thickness) CT scan obtained at level of right inferior pulmonary vein shows an aspergilloma showing air-crescent sign within a dilated bronchus (*arrows*) in left lower lobe. (**b**) Gross pathology of resected specimen (left lower lobectomy) demonstrates a soft yellow-gray lesion (*arrows*) within a dilated bronchus. Air is located between the lesion and airway wall, and the air is the source of air-crescent sign on CT scan. (**c**) Scanning view exhibits a dilated bronchus (*arrows*) harboring a fungus ball (*arrowheads*). (**d**) High-magnification (×100) photomicrograph discloses a part of aspergilloma consisting of dense clump of fungal hyphae (*arrowheads*). Bronchial wall shows chronic inflammation (*open arrow*)

muscular and elastic coats are destroyed on the side nearer to the cavity [14].

## Symptoms and Signs

Hemoptysis is the usual presenting symptom and may be life-threatening when it is massive [15]. Otherwise, respiratory symptoms including cough and dyspnea are due to the underlying disease.

## CT Findings

Rasmussen's aneurysm is a focal dilatation of one of the pulmonary segmental arteries adjacent to tuberculous parenchymal change or chronic tuberculous cavity and is seen as avidly enhancing nodules located within the walls of tuberculous cavity [16] (Fig. 14.3).

## CT–Pathology Comparisons

Rasmussen's aneurysm is caused by weakening of the pulmonary artery wall from adjacent cavitary tuberculosis. Progressive weakening and fibrin replacement of the arterial wall result in pseudoaneurysm formation, and subsequent rupture with hemorrhage.

## Patient Prognosis

Prognosis of Rasmussen's aneurysm is not well known since it is a rare disease.

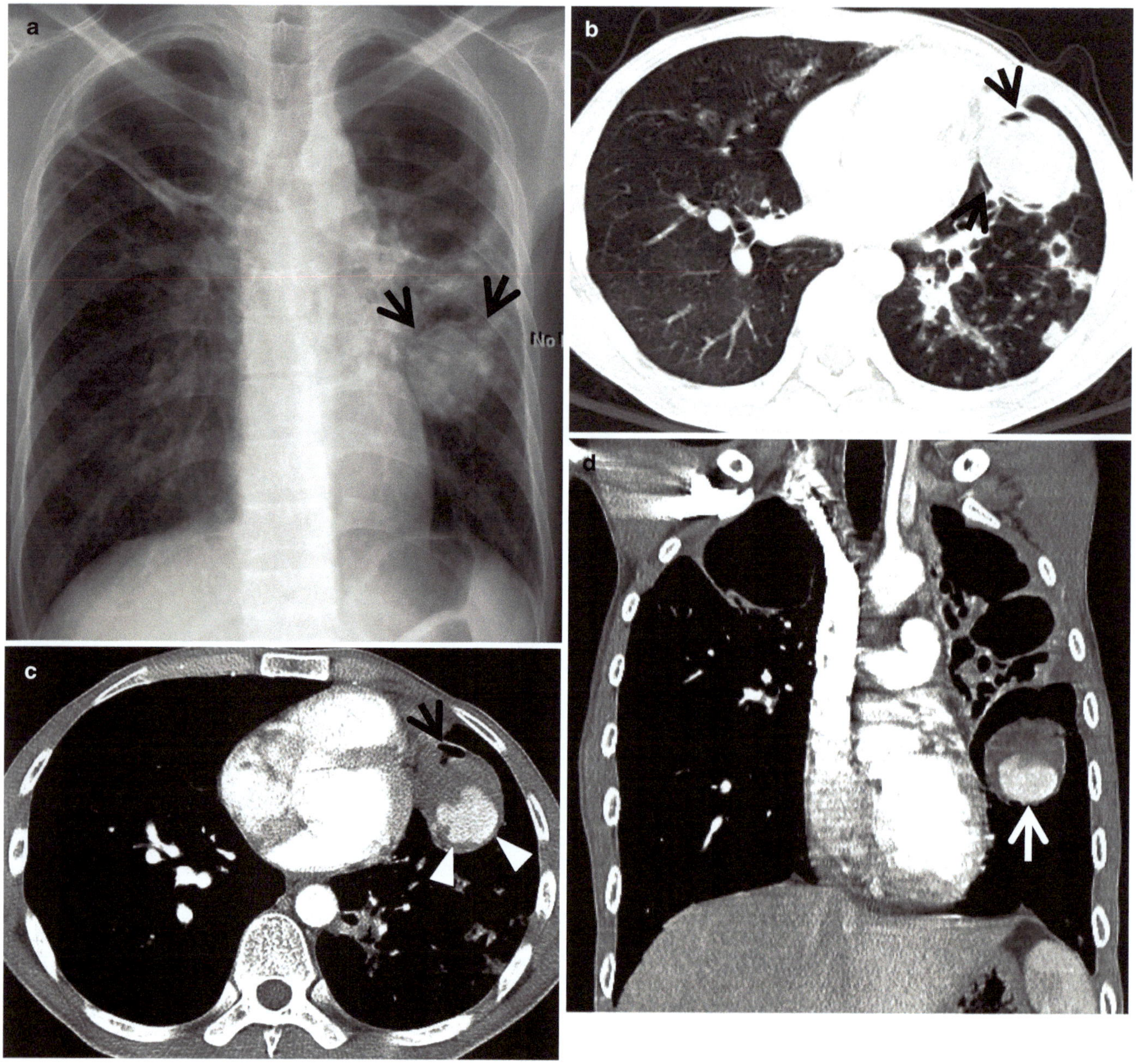


**Fig. 14.3** Air-crescent sign in a Rasmussen's aneurysm in a 34-year-old man. (**a**) Chest radiograph shows destructive tuberculous lesions in the bilateral upper lung zones in which bullae are also seen. Also note a mass showing air-crescent sign (*arrows*). (**b**) Lung window image of thin-section (2.5-mm section thickness) CT scan obtained at level of right inferior pulmonary vein shows a soft tissue mass depicting air-crescent sign (*arrows*) in lingular division of left upper lobe. Also note tuberculous lesions appearing as cavitating and noncavitating nodules in the left lung and right middle lobe. (**c**) Mediastinal window image of enhanced CT scan obtained at same level to (a) demonstrates a highly enhancing lesion of aneurysm (*arrowheads*) with surrounding air crescent (*arrow*). (**d**) Coronal reformatted image (2.0-mm section thickness) exhibits the aneurysm (*arrow*). (**e**) Left pulmonary angiogram discloses the aneurysm (*arrow*) more clearly

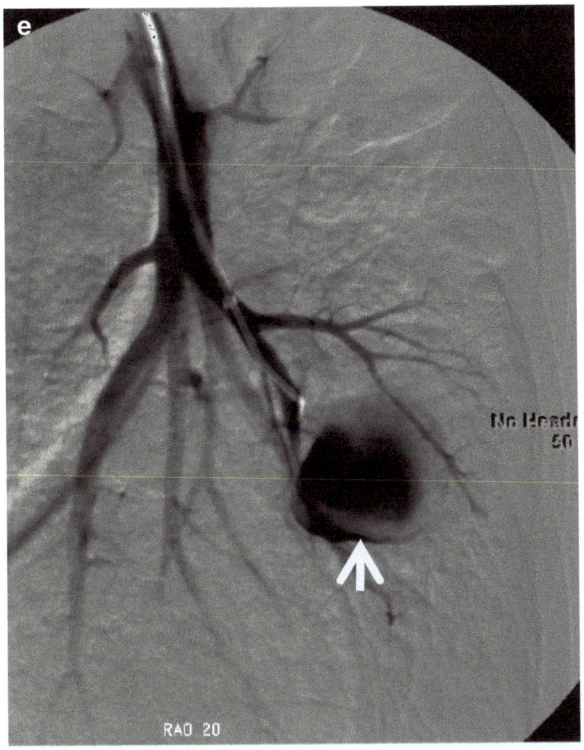


**Fig. 14.3** (continued)

**Table 14.1** Common diseases manifesting as air-crescent sign

| Disease | Key points for differential diagnosis |
|---|---|
| Aspergilloma | Intracavitary non-enhancing soft tissue mass with air-crescent sign |
| Angioinvasive pulmonary aspergillosis | Retraction of infracted lung, CT halo sign |
| Tuberculosis | |
| Rasmussen's aneurysm | Focal dilatation of one of the pulmonary segmental arteries adjacent to tuberculous cavity |
| ANCA-associated granulomatous vasculitis | Multiple, bilateral, subpleural nodules, or masses |
| Complicated hydatid disease | Water-lily sign, homogeneous water density |
| Hematoma<br>Lung abscess<br>Necrotic lung cancer | |

*Note*: *ANCA* antineutrophil cytoplasmic antibody

## References


1. Hansell DM, Bankier AA, MacMahon H, McLoud TC, Muller NL, Remy J. Fleischner Society: glossary of terms for thoracic imaging. Radiology. 2008;246:697–722.
2. Collins J. CT signs and patterns of lung disease. Radiol Clin North Am. 2001;39:1115–35.
3. Ungaro R, Saab S, Almond CH, Kumar S. Solitary peripheral pulmonary artery aneurysms. Pathogenesis and surgical treatment. J Thorac Cardiovasc Surg. 1976;71:566–71.
4. Kim MJ, Lee KS, Kim J, Jung KJ, Lee HG, Kim TS. Crescent sign in invasive pulmonary aspergillosis: frequency and related CT and clinical factors. J Comput Assist Tomogr. 2001;25:305–10.
5. Chung MP, Yi CA, Lee HY, Han J, Lee KS. Imaging of pulmonary vasculitis. Radiology. 2010;255:322–41.
6. Park Y, Kim TS, Yi CA, Cho EY, Kim H, Choi YS. Pulmonary cavitary mass containing a mural nodule: differential diagnosis between intracavitary aspergilloma and cavitating lung cancer on contrast-enhanced computed tomography. Clin Radiol. 2007;62:227–32.
7. Beggs I. The radiology of hydatid disease. AJR Am J Roentgenol. 1985;145:639–48.
8. Saksouk FA, Fahl MH, Rizk GK. Computed tomography of pulmonary hydatid disease. J Comput Assist Tomogr. 1986;10:226–32.
9. Riscili BP, Wood KL. Noninvasive pulmonary Aspergillus infections. Clin Chest Med. 2009;30:315–35, vii.
10. Franquet T, Muller NL, Gimenez A, Guembe P, de La Torre J, Bague S. Spectrum of pulmonary aspergillosis: histologic, clinical, and radiologic findings. Radiographics. 2001;21:825–37.
11. Franquet T, Gimenez A, Cremades R, Domingo P, Plaza V. Spontaneous reversibility of "pleural thickening" in a patient with

semi-invasive pulmonary aspergillosis: radiographic and CT findings. Eur Radiol. 2000;10:722–4.
12. Sansom HE, Baque-Juston M, Wells AU, Hansell DM. Lateral cavity wall thickening as an early radiographic sign of mycetoma formation. Eur Radiol. 2000;10:387–90.
13. Aquino SL, Kee ST, Warnock ML, Gamsu G. Pulmonary aspergillosis: imaging findings with pathologic correlation. AJR Am J Roentgenol. 1994;163:811–5.
14. Morgan JM, Morgan AD, Addis B, Bradley GW, Spiro SG. Fatal haemorrhage from mycotic aneurysms of the pulmonary artery. Thorax. 1986;41:70–1.
15. Kim HY, Song KS, Goo JM, Lee JS, Lee KS, Lim TH. Thoracic sequelae and complications of tuberculosis. Radiographics. 2001;21:839–58; discussion 859–60.
16. Picard C, Parrot A, Boussaud V, et al. Massive hemoptysis due to Rasmussen aneurysm: detection with helicoidal CT angiography and successful steel coil embolization. Intensive Care Med. 2003;29:1837–9.

# 15 Signet Ring Sign

## Definition

The signet ring sign is a combination resembling a signet (or pearl) ring, which is composed of a ring-shaped opacity representing a dilated bronchus in cross section and a smaller adjacent opacity representing its pulmonary artery [1] (Fig. 15.1). Normally, the diameter of a bronchus is equal to the diameter of the adjacent pulmonary artery. The signet ring sign occurs when the bronchoarterial ratio is increased. It is the basic CT sign of bronchiectasis.

## Diseases Causing the Sign

Although the signet ring sign is the basic CT sign of bronchiectasis, it can also be seen in diseases characterized by abnormal reduced pulmonary arterial flow (e.g., *proximal interruption of pulmonary artery* or chronic thromboembolism) (Fig. 15.2) (Table 15.1).

## Distribution

Refer to section "Airway Disease (Bronchiectasis and Bronchiolectasis)" in Chap. 13.

## Clinical Considerations

Clinical considerations of diseases associated with bronchiectasis also refer to section "Airway Disease (Bronchiectasis and Bronchiolectasis)" in Chap. 13.

Proximal interruption of the right pulmonary artery (Fig. 15.2) is usually associated with other congenital cardiac malformations such as ventricular septal defects, the tetralogy of Fallot, coarctation of the aorta, subvalvular aortic stenosis, transposition of the great vessels, scimitar syndrome, and aortopulmonary fistula.

**Key Points for Differential Diagnosis**

1. It is an adjunct finding that can help in differentiating bronchiectasis from other cystic lung lesions [2]. Accompanying findings such as peribronchial thickening, lack of bronchial tapering, and visualization of bronchi within 1 cm of the pleura are all contributing findings to confirming the diagnosis of bronchiectasis.
2. In proximal interruption of the pulmonary artery, cylindrical dilatation of the proximal segmental or subsegmental bronchi is frequently seen, which is completely different from the postinfectious bronchiectasis (peripheral in distribution).

## Proximal Interruption of the Right Pulmonary Artery

### Pathology and Pathogenesis

Proximal interruption of the right pulmonary artery is an uncommon developmental anomaly. The term interruption is used in preference to absence of a pulmonary artery, since the portion of the vessel that is in the lung is usually intact and patent. In proximal interruption, the pulmonary artery ends blindly at the hilum, and blood is supplied to the lung through collateral systemic vessels, mainly bronchial arteries but also transpleural branches of the intercostal, internal mammary, subclavian, and innominate arteries [3].

### Symptoms and Signs

Recurrent pulmonary infection, hemorrhage, and mild dyspnea on exertion are the most common symptoms of this abnormality [4]. Few patients remain asymptomatic.

K.S. Lee et al., *Radiology Illustrated: Chest Radiology*, Radiology Illustrated,
DOI 10.1007/978-3-642-37096-0_15, © Springer-Verlag Berlin Heidelberg 2014

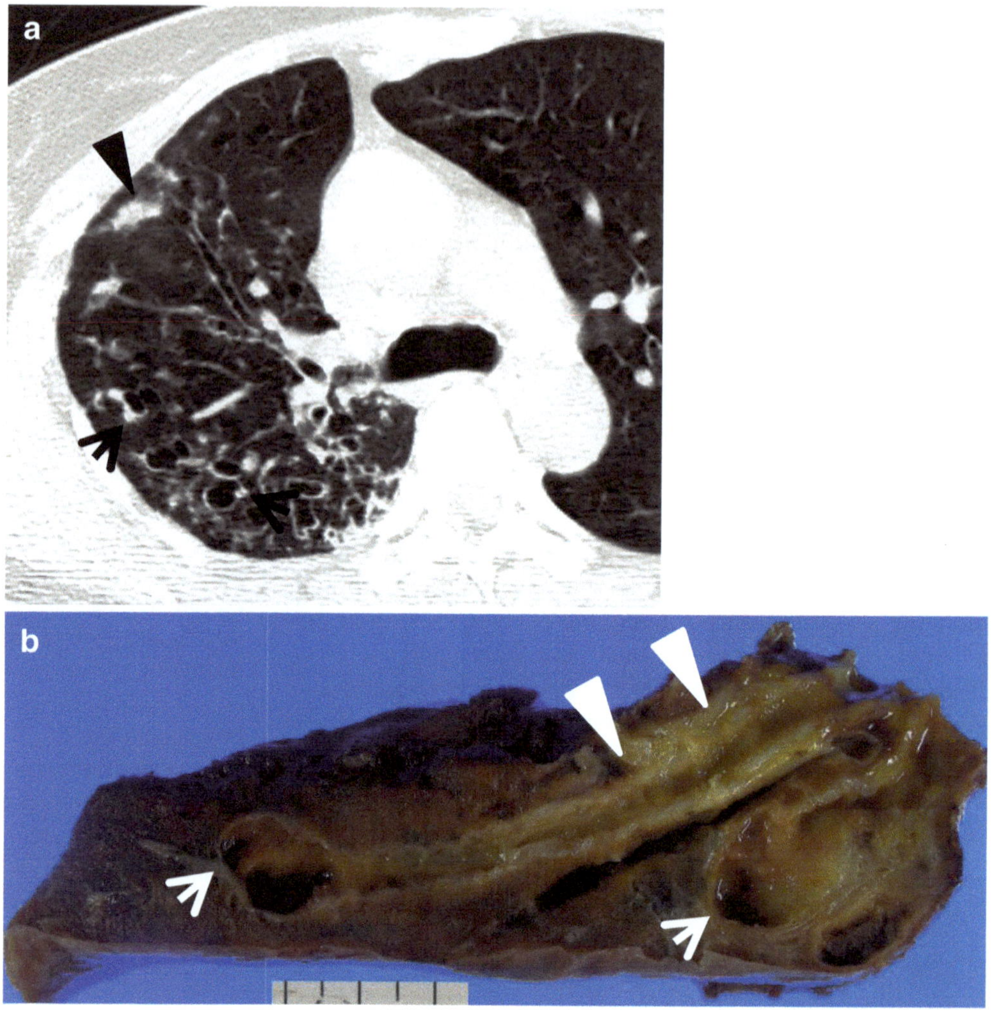


**Fig. 15.1** Bronchiectasis showing signet ring sign in a 44-year-old man. (**a**) Lung window image of CT scan (2.5-mm section thickness) obtained at level of the right upper lobar bronchus shows dilated bronchi showing signet ring sign (*arrows*) in right upper lobe. Also note mucus plugging (*arrowhead*) in dilated bronchi. (**b**) Gross pathologic specimen obtained with right upper lobectomy discloses cylindrical bronchiectasis and distal cystic changes (*arrows*, cystic bronchiectasis). Also note thickened bronchial wall (*arrowheads*) with active inflammation

Hemoptysis attributable to the rupture of hypertrophied collateral vessels occurs in about 10 % of cases.

## CT Findings

Vascular CT findings of proximal interruption of the right pulmonary artery include complete absence of the mediastinal portion of the right main pulmonary artery and enlarged collateral vessels [5] (Fig. 15.2). Parenchymal CT findings include reticular lesions, septal thickening, subpleural consolidation, cystic lung change, bronchial dilatation, and accompanying small systemic artery to constitute signet ring sign (Fig. 15.2), bronchial wall thickening, bronchiectasis, and pleural thickening associated with hypertrophied systemic collateral vessels [6].

## CT–Pathology Comparisons

Smooth septal thickening is usually associated with engorged veins, lymphatics, or interstitial edema [7]. Cystic lung changes postulate that a pressure gradient between the systemic and the pulmonary arteries or high oxygen saturation level may induce lung injury such as ischemia, infarction or bleeding, and inflammatory change resulting in cystic lung change. Subpleural consolidation may be related to small pulmonary infarcts associated with decreased pulmonary circulation and pleural thickening is associated with the development of systemic vessels crossing the pleura. Similar to chronic thromboembolism, decreased pulmonary artery size may allow a reciprocal dilatation of the airways, because they are enclosed within the same bronchovascular connective tissue sheath [6].

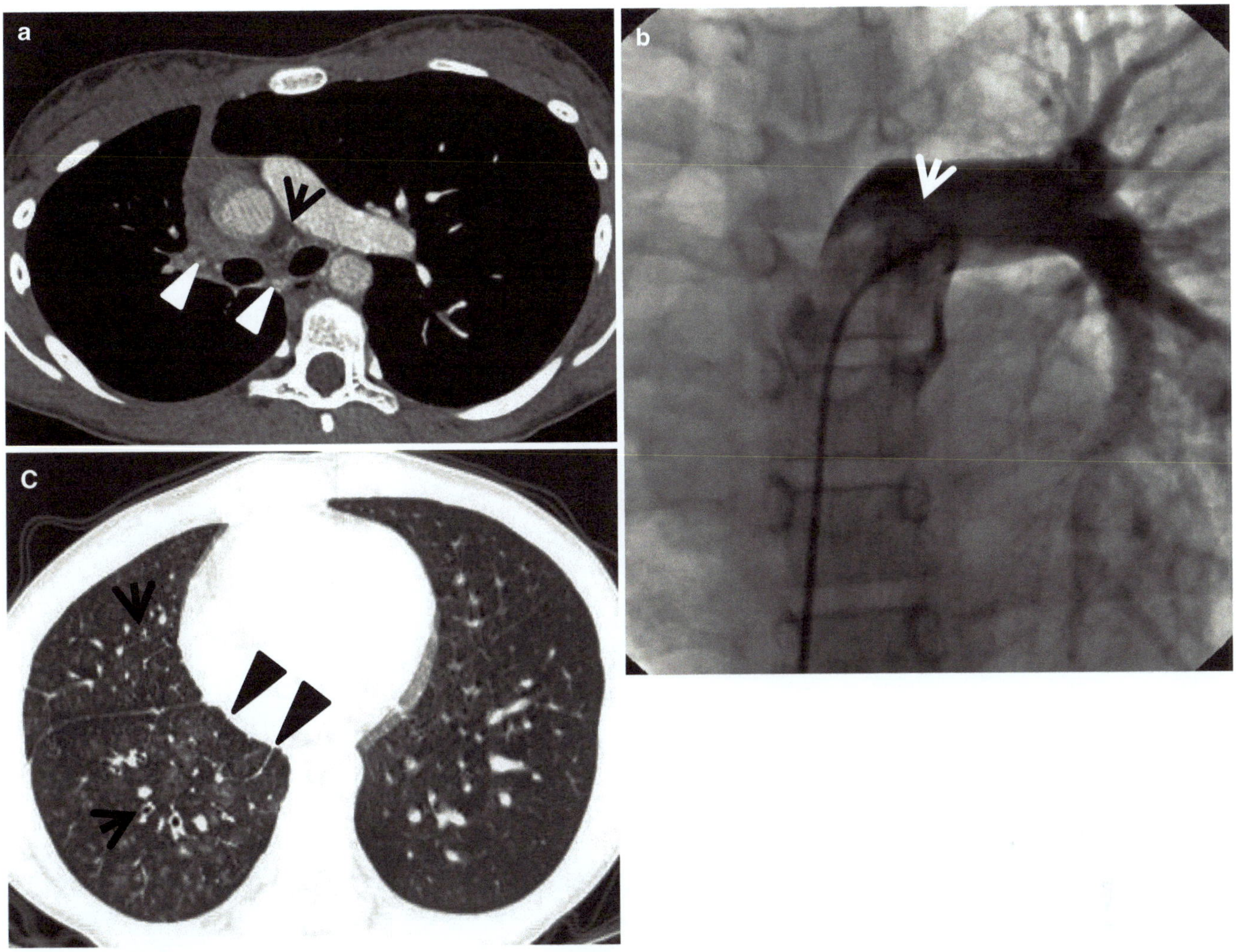


**Fig. 15.2** Proximal interruption of pulmonary artery showing signet ring sign in a 10-year-old girl. (**a**) Mediastinal window image of enhanced CT scan (5.0-mm section thickness) obtained at level of the main bronchi shows interruption of right proximal pulmonary artery (*arrow*) within pericardium. Also note hypertrophied right bronchial artery and branches (*arrowheads*). (**b**) Conventional pulmonary angiograph demonstrates interrupted right proximal pulmonary artery (*arrow*). (**c**) Lung window image obtained at ventricular level displays signet ring sign (*arrows*) constituted by dilated bronchus and accompanying small systemic artery in the right lung. Also note smooth interlobular septal thickening (*arrowheads*) and centrilobular ground-glass opacity nodules (due to aspirated blood with hemoptysis) in the right lung

**Table 15.1** Common diseases manifesting as signet ring sign

| Disease | Key points for differential diagnosis |
|---|---|
| Bronchiectasis | Bronchial dilatation with peribronchial thickening |
| Proximal interruption of pulmonary artery | Complete absence of the mediastinal portion of the right main pulmonary artery, septal thickening |

## Patient Prognosis

Pulmonary hypertension affects 19–25 % of patients with pulmonary artery interruption and is the most important determinant of the prognosis [4].

## References

1. Hansell DM, Bankier AA, MacMahon H, McLoud TC, Muller NL, Remy J. Fleischner Society: glossary of terms for thoracic imaging. Radiology. 2008;246:697–722.
2. Marshall GB, Farnquist BA, MacGregor JH, Burrowes PW. Signs in thoracic imaging. J Thorac Imaging. 2006;21:76–90.
3. Castaner E, Gallardo X, Rimola J, et al. Congenital and acquired pulmonary artery anomalies in the adult: radiologic overview. Radiographics. 2006;26:349–71.
4. Bouros D, Pare P, Panagou P, Tsintiris K, Siafakas N. The varied manifestation of pulmonary artery agenesis in adulthood. Chest. 1995;108:670–6.
5. Morgan PW, Foley DW, Erickson SJ. Proximal interruption of a main pulmonary artery with transpleural collateral vessels: CT and MR appearances. J Comput Assist Tomogr. 1991;15:311–3.
6. Ryu DS, Spirn PW, Trotman-Dickenson B, et al. HRCT findings of proximal interruption of the right pulmonary artery. J Thorac Imaging. 2004;19:171–5.
7. Aquino SL, Kee ST, Warnock ML, Gamsu G. Pulmonary aspergillosis: imaging findings with pathologic correlation. AJR Am J Roentgenol. 1994;163:811–5.

# Part II

# Diffuse Lung Diseases

# 16 Interlobular Septal Thickening

## Smooth Septal Thickening

### Definition

Interlobular septa are sheetlike structures 10–20-mm long that form the border of the secondary pulmonary lobules. The septa are usually perpendicular to the pleura in the lung periphery. They are composed of connective tissue and contain lymphatics and pulmonary venules. On CT scans, diseases affecting one of the components of the septa are responsible for thickening and thus cause the septa visible [1] (Figs. 16.1 and 16.2).

### Diseases Causing the Pattern

The diseases causing smooth interlobular septal thickening include *pulmonary edema* (Fig. 16.2), pulmonary lymphangitic carcinomatosis (PLC), lung involvement of lymphoma or leukemia (Fig. 16.1), diffuse alveolar hemorrhage (DAH), pneumonias, and *lipid storage disease* (*Niemann–Pick disease*) [2] (Fig. 16.3).

The septa may show irregular thickening in pulmonary fibrosis.

### Distribution

In most diseases, lung abnormalities show random and patchy and extensive distribution. In PLC, distribution may be unilateral or bilateral, focal or diffuse, and symmetric or asymmetric. In Niemann–Pick disease, lesions may initially involve only the base and progress to the entire lung [2]. Also in pulmonary fibrosis, the lesions usually start in the lower lung zones to spread to the middle and upper lung zones.

### Clinical Considerations

Impaired cardiac function (heart failure or atrial fibrillation) and fluid overload (e.g., for chemotherapy) in the condition of hampered cardiac function are the most common cause of interstitial pulmonary edema [3]. The most common primary cancer sites related to PLC are the breasts, lungs, colon, and the stomach [4]. Niemann–Pick disease is caused by an inherited defect in the production of sphingomyelinase, resulting in the deposition of sphingomyelin in the liver, spleen, lungs, bone marrow, and brain. Pulmonary involvement can be asymptomatic or severe enough to cause respiratory failure. The disease is characterized histopathologically by the aggregates of large foamy cells (NP cells) in the alveolar septa, bronchial wall and the pleura, thus causing ground-glass opacity (GGO) in the upper lung zones and interlobular septal thickening in the lower lung zones [2].

K.S. Lee et al., *Radiology Illustrated: Chest Radiology*, Radiology Illustrated,
DOI 10.1007/978-3-642-37096-0_16, © Springer-Verlag Berlin Heidelberg 2014

**Key Points for Differential Diagnosis**

| | Distribution | | | | | | | | | | | |
|---|---|---|---|---|---|---|---|---|---|---|---|---|
| | Zones | | | | | | | | Clinical presentations | | | |
| Diseases | U | M | L | SP | C | R | BV | R | Acute | Subacute | Chronic | Others |
| Pulmonary edema | + | + | + | | | + | | + | + | | | With or without parenchymal opacity |
| PLC | + | + | + | | | + | | + | | + | + | May be nodular in progressed stage |
| DAH | + | + | + | | | + | | + | + | | | With parenchymal opacity, subpleural or apical sparing |
| Pneumonia | + | + | + | | | + | | + | + | | | With parenchymal opacity |
| Niemann–Pick disease | | | + | | | + | | + | | | + | With ground-glass opacity in upper lung zone |
| IPF | | + | + | + | | | | + | | | + | Irregular septal thickening with HC or TE |

*Note*: *PLC* pulmonary lymphangitic carcinomatosis, *DAH* diffuse alveolar hemorrhage, *IPF* idiopathic pulmonary fibrosis, *U* upper, *M* middle, *L* lower, *SP* subpleural, *C* central, *R* random, *BV* peribronchovascular, *HC* honeycombing, *TE* traction bronchiectasis

## Pulmonary Edema

### Pathology and Pathogenesis

Pulmonary edema can result from hemodynamic disturbances or from direct increases in capillary permeability due to alveolar microvascular injury. In hemodynamic cause of pulmonary edema (left-sided heart failure), it is characterized by heavy, wet lungs, due to fluid accumulation initially in basal regions (dependent edema). Histologically, alveolar capillaries are engorged and granular pink precipitate in alveolar spaces is seen. In long-standing cases of pulmonary congestion (mitral stenosis), many hemosiderin-laden macrophages appear in the alveolar spaces and the soggy lungs become firm and brown [5].

### Symptoms and Signs

The clinical manifestations of pulmonary edema vary with its severity. Initial symptoms are dyspnea, cough, and tachypnea. Patients can complain of mild pedal edema during the day and paroxysmal nocturnal dyspnea. Wheezing may be heard. Once alveolar flooding has occurred, patients have severe dyspnea, tachypnea, and cough with frothy or blood-tinged sputum. Crackles and rhonchi are heard over the chest. Cheyne–Stokes respiration is common in severe congestive heart failure.

### CT Findings

The thin-section CT (TSCT) findings of pulmonary interstitial edema consist of thickening of the interlobular septa, interlobular fissures, and the peribronchovascular connective tissue (peribronchial cuffing) [6, 7] (Fig. 16.2). The interlobular septal thickening is smooth and uniform, except for a focal nodular appearance due to prominent septal veins. Another common finding is the areas of GGO. These opacities can be diffuse or patchy in distribution and usually involve mainly the perihilar and the dependent lung regions. In cases of alveolar edema, areas of GGO and consolidation involving mainly the perihilar and dependent lung regions are seen on TSCT [6].

### CT-Pathology Comparisons

The earliest manifestation of hydrostatic pulmonary edema is the expansion of connective tissue spaces around conducting airways, their accompanying vessels, and the interlobular septa. Accumulation of fluid within peribronchovascular interstitial tissue and interlobular septa results in peribronchial cuffing and thickening of interlobular septa [8]. Because the pleural connective tissue is in continuity with that of the interlobular septa, accumulation of fluid in the interlobular septa is often associated with thickening of the interlobular fissures. The areas of GGO seen in pulmonary interstitial edema are related to the presence of thickened alveolar walls. If alveoli are filled with fluid, airspace edema appears as areas of GGO and consolidation.

### Patient Prognosis

Treatment of pulmonary edema requires adequate life support followed by specific therapy directed at the factors leading to pulmonary edema. Oxygen supplementation and lung-protective mechanical ventilation may be necessary.

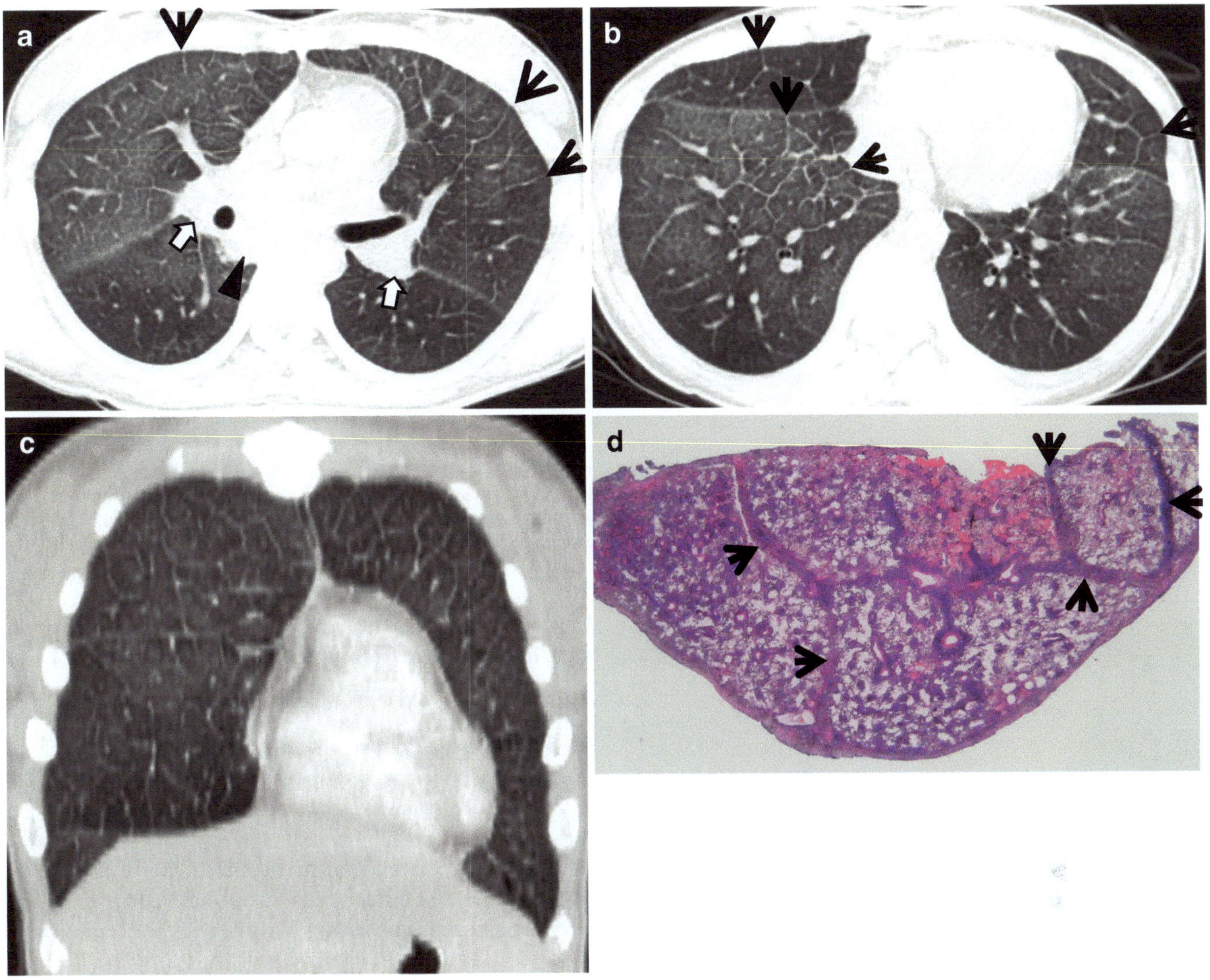


**Fig. 16.1** Smooth interlobular septal thickening with lymphomatous involvement of the lungs in a 27-year-old woman with diffuse large B-cell lymphoma. (**a**, **b**) Lung window of CT scans (5.0-mm section thickness) obtained at levels of bronchus intermedius (**a**) and suprahepatic superior vena cava (**b**), respectively, shows diffuse ground-glass opacity with smooth interlobular septal thickening (*arrows*) in both lungs, particularly in anterior lungs. Also note enlarged lymph nodes in bilateral hila (*open arrows* in **a**) and in subcarcinal area (*arrowhead* in **a**). (**c**) Coronal reformatted image (5.0-mm section thickness) also demonstrates diffuse ground-glass opacity with smooth interlobular septal thickening in both lungs. (**d**) Low-magnification (×40) photomicrograph of pathologic specimen obtained from right upper lobe from a different patient (a 52-year-old man with marginal zone B-cell lymphoma) discloses smooth interlobular septal thickening (*arrows*). Also note thickened alveolar walls. In this patient, thin-section CT scan showed localized area of ground-glass opacity containing internal smooth interlobular septal thickening (not shown here)

Pharmacologic measures to reduce edema accumulation, such as with diuretics, inotropic agents, and vasodilators, can be used.

## Niemann–Pick Disease

### Pathology and Pathogenesis

Niemann–Pick types A and B (NPA and NPB), also called acid sphingomyelinase deficiency, are caused by the deficiency of a specific enzyme, acid sphingomyelinase. The characteristic microscopic feature is an infiltration of lipid-storing foam histiocytes, usually seen within the alveoli, the alveolar walls, and the lymphatic interlobular and subpleural spaces, while the pulmonary architecture remains normal [2].

### Symptoms and Signs

The adult form of Niemann–Pick disease (NPB), which appears during the second and third decades, is relatively benign, presenting with hepatosplenomegaly, hemostatic defects, and, occasionally, cerebellar ataxia. Interstitial lung disease is usually asymptomatic [9].

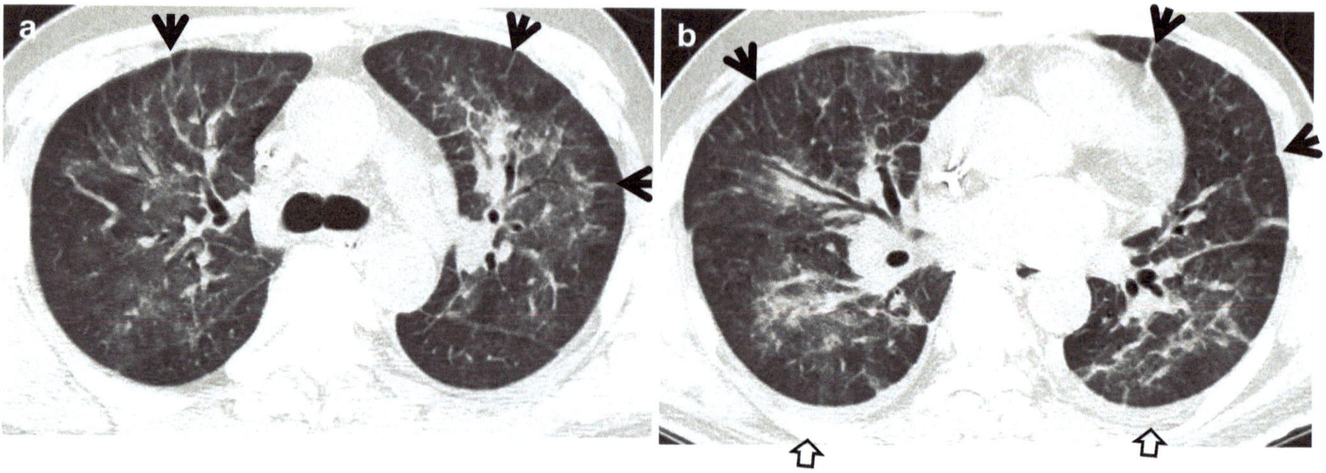


Fig. 16.2 Smooth interlobular septal thickening associated with overhydration interstitial pulmonary edema in a 59-year-old man who has mantle cell lymphoma. Patient received hydration before chemotherapy. (**a**, **b**) Lung window of CT scans (2.5-mm section thickness) obtained at levels of azygos arch (**a**) and lower lobar bronchi (**b**), respectively, shows diffuse ground-glass opacity with smooth interlobular septal thickening (*arrows*) in both lungs, particularly in the anterior lungs. Also note bilateral pleural effusions (*open arrows* in **b**), small in amount. Lung lesions disappeared with diuretic therapy

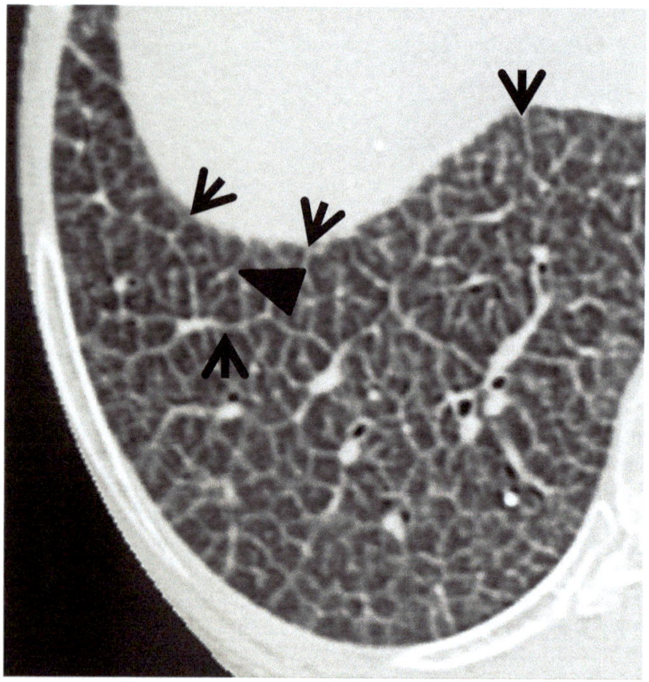

Fig. 16.3 Niemann–Pick disease (lipid storage disease) in a 39-year-old woman. Targeted view of the right lung at level of the liver dome shows thickened interlobular septa (*arrows*) along with thickened intralobular lines (*arrowhead*). Also note background ground-glass opacity in lung parenchyma

## CT Findings

TSCT demonstrates patchy bilateral areas of GGO, smooth thickening of the interlobular septa, and smooth intralobular lines [2, 10] (Fig. 16.3). The abnormalities may be diffuse but tend to involve mainly the lower lung zones. Hepatosplenomegaly and peripheral lymph node enlargement are common.

## CT-Pathology Comparisons

Pathologically, aggregates of large foamy cells (NP cell) are present in the parenchyma of many organs [11]. Areas of GGO on CT are related to the partial filling of the alveoli with NP cells and diffuse endogenous lipid pneumonia, and interlobular septal thickening is related to the accumulation of NP cells in the interlobular septa [2].

## Patient Prognosis

Various therapeutic approaches, including enzyme replacement therapy, gene therapy, and stem cell transplantation, have been tried for this disorder. Neurodegeneration in patients with NPA proceeds rapidly and leads to death within 3 years, while those with NPB have little or no neurodegeneration and frequently survive into adulthood.

# Nodular Septal Thickening

## Definition

Interlobular septa are the sheetlike structures of 10–20-mm length that form the border of the secondary pulmonary lobules. The septa are usually perpendicular to the pleura in the lung periphery. They are composed of connective tissue and contain lymphatics and pulmonary venules. Nodular thickening of the interlobular septa may be caused by the disease involving the lymphatics within the septa (Figs. 16.4, 16.5, and 16.6).

## Diseases Causing the Pattern

The diseases causing nodular interlobular septal thickening include *pulmonary lymphangitic carcinomatosis* (*PLC*) [4] (Figs. 16.4 and 16.5) and pulmonary sarcoidosis [12] (Fig. 16.6). In silicosis and amyloidosis, nodular interlobular septal thickening may be occasionally associated [13, 14] (please also note section "Small Nodules with Perilymphatic Distribution" in Chap. 18).

## Distribution

In most diseases, lung abnormalities show random or patchy and extensive distribution. In PLC, distribution may be unilateral or bilateral, focal or diffuse, and symmetric or asymmetric. In silicosis, the lesions show typically upper and middle lung zone predominance as in sarcoidosis. However, in sarcoidosis, the abnormalities may involve the whole lung without zonal predominance. In amyloidosis, the lesions usually show lower lung zone predominance.

## Clinical Considerations

The most common primary cancer sites related to PLC are the breasts, lungs, colon, and the stomach [4]. The presence of occupational exposure history to coal dusts or silica renders a diagnosis of pneumoconiosis. Patients with pulmonary sarcoidosis usually have no specific symptoms. The disease may be suspected with abnormal chest radiographs. Conversely patients with pulmonary sarcoidosis may have fatigue, fever, weight loss, dry cough, or shortness of breath. Up to 20 % of individuals with sarcoidosis develop skin problems such as rash or nodules. Eye symptoms such as blurred vision, pain, and photosensitivity may occur occasionally in sarcoidosis. Amyloidosis is a heterogeneous group of disorder characterized by accumulation of B-pleated sheets of insoluble proteins (amyloid). The deposition of amyloid in the lung is common in systemic amyloidosis, either in primary systemic disease or secondary to systemic disease processes such as chronic renal failure, chronic infections, rheumatoid arthritis, tuberculosis, syphilis, osteomyelitis, or inflammatory bowel disease [2].

### Key Points for Differential Diagnosis

| | Distribution | | | | | | | | | | | |
|---|---|---|---|---|---|---|---|---|---|---|---|---|
| | Zones | | | | | | | | Clinical presentations | | | |
| Diseases | U | M | L | SP | C | R | BV | R | Acute | Subacute | Chronic | Others |
| PLC | + | + | + | | | + | | + | | + | + | Nodular thickening in progressed stage |
| Sarcoidosis | + | + | ± | | | + | + | | | | + | With parenchymal opacity or small nodules of perilymphatic distribution |
| Silicosis | + | + | | | | + | | + | | | + | With small nodules of perilymphatic distribution |
| Amyloidosis | | | + | + | | | | + | | | + | With parenchymal opacity or small nodules of perilymphatic distribution |

*Note*: *PLC* pulmonary lymphangitic carcinomatosis, *U* upper, *M* middle, *L* lower, *SP* subpleural, *C* central, *R* random, *BV* bronchovascular

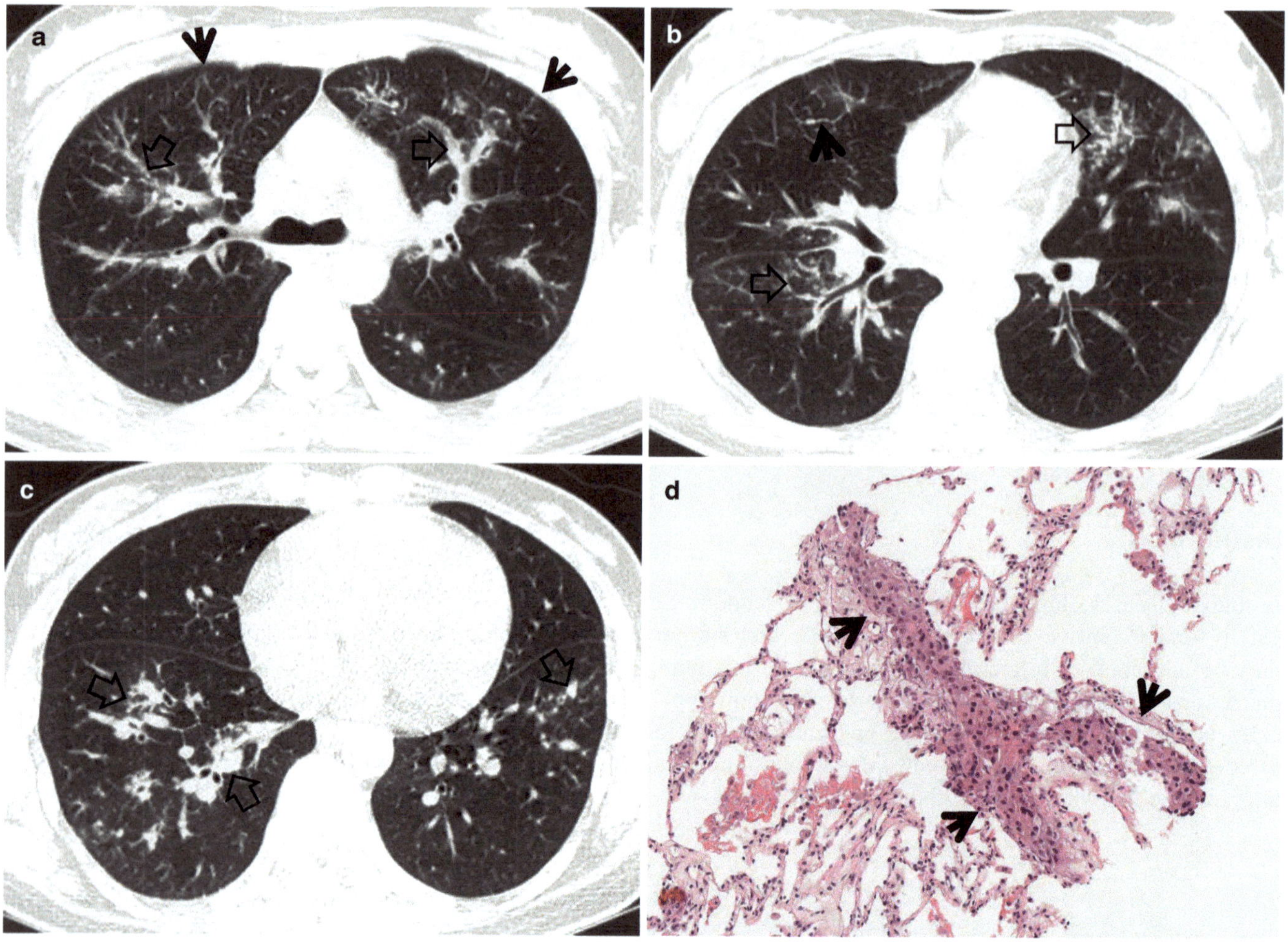


**Fig. 16.4** Pulmonary lymphangitic carcinomatosis in a 35-year-old woman with poorly differentiated tubular adenocarcinoma of the stomach. (**a**–**c**) Lung window images of thin-section (2.5-mm section thickness) CT scans obtained at levels of right upper (**a**) and middle (**b**) lobar bronchi and basal segmental bronchi (**c**), respectively, show smooth and nodular (*arrows*) thickening of interlobular septa. Also note thickening of axial interstitium (*open arrows*). (**d**) High-magnification photomicrograph (×200) of transbronchial lung biopsy specimen obtained from a different patient discloses tumor cells (*arrows*) packing lymphatics in interstitium which causes smooth or nodular thickening of interlobular septum on CT scan

## Pulmonary Lymphangitic Carcinomatosis

### Pathology and Pathogenesis

PLC is a condition of metastatic carcinoma involving the lung, primarily within lymphatics. The tumor type is most often adenocarcinoma. Variable amounts of tumor may be present throughout the lung, involving the interstitium of the alveolar walls, the air spaces themselves, and the lumens of small muscular pulmonary arteries [4, 15] (Fig. 16.4).

### Symptoms and Signs

Because of the large degree of reserve in pulmonary function, patients may present with minimal or no respiratory symptoms. Nonspecific symptoms of cough, dyspnea, or chest pain can result from extensive lymphatic infiltration. Severe dyspnea with hypoxemia can be found as the disease progresses.

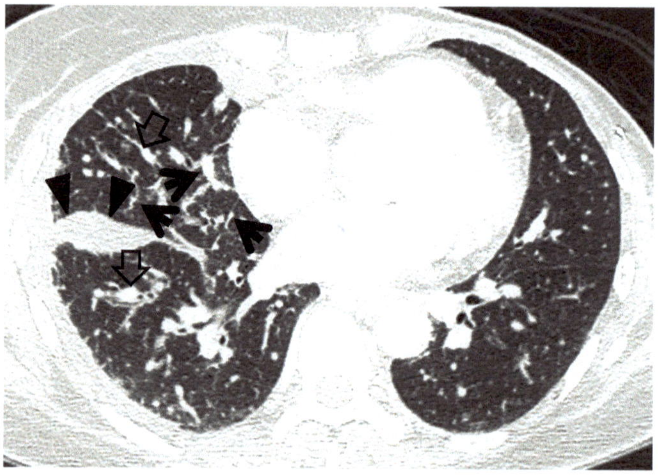

**Fig. 16.5** Pulmonary lymphangitic carcinomatosis in a 52-year-old woman with breast cancer who underwent left mastectomy. Lung window image of thin-section (1.0-mm section thickness) CT obtained at level of right inferior pulmonary vein shows nodular and band-like interlobular septal thickening (*arrows*), particularly in the right lung. Also note axial interstitial thickening (*open arrows*) of the right lung as compared with the left lung. Right major fissural effusion (*arrowheads*) is noticed

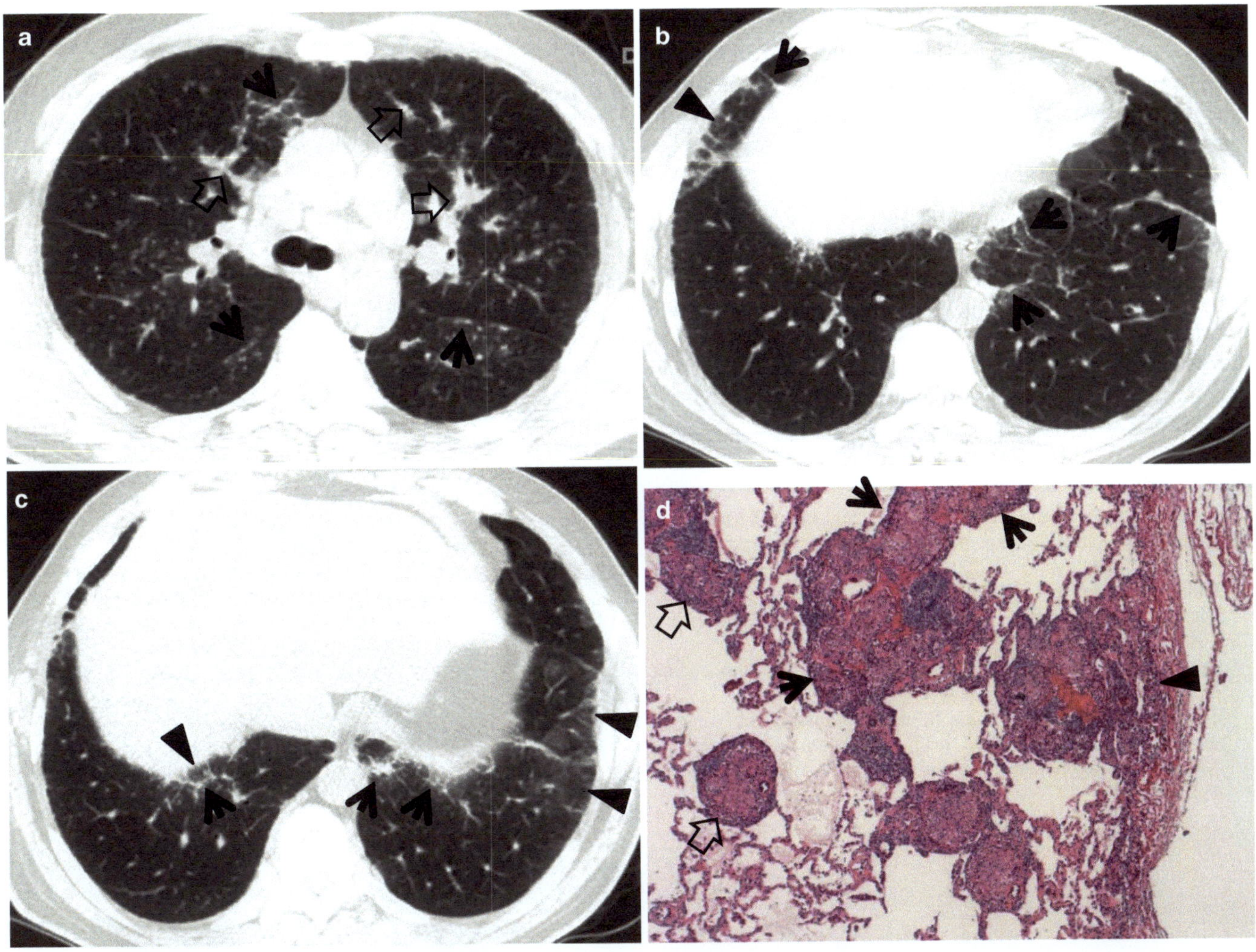


**Fig. 16.6** Nodular septal thickening in a 53-year-old man with pulmonary sarcoidosis. (**a–c**) Lung window images of thin-section (1.5-mm section thickness) CT scans obtained at levels of the main bronchi (**a**), liver dome (**b**), and suprahepatic inferior vena cava (**c**), respectively, show nodular (*arrows*) thickening of interlobular septa and interlobular fissure, axial interstitial thickening (*open arrows*), and patchy areas of ground-glass opacity (*arrowheads*) in both lungs. (**d**) High-magnification (×100) photomicrograph of surgical lung biopsy obtained from a different patient discloses noncaseating granulomas located in interlobular septum (*arrows*), alveolar walls (*open arrows*), and subpleural interstitium (*arrowhead*). Granulomas in interlobular septum constitute nodular interlobular septum on CT scan

## CT Findings

The characteristic HRCT findings of PLC consist of smooth or nodular thickening of the interlobular septa and peribronchovascular interstitium with preservation of normal lung architecture [4, 15] (Figs. 16.4 and 16.5). Tumor spread in the pleural interstitial tissue lead to smooth or nodular thickening of the interlobular fissures (Fig. 16.5). The abnormalities may be initially subtle, but tend to progress to extensive bilateral disease associated with areas of ground-glass opacity (Figs. 16.4 and 16.5). Pleural effusion and hilar or mediastinal lymph node enlargement are seen in 30–40 % of patients (Fig. 16.5).

## CT-Pathology Comparisons

Thickening of the interlobular septa and the peribronchovascular interstitium on CT is pathologically related to tumor cell infiltration, desmoplastic reaction, and edema caused by lymphatic obstruction [4] (Fig. 16.4). Tumor infiltration and edema in the pleural interstitial tissue lead to thickening of interlobular fissures. Diffuse ground-glass opacity areas seen in the progressed disease are caused by pulmonary edema.

## Patient Prognosis

Although prognosis of PLC largely depends on the malignancy of origin, the overall outcome of the patients is dismal unless they are curable cancers with aggressive multimodal therapy.

## References


1. Hansell DM, Bankier AA, MacMahon H, McLoud TC, Muller NL, Remy J. Fleischner Society: glossary of terms for thoracic imaging. Radiology. 2008;246:697–722.
2. Chung MJ, Lee KS, Franquet T, Muller NL, Han J, Kwon OJ. Metabolic lung disease: imaging and histopathologic findings. Eur J Radiol. 2005;54:233–45.
3. Ware LB, Matthay MA. Clinical practice. Acute pulmonary edema. N Engl J Med. 2005;353:2788–96.
4. Johkoh T, Ikezoe J, Tomiyama N, et al. CT findings in lymphangitic carcinomatosis of the lung: correlation with histologic findings and pulmonary function tests. AJR Am J Roentgenol. 1992;158:1217–22.
5. Husain AN. Chapter 15. The lung. In: Maitra A, Kumar V, editors. Robbins and Cotran pathologic basis of disease. International edition, 8th ed. Philadelphia: Saunders/Elsevier; 2010. p. 706.
6. Primack SL, Muller NL, Mayo JR, Remy-Jardin M, Remy J. Pulmonary parenchymal abnormalities of vascular origin: high-resolution CT findings. Radiographics. 1994;14:739–46.
7. Storto ML, Kee ST, Golden JA, Webb WR. Hydrostatic pulmonary edema: high-resolution CT findings. AJR Am J Roentgenol. 1995;165:817–20.
8. Bessis L, Callard P, Gotheil C, Biaggi A, Grenier P. High-resolution CT of parenchymal lung disease: precise correlation with histologic findings. Radiographics. 1992;12:45–58.
9. Schuchman EH. The pathogenesis and treatment of acid sphingomyelinase-deficient Niemann-Pick disease. Int J Clin Pharmacol Ther. 2009;47 Suppl 1:S48–57.
10. Mendelson DS, Wasserstein MP, Desnick RJ, et al. Type B Niemann-Pick disease: findings at chest radiography, thin-section CT, and pulmonary function testing. Radiology. 2006; 238:339–45.
11. Nicholson AG, Florio R, Hansell DM, et al. Pulmonary involvement by Niemann-Pick disease. A report of six cases. Histopathology. 2006;48:596–603.
12. Murdoch J, Muller NL. Pulmonary sarcoidosis: changes on follow-up CT examination. AJR Am J Roentgenol. 1992;159:473–7.
13. Bergin CJ, Muller NL. CT in the diagnosis of interstitial lung disease. AJR Am J Roentgenol. 1985;145:505–10.
14. Chong S, Lee KS, Chung MJ, Han J, Kwon OJ, Kim TS. Pneumoconiosis: comparison of imaging and pathologic findings. Radiographics. 2006;26:59–77.
15. Munk PL, Muller NL, Miller RR, Ostrow DN. Pulmonary lymphangitic carcinomatosis: CT and pathologic findings. Radiology. 1988;166:705–9.

# 17 Honeycombing

## Honeycombing with Subpleural or Basal Predominance

### Definition

Pathologically, honeycombing (HC) represents destroyed and fibrotic lung tissue containing numerous cystic airspaces with thick fibrous walls [1] (Fig. 17.1). In addition, HC on pathology is characterized by cysts usually measuring <1 mm, often below the resolution of CT, and therefore not necessarily concordant with macroscopic HC seen on CT images. On thin-section CT (TSCT) scans, the appearance is of clustered cystic air spaces, typically of comparable diameters on the order of 3–10 mm but occasionally as large as 25 mm [2] (Fig. 17.1b). Some researchers may consider HC as a multilayer cluster of cysts with shared walls, but others may recognize a single layer cluster of cysts [3] (Fig. 17.1c).

### Diseases Causing the Pattern

Cystic structures of HC on transverse CT images consist of either dilated peripheral bronchioles or alveolar ducts, surrounded by several in-folded layers of thickened alveolar septa (a true HC cyst) or tangential view of traction bronchiectasis (TB). In *idiopathic pulmonary fibrosis (IPF) and usual interstitial pneumonia (UIP)* (Figs. 17.1 and 17.2), cystic structures are mainly composed of true HC cysts in the peripheral portion of the lungs, while most cystic structures in patients with *nonspecific interstitial pneumonia (NSIP)* (Fig. 17.3) seem to be tangential views of TB [4]. Of course, even in patients with NSIP, main cysts of HC are the true HC cysts as in IPF/UIP. Honeycombing has been reported in up to 40 % of NSIP [5]. HC may be observed in approximately 10 % of patients with *asbestosis* (Fig. 17.4) along with findings of irregular interlobular septal thickening, intralobular interstitial thickening, subpleural dot-like or branching opacity, and ground-glass opacity (GGO), not to mention of pleural plaques [6].

### Distribution

In most diseases, lung abnormalities show lower lung zone and subpleural-distribution predominance. In NSIP, abnormalities may be located along the bronchovascular bundles and may demonstrate subpleural sparing [7].

### Clinical Considerations

The identification of HC is essential for making the certain CT diagnosis of UIP and for predicting patient prognosis with fibrotic IIPs [8].

Even in cases of fibrotic idiopathic interstitial pneumonias (IIPs) with little HC, serial CT reveals an increase in the extent of HC and reticulation and a decrease in the extent of GGO. Overall extent of lung fibrosis on the baseline CT examination appears predictive of survival in fibrotic IIPs with little HC [9].

Measuring a fibrotic score (the extent of reticulation plus HC) at TSCT helps predict patient prognosis. In other words, patients with UIP or fibrotic NSIP who have a high fibrotic score determined at thin-section CT and a low DLco level have a high death risk [10].

HC mimickers at CT are paraseptal emphysema and TB of varying severity. NSIP may simulate UIP at CT in the presence of emphysema [11]. Any fibrotic interstitial pneumonia with concurrent emphysema may cause problems in CT interpretation [12].

K.S. Lee et al., *Radiology Illustrated: Chest Radiology*, Radiology Illustrated,
DOI 10.1007/978-3-642-37096-0_17, © Springer-Verlag Berlin Heidelberg 2014

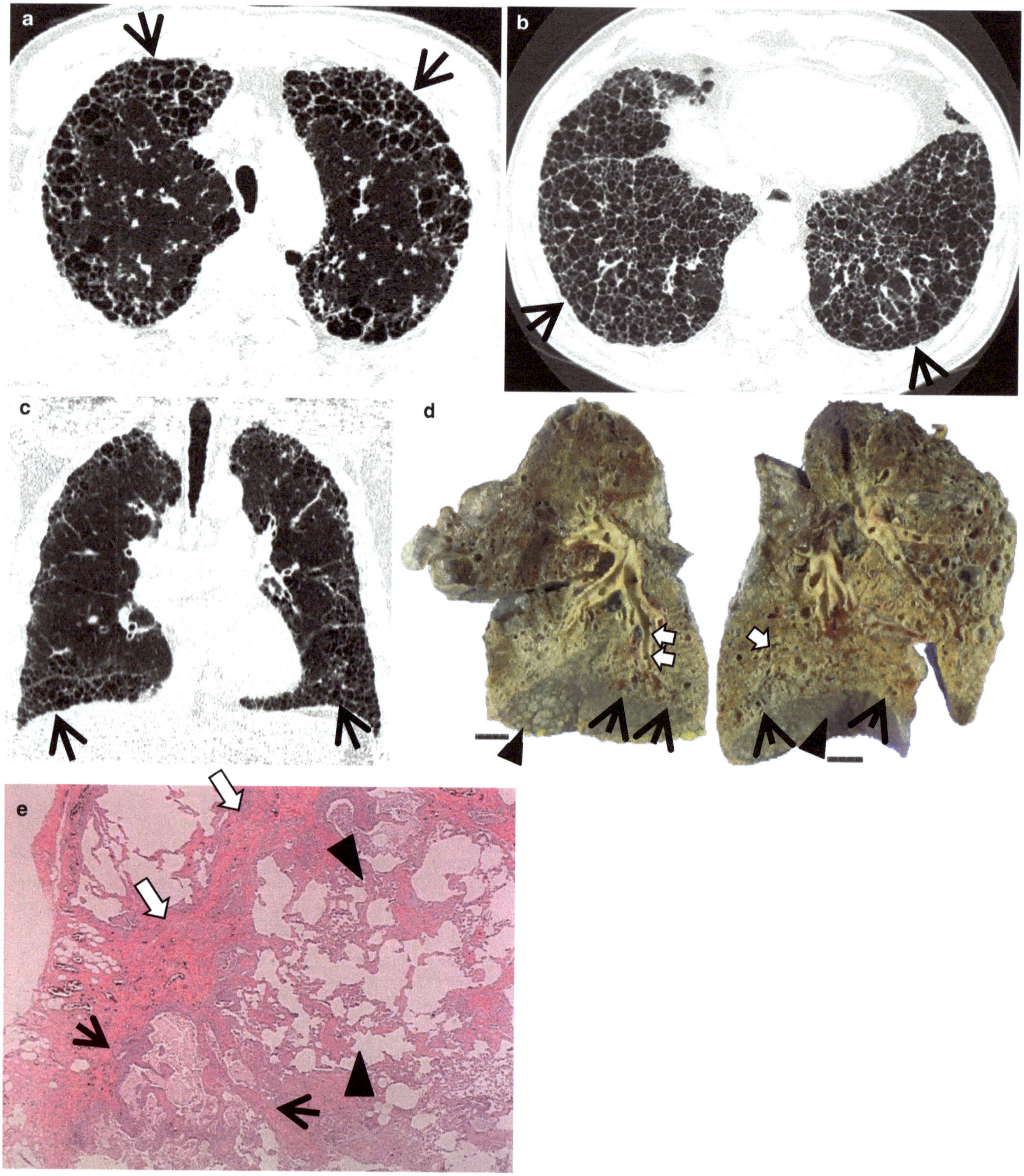


**Fig. 17.1** Typical honeycomb cysts in a 50-year-old man with usual interstitial pneumonia. (**a**, **b**) Lung window images of thin-section (1.5-mm section thickness) CT scans obtained at levels of aortic arch (**a**) and liver dome (**b**), respectively, show back-to-back cysts (*arrows*) in subpleural regions of both lungs. Cysts are at least two layers or more in both lungs. (**c**) Coronal reformatted image (2.0-mm section thickness) demonstrates subpleural honeycomb cysts (*arrows*) in both lungs. (**d**) Explanted lungs from a different patient who suffered from acute exacerbation of usual interstitial pneumonia depict consolidative lower lobes (*arrowheads*) through which honeycomb cysts (*arrows*) are visualized. Also note traction bronchiectasis (*open arrows*). (**e**) High-magnification (× 200) photomicrograph discloses combined findings of honeycomb cysts filled with mucus (*arrows*), interstitial fibrosis (*open arrows*), and inflammatory cell infiltration (*arrowheads*)

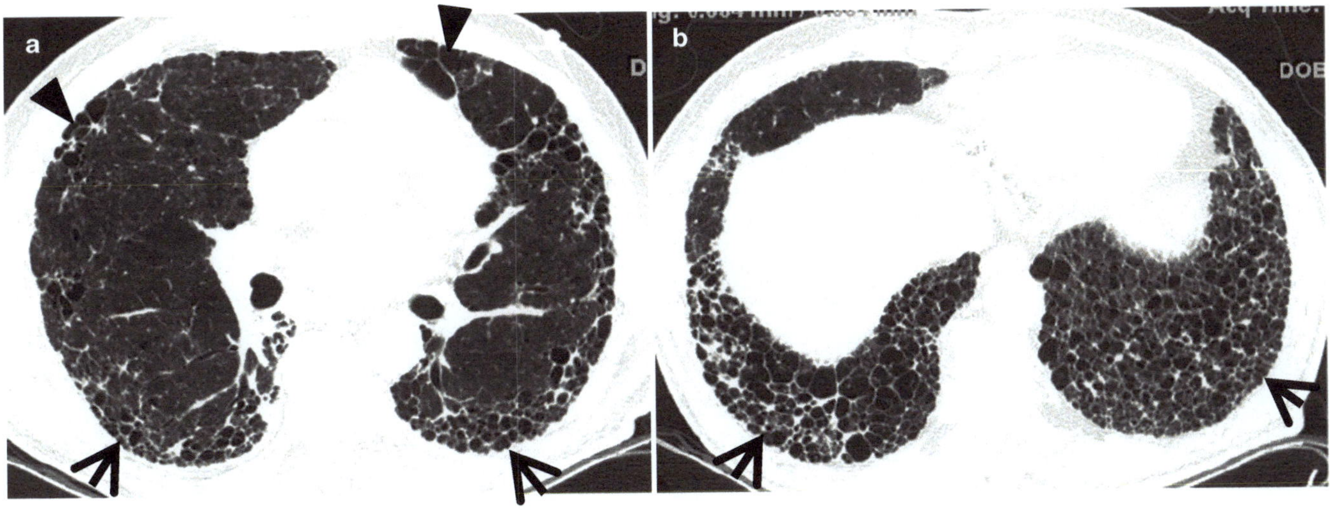


**Fig. 17.2** Typical honeycomb cysts in a 58-year-old man with usual interstitial pneumonia. (**a**, **b**) Lung window images of thin-section (1.5-mm section thickness) CT scans obtained at levels of distal bronchus intermedius (**a**) and liver dome (**b**), respectively, show back-to-back cysts (*arrows*) in subpleural regions of both lungs. Most cysts are at least two layers or more in both lungs. Also note some areas of pulmonary emphysema (*arrowheads*) in anterior lungs of the middle lung zones

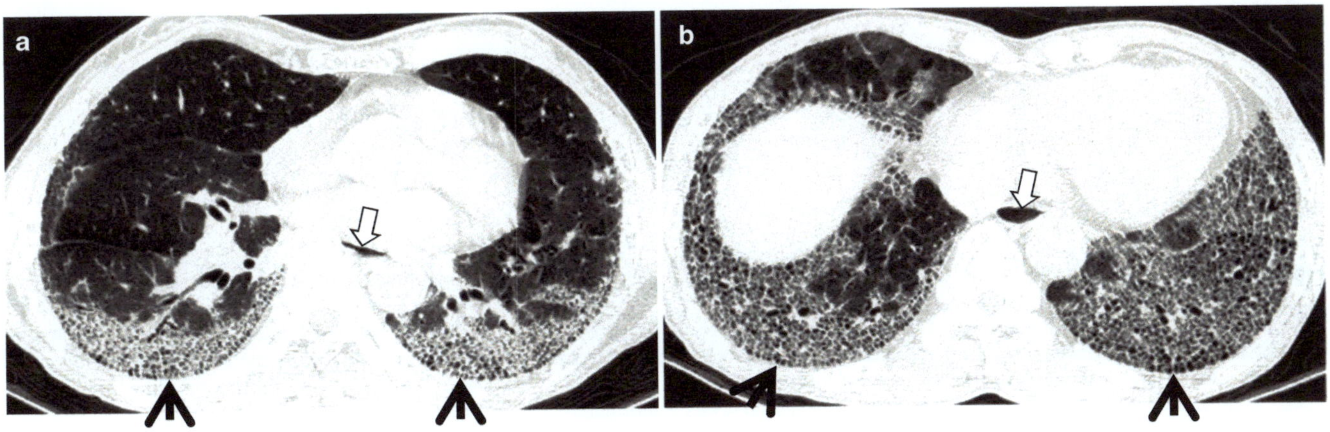


**Fig. 17.3** Honeycomb cysts in a 67-year-old woman with progressive systemic sclerosis (PSS)-associated nonspecific interstitial pneumonia. (**a**, **b**) Lung window images of thin-section (1.5-mm section thickness) CT scans obtained at levels of inferior pulmonary veins (**a**) and liver dome (**b**), respectively, show honeycomb cysts (*arrows*) seen through ground-glass opacity in bilateral lower lung zones. Patient had acute exacerbation of pulmonary fibrosis and, thus, had accompanying ground-glass opacity with background honeycomb cysts. Also note distal esophageal dilatation with air filling (*open arrows*) owing to esophageal involvement of PSS

### Key Points for Differential Diagnosis

| | Distribution | | | | | | | | | | | |
|---|---|---|---|---|---|---|---|---|---|---|---|---|
| | Zones | | | | | | | | Clinical presentations | | | |
| Diseases | U | M | L | SP | C | R | BV | R | Acute | Subacute | Chronic | Others |
| IPF/UIP | | + | + | + | | | | + | | | + | |
| NSIP | | + | + | + | + | | + | + | | + | + | Female predominance; subpleural sparing and along BV bundles |
| Asbestosis | | + | + | + | | | | + | | | + | Exposure history and pleural plaques; with subpleural dot-like or branching opacity and subpleural lines |

*Note*: *IPF* idiopathic pulmonary fibrosis, *UIP* usual interstitial pneumonia, *NSIP* nonspecific interstitial pneumonia, *U* upper, *M* middle, *L* lower, *SP* subpleural, *C* central, *R* random, *BV* bronchovascular

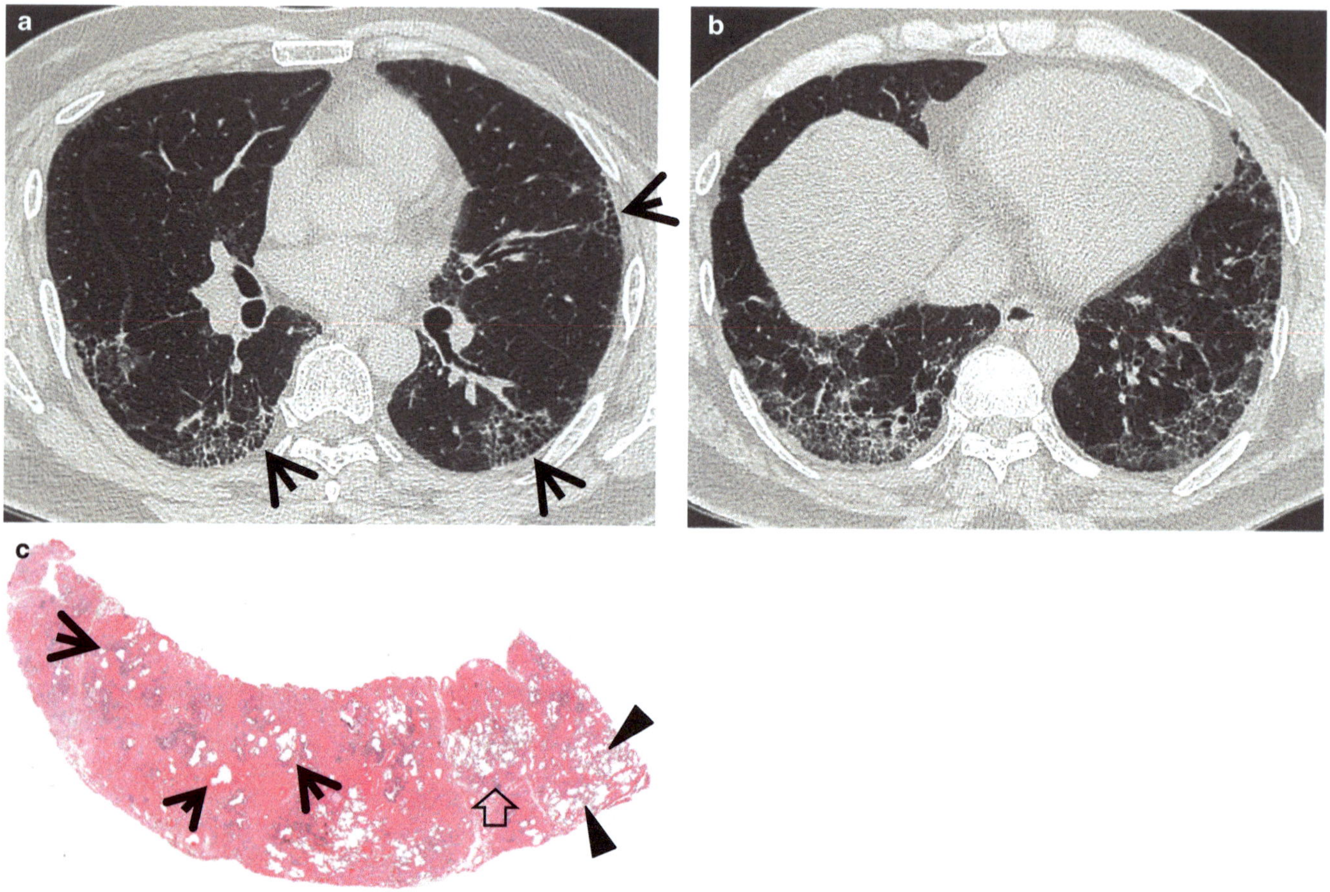


**Fig. 17.4** Honeycomb cysts in a 39-year-old man with asbestosis who is working in a building demolition place. (**a**, **b**) Lung window images of thin-section (1.5-mm section thickness) CT scans obtained at levels of right middle lobar bronchus (**a**) and liver dome (**b**), respectively, show reticulation and ground-glass opacity in subpleural regions of lower lung zones. Also note scattered areas of honeycomb cysts (*arrows*). (**c**) Low-magnification (×40) photomicrograph of surgical biopsy specimen obtained from right lower lobe discloses pulmonary fibrosis of usual interstitial pneumonia pattern with large area of irregular interstitial fibrosis including microscopic honeycombing (*arrows*), few areas of chronic inflammatory cell infiltration (*open arrow*), and normal lung areas (*arrowheads*)

## Idiopathic Pulmonary Fibrosis/Usual Interstitial Pneumonia

### Pathology and Pathogenesis

In a typical case, the lungs are shrunken and firm when removed at autopsy or explanted. The lower lobes are most severely affected, with the pleura having a finely nodular "cobblestone" pattern, resembling that of a cirrhotic liver. Pleural fibrosis is uncommon, in contrast to asbestosis. The cut surface of the lung shows fibrosis and a variable degree of "honeycombing," which is most marked beneath the pleura (Fig. 17.1). The cardinal features of UIP are subpleural and paraseptal predominance, patchy parenchymal involvement, fibrosis leading to loss of architecture, fibroblastic foci adjacent to the established fibrosis indicative of progressive disease, only mild to moderate chronic interstitial inflammation, and an absence of any causal feature such as inorganic dust, granulomas, or accumulations of Langerhans cells [13].

### Symptoms and Signs

IPF occurs in middle-aged and elderly adults (median age at diagnosis 66 years, range 55–75 years) [14]. Dry cough and slowly progressive dyspnea on exertion are the cardinal symptoms of IPF. Systemic symptoms, such as fever and weight loss, are rare. Patients may be asymptomatic at the early stage of IPF. Finger clubbing is found in more than 50 % of the patients. Bibasilar fine inspiratory crackle, so-called Velcro-like rale, is heard on chest auscultation.

### CT Findings

The characteristic HRCT findings of UIP consist of intralobular lines and honeycombing involving mainly the subpleural regions and lung bases [15] (Figs. 17.1 and 17.2). The intralobular interstitial thickening also results in the presence of irregular interfaces between the lung and pulmonary vessels, bronchi, and pleural surfaces. The bronchioles and bronchi in the areas of fibrosis are often dilated and tortuous (traction bronchiolectasis and bronchiectasis). Parenchymal involvement is typically patchy on HRCT, with areas of normal and markedly abnormal lung often present in the same lobe. Other findings of UIP on HRCT include irregular thickening of interlobular septa and patchy areas of GGO. On HRCT, the overall extent of fibrosis (reticulation and honeycombing) has been consistently shown to correlate with disease severity parameters on pulmonary function tests and prognosis [10]. Recently, the extent of honeycombing at baseline as well as its progression on sequential follow-up CT scan is demonstrated as an important prognostic determinant in patients of fibrotic interstitial pneumonia, including UIP and fibrotic NSIP [9].

### CT–Pathology Comparisons

Histologically, UIP shows a variable degree of interstitial inflammation and fibrosis [13]. As disease becomes more severe, alveoli are replaced by fibrous tissue. Contraction of this tissue results in the dilatation of respiratory bronchioles and alveolar ducts, leading to the formation of honeycombing cysts. The intralobular lines reflect the presence of interstitial fibrosis. Interlobular septal thickening reflects the presence of fibrosis in the periphery of the secondary lobules and patchy areas of GGO reflects areas of inflammation or fibrosis. Patchy parenchymal involvement on HRCT reflects histologic features of heterogeneous appearance in which areas of fibrosis with scarring and honeycombing alternate with areas of less affected or normal parenchyma.

### Patient Prognosis

IPF is a chronic, progressive, irreversible, and usually fatal lung disease. There is no therapy proven to be effective [16]. Median survival has been reported to be 2–5 years. Lung transplantation remains the last therapeutic option.

## Nonspecific Interstitial Pneumonia

### Pathology and Pathogenesis

It is a uniform-appearing, cellular interstitial pneumonia characterized by a lymphoplasmacytic infiltrate within the alveolar septa. Varying amounts of fibrosis consisting predominantly of collagen are admixed with the chronic inflammation, and cases can be divided into cellular and fibrotic variants. Patchy intra-alveolar macrophage accumulation and small foci of intraluminal fibrosis resembling BOOP may occur but are always overshadowed by the more extensive interstitial pneumonia [17].

### Symptoms and Signs

Cough and dyspnea are the most common symptoms in patients with idiopathic NSIP [14]. The duration of respiratory symptoms is around 6 months, which is shorter than in IPF. Median age of NSIP is 52 years (range 26–73). Finger clubbing can be observed but is less frequent than in IPF.

### CT Findings

The most common HRCT findings of NSIP consist of lower lobe, peripherally predominant, and GGO with reticular abnormality, traction bronchiectasis, and lower lobe volume loss [5]. Honeycombing and consolidation are relatively uncommon. The reported prevalence of honeycombing ranges from 0 to 44 % (Fig. 17.3). The HRCT pattern of NSIP may overlap with those of cryptogenic organizing pneumonia (COP), desquamative interstitial pneumonia, and UIP. The parenchymal abnormalities of NSIP, including reticular pattern, traction bronchiectasis, and GGO, may be reversible on follow-up exam. Although differentiation from UIP is very difficult, NSIP is characterized by lack of honeycombing, more GGO, and a finer reticular pattern than UIP. Moreover, in NSIP, relative subpleural sparing [7] or distribution of reticulation along the central bronchovascular bundles is more frequently observed. On recent comparative study of NSIP and UIP at long-term follow-up, 28 % of patients with initial CT findings suggestive of NSIP progressed to features suggestive of IPF/UIP on follow-up CT scans [7].

### CT–Pathology Comparisons

Areas of GGO with or without reticular abnormality or traction bronchiectasis on CT correspond histologically to the areas of interstitial thickening caused by varying degrees of interstitial inflammation or fibrosis showing temporal uniformity [18]. The areas of consolidation are related to the areas of COP, foamy cell collections in alveolar spaces or foci of honeycombing in which the cystic spaces are filled with mucus.

### Patient Prognosis

Prognosis of idiopathic NSIP is much better than IPF. The 5-year and 10-year survival of the patients with idiopathic NSIP has been reported to be 82.3 and 73.2 %, respectively [14]. Cellular NSIP shows a much better survival than fibrotic NSIP. Corticosteroids with or without immunomodulatory drugs such as azathioprine and cyclophosphamide are the main drugs for the treatment.

## Asbestosis

### Pathology and Pathogenesis

Asbestosis is defined as diffuse pulmonary fibrosis caused by the inhalation of excessive amounts of asbestos fibers. Histologically, asbestosis is characterized by discrete foci of fibrosis in the walls of respiratory bronchioles accompanied by asbestos bodies. As the fibrotic process progresses, it extends distally to the alveolar ducts and proximally to the membranous (terminal) bronchioles. The fibrosis also extends radially to involve alveolar septa distant from the respiratory bronchiole. In the most advanced cases, honeycomb fibrosis is present. The hallmark of asbestos exposure is the asbestos body, namely, a rodlike, beaded, or dumbbell-shaped structure with golden-brown coating and a thin, translucent core. Detection of asbestos bodies may be facilitated by the use of iron stains, which impart a deep blue color. Pleural plaques consist of layers of acellular hyalinized collagen, arranged in a "basket weave" pattern, or appear as compact layers of collagen. A mild lymphocytic infiltrate sometimes accompanies the fibrosis [19].

### Symptoms and Signs

Clinically, asbestosis manifests as dry cough, dyspnea, fine inspiratory crackles on auscultation, and a restrictive defect in pulmonary function test with or without finger clubbing [15]. Sputum production and wheezing are less common. Patients may be asymptomatic in mild cases.

### CT Findings

HRCT with the patient prone is the most sensitive imaging technique to detect asbestosis. Findings in early disease include subpleural dots or branching structures, intralobular lines, thickened interlobular septa, subpleural curvilinear lines, pleura-based irregular small nodules, patchy areas of GGO, and small, cystic spaces [17] (Fig. 17.4). These abnormalities tend to involve mainly the dorsal subpleural regions of lower lobes. Honeycombing is a common finding in advanced-stage disease. On comparative study of asbestosis and IPF, subpleural dot-like or branching opacities, curvilinear lines, band-like opacities, and air trapping are more common in asbestosis, whereas honeycombing, visible bronchioles, and bronchiectasis within consolidation are more common in IPF [6]. However, the presence of parietal pleural thickening in association with lung fibrosis is the most important feature differentiating asbestosis from IPF.

### CT–Pathology Comparisons

HRCT-pathology correlation studies have shown that subpleural dots and branching structures correspond to peribronchiolar fibrosis [20]. Extension of fibrous tissue into the parenchyma between affected bronchioles results in pleura-based nodular irregularities. Thickened interlobular septa on HRCT may correspond to the fibrosis of the septa themselves or to fibrosis in the periphery of lobule. GGOs are related to mild alveolar wall fibrosis. In the most severe cases, diffuse interstitial fibrosis leads to parenchymal remodeling and honeycombing.

### Patient Prognosis

No specific treatment is available other than prevention of further exposure to asbestos, smoking cessation, and treatment for coexisting chronic obstructive pulmonary disease and cor pulmonale if present. The prognosis of asbestosis is highly variable and depends on the extent of lung involvement. Development of lung cancer or pleural tumor should be closely monitored.

## Honeycombing with Upper Lung Zone Predominance

### Definition

Pathologically, honeycombing (HC) represents destroyed and fibrotic lung tissue containing numerous cystic airspaces with thick fibrous walls [1]. In addition, HC on pathology is characterized by cysts usually measuring <1 mm, often below the resolution of CT, and therefore not necessarily concordant with macroscopic HC seen on CT images. On thin-section CT (TSCT) scans, the appearance is of clustered cystic air spaces, typically of comparable diameters on the order of 3–10 mm but occasionally as large as 25 mm [2] (Please refer to section "Honeycombing with Subpleural or Basal Predominance") (Fig. 17.5).

### Diseases Causing the Pattern and Distribution

In *familial idiopathic pulmonary fibrosis (IPF)*, honeycombing (HC) is seen in approximately one-third of patients, and lung lesions demonstrate still lower lung zone predominance (67 %, 6 of 9 patients). However, upper lung zone predominance (33 %) is higher than non-familial usual interstitial pneumonia (UIP) [21] (Fig. 17.5).

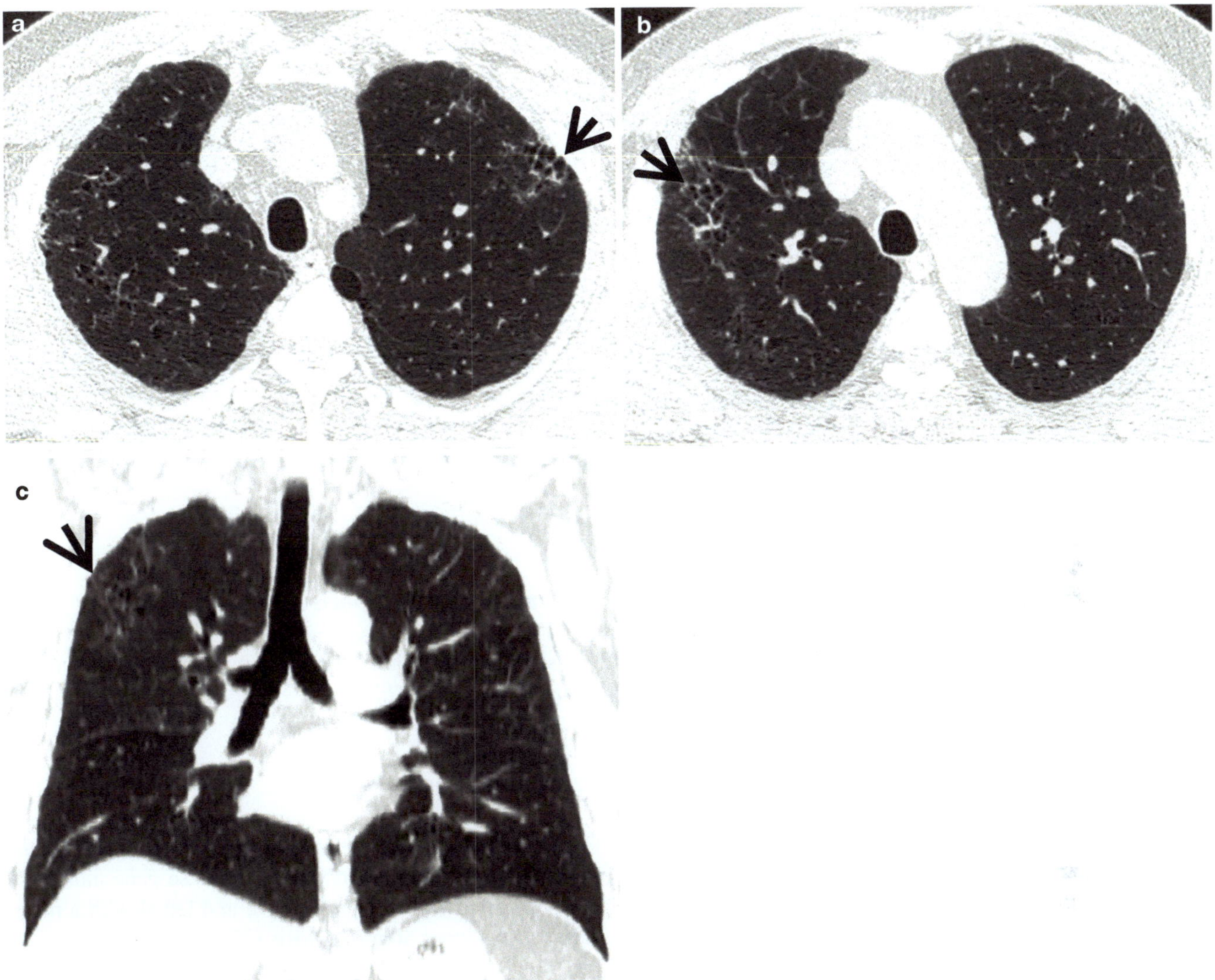


**Fig. 17.5** Biopsy-proven usual interstitial pneumonia showing upper lung zone-predominant honeycomb cysts in a 51-year-old man. Patient did not have family history for usual interstitial pneumonia.(**a**, **b**) Lung window images of thin-section (1.5-mm section thickness) CT scans obtained at levels of great vessels (**a**) and aortic arch (**b**), respectively, show patchy areas of honeycomb cysts (*arrows*) in both lungs with upper lung zone predominance. (**c**) Coronal reformatted image (2.0-mm section thickness) demonstrates upper lung zone-predominant honeycomb cysts (*arrow*)

According to a study, HC is seen in approximately 60 % of patients with *chronic hypersensitivity pneumonia (HP)* with upper lung zone predominance [22]. In *advanced fibrotic sarcoidosis*, traction bronchiectasis, HC, other types of cystic destruction, bullae, and paracicatricial emphysema are encountered, mainly in middle or upper lung zone predominance [23].

## Distribution

In all three categories of diseases, the various patterns of lung abnormalities including HC demonstrate upper lung zone predominance.

## Clinical Considerations

The clinical presentation in familial IPF is similar to those in nonfamilial IPF and consists of dry cough and progressive dyspnea. Survival in this group of patients is considerably longer, with a 5-year survival rate of 67 % [21].

Although HC is seen in approximately 60 % patients with chronic HP, the HC is not a discriminating factor of the disease from UIP or fibrotic nonspecific interstitial pneumonia [22].

In end-stage fibrotic sarcoidosis, there distinct patterns of lung lesion distribution are seen; the bronchial distortion pattern (47 % of patients) with or without coexisting masses, the HC pattern (29 %), and the linear pattern (24 %). The patterns are associated with different functional profiles [24].

**Key Points for Differential Diagnosis**

| Diseases | Distribution | | | | | | | | Clinical presentations | | | Others |
|---|---|---|---|---|---|---|---|---|---|---|---|---|
| | Zones | | | | | | | | | | | |
| | U | M | L | SP | C | R | BV | R | Acute | Subacute | Chronic | |
| Familial IPF | + | + | + | + | | | | + | | | + | HC and upper lung zone predominance, respectively, are seen in one-third of patients |
| Chronic HP | + | + | | | | + | | + | | | + | Lobular area of mosaic attenuation and small centrilobular nodules |
| Advanced fibrotic sarcoidosis | + | + | | + | | + | | + | | | + | Associated hilar or mediastinal lymph node enlargement |

*Note*: *IPF* idiopathic pulmonary fibrosis, *HP* hypersensitivity pneumonitis, *U* upper, *M* middle, *L* lower, *SP* subpleural, *C* central, *R* random, *BV* bronchovascular, *HC* honeycombing

## Idiopathic Familial Pulmonary Fibrosis

### Pathology and Pathogenesis

There is a small subset of patients with IPF who have a history of unexplained lung disease in first-degree relatives. This form of pulmonary fibrosis has been referred to as familial IPF or familial interstitial pneumonia. Genetic analysis was performed in search of the mechanism underlying familial IPF, and telomerase germ line mutations were identified in 8 %. The role of telomerase mutations was hypothesized to be a function of excess telomere shortening over time, resulting in cellular dysfunction and premature cell death [25].

### Symptoms and Signs

The clinical features of familial IPF are indistinguishable from sporadic form of IPF, but the age at diagnosis is significantly younger [26].

### CT Findings

Like sporadic IPF, characteristic thin-section CT (TSCT) findings of familial IPF include areas of ground-glass opacity (GGO), intralobular reticular opacity, irregular thickening of the interlobular septa, traction bronchiectasis, and small foci of consolidation. HC is seen in approximately one-third of patients, and lung lesions demonstrate still lower lung zone predominance (67 %, 6 of 9 patients). However, upper lung zone predominance (33 %) is higher than nonfamilial IPF [21] (Fig. 17.5).

### CT–Pathology Comparisons

Please, refer to section "Honeycombing with Subpleural or Basal Predominance".

### Patient Prognosis

Overall prognosis of familial IPF is not well known, but pulmonary fibrosis associated with telomerase gene mutations has been reported to be progressive and lethal with a mean survival of 3 years after diagnosis [27].

## Chronic Hypersensitivity Pneumonia

### Pathology and Pathogenesis

The fibrosis pattern in chronic HP, which exhibits a predominantly UIP-like pattern histologically, is characterized by centrilobular fibrosis, bridging fibrosis, and intraluminal fibrosis, in addition to the subpleural and paraseptal fibrosis that is seen commonly in UIP cases. Bronchiolar alterations in patients with chronic HP are characterized by lymphoid aggregates, occasional granulomas or giant cells, and fibroblastic foci in the respiratory bronchioles [28].

### Symptoms and Signs

Chronic HP manifests as slowly progressive shortness of breath, cough, fatigue, malaise, and weight loss [29]. It frequently results in severe irreversible physiologic impairment due to lung fibrosis. History of acute episodes of HP is usually absent or unrecognized. Digital clubbing may be seen in advanced fibrotic HP.

### CT Findings

The radiologic findings of chronic HP are characterized by the presence of fibrosis, although evidence of active disease is often present. TSCT findings of chronic HP include intralobular interstitial thickening, irregular interlobular septal thickening, traction bronchiectasis, and HC superimposed on findings of subacute HP such as bilateral patchy areas of GGO, poorly defined small centrilobular nodules, and lobular areas of mosaic attenuation on inspiratory images and of air trapping on expiratory CT images [30]. Chronic HP may closely mimic UIP and fibrotic NSIP. The TSCT features that best differentiated chronic HP from UIP and NSIP are the presence of lobular areas of mosaic attenuation and centrilobular small nodules and the lack of lower zone predominance of HC [22].

### CT–Pathology Comparisons

Histologic features of chronic HP comprise overlapping UIP-like pattern, a NSIP-like pattern, organizing pneumonia pattern, centrilobular fibrosis, or bridging fibrosis (continuous fibrosis between the centrilobular and subpleural location) with or without granuloma [31].

### Patient Prognosis

Avoidance of further exposure to potential antigen is crucial in the management. Corticosteroids can be tried, but patients with chronic HP often progress to irreversible pulmonary fibrosis and about 30 % of them die within a few years of diagnosis. In general, the risk of mortality increases with evidence of fibrosis in lung biopsy or TSCT or with a more severe respiratory impairment on pulmonary function tests [32].

## End-stage Fibrotic Pulmonary Sarcoidosis

### Pathology and Pathogenesis

The characteristic histopathologic lesion of pulmonary sarcoidosis is the non-necrotizing granuloma, typically occurring within areas of sclerotic fibrosis. In sarcoidosis, small granulomas have a tendency to coalesce to form larger nodular lesions, all embedded in refractile eosinophilic collagen. Granulomas are distributed along lymphatic routes in the pleura, within the intralobular septa, and along the bronchovascular bundles. Multinucleate giant cells are characteristically present in the disease, often accompanied by a variety of distinctive cytoplasmic inclusions (*e.g.*, Schaumann bodies, asteroid bodies). Spontaneous resolution is common, suggesting that the granulomas often resolve but in other patients healing is by fibrosis, often with HC [33].

### Symptoms and Signs

Patients with end-stage fibrocystic pulmonary sarcoidosis commonly show varying degree of severe restrictive and obstructive pulmonary functional impairment. They complain of marked dyspnea and signs of right heart failure, especially lower extremity edema.

### CT Findings

TSCT findings of end-stage fibrotic pulmonary sarcoidosis include reticular opacity, traction bronchiectasis, architectural distortion, fibrotic cysts, bullae, and paracicatricial emphysema [34]. Occasionally, HC-like cysts are seen, which are most commonly distributed in the subpleural regions of the middle and upper lung zones, whereas the lung bases are usually spared [24]. Distribution and location of fibrosis and HC-like cysts are the differential diagnostic points from UIP.

### CT–Pathology Comparisons

Obstruction of lobar or segmental bronchi by either wall fibrosis or accumulation of granulomas may result in parenchymal distortion and cyst formation.

### Patient Prognosis

End-stage pulmonary sarcoidosis with cor pulmonale may warrant supplemental oxygen, diuretics, and bronchodilators for airway obstruction. Lung transplantation has been performed successfully [35].

## References


1. Arakawa H, Honma K. Honeycomb lung: history and current concepts. AJR Am J Roentgenol. 2011;196:773–82.
2. American Thoracic Society, European Respiratory Society. American Thoracic Society/European Respiratory Society International Multidisciplinary Consensus Classification of the Idiopathic Interstitial Pneumonias. This joint statement of the American Thoracic Society (ATS), and the European Respiratory Society (ERS) was adopted by the ATS board of directors, June 2001 and by the ERS Executive Committee, June 2001. Am J Respir Crit Care Med. 2002;165:277–304.

3. Akira M, Sakatani M, Ueda E. Idiopathic pulmonary fibrosis: progression of honeycombing at thin-section CT. Radiology. 1993;189: 687–91.
4. Watadani T, Sakai F, Johkoh T, et al. Interobserver variability in the CT assessment of honeycombing in the lungs. Radiology. 2013;266: 936–44.
5. Kligerman SJ, Groshong S, Brown KK, Lynch DA. Nonspecific interstitial pneumonia: radiologic, clinical, and pathologic considerations. Radiographics. 2009;29:73–87.
6. Akira M, Yamamoto S, Inoue Y, Sakatani M. High-resolution CT of asbestosis and idiopathic pulmonary fibrosis. AJR Am J Roentgenol. 2003;181:163–9.
7. Silva CI, Muller NL, Hansell DM, Lee KS, Nicholson AG, Wells AU. Nonspecific interstitial pneumonia and idiopathic pulmonary fibrosis: changes in pattern and distribution of disease over time. Radiology. 2008;247:251–9.
8. Flaherty KR, Toews GB, Travis WD, et al. Clinical significance of histological classification of idiopathic interstitial pneumonia. Eur Respir J. 2002;19:275–83.
9. Lee HY, Lee KS, Jeong YJ, et al. High-resolution CT findings in fibrotic idiopathic interstitial pneumonias with little honeycombing: serial changes and prognostic implications. AJR Am J Roentgenol. 2012;199:982–9.
10. Shin KM, Lee KS, Chung MP, et al. Prognostic determinants among clinical, thin-section CT, and histopathologic findings for fibrotic idiopathic interstitial pneumonias: tertiary hospital study. Radiology. 2008;249:328–37.
11. Akira M, Inoue Y, Kitaichi M, Yamamoto S, Arai T, Toyokawa K. Usual interstitial pneumonia and nonspecific interstitial pneumonia with and without concurrent emphysema: thin-section CT findings. Radiology. 2009;251:271–9.
12. Cottin V, Nunes H, Brillet PY, et al. Combined pulmonary fibrosis and emphysema: a distinct underrecognised entity. Eur Respir J. 2005; 26:586–93.
13. Raghu G, Collard HR, Egan JJ, et al. An official ATS/ERS/JRS/ALAT statement: idiopathic pulmonary fibrosis: evidence-based guidelines for diagnosis and management. Am J Respir Crit Care Med. 2011;183:788–824.
14. King Jr TE, Pardo A, Selman M. Idiopathic pulmonary fibrosis. Lancet. 2011;378:1949–61.
15. Muller NL, Coiby TV. Idiopathic interstitial pneumonias: high-resolution CT and histologic findings. Radiographics. 1997;17: 1016–22.
16. Travis WD, Hunninghake G, King Jr TE, et al. Idiopathic nonspecific interstitial pneumonia: report of an American Thoracic Society project. Am J Respir Crit Care Med. 2008;177:1338–47.
17. Katzenstein AL, Myers JL. Nonspecific interstitial pneumonia and the other idiopathic interstitial pneumonias: classification and diagnostic criteria. Am J Surg Pathol. 2000;24:1–3.
18. Kim TS, Lee KS, Chung MP, et al. Nonspecific interstitial pneumonia with fibrosis: high-resolution CT and pathologic findings. AJR Am J Roentgenol. 1998;171:1645–50.
19. Roggli VL, Gibbs AR, Attanoos R, et al. Pathology of asbestosis-an update of the diagnostic criteria: report of the asbestosis committee of the college of American pathologists and pulmonary pathology society. Arch Pathol Lab Med. 2010;134:462–80.
20. Akira M, Yamamoto S, Yokoyama K, et al. Asbestosis: high-resolution CT-pathologic correlation. Radiology. 1990;176: 389–94.
21. Nishiyama O, Taniguchi H, Kondoh Y, et al. Familial idiopathic pulmonary fibrosis: serial high-resolution computed tomography findings in 9 patients. J Comput Assist Tomogr. 2004;28:443–8.
22. Silva CI, Muller NL, Lynch DA, et al. Chronic hypersensitivity pneumonitis: differentiation from idiopathic pulmonary fibrosis and nonspecific interstitial pneumonia by using thin-section CT. Radiology. 2008;246:288–97.
23. Nunes H, Uzunhan Y, Gille T, Lamberto C, Valeyre D, Brillet PY. Imaging of sarcoidosis of the airways and lung parenchyma and correlation with lung function. Eur Respir J. 2012;40:750–65.
24. Abehsera M, Valeyre D, Grenier P, Jaillet H, Battesti JP, Brauner MW. Sarcoidosis with pulmonary fibrosis: CT patterns and correlation with pulmonary function. AJR Am J Roentgenol. 2000;174: 1751–7.
25. Armanios MY, Chen JJ, Cogan JD, et al. Telomerase mutations in families with idiopathic pulmonary fibrosis. N Engl J Med. 2007;356:1317–26.
26. van Moorsel CH, van Oosterhout MF, Barlo NP, et al. Surfactant protein C mutations are the basis of a significant portion of adult familial pulmonary fibrosis in a Dutch cohort. Am J Respir Crit Care Med. 2010;182:1419–25.
27. Diaz de Leon A, Cronkhite JT, Katzenstein AL, et al. Telomere lengths, pulmonary fibrosis and telomerase (TERT) mutations. PLoS One. 2010;5:e10680.
28. Takemura T, Akashi T, Kamiya H, et al. Pathological differentiation of chronic hypersensitivity pneumonitis from idiopathic pulmonary fibrosis/usual interstitial pneumonia. Histopathology. 2012;61: 1026–35.
29. Selman M, Buendia-Roldan I. Immunopathology, diagnosis, and management of hypersensitivity pneumonitis. Semin Respir Crit Care Med. 2012;33:543–54.
30. Hansell DM, Wells AU, Padley SP, Muller NL. Hypersensitivity pneumonitis: correlation of individual CT patterns with functional abnormalities. Radiology. 1996;199:123–8.
31. Takemura T, Akashi T, Ohtani Y, Inase N, Yoshizawa Y. Pathology of hypersensitivity pneumonitis. Curr Opin Pulm Med. 2008;14: 440–54.
32. Hanak V, Golbin JM, Hartman TE, Ryu JH. High-resolution CT findings of parenchymal fibrosis correlate with prognosis in hypersensitivity pneumonitis. Chest. 2008;134:133–8.
33. Rosen Y, Athanassiades TJ, Moon S, Lyons HA. Nongranulomatous interstitial pneumonitis in sarcoidosis. Relationship to development of epithelioid granulomas. Chest. 1978;74:122–5.
34. Baughman RP, Winget DB, Bowen EH, Lower EE. Predicting respiratory failure in sarcoidosis patients. Sarcoidosis Vasc Diffuse Lung Dis. 1997;14:154–8.
35. Shlobin OA, Nathan SD. Management of end-stage sarcoidosis: pulmonary hypertension and lung transplantation. Eur Respir J. 2012; 39:1520–33.

# Small Nodules

# 18

## Small Nodules with Centrilobular Distribution

### Definition

Small nodules, usually less than 10 mm in diameter, are regarded to be centrilobular when the nodules are separated from pleural surfaces or the interlobular septa by a distance of several millimeters, usually centered 4–10 mm from the pleural or fissural surfaces or from interlobular septa [1, 2]. They are frequently associated with centrilobular branching nodular structures, thus forming the so-called tree-in-bud sign (Figs. 18.1 and 18.2) (see also Chap. 9). The small nodules represent lesions involving the small airways. However, vascular lesions involving the arterioles and capillaries may simulate the centrilobular small nodules and branching nodular structures (vascular tree-in-bud sign) [1, 3, 4] (Fig. 18.3).

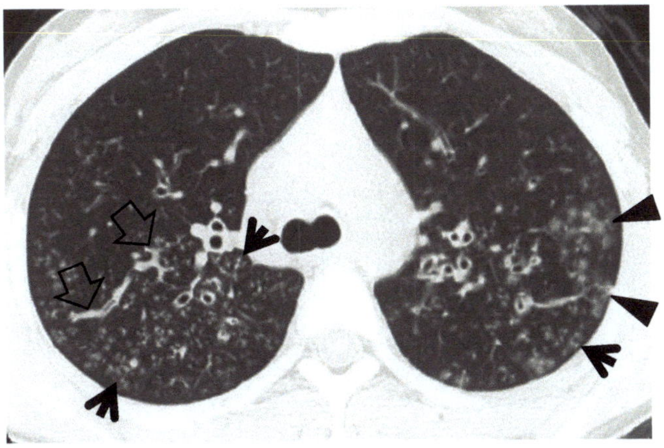

**Fig. 18.1** Cystic fibrosis in a 21-year-old woman. Lung window image of CT scan (2.5-mm section thickness) obtained at level of azygos arch shows well-defined (*arrows*) and poorly defined (*arrowheads*) tree-in-bud sign in both upper lobes. Also note mucus plugging (*open arrows*) in medium-sized airways

### Diseases Causing the Pattern

The diseases manifesting small nodules of centrilobular distribution or tree-in-bud signs include infectious bronchiolitis including *Haemophilus influenzae* pneumonia and *Mycoplasma pneumoniae* pneumonia [5] (Fig. 18.4), bronchogenic dissemination of pulmonary tuberculosis [6, 7] or the *nodular bronchiectatic form of nontuberculous mycobacterial (NTM) pulmonary disease* [8, 9] (Fig. 18.5), *diffuse panbronchiolitis (DPB)* [10] (Fig. 18.6), subacute hypersensitivity pneumonitis, *follicular bronchiolitis* [11] (Fig. 18.7) or bronchus-associated lymphoid tissue lymphoma [12], and cystic fibrosis [13].

Vascular tree-in-bud sign may be seen in *pulmonary tumor embolism* [3] or localized lymphangitic carcinomatosis (Figs. 18.3 and 18.8), foreign-body-induced necrotizing vasculitis or necrotizing pulmonary vasculitis in systemic lupus erythematosus [4, 6], and localized pulmonary lymphatic metastasis [14].

### Distribution

In infectious bronchiolitis and DPB, the small nodules or tree-in-bud signs show middle and lower lung zone predominance. In particular, the small nodules in DPB depict symmetric and subpleural distribution along with bronchiectasis [10]. They are random and patchy in distribution in bronchogenic dissemination of tuberculosis, hypersensitivity pneumonitis, and follicular bronchiolitis or bronchus-associated lymphoid tissue lymphoma or follicular bronchiolitis. Right middle lobe and lingular division of the left upper lobe are typical location of nodular bronchiectatic form of nontuberculous mycobacterial pulmonary disease. Other lobes such as right upper lobe and both lower lobes may have lesions of tree-in-bud signs (pathologic cellular bronchiolitis). The lesions of bronchiectasis and cellular bronchiolitis (tree-in-bud signs) in the disease are asymmetrically distributed, differently from DPB [8, 9].

K.S. Lee et al., *Radiology Illustrated: Chest Radiology*, Radiology Illustrated,
DOI 10.1007/978-3-642-37096-0_18, © Springer-Verlag Berlin Heidelberg 2014

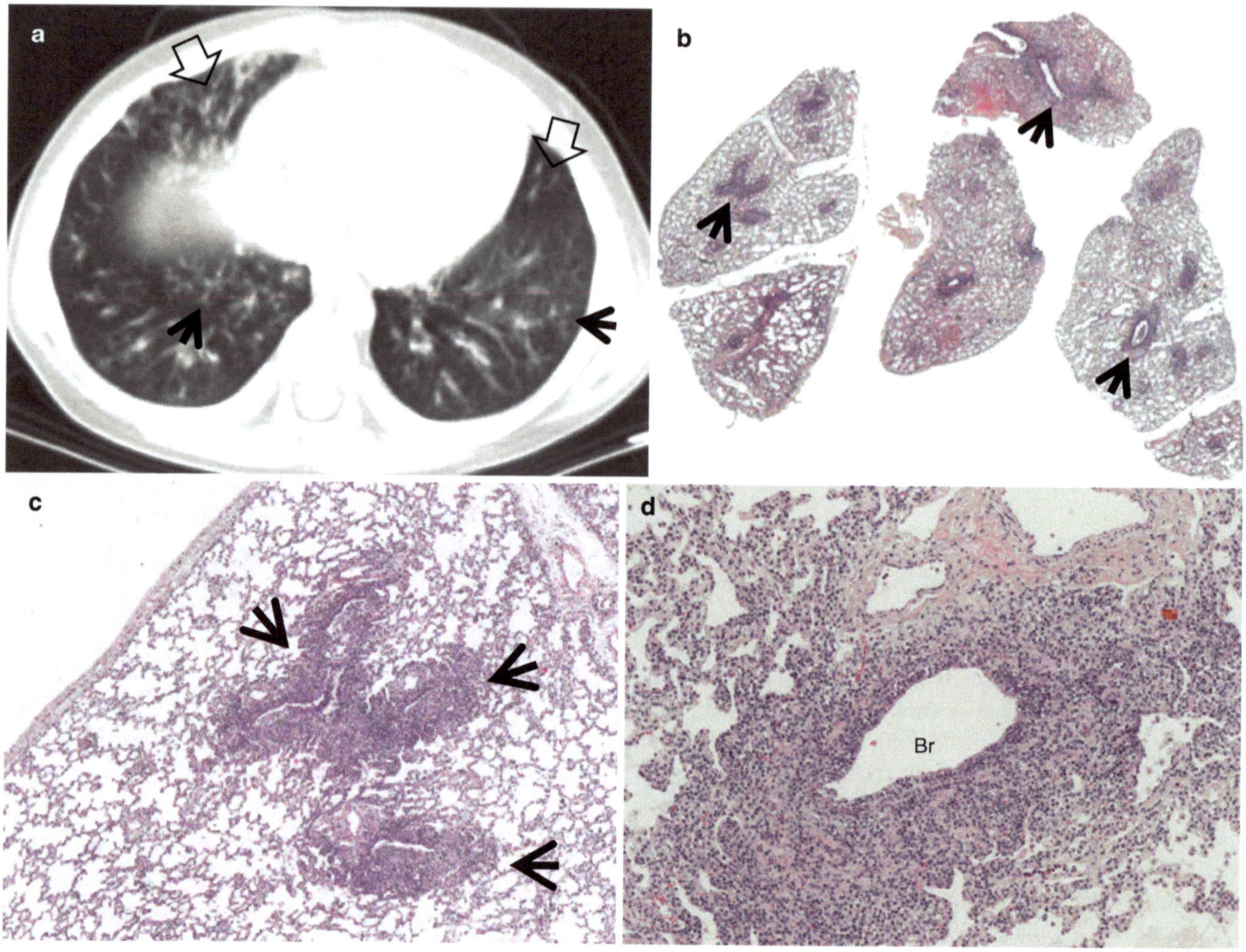


**Fig. 18.2** Infectious bronchiolitis showing tree-in-bud signs in a 3-year-old boy. (**a**) Lung window image of CT scan (5.0-mm section thickness) obtained at level of liver dome shows tree-in-bud signs (*arrows*) in both lower lobes. Also note bronchiectasis (*open arrows*) in bottom of right middle lobe and lingular division of left upper lobe. (**b**) Low-magnification (×10) photomicrograph of surgical biopsy specimen obtained from right lower lobe demonstrates bronchiolocentric (*arrows*) dense inflammatory cell (cellular) infiltration. (**c**) High-magnification (×100) photomicrography exhibits more clearly bronchiolocentric (*arrows*) dense inflammatory cell infiltration. (**d**) High-magnification (×200) photomicrograph discloses thickened bronchiolar wall with dense lymphoplasma cell infiltration and expansion of subepithelial connective tissue. *Br* bronchiole

In tumor thrombotic microangiopathy, necrotizing vasculitis, and localized lymphatic metastasis, the vascular tree-in-bud sings demonstrate lower lung zone and subpleural predominance.

## Clinical Considerations

Chronic maxillary sinusitis is usually associated with DPB. Follicular bronchiolitis is a kind of lymphoproliferative disease. Therefore, the disease is frequently associated with rheumatoid arthritis, mixed collagen vascular disorders, autoimmune disorders, or acquired immunodeficiency syndrome [11]. Patient diagnosis of cystic fibrosis may be confirmed with positive chloride sweat test in all cases. As in DPB, maxillary sinusitis is frequently associated and the sinusitis may be used as a surrogate model for gene therapy [15].

Pulmonary tumor thrombotic microangiopathy is infrequently seen in a patient with gastric cancer [16], ovarian cancer, or lung invasive adenocarcinoma. In tumor thrombotic microangiopathy, hypoxemia is severe and patient complains of progressive dyspnea.

**Key Points for Differential Diagnosis**

| | Distribution | | | | | | | | | | | |
|---|---|---|---|---|---|---|---|---|---|---|---|---|
| | Zones | | | | | | | | Clinical presentations | | | |
| Diseases | U | M | L | SP | C | R | BV | R | Acute | Subacute | Chronic | Others |
| Infectious bronchiolitis | | + | + | | | + | | + | + | | | |
| Bronchogenic dissemination of TB | + | + | + | | | + | | + | + | + | | With or without parenchymal opacity (TB) |
| NTM disease | | + | + | | | + | | + | | | + | With bronchiectasis, mainly in RML and Li division of LUL |
| DPB | | + | + | + | | | | + | | | + | Sinusitis, bilateral symmetric distribution with bronchiectasis |
| HP | + | + | + | | | + | | + | | + | | With parenchymal diffuse ground-glass opacity |
| Follicular bronchiolitis | + | + | + | | | + | + | + | | + | + | Underlying condition such as collagen vascular disease or immunosuppressive disease |
| Cystic fibrosis | + | + | | + | | | | + | | | + | With bronchiectasis |
| TTM | | | + | + | | | | + | | | + | Underlying malignancy such as gastric, ovarian, or lung cancer |

*Note*: *TB* tuberculosis, *NTM* nontuberculous mycobacterial, *DPB* diffuse panbronchiolitis, *HP* hypersensitivity pneumonitis, *TTM* tumor thrombotic microangiopathy, *U* upper, *M* middle, *L* lower, *SP* subpleural, *C* central, *R* random, *BV* bronchovascular, *RML* right middle lobe, *Li* lingular division, *LUL* left upper lobe

## *Mycoplasma Pneumoniae* Pneumonia

### Pathology and Pathogenesis

*Mycoplasmas* are the smallest (0.2–0.8 μm) free-living bacteria, but they lack a true cell wall. They are facultative anaerobes, except for *Mycoplasma pneumoniae*, the most common pulmonary pathogen, which is a strict aerobe. Although it is primarily an infection of young adults, it can attack the elderly. The most common clinical syndrome is tracheobronchitis, with one-third of patients developing a mild but persistent pneumonia. Mycoplasma pneumonia is rarely biopsied, because positive cold agglutinin and specific complement fixation antigen assays establish the diagnosis. Biopsied cases show lymphocytic or neutrophilic bronchiolitis with alveolar wall inflammation and fibrinous exudates [17].

### Symptoms and Signs

*Mycoplasma pneumoniae* pneumonia closely resembles typical pneumonia in the clinical manifestations, such as fever, cough, and purulent sputum. However, patients with *Mycoplasma pneumoniae* pneumonia commonly have upper respiratory tract manifestations (otitis, bullous myringitis, and mild nonexudative pharyngitis). Extrapulmonary features, such as unexplained watery diarrhea, thrombocytosis, and hemolysis, are also common.

### CT Findings

Common thin-section CT (TSCT) findings include centrilobular small nodules and branching linear opacity lesions (tree-in-bud pattern) in a patchy distribution, bronchial wall thickening, and areas of ground-glass opacity (GGO) and consolidation in a lobular or segmental distribution [18, 19] (Fig. 18.4). The abnormalities tend to have a patchy unilateral or asymmetric bilateral distribution, but may be diffuse. Another common abnormality is thickening of the peribronchial interstitium. The CT findings of Mycoplasma pneumonia in children include lobar or segmental consolidation with pleural effusion and regional lymphadenopathy and mild volume loss similar to those of bacterial lobar pneumonia [19]. Most patients with Mycoplasma pneumonia recover

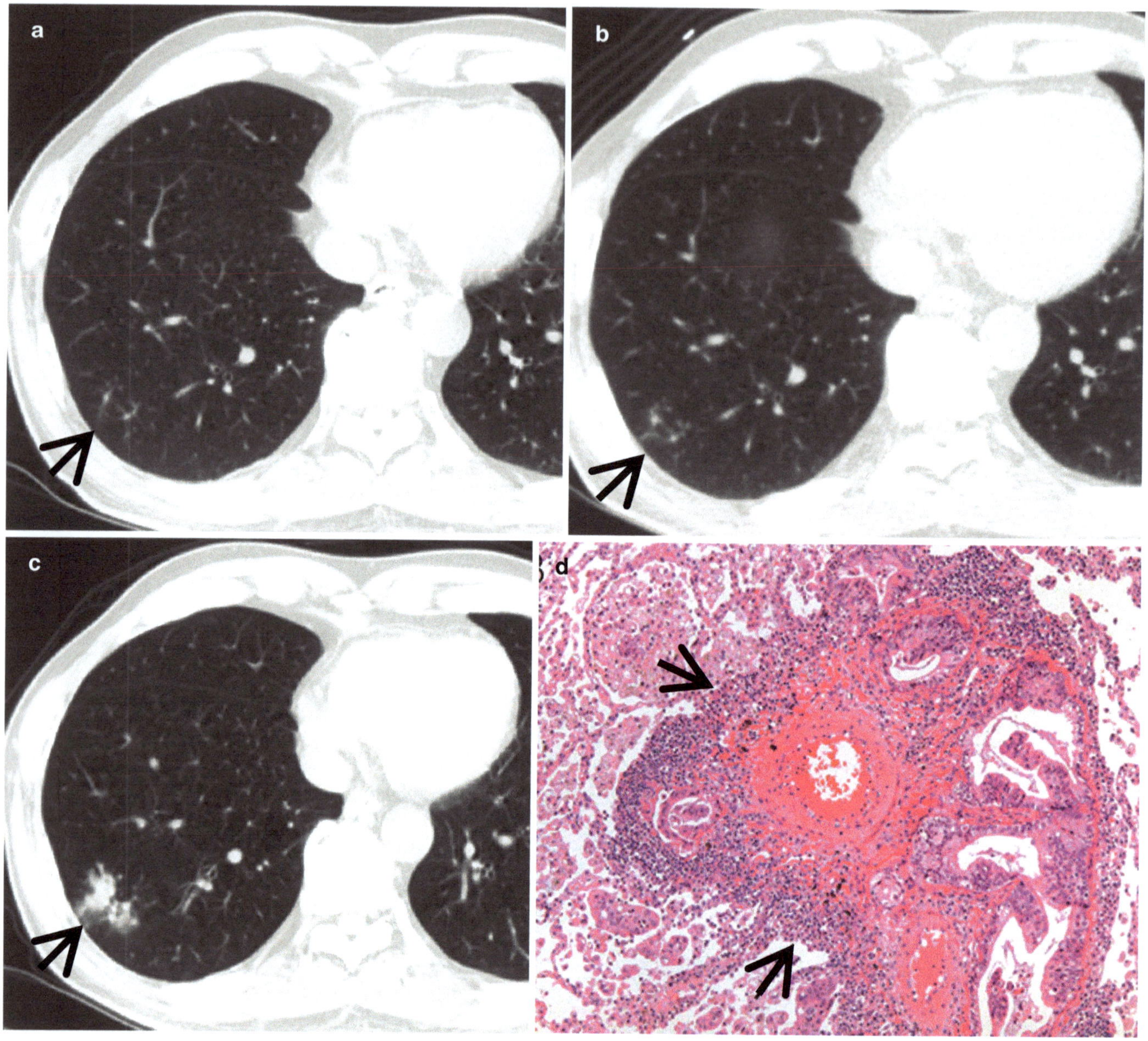


**Fig. 18.3** Lymphangitic metastasis along bronchovascular bundles manifesting as vascular tree-in-bud sign in a 59-year-old man who has pancreas head cancer. (**a**–**c**) Lung window images of serial CT scans obtained at same level over the follow-up period of 6 months show evolving lung lesion from tree-in-bud sign (*arrows* in **a** and **b**) to localized area of lobular consolidation or a poorly defined nodule (*arrow* in **c**) in the right lower lobe. (**d**) High-magnification photomicrograph of surgical lung biopsy obtained from right lower lobe and at similar time to (**c**) discloses tumor cells (*arrows*) tracking arteriolar walls (definition-wise, lymphangitic tumor spread). Please note patent arteriolar lumen without cancer cells

completely; however, a small percentage, particularly children, develops bronchiectasis and bronchiolitis obliterans [20].

## CT–Pathology Comparisons

Centrilobular small nodules and branching linear opacity lesions on TSCT reflect the presence of cellular inflammatory bronchiolitis. Lobular or segmental consolidation is related to pneumonia caused by extension of infection and concomitant inflammatory reaction into the parenchyma adjacent to the airways [17].

## Patient Prognosis

Treatment response is good if timely diagnosed and treated with effective antibiotics, but severe adult respiratory distress syndrome and macrolide-resistant *Mycoplasma pneumonia* have been reported [21].

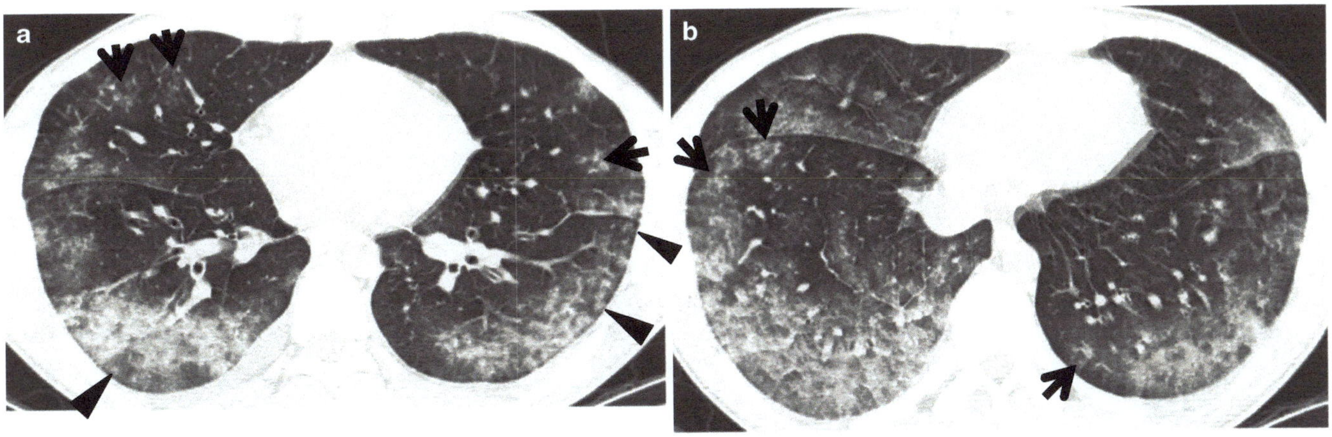


**Fig. 18.4** *Mycoplasma pneumoniae* pneumonia in a 2-year-old man. (**a**, **b**) Lung window images of CT scans (2.5-mm section thickness) obtained at levels of cardiac ventricle (**a**) and suprahepatic inferior vena cava (**b**), respectively, show extensive ground-glass opacity in both lungs. Also note poorly formed centrilobular small nodules (*arrowheads*) and tree-in-bud signs (*arrows*) in both lungs

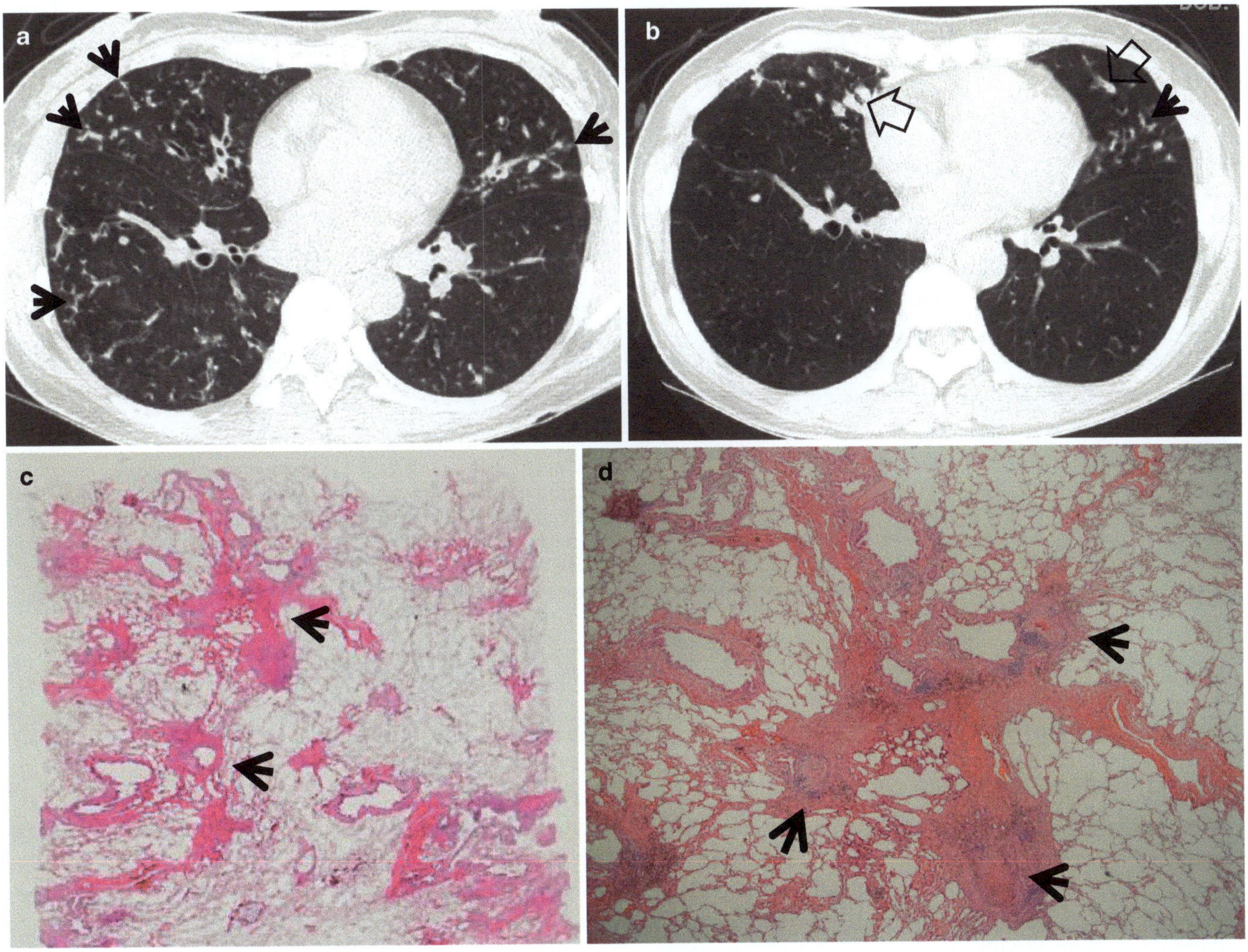


**Fig. 18.5** *Mycobacterium intracellulare* pulmonary disease in a 53-year-old woman. (**a**, **b**) Lung window images of consecutive CT scans (2.5-mm section thickness) obtained at level of inferior pulmonary veins show tree-in-bud signs (*arrows*) in both lungs. Also note bronchiectasis with (*open arrows*) or without mucus plugging especially in right middle lobe and lingular division of left upper lobe. (**c**) Low-magnification photomicrograph (×40) of pathologic specimen obtained from a different patient with nontuberculous mycobacterial pulmonary disease exhibits bronchiolocentric (membranous bronchiole, *arrows*) chronic inflammation, fibrosis, and granuloma formation. (**d**) High-magnification photomicrograph (×100) discloses granulomas (*arrows*) with surrounding chronic inflammation and fibrosis along membranous bronchioles

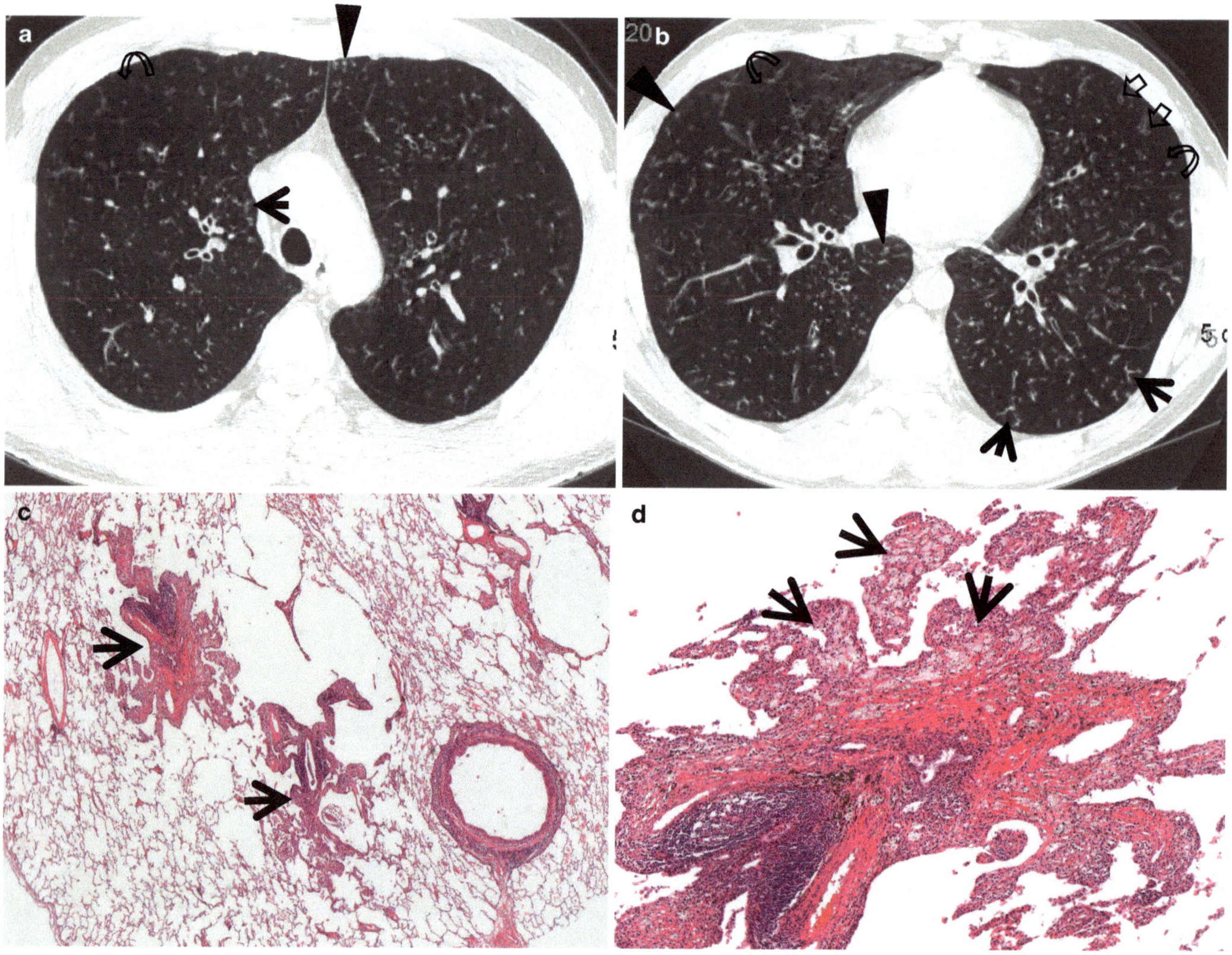


**Fig. 18.6** Diffuse panbronchiolitis in a 38-year-old man. (**a**, **b**) Lung window images of thin-section CT scans (1.5-mm section thickness) obtained at levels of aortic arch (**a**) and right inferior pulmonary vein (**b**), respectively, show small centrilobular nodules (*arrowheads*), tree-in-bud signs (*arrows*), bronchiolectasis (*open arrows*), and area of mosaic attenuation (*curved arrows*) in both lungs. (**c**) Low-magnification (×40) photomicrograph of surgical lung biopsy obtained from right lower lobe demonstrates marked membranous bronchiolar wall thickening (*arrows*) with lymphocytes and macrophages. (**d**) A more closer look (×100) of the inflamed bronchiole discloses bronchiolar wall thickening with chronic inflammatory cell infiltration and patchy aggregates of fibrosis. Surrounding alveolar walls contain many foamy macrophages (*arrows*)

## Nontuberculous Mycobacterial Pulmonary Disease

### Pathology and Pathogenesis

Chronic progressive disease also resembles tuberculosis, with upper lobe thin-walled cavities and granulomatous inflammation, with or without caseous necrosis. This presentation most often is seen in patients with underlying chronic lung disease such as chronic obstructive pulmonary disease (COPD), bronchiectasis, cystic fibrosis, pneumoconiosis, reflux disease, or preexisting cavitary lung disease of any cause. The differentiation of tuberculosis from NTM disease could not be accurately made based solely on the histologic features (Fig. 18.5). However, the airway-centered tendency of NTM reflects an airborne etiology, and this could be correlated with the classification according to the radiologic findings. In addition, coexisting constitutional lung diseases, and especially bronchiectasis, were suspected to be predisposing conditions for NTM organisms to colonize and progress to true NTM pulmonary disease [22].

### Symptoms and Signs

NTM lung infection presents with diverse manifestations. Symptoms of bronchiectasis including cough, sputum production, and hemoptysis can occur. Tuberculosis-like

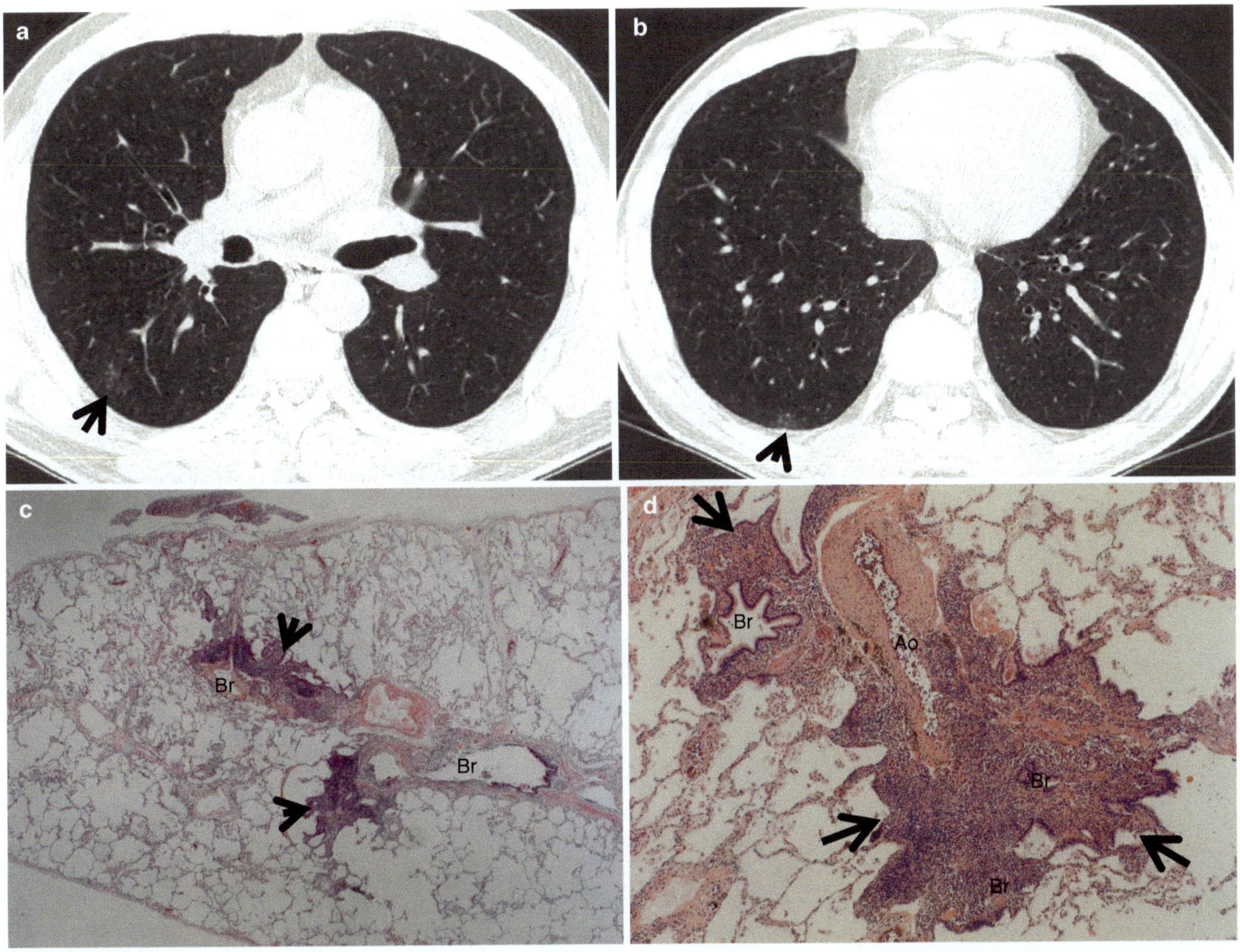


**Fig. 18.7** Follicular bronchiolitis in a 61-year-old man with Sjögren's syndrome. (**a**, **b**) Lung window images of thin-section CT scans (1.5-mm section thickness) obtained at levels of aortic arch (**a**) and right inferior pulmonary vein (**b**), respectively, show small centrilobular nodules and branching nodular structures (tree-in-bud signs, *arrows*) in superior and posterior basal segments of right lower lobe. (**c**) Low-magnification (×40) photomicrograph of surgical biopsy specimen obtained from right lower lobe demonstrates bronchiolocentric (*Br*) inflammatory lesions (*arrows*). (**d**) High-magnification (×200) photomicrograph discloses narrowed or obliterated bronchiolar lumen (*Br*) owing to dense lymphocyte infiltrates (*arrows*). *Ao* arteriole

symptoms, such as fatigue, weight loss, night sweating, and fever, are not uncommon. Some patients may be asymptomatic.

## CT Findings

The most common TSCT findings of nodular bronchiectatic form of NTM pulmonary disease include centrilobular small nodules or tree-in-bud pattern, with tubular bronchiectasis, usually in right middle lobe, the lingular segment of left upper lobe, and both the lower lobes [8, 9] (Fig. 18.5). TSCT findings of bronchiectasis and bronchiolitis involving more than five lobes, especially when associated with lobular consolidation or a cavity, are highly suggestive of NTM pulmonary disease [9].

## CT–Pathology Comparisons

Centrilobular small nodules, tree-in-bud pattern, and bronchiectasis correspond histopathologically to bronchiectasis and bronchiolar and peribronchiolar inflammation with or without granuloma formation [8]. NTM pulmonary disease is mainly a bronchocentric or bronchiolocentric inflammatory process [23]. It begins with bronchial or bronchiolar wall thickening and develops into peribronchial or peribronchiolar thickening or a peribronchial nodule. Nodular bronchiectatic form of NTM disease on TSCT represents this stage of inflammation mainly involving small airways. During the inflammatory process, the central necrotic portion with destroyed bronchial wall and cartilage seems to be ulcerated and detached into the airway. In this circumstance, the central patent bronchus disposes of the detached central necrotic

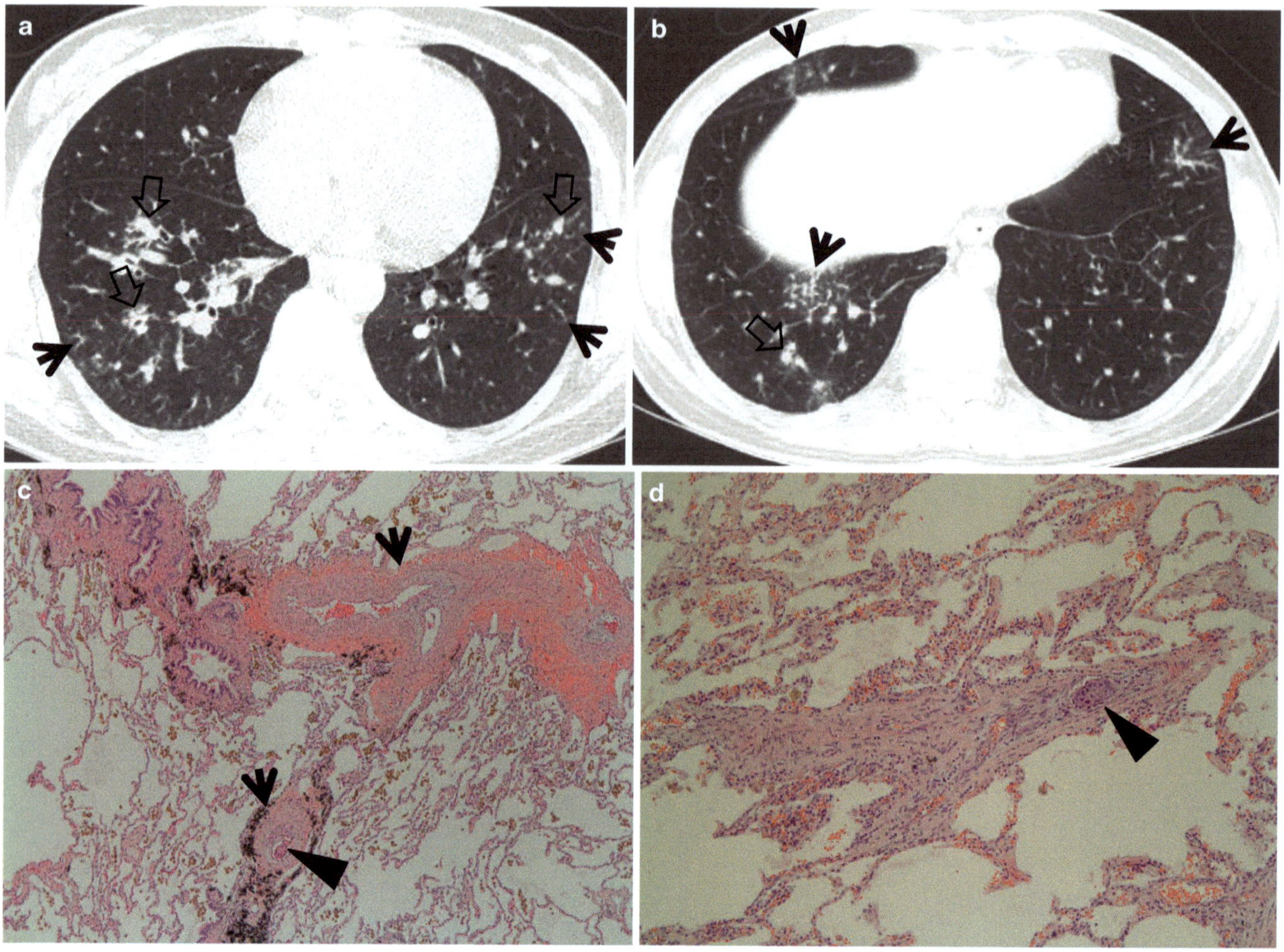


**Fig. 18.8** Tumor emboli and lymphangitic carcinomatosis along bronchovascular bundles showing vascular tree-in-bud signs in a 34-year-old woman with gastric cancer. (**a**, **b**) Lung window images of thin-section CT scans (1.5-mm section thickness) obtained at levels of cardiac ventricle (**a**) and liver dome (**b**), respectively, show thickened axial interstitium (bronchovascular bundles) (*open arrows*) and several foci of tree-in-bud signs (*arrows*) in both lungs. (**c**) High-magnification (×100) photomicrograph of surgical lung biopsy specimen from another patient demonstrates dilated arterioles (*arrows*) with thickened wall. Please note intravascular tumor emboli (*arrowhead*). There are many hemosiderin-laden macrophages in alveolar spaces. (**d**) Another photomicrograph (×100) discloses an arteriole with thick wall containing intraluminal tumor emboli (*arrowhead*)

debris, thus resulting in cavity formation and bronchogenic spread of the infection. Cavitary form of NTM infection on TSCT represents this stage of inflammation mainly involving relatively large airways and more extensive inflammation.

### Patient Prognosis

Making a diagnosis of NTM lung disease does not necessitate the institution of therapy. Decision to treat or not should be based on the potential risk and benefit of long-term medical therapy and on the species of NTM [24]. In particular, *Mycobacterium abscessus* infection is quite resistant to medical therapy [25]. Surgical resection is the one of the treatment options if the lung lesion is localized.

## Diffuse Panbronchiolitis

### Pathology and Pathogenesis

DPB is a distinctive inflammatory condition characterized by chronic bronchiolitis associated with prominent interstitial vacuolated or "foamy" histiocytes in a peribronchiolar distribution. A genetic susceptibility has been well documented over the years and has been identified as a human leukocyte antigen (HLA)-associated major susceptibility gene [26].

### Symptoms and Signs

Common symptoms of DPB are persistent cough, large amount of purulent sputum, and progressive exertional dyspnea [27]. Wheezing and crackles are heard. Superimposed pneumonia can occur. More than 80 % of patients have a history or coexistence of chronic paranasal sinusitis.

### CT Findings

The characteristic TSCT findings include centrilobular small nodules and branching linear opacity lesions, bronchiolectasis, bronchiectasis, and mosaic areas of decreased parenchymal attenuation [10] (Fig. 18.6). The presence of these findings is related to the stage of disease: the earliest manifestation consists of centrilobular small nodules, followed by branching opacity lesions that connect to the nodules, followed by bronchiolectasis and, eventually, bronchiectasis. Cystic bronchiectasis may be seen in the late stage [28]. The nodular bronchiectatic form of nontuberculous mycobacterial lung disease and DPB shows similar imaging findings. However, the number of lobes involved with bronchiectasis and cellular bronchiolitis on TSCT are more numerous in DPB patients [29].

### CT–Pathology Comparisons

TSCT findings of centrilobular small nodules and branching linear opacity lesions, bronchiolectasis, and bronchiectasis have been shown to correspond to bronchiolar wall and peribronchiolar inflammation and fibrosis, bronchiolar dilatation with the presence of intraluminal secretions, and dilated air-filled bronchioles. Mosaic areas of decreased parenchymal attenuation are related to air trapping caused by bronchiolar narrowing in the subpleural areas [10].

### Patient Prognosis

Long-term low-dose erythromycin therapy is effective for DPB with a 5-year survival rate of 91 % [30]. Prognosis is poor in the advanced cases with extensive bronchiectasis or respiratory failure.

## Follicular Bronchiolitis

### Pathology and Pathogenesis

Follicular bronchiolitis is characterized by lymphoid follicles containing reactive germinal centers in the walls of bronchioles and occasionally pleura, especially in patients with rheumatoid arthritis (Fig. 18.7). There may be postobstructive changes such as mucostasis and organizing pneumonia and absence of significant lymphoid infiltrate in the adjacent lung parenchyma [31].

### Symptoms and Signs

Presenting symptoms include cough, dyspnea, fever, recurrent pneumonia, weight loss, and fatigue [32]. Since follicular bronchiolitis is commonly associated with underlying systemic diseases such as immunodeficiencies and connective tissue diseases, particularly rheumatoid arthritis and Sjögren's syndrome, clinical manifestations of underlying disease can be found.

### CT Findings

The main TSCT findings of follicular bronchiolitis include bilateral centrilobular small nodules and peribronchiolar nodules [11] (Fig. 18.7). Most nodules measure less than 3 mm in diameter but occasionally are as large as 1–2 cm in diameter. Other findings include patchy GGO areas, bronchial wall thickening, and patchy areas of low attenuation.

### CT–Pathology Comparisons

Centrilobular small nodules and peribronchiolar nodules on TSCT reflect peribronchiolar inflammation and coalescent germinal centers [11].

### Patient Prognosis

The management of follicular bronchiolitis is principally directed at the underlying disease. Corticosteroids and azathioprine therapy have been used with some success in those with progressive follicular bronchiolitis. Prognosis is generally favorable but depends on the underlying condition and the age at the time of biopsy [32].

## Pulmonary Tumor Embolism

### Pathology and Pathogenesis

Tumor emboli are common in the lungs. A few of them survive to form metastatic deposits but most die very soon after arriving in the lungs: the embolus then becomes enclosed by platelets and finally undergoes organization. Occlusion of the pulmonary arteries may be due to tumor alone, or the tumor may promote thrombosis, organization of which results in fibrocellular intimal thickening, the so-called carcinomatous thrombotic microangiopathy (tumor thrombotic microangiopathy, TTM) or vascular intimal carcinomatosis [33].

### Symptoms and Signs

The most common presenting complaint is dyspnea, in 57–100 % of cases [34]. Clinical symptoms and signs of pulmonary tumor embolism include subacute and progressive dyspnea, tachypnea, tachycardia, and hypoxemia. Right heart failure is present in 15–20 % of cases.

### CT Findings

CT findings of pulmonary tumor embolism include peripheral wedge-shaped opacity, filling defects in the central pulmonary arteries, dilated and beaded peripheral pulmonary arteries, and nodular and branching centrilobular small nodules (tree-in-bud pattern) [35, 36] (Fig. 18.8).

### CT–Pathology Comparisons

Vascular tree-in-bud sign are caused by the filling of centrilobular arteries with tumor cells themselves or thrombotic microangiopathy characterized by extensive fibrocellular intimal hyperplasia of small pulmonary arteries initiated by tumor microemboli [35]. Dilated and beaded peripheral pulmonary arteries reflect intravascular tumor emboli or microangiopathy (fibrocellular intimal hyperplasia) [36]. Peripheral wedge-shaped opacity distal to some of the dilated pulmonary arteries suggests pulmonary infarct.

### Patient Prognosis

There is no specific treatment if pulmonary tumor embolism is diagnosed antemortem. There have been case reports of survival if the tumor is highly responsive to chemotherapy (e.g., choriocarcinoma, Wilms' tumor, renal cell carcinoma, gastric cancer) [37].

## Small Nodules with Perilymphatic Distribution

### Definition

Small nodules are considered perilymphatic when the nodules are predominant in relation to the subpleural location, interlobular septa, and centrilobular core structures as well. The nodules may be observed along the parahilar bronchovascular bundles [1]. The distinction between perilymphatic and random distribution is usually determined by observing patchy versus random and the presence of thickening or nodularity of the bronchovascular bundles (Fig. 18.9). Namely, the patchy distribution and the presence of interstitial thickening or nodularity favor the decision of perilymphatic distribution, whereas random distribution and normal or smooth bronchovascular bundles suggest random distribution [2].

### Diseases Causing the Pattern

Perilymphatic small nodules are observed in patients with *pneumoconiosis* (Fig. 18.10), *pulmonary sarcoidosis* (Figs. 18.9 and 18.11), lymphangitic carcinomatosis, and *pulmonary alveoloseptal amyloidosis* [1] (Fig. 18.12).

### Distribution

In pneumoconiosis, small nodules show upper and middle lung zone predominance. Also in sarcoidosis, the lesions usually show upper and middle lung zone predominance but may show no zonal predominance. Lymphangitic carcinomatosis demonstrates middle and lower lung zone predominance as is the case in amyloidosis [38].

### Clinical Considerations

The presence of occupational exposure history to coal dusts or silica renders a diagnosis of pneumoconiosis. Patients with pulmonary sarcoidosis usually have no specific symptoms. The disease may be suspected with abnormal chest radiographs. Conversely patients with pulmonary sarcoidosis may have fatigue, fever, weight loss, dry cough, or shortness of breath. Up to 20 % of individuals with sarcoidosis develop skin problems such as rash or nodules. Eye symptoms such as blurred vision, pain, and photosensitivity may occur occasionally in sarcoidosis. The most common primary cancer sites related to PLC are the breasts, lungs, colon, and the stomach [39].

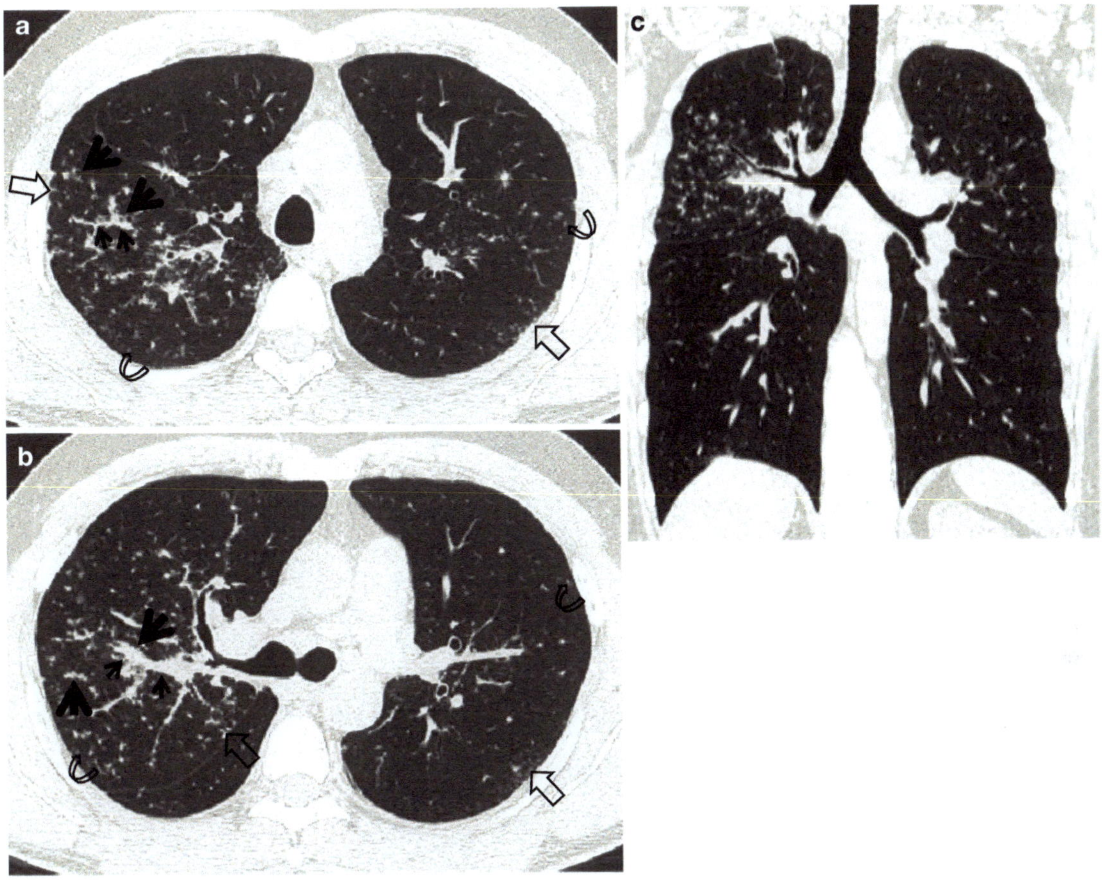


**Fig. 18.9** Pulmonary sarcoidosis manifesting perilymphatic nodules in a 31-year-old man. (**a**, **b**) Lung window images of thin-section (1.0-mm section thickness) CT scans obtained at levels of aortic arch (**a**) and right upper lobar bronchus (**b**), respectively, show small nodules along bronchovascular bundles (*arrows*), subpleural lungs (*open arrows*), and in centrilobular areas (*curved arrows*). Also note thickening of bronchovascular bundles (*small arrows*) indicative of perilymphatic lesions of sarcoidosis. (**c**) Coronal reformatted image (2.0-mm section thickness) demonstrates upper lung zone predominance of perilymphatic nodular lesions

**Key Points for Differential Diagnosis**

| | Distribution | | | | | | | | Clinical presentations | | | |
|---|---|---|---|---|---|---|---|---|---|---|---|---|
| | Zones | | | | | | | | | | | |
| Diseases | U | M | L | SP | C | R | BV | R | Acute | Subacute | Chronic | Others |
| Pneumoconiosis | + | + | | | | + | | + | | | + | |
| Sarcoidosis | + | + | ± | | | + | + | | | + | + | Usually associated with lymph node sarcoidosis |
| PLC | | + | + | | | + | | + | | + | + | With smooth or nodular interlobular septal thickening |
| Pulmonary amyloidosis | | + | + | + | | | | + | | | + | May show internal calcifications |

*Note*: *PLC* pulmonary lymphangitic carcinomatosis, *U* upper, *M* middle, *L* lower, *SP* subpleural, *C* central, *R* random, *BV* bronchovascular

## Pneumoconiosis

### Pathology and Pathogenesis

Pneumoconiosis is defined as permanent alteration of the lung structure due to the inhalation of mineral dust and the tissue reactions of the lung to its presence, excluding bronchitis and emphysema. To reach the lung, dust particles have to be very small. Particle density and shape also affect the aerodynamic properties of dust. Host factors such as airflow characteristics, airway branching patterns, and airway disease also affect dust deposition [40].

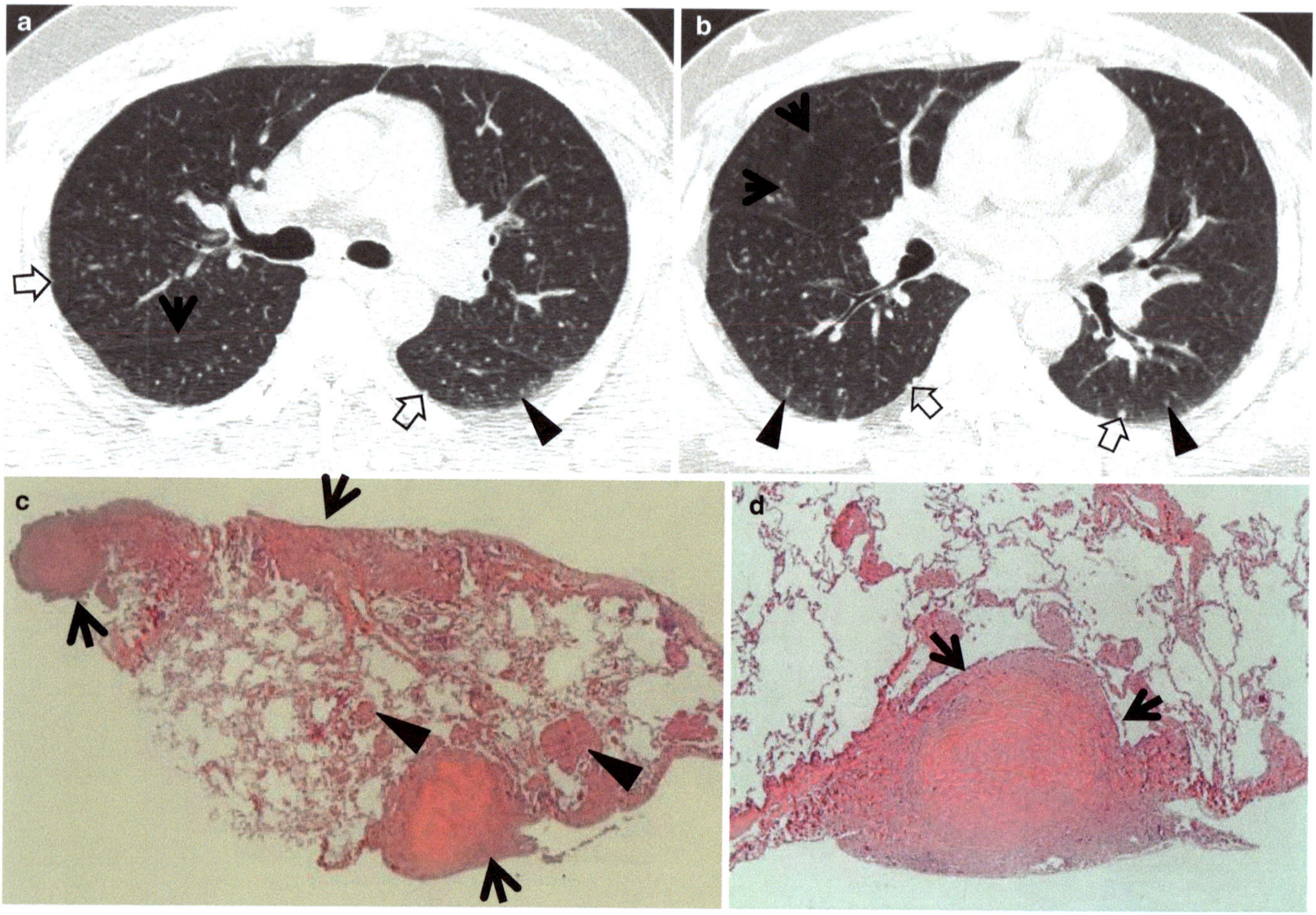


**Fig. 18.10** Pneumoconiotic nodules showing perilymphatic distribution in a 32-year-old building demolition worker. (**a**, **b**) Lung window images of thin-section (1.0-mm section thickness) CT scans obtained at levels of right upper lobar bronchus (**a**) and distal bronchus intermedius (**b**), respectively, show small nodules along fissures (*arrows*), subpleural lungs (*open arrows*), and in centrilobular regions (*arrowheads*). (**c**) Low-magnification (×10) photomicrograph of surgical biopsy specimen obtained from right upper lobe demonstrates multiple noncaseating and fibrotic granulomas having perilymphatic distribution; granulomas are located along pleura (*arrows*) and in alveolar walls (*arrowheads*). (**d**) High-magnification (×2,000 photomicrograph discloses a well-circumscribed pneumoconiosis nodule (*arrows*) composed of mature collagen in the central portion, with a peripheral zone of particle-laden macrophages

## Symptoms and Signs

Some patients with pneumoconiosis are asymptomatic and diagnosed incidentally after radiographic screening examination. They may have a dry cough. Shortness of breath is more common at later stages, especially with progressive massive fibrosis. Other patients can present with associated conditions such as tuberculosis and lung cancer.

## CT Findings

On TSCT, the most characteristic feature of pneumoconiosis is the presence of multiple small nodules of 2–5 mm in diameter (Fig. 18.10). The nodules are seen mainly in the centrilobular regions, reflecting their peribronchiolar localization. They are also seen in the subpleural regions and along the interlobular septa because of their perilymphatic distribution [40]. The nodules tend to involve mainly dorsal regions of the upper lobes and are most numerous in the right upper lobe [41].

When nodules coalesce to form opacities larger than 10 mm in diameter, they are called progressive massive fibrosis (PMF). PMF tends to develop in the periphery of the upper and middle lung zones and often appears to migrate gradually toward the hila. Foci of emphysema are often present between the conglomerate mass and the pleura. The opacities are usually bilateral and symmetric.

## CT–Pathology Comparisons

Inhaled inorganic particles that land on the epithelium of the respiratory bronchioles enter the adjacent interstitium, where they accumulate within macrophages. Particles that land in the alveoli in the periphery of the lung also accumulate within macrophages in the

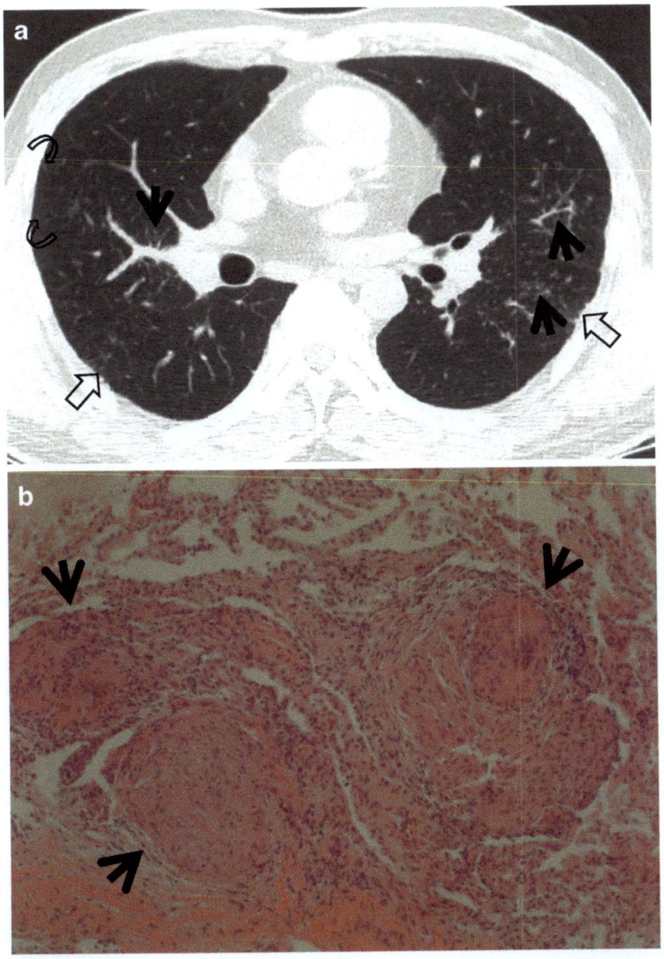


**Fig. 18.11** Pulmonary sarcoidosis depicting perilymphatic nodules in a 36-year-old man. (**a**) Lung window images of CT (2.5-mm section thickness) scan obtained at level of distal bronchus intermedius show small nodules along bronchovascular bundles (*arrows*), subpleural lungs (*open arrows*), and in centrilobular areas (*curved arrows*). (**b**) High-magnification (×200) photomicrograph of transbronchial lung biopsy specimen obtained from lingular division of left upper lobe discloses noncaseating granulomas (*arrows*) located along bronchiole

interstitial tissue of the interlobular septa and pleura. On histopathologic analysis, pneumoconiosis nodules are composed of mature collagen in the central portion, with a peripheral zone of particle-laden macrophages [40] (Fig. 18.10). Therefore, nodules of pneumoconiosis appear as well-circumscribed nodules with perilymphatic distribution on TSCT.

### Patient Prognosis

Patients should generally be removed from further exposure. No proven curative treatment for pneumoconiosis exists. Bronchodilators are considered for symptomatic patients with airflow obstruction. Pneumothorax, cor pulmonale, and respiratory failure should be managed separately.

## Pulmonary Sarcoidosis

### Pathology and Pathogenesis

Classic sarcoidosis shows non-necrotizing granulomatous inflammation distributed primarily along the bronchovascular bundle and lymphatics. The granulomas predominantly involve airway submucosa and the pulmonary interstitium rather than airspaces. Granulomas are well circumscribed and composed of tightly clustered epithelioid histiocytes and occasional multinucleated giant cells with few intervening lymphocytes and other inflammatory cells [42] (Fig. 18.11).

### Symptoms and Signs

Pulmonary sarcoidosis is frequently detected on the screening chest radiograph in an asymptomatic patient. As the lung disease progresses, nonspecific respiratory symptoms including dry cough, exertional dyspnea, and wheezing can occur. Some patients complain of extrapulmonary symptoms and signs such as fever, arthralgia, uveitis, and erythema nodosum skin rash [43].

### CT Findings

The presence of small nodules with perilymphatic distribution is the most common parenchymal disease pattern seen in patients with pulmonary sarcoidosis [44] (Figs. 18.9 and 18.11). TSCT shows sharply defined small (2–4 mm in diameter), rounded nodules, usually with a bilateral and symmetric distribution, predominantly but not invariably in the upper and middle zones. The nodules are found most often in the subpleural and peribronchovascular interstitium and less often in the interlobular septa. Sarcoid nodules may coalesce over time, forming large nodules. Other findings include reticulonodular pattern, parenchymal consolidation, ground-glass opacity, and fibrocystic changes [45].

### CT–Pathology Comparisons

Correlation of TSCT with pathologic findings has shown that sarcoid nodules represent interstitial aggregates of granulomas and associated fibrous tissue [46]. Large nodules represent coalescent granulomas. Ground-glass opacity represents an accumulation of many granulomatous lesions, with or without fibrosis, in the alveolar septa and around the small vessels.

### Patient Prognosis

Treatment of pulmonary sarcoidosis is usually limited to the symptomatic patients. Corticosteroids remain as the principal

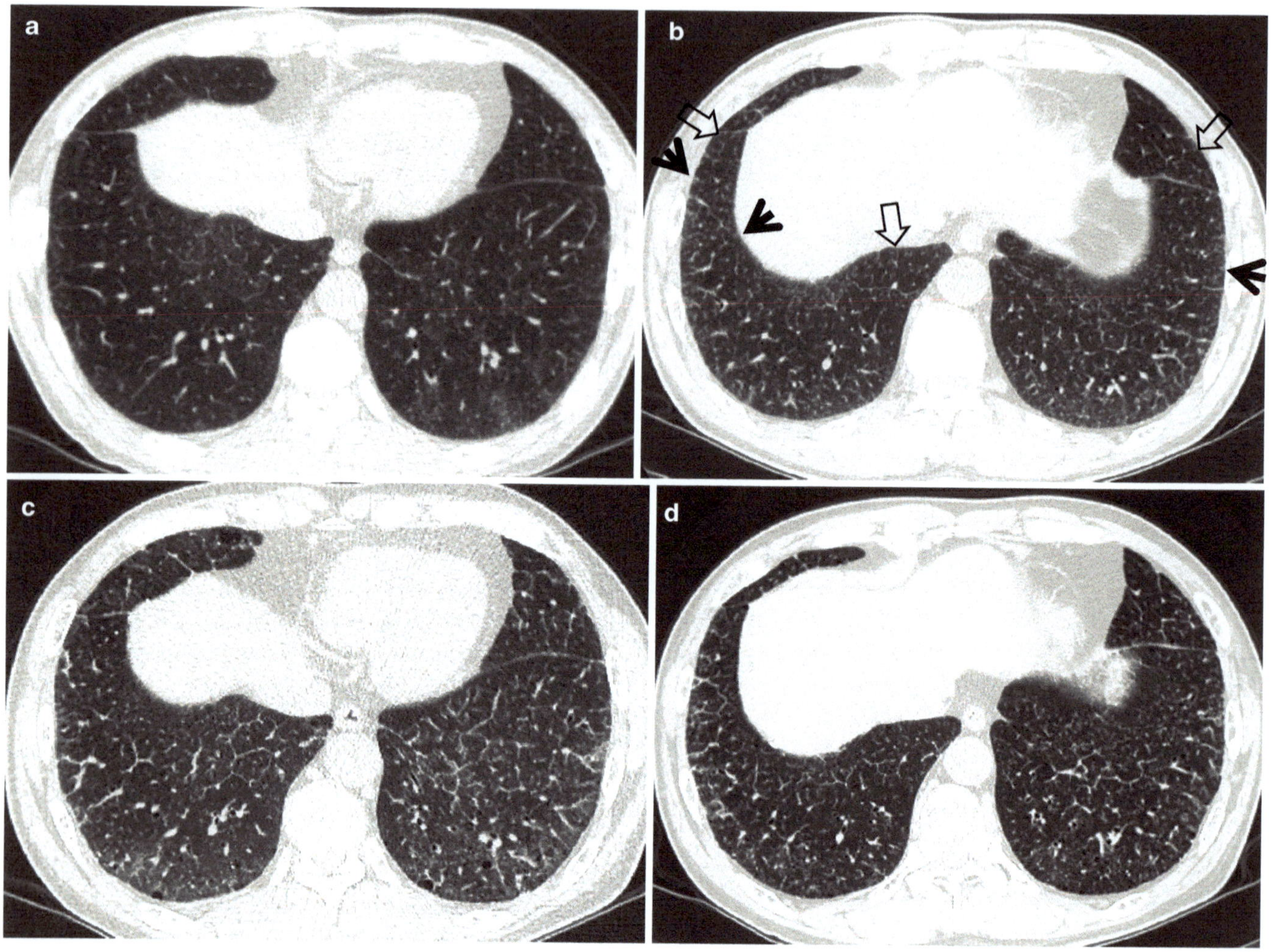


**Fig. 18.12** Alveoloseptal amyloidosis in a 58-year-old man who also has biopsy-proved gastric amyloidosis. (**a**, **b**) Lung window images of consecutive CT (2.5-mm section thickness) scans obtained at level of liver dome show small nodules along pleura (*arrows*) and smooth or mildly nodular thickening of interlobular septa (*open arrows*). Also note areas of ground-glass opacity. (**c**, **d**) CT scans obtained at similar levels to and 40 months after **a** and **b**, respectively, demonstrate progressed disease with increased extent of interlobular septal thickening and small nodules in both lungs. Diffusing capacity at this time was 45 % of expected value

treatment, but infliximab can be useful in treating the refractory cases [47]. Remission occurs for more than half of patients within 5 years of diagnosis with few or no consequences. Up to one-third of patients have persistent disease, leading to significant organ impairment.

## Pulmonary Alveoloseptal Amyloidosis

### Pathology and Pathogenesis

Amyloidosis is the extracellular deposition of misfolded proteins in beta-pleated sheets. Primary pulmonary amyloidosis (PPA) is amyloid deposition in the respiratory tract without associated systemic amyloidosis. There are two main types of PPA: tracheobronchial amyloidosis and nodular amyloidosis, the deposition of balls of amyloid (usually composed of lambda light chain) within the lung parenchyma. Secondary pulmonary amyloidosis is amyloid deposition in lung parenchyma and around blood vessels in patient with systemic amyloidosis [48].

### Symptoms and Signs

Pulmonary alveoloseptal amyloidosis manifests as interstitial lung disease. Patients are often symptomatic with dry cough and slowly progressive dyspnea on exertion. Hemoptysis is rare.

### CT Findings

Common TSCT findings of alveoloseptal amyloidosis include reticular opacity, interlobular septal thickening, and small nodules. Small nodules (2–4 mm diameter) are usually multiple and subpleural (Fig. 18.11). Less common findings are ground-glass opacity, traction bronchiectasis, and honeycombing [49, 50].

### CT–Pathology Comparisons

TSCT findings of alveoloseptal amyloidosis are caused by the deposition of amyloid in the parenchymal interstitium and in the media of small blood vessels.

### Patient Prognosis

Pulmonary involvement is not a major contributor to death in systemic amyloidosis, and the median survival of patients with clinically overt lung deposition is about 16 months [51].

## Small Nodules with Random (Miliary) Distribution

### Definition

Small nodular lesions considered random in distribution when the nodules did not show either a centrilobular or a perilymphatic distribution. In other words, they are uniform and even in distribution without a consistent or predominant relationship to any anatomic structures [1]. In random distribution, the small nodules are diffusely seen in all lobes of both lungs and affect the lungs either equally or symmetrically. There is no thickening in the interstitium, both axially (peribronchovascular) and peripherally (interlobular septa) [2] (Fig. 18.13).

### Diseases Causing the Pattern

*Miliary tuberculosis* (TB) (Fig. 18.14) and *miliary metastases* (Fig. 18.15) are the two most common conditions that manifest random nodules in both lungs [1]. Small nodules of random distribution can also be observed in disseminated fungal (*e.g.*, *Candida* albicans and cryptococcosis) and viral pneumonias and in sarcoidosis [52, 53].

### Distribution

In most diseases, lung abnormalities show random and diffuse in distribution. In sarcoidosis, the miliary nodules may show peripheral (subpleural) distribution [53].

### Clinical Considerations

The small miliary lung nodules in miliary TB may be associated with diffuse ground-glass opacity (GGO) (acute lung injury) [54] or cystic lung lesions [53, 55]. Lung adenocarcinoma is one of primary cancers that are associated with miliary pulmonary dissemination of the cancer. Therefore, the primary lung adenocarcinoma per se is seen through miliary metastatic lung nodules [56].

**Key Points for Differential Diagnosis**

| | Distribution | | | | | | | | | | | |
|---|---|---|---|---|---|---|---|---|---|---|---|---|
| | Zones | | | | | | | | Clinical presentations | | | |
| Diseases | U | M | L | SP | C | R | BV | R | Acute | Subacute | Chronic | Others |
| Miliary tuberculosis | + | + | + | | | + | | + | + | | | Diffuse ground-glass opacity, cystic lung lesions |
| Miliary metastases | + | + | + | | | + | | + | | + | + | Nodules may show cavitation |
| Sarcoidosis | + | + | + | + | | + | | + | | + | | With interlobular septal thickening or interlobar fissural thickening |

*Note*: *U* upper, *M* middle, *L* lower, *SP* subpleural, *C* central, *R* random, *BV* bronchovascular

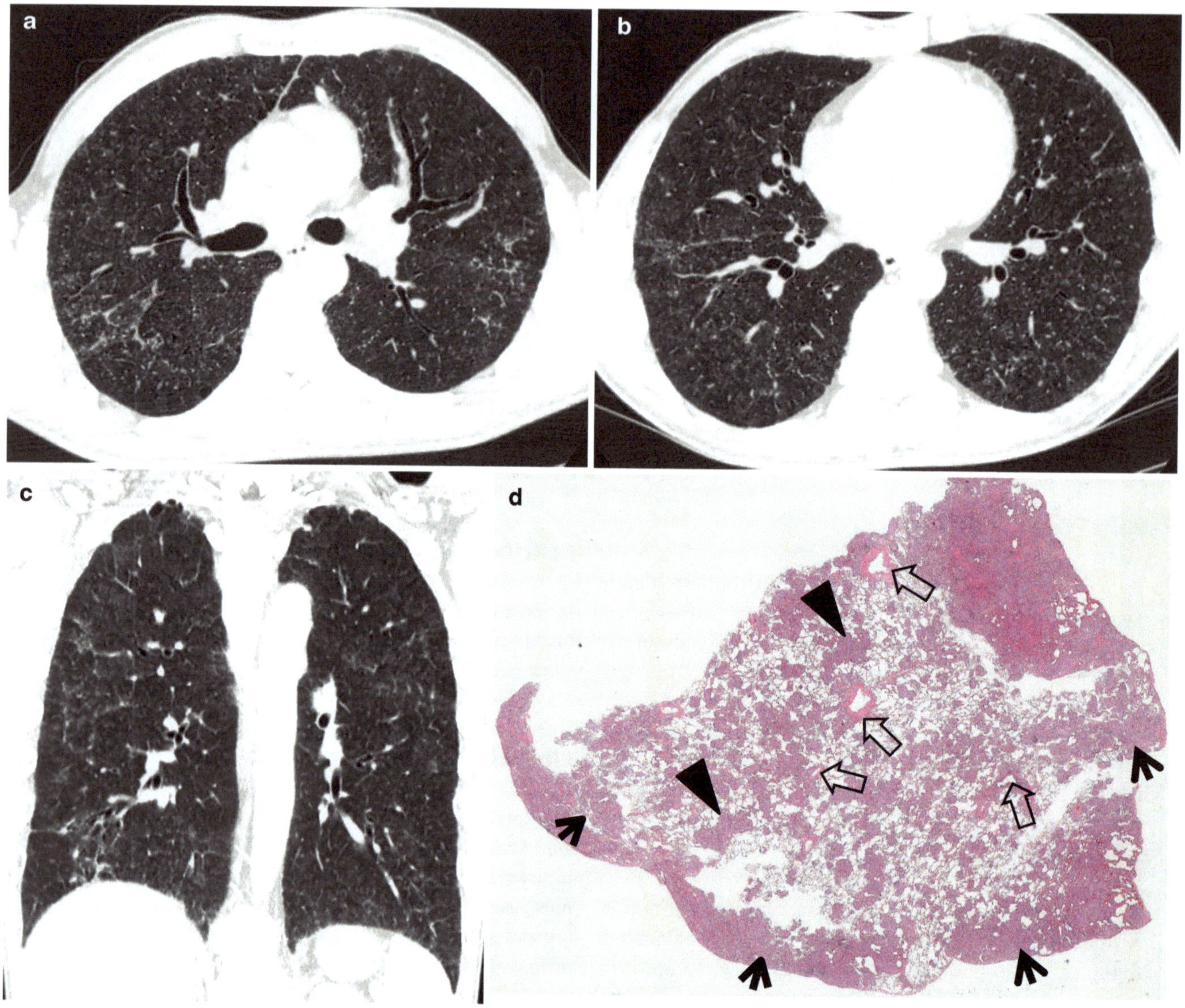


**Fig. 18.13** Miliary sarcoidosis in a 47-year-old man. (**a**, **b**) Lung window images of thin-section (1.5-mm section thickness) CT scans obtained at levels of right upper lobar bronchus (**a**) and inferior pulmonary veins (**b**), respectively, show randomly distributed innumerable small nodules in both lungs. Also note diffuse ground-glass opacity in background lungs. (**c**) Coronal reformatted image (2.0-mm section thickness) demonstrates randomly distributed small nodules and ground-glass opacity in both lungs. (**d**) Low-magnification photomicrograph of surgical biopsy specimen obtained from the right upper lobe discloses small, noncaseating, and uniform granulomas having random (subpleural [*arrows*], along bronchovascular bundles [*open arrows*], and in alveolar walls [*arrowheads*]) distribution

## Miliary Tuberculosis

### Pathology and Pathogenesis

When many bacilli enter the circulation simultaneously with subsequent massive hematogenous dissemination, generalized miliary TB develops. Many are filtered out in the pulmonary capillaries to give origin to a preponderance of the miliary tubercles in the lungs. Histologically, a multinucleate giant cell commonly forms the center and is enclosed by a zone of epithelioid macrophages and an outer shell of lymphocytes [57] (Fig. 18.14).

### Symptoms and Signs

Acute miliary TB has a severe and rapidly progressive course, usually after acute infection in young adults. Nonreactive TB develops slowly in older adults with disease reactivation. The most common symptoms of military TB are nonspecific.

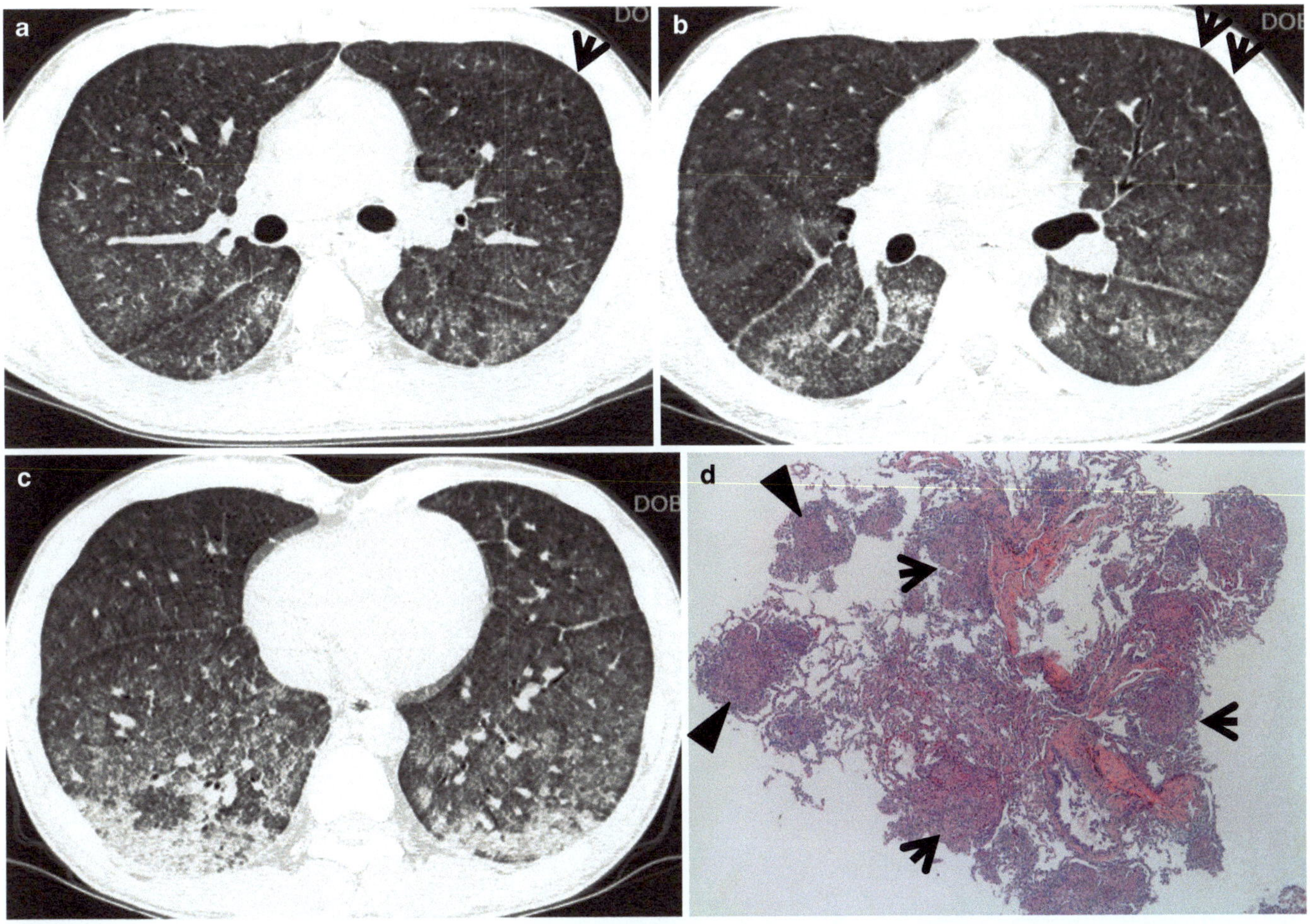


**Fig. 18.14** Miliary tuberculosis manifesting as acute lung injury in a 27-year-old man who is complaining of dyspnea. (**a–c**) Lung window images of thin-section (1.5-mm section thickness) CT scans obtained at levels of main bronchi (**a**), right bronchus intermedius (**b**), and cardiac ventricle (*arrows*) (**c**), respectively, show randomly distributed innumerable small nodules with background diffuse ground-glass opacity in both lungs. Also note interlobular septal thickening (*arrows*) and consolidative lesions in dependent portion of the lower lung zones. (**d**) High-magnification (×100) photomicrograph of transbronchial lung biopsy specimen obtained from the right upper lobe discloses multiple granulomas located along bronchiole (*arrows*) and in alveolar walls (*arrowheads*)

Constitutional symptoms including fever, anorexia, weight loss, and night sweats are common. Cough and dyspnea are present more than two-third of patients [58]. Fulminant disease including ARDS and septic shock has been described. Hepatomegaly and splenomegaly are frequently found.

## CT Findings

The most common characteristic TSCT finding of miliary TB is innumerable miliary nodules, variable in size from 1 to 3 mm in diameter [59, 60] (Fig. 18.14). The size and profusion of nodules are not significantly different in the upper, middle, lower lung zones, and the nodules have diffuse random distribution in the horizontal plane and within the secondary pulmonary lobule as well. GGO is the second most common finding of miliary TB [54] and reticular pattern of diffuse intralobular lines and interlobular septal thickening has also been frequently described in miliary TB [59] (Fig. 18.14). The extent is variable and the distribution is random. Other findings include large nodules, necrotic lymph node, and pleural effusion.

## CT–Pathology Comparisons

Each focus of miliary infection results in local granulomas that, when well developed, consist of a relatively well-delimited rim of epithelioid histiocytes and fibrous tissue [60] (Fig. 18.13). They appear as both sharply and poorly defined nodules on TSCT. The diversity of the margins presumably reflects the presence of some degree of active inflammation within the center of lobules secondarily affecting adjacent airspaces and thus resulting in poorly marginated nodules. Areas of GGO represent small granulomas resulting in minimal thickening of the alveolar walls and septal interstitium or partly filled alveolar lumen with fluid,

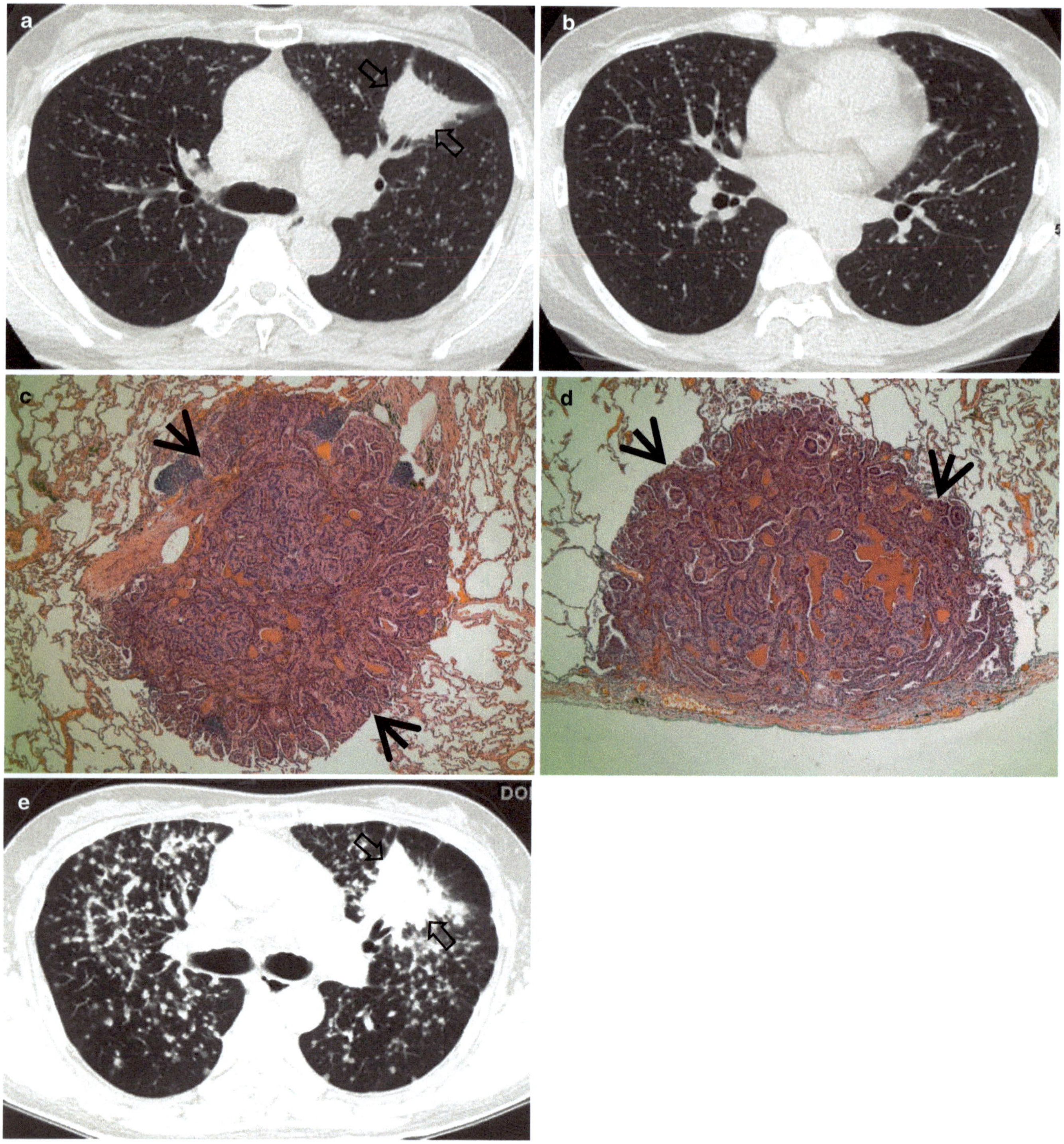


**Fig. 18.15** Miliary metastases in a 60-year-old woman who has lung adenocarcinoma. (**a**, **b**) Lung window images of CT (2.5-mm section thickness) scans obtained at levels of right upper lobar bronchus (**a**) and basal trunk (**b**), respectively, show a primary lung cancer (*open arrows*) in the left upper lobe and randomly distributed innumerable small nodules in both lungs. Also note diffuse ground-glass opacity in background lungs. (**c**, **d**) High-magnification photomicrographs of surgical lung biopsy obtained from a different patient with lung military metastases discloses tumor nodules located along bronchovascular bundle (*arrows* in **c**) and along the pleura (*arrows* in **d**). (**e**) Six-month follow-up CT exhibits progressed disease with increased size of primary mass (*open arrows*) in the left upper lobe and increased size and number of metastatic nodules

macrophages, neutrophils, or amorphous material [59]. Histopathologically, diffuse interstitial inflammatory infiltrates and innumerable tiny granulomas scattered throughout the pulmonary interstitium account for diffuse intralobular lines and interlobular septal thickening [52].

### Patient Prognosis

Miliary TB is uniformly fatal if not treated. Anti-TB treatment for at least 9–12 months is recommended. Adjunctive treatment with corticosteroids may be useful for those with refractory hypoxemia. The mortality related to miliary TB is about 25–39 % in adults patients [58]. Delay in the diagnosis or commencement of treatment appears to be an important cause of mortality.

## Miliary Metastasis

### Pathology and Pathogenesis

The nodules, usually dense and well defined, tend to appear evenly distributed (Fig. 18.15). Individual nodules may have feeding vessels consistent with their hematogenous origin [61].

### Symptoms and Signs

In patients with miliary metastasis, clinical manifestations are nonspecific. Cough and dyspnea are the most common respiratory symptoms. Symptoms related to primary cancer can be seen. Anorexia, weight loss, and general weakness are also common.

### CT Findings

On CT, miliary metastasis appears as multiple small nodules of a few millimeters in diameter [62]. They are usually of varying in size. The nodules tend to be most numerous in the outer third of the lungs, particularly the subpleural regions of the lower lung zones, and have a random distribution within the secondary pulmonary lobules (Fig. 18.15).

### CT–Pathology Comparisons

Hematogenous metastatic pulmonary nodules usually begin to proliferate from tumor emboli in arterioles or capillaries; they tend to have a peripheral distribution in the lungs and a random distribution within the secondary pulmonary lobules [62, 63] (Fig. 18.15).

### Patient Prognosis

Prognosis is very poor unless the primary tumor is highly responsive to anticancer chemotherapy.

## References


1. Lee KS, Kim TS, Han J, et al. Diffuse micronodular lung disease: HRCT and pathologic findings. J Comput Assist Tomogr. 1999;23:99–106.
2. Gruden JF, Webb WR, Naidich DP, McGuinness G. Multinodular disease: anatomic localization at thin-section CT–multireader evaluation of a simple algorithm. Radiology. 1999;210:711–20.
3. Han D, Lee KS, Franquet T, et al. Thrombotic and nonthrombotic pulmonary arterial embolism: spectrum of imaging findings. Radiographics. 2003;23:1521–39.
4. Chung MP, Yi CA, Lee HY, Han J, Lee KS. Imaging of pulmonary vasculitis. Radiology. 2010;255:322–41.
5. Hwang JH, Kim TS, Lee KS, et al. Bronchiolitis in adults: pathology and imaging. J Comput Assist Tomogr. 1997;21:913–9.
6. Lee KS, Kim YH, Kim WS, Hwang SH, Kim PN, Lee BH. Endobronchial tuberculosis: CT features. J Comput Assist Tomogr. 1991;15:424–8.
7. Im JG, Itoh H, Shim YS, et al. Pulmonary tuberculosis: CT findings–early active disease and sequential change with antituberculous therapy. Radiology. 1993;186:653–60.
8. Jeong YJ, Lee KS, Koh WJ, Han J, Kim TS, Kwon OJ. Nontuberculous mycobacterial pulmonary infection in immunocompetent patients: comparison of thin-section CT and histopathologic findings. Radiology. 2004;231:880–6.
9. Koh WJ, Lee KS, Kwon OJ, Jeong YJ, Kwak SH, Kim TS. Bilateral bronchiectasis and bronchiolitis at thin-section CT: diagnostic implications in nontuberculous mycobacterial pulmonary infection. Radiology. 2005;235:282–8.
10. Nishimura K, Kitaichi M, Izumi T, Itoh H. Diffuse panbronchiolitis: correlation of high-resolution CT and pathologic findings. Radiology. 1992;184:779–85.
11. Howling SJ, Hansell DM, Wells AU, Nicholson AG, Flint JD, Muller NL. Follicular bronchiolitis: thin-section CT and histologic findings. Radiology. 1999;212:637–42.
12. Bae YA, Lee KS, Han J, et al. Marginal zone B-cell lymphoma of bronchus-associated lymphoid tissue: imaging findings in 21 patients. Chest. 2008;133:433–40.
13. Bhalla M, Turcios N, Aponte V, et al. Cystic fibrosis: scoring system with thin-section CT. Radiology. 1991;179:783–8.
14. Moon JW, Lee HY, Han J, Lee KS. Tree-in-bud sign as a manifestation of localized pulmonary lymphatic metastasis from a pancreas cancer. Intern Med. 2011;50:3027–9.
15. Wagner JA, Nepomuceno IB, Shah N, et al. Maxillary sinusitis as a surrogate model for CF gene therapy clinical trials in patients with antrostomies. J Gene Med. 1999;1:13–21.
16. Miyano S, Izumi S, Takeda Y, et al. Pulmonary tumor thrombotic microangiopathy. J Clin Oncol. 2007;25:597–9.
17. Rollins S, Colby T, Clayton F. Open lung biopsy in Mycoplasma pneumoniae pneumonia. Arch Pathol Lab Med. 1986;110:34–41.
18. Reittner P, Muller NL, Heyneman L, et al. Mycoplasma pneumoniae pneumonia: radiographic and high-resolution CT features in 28 patients. AJR Am J Roentgenol. 2000;174:37–41.
19. Lee I, Kim TS, Yoon HK. Mycoplasma pneumoniae pneumonia: CT features in 16 patients. Eur Radiol. 2006;16:719–25.
20. Kim CK, Chung CY, Kim JS, Kim WS, Park Y, Koh YY. Late abnormal findings on high-resolution computed tomography after Mycoplasma pneumonia. Pediatrics. 2000;105:372–8.

21. Marrie TJ, Costain N, La Scola B, et al. The role of atypical pathogens in community-acquired pneumonia. Semin Respir Crit Care Med. 2012;33:244–56.
22. Song HJ, An JS, Han J, Koh WJ, Kim HK, Choi YS. Pathologic findings of surgically resected nontuberculous mycobacterial pulmonary infection. Korean J Pathol. 2010;44:56–62.
23. Kim TS, Koh WJ, Han J, et al. Hypothesis on the evolution of cavitary lesions in nontuberculous mycobacterial pulmonary infection: thin-section CT and histopathologic correlation. AJR Am J Roentgenol. 2005;184:1247–52.
24. Griffith DE, Aksamit TR. Bronchiectasis and nontuberculous mycobacterial disease. Clin Chest Med. 2012;33:283–95.
25. Koh WJ, Jeon K, Lee NY, et al. Clinical significance of differentiation of Mycobacterium massiliense from Mycobacterium abscessus. Am J Respir Crit Care Med. 2011;183:405–10.
26. Iwata M, Colby TV, Kitaichi M. Diffuse panbronchiolitis: diagnosis and distinction from various pulmonary diseases with centrilobular interstitial foam cell accumulations. Hum Pathol. 1994;25:357–63.
27. Kudoh S, Keicho N. Diffuse panbronchiolitis. Clin Chest Med. 2012;33:297–305.
28. Akira M, Kitatani F, Lee YS, et al. Diffuse panbronchiolitis: evaluation with high-resolution CT. Radiology. 1988;168:433–8.
29. Park HY, Suh GY, Chung MP, et al. Comparison of clinical and radiographic characteristics between nodular bronchiectatic form of nontuberculous mycobacterial lung disease and diffuse panbronchiolitis. J Korean Med Sci. 2009;24:427–32.
30. Kudoh S, Azuma A, Yamamoto M, Izumi T, Ando M. Improvement of survival in patients with diffuse panbronchiolitis treated with low-dose erythromycin. Am J Respir Crit Care Med. 1998;157:1829–32.
31. Yousem SA, Colby TV, Carrington CB. Follicular bronchitis/bronchiolitis. Hum Pathol. 1985;16:700–6.
32. Aerni MR, Vassallo R, Myers JL, Lindell RM, Ryu JH. Follicular bronchiolitis in surgical lung biopsies: clinical implications in 12 patients. Respir Med. 2008;102:307–12.
33. Sato Y, Marutsuka K, Asada Y, Yamada M, Setoguchi T, Sumiyoshi A. Pulmonary tumor thrombotic microangiopathy. Pathol Int. 1995;45:436–40.
34. Roberts KE, Hamele-Bena D, Saqi A, Stein CA, Cole RP. Pulmonary tumor embolism: a review of the literature. Am J Med. 2003;115:228–32.
35. Franquet T, Gimenez A, Prats R, Rodriguez-Arias JM, Rodriguez C. Thrombotic microangiopathy of pulmonary tumors: a vascular cause of tree-in-bud pattern on CT. AJR Am J Roentgenol. 2002;179:897–9.
36. Shepard JA, Moore EH, Templeton PA, McLoud TC. Pulmonary intravascular tumor emboli: dilated and beaded peripheral pulmonary arteries at CT. Radiology. 1993;187:797–801.
37. Bassiri AG, Haghighi B, Doyle RL, Berry GJ, Rizk NW. Pulmonary tumor embolism. Am J Respir Crit Care Med. 1997;155:2089–95.
38. Graham CM, Stern EJ, Finkbeiner WE, Webb WR. High-resolution CT appearance of diffuse alveolar septal amyloidosis. AJR Am J Roentgenol. 1992;158:265–7.
39. Johkoh T, Ikezoe J, Tomiyama N, et al. CT findings in lymphangitic carcinomatosis of the lung: correlation with histologic findings and pulmonary function tests. AJR Am J Roentgenol. 1992;158:1217–22.
40. Fujimura N. Pathology and pathophysiology of pneumoconiosis. Curr Opin Pulm Med. 2000;6:140–4.
41. Remy-Jardin M, Remy J, Farre I, Marquette CH. Computed tomographic evaluation of silicosis and coal workers' pneumoconiosis. Radiol Clin North Am. 1992;30:1155–76.
42. Mitchell DN, Scadding JG, Heard BE, Hinson KF. Sarcoidosis: histopathological definition and clinical diagnosis. J Clin Pathol. 1977;30:395–408.
43. Baughman RP, Culver DA, Judson MA. A concise review of pulmonary sarcoidosis. Am J Respir Crit Care Med. 2011;183:573–81.
44. Brauner MW, Grenier P, Mompoint D, Lenoir S, de Cremoux H. Pulmonary sarcoidosis: evaluation with high-resolution CT. Radiology. 1989;172:467–71.
45. Criado E, Sanchez M, Ramirez J, et al. Pulmonary sarcoidosis: typical and atypical manifestations at high-resolution CT with pathologic correlation. Radiographics. 2010;30:1567–86.
46. Nishimura K, Itoh H, Kitaichi M, Nagai S, Izumi T. Pulmonary sarcoidosis: correlation of CT and histopathologic findings. Radiology. 1993;189:105–9.
47. Baughman RP, Drent M, Kavuru M, et al. Infliximab therapy in patients with chronic sarcoidosis and pulmonary involvement. Am J Respir Crit Care Med. 2006;174:795–802.
48. Bhargava P, Rushin JM, Rusnock EJ, et al. Pulmonary light chain deposition disease: report of five cases and review of the literature. Am J Surg Pathol. 2007;31:267–76.
49. Pickford HA, Swensen SJ, Utz JP. Thoracic cross-sectional imaging of amyloidosis. AJR Am J Roentgenol. 1997;168:351–5.
50. Chung MJ, Lee KS, Franquet T, Muller NL, Han J, Kwon OJ. Metabolic lung disease: imaging and histopathologic findings. Eur J Radiol. 2005;54:233–45.
51. Utz JP, Swensen SJ, Gertz MA. Pulmonary amyloidosis. The Mayo Clinic experience from 1980 to 1993. Ann Intern Med. 1996;124:407–13.
52. McGuinness G, Naidich DP, Jagirdar J, Leitman B, McCauley DI. High resolution CT findings in miliary lung disease. J Comput Assist Tomogr. 1992;16:384–90.
53. Voloudaki AE, Tritou IN, Magkanas EG, Chalkiadakis GE, Siafakas NM, Gourtsoyiannis NC. HRCT in miliary lung disease. Acta Radiol. 1999;40:451–6.
54. Choi D, Lee KS, Suh GY, et al. Pulmonary tuberculosis presenting as acute respiratory failure: radiologic findings. J Comput Assist Tomogr. 1999;23:107–13.
55. Ko KS, Lee KS, Kim Y, Kim SJ, Kwon OJ, Kim JS. Reversible cystic disease associated with pulmonary tuberculosis: radiologic findings. Radiology. 1997;204:165–9.
56. Laack E, Simon R, Regier M, et al. Miliary never-smoking adenocarcinoma of the lung: strong association with epidermal growth factor receptor exon 19 deletion. J Thorac Oncol. 2011;6:199–202.
57. Lalvani A. Diagnosing tuberculosis infection in the 21st century: new tools to tackle an old enemy. Chest. 2007;131:1898–906.
58. Sharma SK, Mohan A, Sharma A, Mitra DK. Miliary tuberculosis: new insights into an old disease. Lancet Infect Dis. 2005;5:415–30.
59. Hong SH, Im JG, Lee JS, Song JW, Lee HJ, Yeon KM. High resolution CT findings of miliary tuberculosis. J Comput Assist Tomogr. 1998;22:220–4.
60. Jeong YJ, Lee KS. Pulmonary tuberculosis: up-to-date imaging and management. AJR Am J Roentgenol. 2008;191:834–44.
61. Seo JB, Im JG, Goo JM, Chung MJ, Kim MY. Atypical pulmonary metastases: spectrum of radiologic findings. Radiographics. 2001;21:403–17.
62. Murata K, Takahashi M, Mori M, et al. Pulmonary metastatic nodules: CT-pathologic correlation. Radiology. 1992;182:331–5.
63. Hirakata K, Nakata H, Nakagawa T. CT of pulmonary metastases with pathological correlation. Semin Ultrasound CT MR. 1995;16:379–94.

# 19 Multiple Nodular or Mass(-like) Pattern

## Definition

When the lesions of lung opacification appear with discrete margin, we call them multiple nodules or masses (please also note section "Patchy and Nodular Consolidation" in Chap. 3) (Figs. 19.1 and 19.2).

## Diseases Causing the Pattern

*Pulmonary metastases* (Fig. 19.2) are the most common cause of multiple nodules or masses. *Lymphoproliferative diseases* (Fig. 19.3), particularly in the secondary involvement of the lungs in Hodgkin lymphoma or non-Hodgkin lymphoma, may also manifest multiple nodules or masses [1]. *Pulmonary epithelioid hemangioendothelioma* (Fig. 19.4), which is a low- to intermediate-grade vascular neoplasm, can manifest multiple nodules. Rheumatoid nodules, *amyloidomas* (Fig. 19.5), sarcoidosis, *pulmonary vasculitis including ANCA-associated granulomatous vasculitis (former Wegner's granulomatosis)* (Fig. 19.6), fungal infection (Fig. 19.7) or nocardiosis, and septic emboli are the benign inflammatory or infectious causes of multiple pulmonary nodules. Pulmonary Langerhans cell histiocytosis (eosinophilic granuloma) also manifests multiple variable-sized cavitating or noncavitating nodules with cystic lung lesions.

## Distribution

Lesions in abovementioned diseases show random distribution.

## Clinical Considerations

The presence of multiple nodules or masses in both lungs in a patient with extrathoracic malignancy or primary lung cancer suggests the diagnosis of pulmonary metastases or

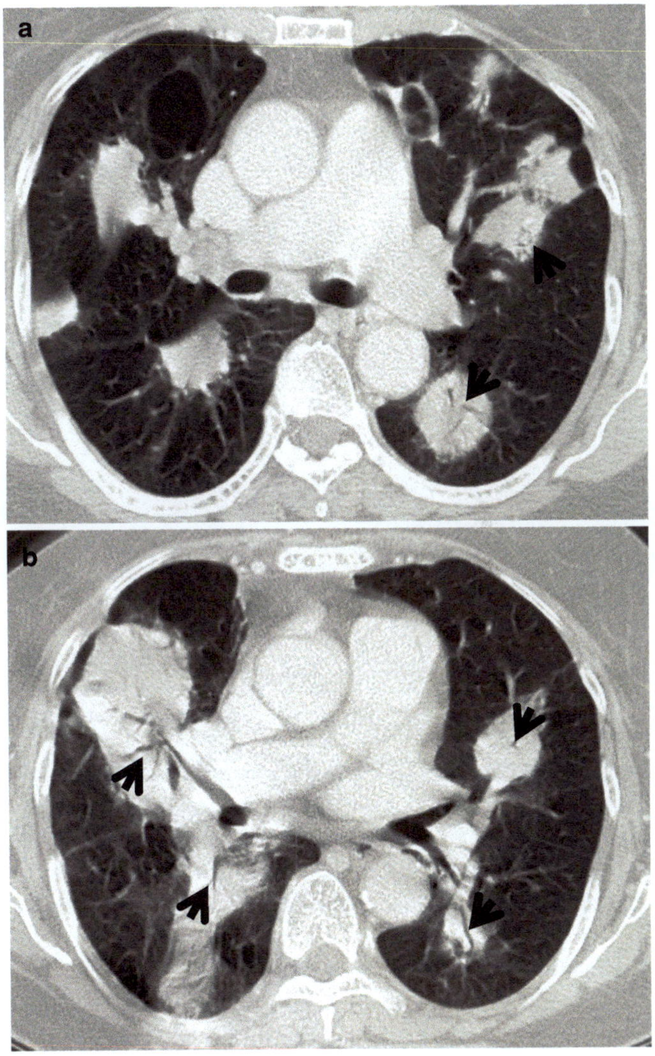


**Fig. 19.1** Marginal zone B-cell lymphoma manifesting as multiple masses in both lungs in a 73-year-old woman. (**a**, **b**) Lung window images of CT scans (2.5-mm section thickness) obtained at levels of distal main bronchi (**a**) and right middle lobar bronchus (**b**), respectively, show multiple masses in both lungs. Mass contain internal CT air-bronchogram sign (*arrows*). Also note thin-walled air-filled cyst in bottom of right upper lobe. Histopathologic evaluation of ore biopsy obtained from a mass suggested extranodal marginal zone lymphoma or lymphoplasmacytic lymphoma

K.S. Lee et al., *Radiology Illustrated: Chest Radiology*, Radiology Illustrated,
DOI 10.1007/978-3-642-37096-0_19, © Springer-Verlag Berlin Heidelberg 2014

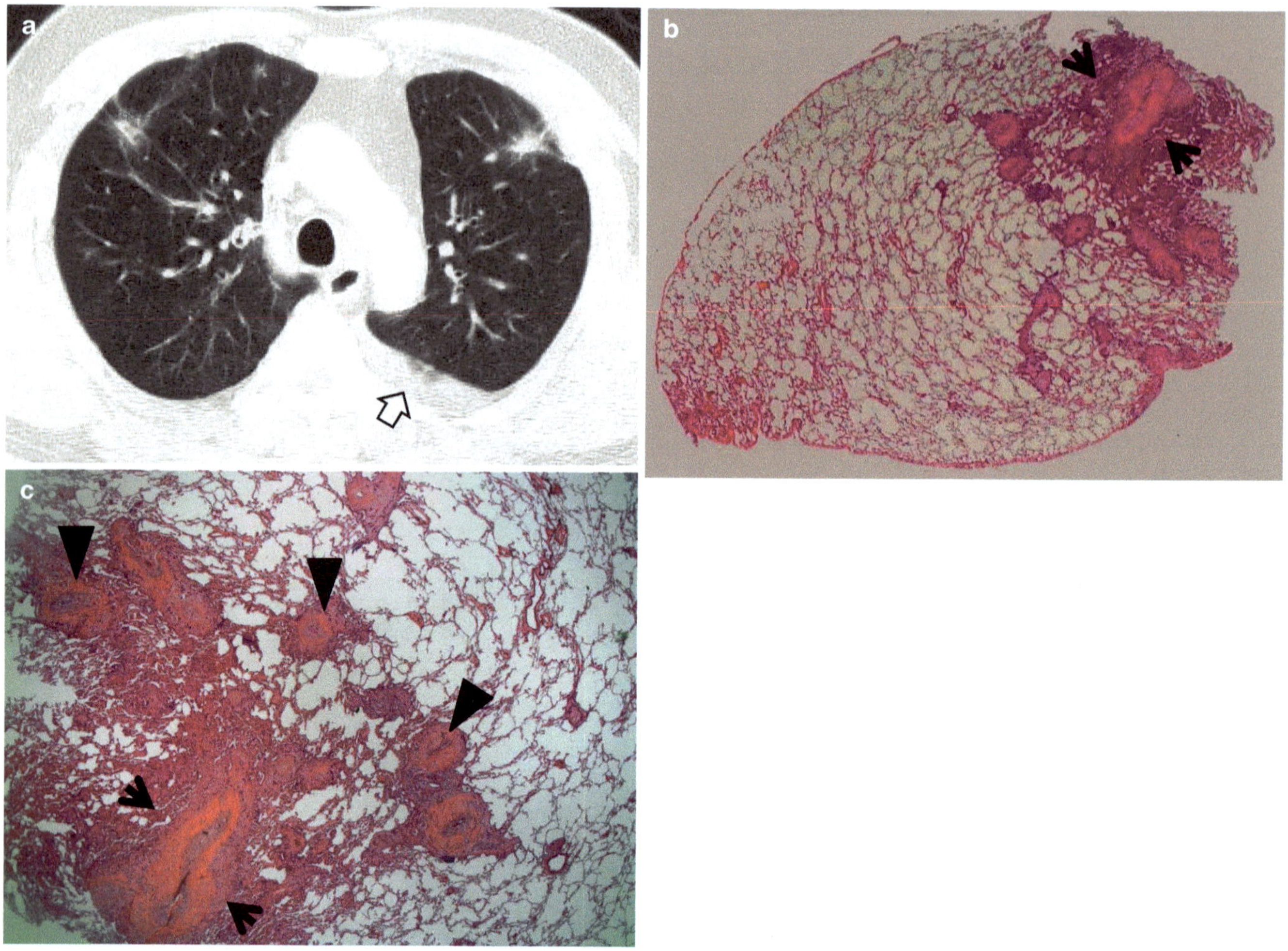


**Fig. 19.2** Pulmonary metastases from a breast cancer in a 62-year-old man. (**a**) Lung window of CT scan (5.0-mm section thickness) obtained at level of aortic arch shows multiple variable-sized poorly defined nodules in both upper lobes. Also note left pleural effusion (*open arrow*). (**b**) Low-magnification (×40) photomicrograph of pathologic specimen obtained from right upper lobe with wedge resection demonstrates a predominant nodule (*arrows*) and surrounding malignant satellite nodules. (**c**) High-magnification (×100) photomicrograph discloses duct-forming adenocarcinoma (*arrows*) with lymphangitic tumor spread. Also note pulmonary arterial invasion (*arrowheads*)

lung-to-lung metastases. Pulmonary nodules in a patient with rheumatoid arthritis may favor the diagnosis of necrobiotic nodules (rheumatoid nodules). Approximately 15–20 % of patients with pulmonary epithelioid hemangioendothelioma (EH) have a hepatic involvement. Pulmonary EH manifesting as multiple nodules have a relatively good prognosis, whereas the disease manifesting as reticulonodular lesions or diffuse infiltrative pleural thickening have aggressive clinical courses. Lung nodules in a patient with chronic inflammatory disease (e.g., Sjögren's syndrome) or systemic lymphoproliferative disorders and plasma cell dyscrasias (e.g., multiple myeloma) may suggest the presence of amyloidomas [2]. Nocardiosis is a disease in patients with underlying diabetes or chronic kidney disease [3]. Common predisposing factors for septic embolism include tricuspid valve endocarditis with or without IV drug addiction, alcoholism, skin infection, and peripheral septic thrombophlebitis [4]. Airway invasive pulmonary aspergillosis is a disease in immunocompromised patients (those who have hematologic malignancy and who underwent hematopoietic stem cell transplantation) particularly whose peripheral blood absolute neutrophil count is <500 cells/μL (neutropenia). Cryptococcosis is an indolent lung infection in mildly immunocompromised patients [5]. Generalized symptoms and signs, such as diffuse alveolar hemorrhage, acute glomerulonephritis, chronic refractory sinusitis or rhinorrhea, imaging findings of nodules or cavities, and multisystemic disease, precede typical imaging findings in pulmonary vasculitis [6].

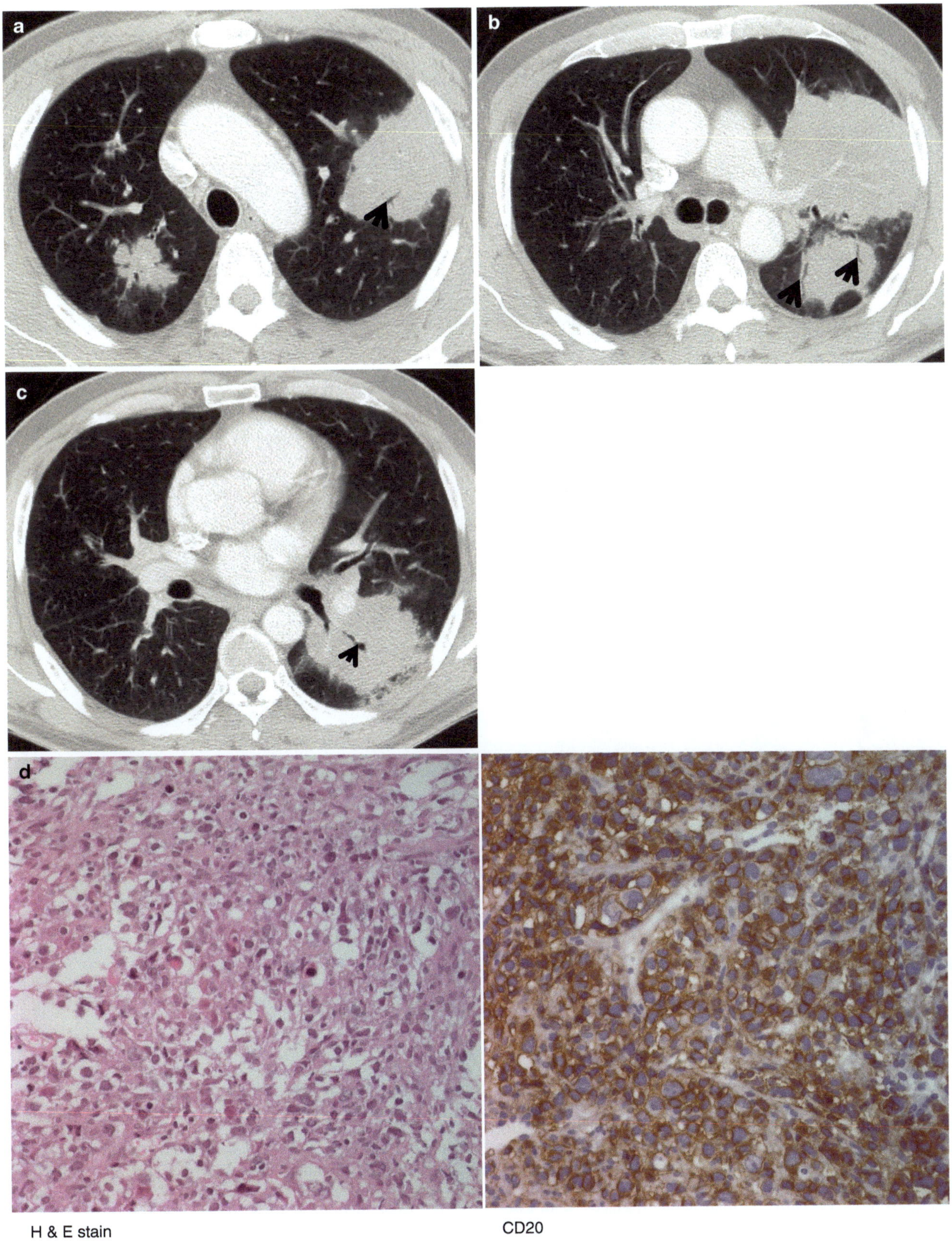


**Fig. 19.3** Diffuse large B-cell lymphoma involving lung parenchyma in a 48-year-old man who is complaining of febrile sense, cough, and dyspnea. (**a**–**c**) Lung window images of CT scans (2.5-mm section thickness) obtained at levels of aortic arch (**a**), main bronchi (**b**), and bronchus intermedius (**c**), respectively, show multiple variable-sized nodules and masses in both lungs. Lesions typically have bronchovascular distribution. Also note CT air-bronchogram signs (*arrows*) within mass lesions. (**d**) Photomicrographs of H & E staining (*left*) and immunohistochemical staining of CD20 (*right*), respectively, disclose atypical, pleomorphic, and large lymphoid cells and reactive to CD20. These findings are compatible with large B-cell lineage lymphoma

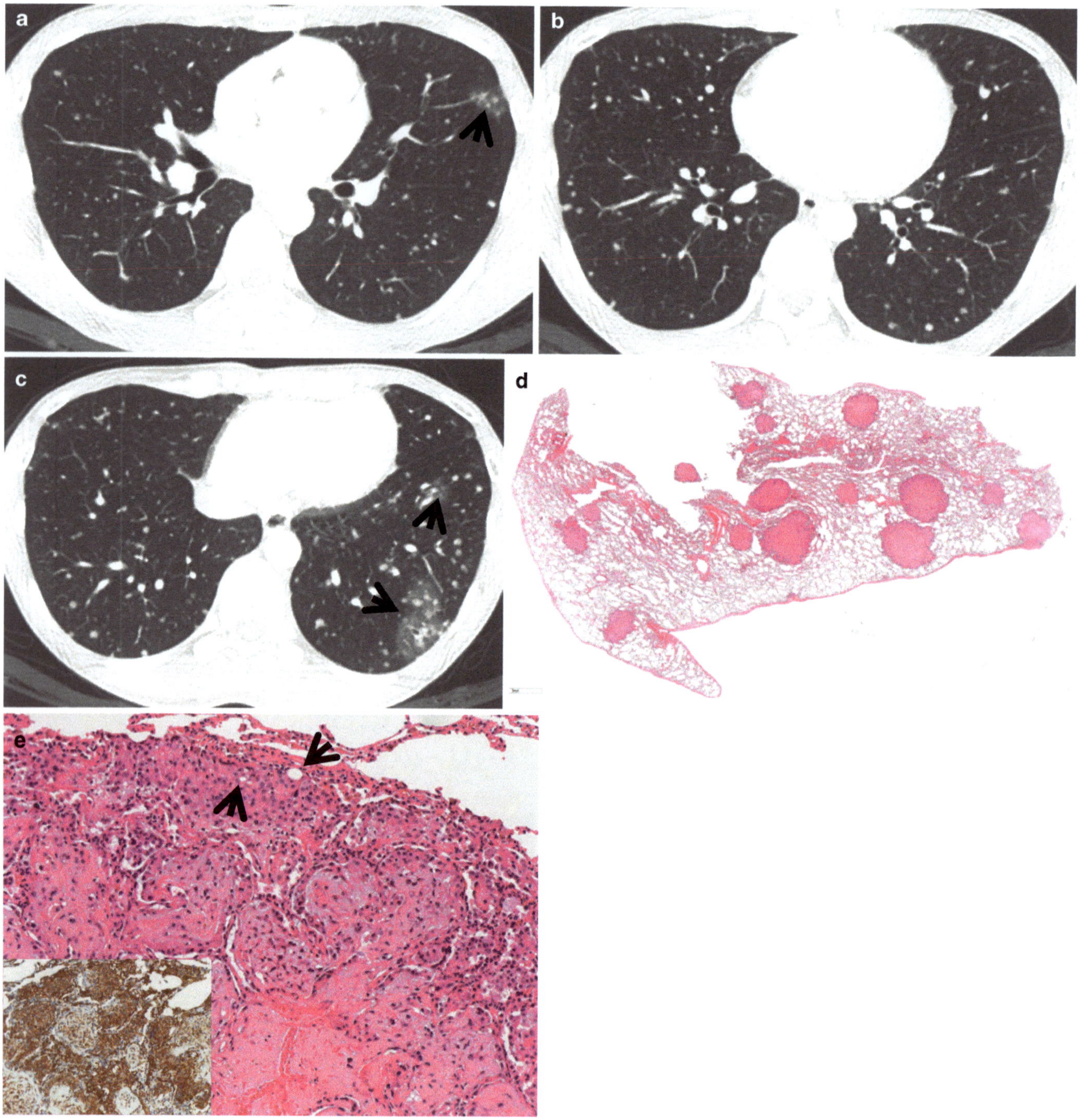


**Fig. 19.4** Epithelioid hemangioendothelioma appearing as multiple innumerable pulmonary nodules in both lungs in a 22-year-old man. (**a–c**) Lung window images of CT scans (2.5-mm section thickness) obtained at levels of right middle lobar bronchus (**a**), cardiac ventricle (**b**), and suprahepatic inferior vena cava (**c**), respectively, show multiple variable-sized small nodules in both lungs. Nodules show random distribution. Also note surrounding ground-glass opacity (*arrows*) in some nodules, suggestive of associated hemorrhage. (**d**) Low-magnification (×40) photomicrograph exhibits multiple nodules having central sclerotic and peripheral mild cellular (epithelioid endothelial proliferation) components. Nodules are distributed randomly. (**e**) High-magnification (×200) photomicrograph discloses abundant eosinophilic stroma and tumor cells containing prominent cytoplasmic vacuoles or intracytoplasmic lumina (*arrows*). *Inset*: positive staining for CD31 indicating endothelial origin of tumor cells

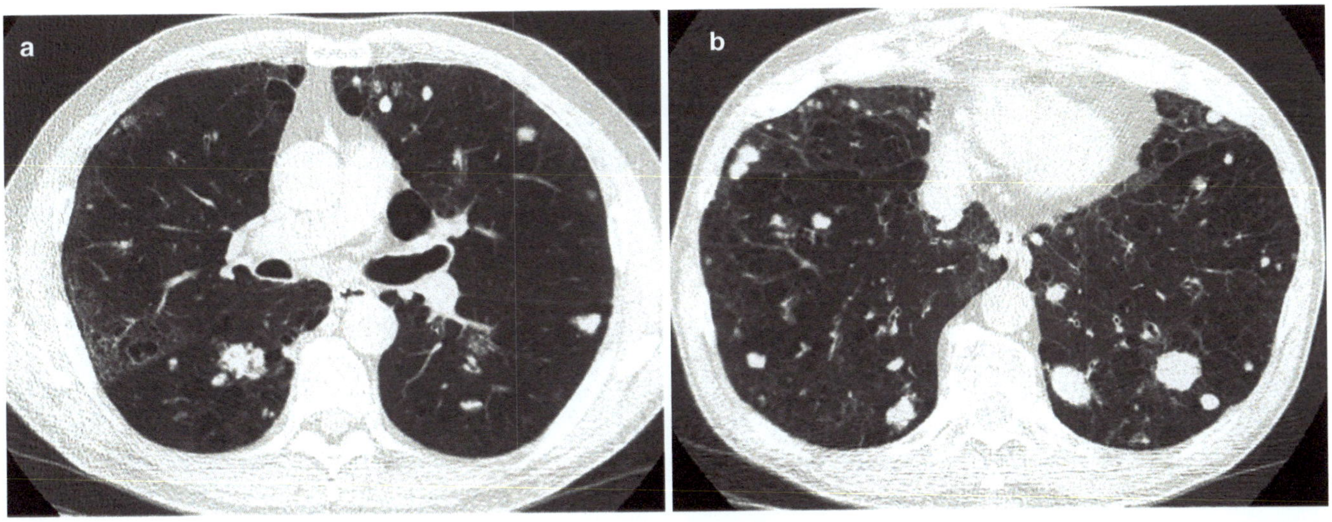

**Fig. 19.5** Biopsy-proven (surgical lung biopsy using video-assisted thoracoscopic surgery) amyloidomas presenting as multiple variable-sized nodules in a 62-year-old man. (**a**, **b**) Lung window images of thin-section (1.5-mm section thickness) CT scans obtained at levels of bronchus intermedius (**a**) and suprahepatic inferior vena cava (**b**), respectively, show multiple lung nodules of different size. Also note accompanying emphysema and bullae in both lungs

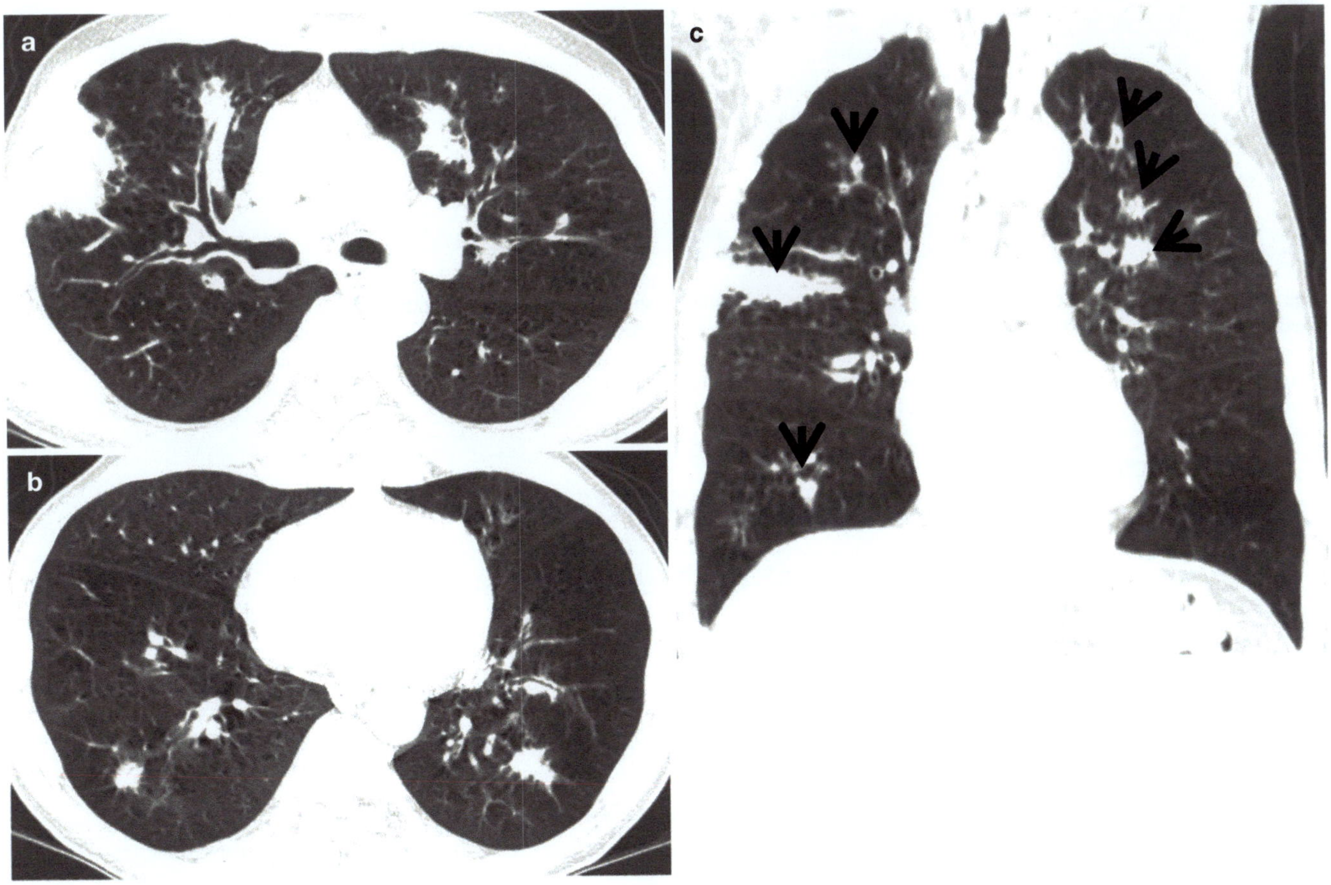

**Fig. 19.6** Antineutrophil cytoplasmic antibody (ANCA)-associated granulomatous vasculitis displaying multiple masses in a 64-year-old man. (**a**, **b**) Lung window images of thin-section (1.5-mm section thickness) CT scans obtained at levels of right upper lobar bronchus (**a**) and cardiac ventricle (**b**), respectively, show multiple variable-sized nodules and masses in both lungs. Lesions are typically located along bronchovascular bundles or subpleural lungs. Also note relatively extensive pulmonary emphysema. (**c**) Coronal reformatted CT image (5.0-mm section thickness) demonstrates nodules or mass (*arrows*) of diverse size in both lungs, which are distributed along bronchovascular bundles. Also note extensive emphysema in both lungs

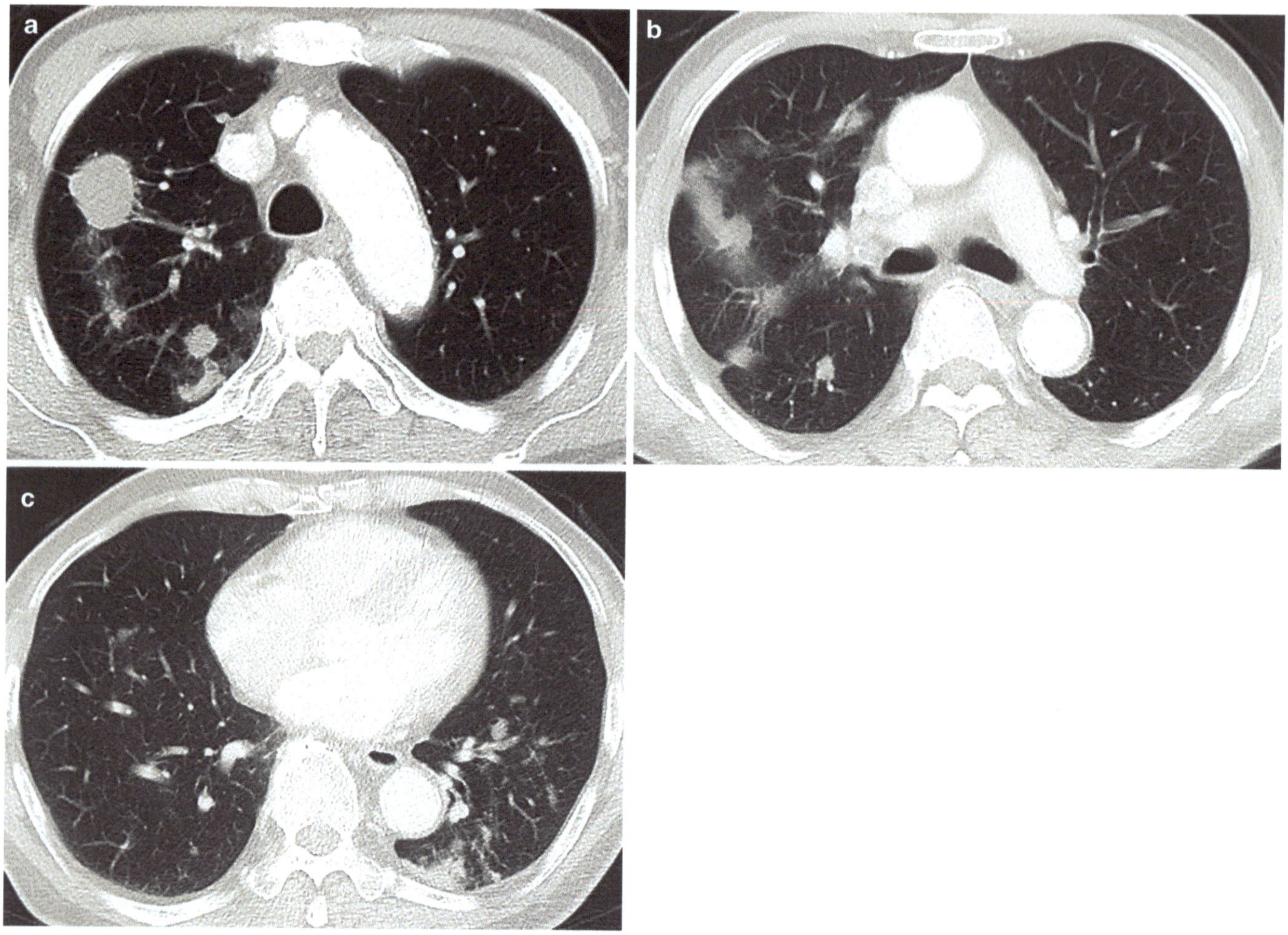


**Fig. 19.7** Pulmonary cryptococcosis manifesting as multiple variable-sized nodules in both lungs in a 72-year-old man. (**a–c**) Lung window images of CT scans (2.5-mm section thickness) obtained at levels of aortic arch (**a**), main bronchi (**b**), and cardiac ventricle (**c**), respectively, show multiple variable-sized nodules and masses in both lungs. Lesions are located along bronchovascular bundles or subpleural lung. Core biopsy from right upper lobe nodule discloses cryptococcal organisms

**Key Points for Differential Diagnosis**

| Diseases | Distribution | | | | | | | | Clinical presentations | | | Others |
|---|---|---|---|---|---|---|---|---|---|---|---|---|
| | Zones | | | | | | | | | | | |
| | U | M | L | SP | C | R | BV | R | Acute | Subacute | Chronic | |
| Pulmonary metastasis | | + | + | + | | + | | + | | | + | Variable-sized nodules |
| Lymphoproliferative disease | | | + | + | | | + | | | + | + | |
| Pulmonary epithelioid hemangioendothelioma | + | + | + | | | + | | + | | | + | Most are less than 1 cm, little or no growth on serial exam |
| Rheumatoid nodules | + | + | | + | | + | | + | | | + | Variable in size, may cavitate, unpredictable natural course |
| Amyloidomas | | | + | + | | | | + | | | + | Internal calcifications (50 %) |
| Sarcoidosis | + | + | | + | | | + | | | | + | Cavitation may occur; mediastinal or hilar LN enlargement, female predominance, African Americans |
| ANCA-associated granulomatous vasculitis | + | + | + | + | | + | + | + | | + | + | Large necrotic area on enhanced scans |
| Fungal infection or nocardiosis | + | + | + | + | | + | | + | + | + | | |
| Septic lung | + | + | + | + | | + | | + | | | | Feeding vessel sign, cavitation |

*Note*: *ANCA* antineutrophil cytoplasmic antibody, *U* upper, *M* middle, *L* lower, *SP* subpleural, *C* central, *R* random, *BV* bronchovascular, *LN* lymph node

## Pulmonary Metastasis

### Pathology and Pathogenesis

Although metastasis to the lung can occur along multiple routes (through pulmonary or bronchial arteries, lymphatics, or airways), the radiologic manifestations of such disease demonstrate considerable overlap. The four patterns of metastatic disease to the lung parenchyma are parenchymal nodules (Fig. 19.2), interstitial thickening (lymphangitic carcinomatosis), tumor emboli with or without pulmonary hypertension or infarction, and airway obstruction from endobronchial tumor [7].

### Symptoms and Signs

Surprisingly, significant number of patients with pulmonary metastasis showing multiple nodules or masses is asymptomatic. Nonspecific symptoms including cough, vague chest discomfort, and dyspnea can result from a very large tumor burden. Hemoptysis can occur. Constitutional symptoms such as weight loss, anorexia, and generalized weakness may be the only manifestation in the absence of respiratory symptoms.

### CT Findings

CT finding of hematogenous pulmonary metastasis consists of multiple nodules (Fig. 19.2). The size of nodules range from a few millimeters to several centimeters in diameter, and nodules are usually of varying size. They tend to be most numerous in the outer third of lungs, particularly the subpleural regions of the lower lung zones, and have a random distribution within the secondary pulmonary lobules [8, 9]. Most nodules are round and have smooth margins. They may be lobulated, however, and have irregular margins. Occasionally, a ground-glass opacity (GGO) halo can be seen in highly vascular or hemorrhagic tumors such as angiosarcoma [10]. Cavitation of nodular metastasis can occur in 4 % of metastases. (Please note section "Cavities" in Chap. 23.) Calcification in nodular metastasis is very uncommon and usually indicates that the primary neoplasm is osteogenic sarcoma, chondrosarcoma, synovial sarcoma, or carcinoma of the colon, ovary, breast, or thyroid [8].

### CT–Pathology Comparisons

The margins of nodular metastases on thin-section CT may depend on their histologic appearance at the growing edge of the tumor [11]. Smooth margins on CT scans correspond to the expanding (tumors that compress the surrounding normal lung) and alveolar space-filling (tumors that infiltrate and fill the alveolar spaces) types, nodules that have poorly defined margins tend to be the alveolar cell type (tumors that grow along the alveolar walls), and those that have irregular margins are predominantly the interstitial proliferation (tumors that infiltrate the interstitium) type. A GGO halo surrounding nodular metastasis reflects the presence of hemorrhage in the parenchyma adjacent to the nodule or the spread of tumor cells along the alveolar walls [8].

### Patient Prognosis

Prognosis of the patients with pulmonary metastasis presenting with multiple nodules or masses is poor unless the primary tumor is highly responsive to anticancer chemotherapy.

## Pulmonary Lymphoma

### Pathology and Pathogenesis

Extranodal marginal zone B-cell lymphoma of bronchial-associated lymphoid tissue (BALT lymphoma) may be the most common type of pulmonary lymphoma and frequently shows nodular interstitial infiltrate of lymphoma cells along bronchovascular bundles and interlobular septa. Sheets of infiltrating lymphoma cells can obliterate underlying lung architecture. Lymphoepithelial lesions, characterized by epithelial infiltration by lymphoma cells, are common [12].

### Symptoms and Signs

Median age of primary pulmonary lymphoma is about 60 years [13]. Patients often present with pulmonary symptoms such as cough, dyspnea, chest discomfort, occasional hemoptysis, or constitutional symptoms. However, a majority of low-grade lymphoma patients are asymptomatic.

### CT Findings

Typical CT findings of primary or secondary pulmonary lymphoma include single or multiple nodules or masses (Fig. 19.3) of mass-like airspace consolidation with air bronchograms [1, 14]. Less common CT findings include interlobular septal thickening, thickening of bronchovascular bundles, centrilobular nodules, and areas of GGO.

### CT–Pathology Comparisons

Multiple nodules or masses on thin-section CT are related to the proliferation of tumor cells within the interstitium and extension of tumor cells into the parenchymal interstitium and airspaces.

### Patient Prognosis

Patients with pulmonary marginal zone B-cell lymphoma usually have limited disease and follow an indolent clinical course with favorable response. Diffuse large B-cell lymphomas are aggressive, but complete remission and long-term survival can be seen, with reported survival time of approximately 8–10 years [15].

## Pulmonary Epithelioid Hemangioendothelioma

### Pathology and Pathogenesis

Pulmonary EH in the lung reveals single or multiple nodules replacing normal lung architecture (Fig. 19.4). These nodules display different stages of development; some show areas of calcification and ossification, while others show a characteristic chondromyxoid background, and still others may show a predominant solid cellular proliferation. Polypoid nodules are arranged within alveolar spaces or are seen infiltrating into interstitial areas. At higher magnification, the tumor cells are seen to be arranged in small nests or cords within the myxoid background (Fig. 19.2). Although necrosis may be seen in a few cases, mitotic activity and cellular pleomorphism are unusual [16, 17].

### Symptoms and Signs

Pulmonary EH is diagnosed incidentally in about half of the patients [18]. Respiratory symptoms including cough, dyspnea, hemoptysis, and chest pain has been described. Weight loss can be seen.

### CT Findings

The most common CT finding of pulmonary EH is the presence of multiple discrete nodules [16, 17] (Fig. 19.4). The nodules range in size up to 2 cm, but most are less than 1 cm in diameter. On serial CT examinations, these lesions have little or no growth. Other findings of pulmonary EH include multiple reticulonodular opacities mimicking hematolymphangitic metastasis and diffuse infiltrative pleural thickening mimicking malignant pleural mesothelioma or diffuse pleural carcinomatosis [19, 20].

### CT–Pathology Comparisons

The tumor cells of pulmonary EH typically spread into adjacent bronchioles and alveolar spaces in a micropolypoid manner, resulting in multiple nodules on CT scans (Fig. 19.4). Infiltrative nodular proliferation of tumor cells within the lumina of small arteries, veins and lymphatics might simulate hematolymphangitic metastases and infiltrative growth pattern of epithelioid tumor cells along the pleura could mimic diffuse malignant pleural mesothelioma [16].

### Patient Prognosis

Surgery can be proposed in cases of unilateral single or multiple nodules. There is no single effective treatment in cases of bilateral multiple nodules. The 5-year survival probability is 60 % (range, 47–71 %). Patients with hemorrhagic symptoms and pleural effusion show a worse survival.

## Amyloidomas

### Pathology and Pathogenesis

Amyloidosis is the extracellular deposition of misfolded proteins in beta-pleated sheets. Amyloidoma is nodular amyloidosis, which presents as single or multiple nodules measuring 1–4 cm in diameter (Fig. 19.5). These are firm, irregular, and yellow to gray. Histologically, amyloid is amorphous eosinophilic material with a foreign-body giant cell reaction. That may have lymphoplasmacytic infiltrate at the periphery of the nodules, calcification, chondrification, or ossification. Please also note section "Honeycombing with Upper Lung Zone Predominance" in Chap. 17.

### Symptoms and Signs

Amyloid nodules in the lung parenchyma are usually an incidental finding that need to be distinguished from neoplasia [21]. Larger nodules can occasionally produce space-occupying effects.

### CT Findings

On CT, amyloidomas appear as nodules with sharp or lobulated margins in a peripheral or subpleural location [22]. Nodules are variable in shape and size, measuring from 0.5 to 15 cm in diameter (Fig. 19.5). The nodules show slow growth often over several years without regression. Calcification is often central or in an irregular pattern within the nodule and is seen in approximately 50 % of cases. Cavitation may occur, but is very rare.

### CT–Pathology Comparisons

Nodular appearance of amyloidoma on CT represent _ replacement of the parenchyma by amyloid admixed with multinucleated giant cells and plasma cells.

### Patient Prognosis

Nodular parenchymal amyloidosis rarely requires intervention or medical therapy.

## ANCA-Associated Granulomatous Vasculitis

### Pathology and Pathogenesis

In classic form of ANCA-associated granulomatous vasculitis, multiple irregular but well-circumscribed masses of various sizes are shown in the lungs. They consist of gray-indurated tissue surrounding a soft, friable, gray, or hemorrhagic necrotic center which may cavitate. Microscopically, the nodules show irregular areas of necrosis surrounded by inflammatory granulation tissue. The outlines of necrotic vessels or other structures may be evident centrally, and there is often extensive karyorrhexis resulting in the accumulation of fine hematoxyphilic nuclear dust. Variable numbers of multinucleate foreign-body or Langerhans giant cells may be seen [23].

### Symptoms and Signs

ANCA-associated granulomatous vasculitis is characterized by necrotizing granulomatous inflammation with the classic triad of upper airway involvement (sinusitis, otitis, ulcerations, bony deformities, subglottic, or bronchial stenosis), lower respiratory tract involvement (cough, chest pain, dyspnea, hemoptysis), and glomerulonephritis (hematuria, RBC casts, proteinuria, azotemia). Constitutional symptoms that include fever, arthralgia, myalgia, and weight loss and ocular involvement are common. Massive pulmonary hemorrhage, although uncommon, is a life-threatening manifestation.

### CT Findings

The most common CT finding at the initial presentation is the presence of multiple, bilateral nodules or masses [6, 24] (Fig. 19.6). The nodules tend to have a random distribution, but they occasionally have a subpleural or peribronchovascular distribution. With progression of disease, the nodules tend to increase in size and number. Cavitation occurs in approximately 50 % of cases. The cavities are usually thick walled and tend to have an irregular, shaggy inner lining. Other common findings include bronchial wall thickening, large airway involvement, airspace consolidation, and areas of GGO. Centrilobular small nodules and a tree-in-bud pattern may be seen in up to 10 % of patients. After treatment, these lesions usually show a decrease in the extent.

### CT–Pathology Comparisons

Nodules or masses on CT represent inflammatory nodules composed of large areas of parenchymal necrosis, granulomatous inflammation, and vasculitis. Airspace consolidation and areas of GGO represent diffuse alveolar hemorrhage caused by necrotizing capillaritis. Centrilobular nodules and the tree-in-bud sign may result from bronchiolar inflammatory changes rather than from vasculitis [24].

### Patient Prognosis

The pharmacologic treatment of vasculitis necessitates the use of cytotoxic medications and systemic corticosteroids. The 5-year survival of ANCA-associated granulomatous vasculitis has been reported to be 74–91 % [25]. Main factors affecting survival are age and target organ damage.

## References

1. Bae YA, Lee KS. Cross-sectional evaluation of thoracic lymphoma. Radiol Clin North Am. 2008;46:253–64. viii.
2. Dacic S, Colby TV, Yousem SA. Nodular amyloidoma and primary pulmonary lymphoma with amyloid production: a differential diagnostic problem. Mod Pathol. 2000;13:934–40.
3. Yoon HK, Im JG, Ahn JM, Han MC. Pulmonary nocardiosis: CT findings. J Comput Assist Tomogr. 1995;19:52–5.
4. Han D, Lee KS, Franquet T, et al. Thrombotic and nonthrombotic pulmonary arterial embolism: spectrum of imaging findings. Radiographics. 2003;23:1521–39.

5. Song KD, Lee KS, Chung MP, et al. Pulmonary cryptococcosis: imaging findings in 23 non-AIDS patients. Korean J Radiol. 2010;11:407–16.
6. Chung MP, Yi CA, Lee HY, Han J, Lee KS. Imaging of pulmonary vasculitis. Radiology. 2010;255:322–41.
7. Crow J, Slavin G, Kreel L. Pulmonary metastasis: a pathologic and radiologic study. Cancer. 1981;47:2595–602.
8. Hirakata K, Nakata H, Nakagawa T. CT of pulmonary metastases with pathological correlation. Semin Ultrasound CT MR. 1995;16:379–94.
9. Murata K, Takahashi M, Mori M, et al. Pulmonary metastatic nodules: CT-pathologic correlation. Radiology. 1992;182:331–5.
10. Primack SL, Hartman TE, Lee KS, Muller NL. Pulmonary nodules and the CT halo sign. Radiology. 1994;190:513–5.
11. Hirakata K, Nakata H, Haratake J. Appearance of pulmonary metastases on high-resolution CT scans: comparison with histopathologic findings from autopsy specimens. AJR Am J Roentgenol. 1993;161:37–43.
12. Nicholson AG, Wotherspoon AC, Diss TC, et al. Pulmonary B-cell non-Hodgkin's lymphomas. The value of immunohistochemistry and gene analysis in diagnosis. Histopathology. 1995;26:395–403.
13. Cadranel J, Wislez M, Antoine M. Primary pulmonary lymphoma. Eur Respir J. 2002;20:750–62.
14. Lee KS, Kim Y, Primack SL. Imaging of pulmonary lymphomas. AJR Am J Roentgenol. 1997;168:339–45.
15. William J, Variakojis D, Yeldandi A, Raparia K. Lymphoproliferative neoplasms of the lung: a review. Arch Pathol Lab Med. 2013;137:382–91.
16. Kim EY, Kim TS, Han J, Choi JY, Kwon OJ, Kim J. Thoracic epithelioid hemangioendothelioma: imaging and pathologic features. Acta Radiol. 2011;52:161–6.
17. Luburich P, Ayuso MC, Picado C, Serra-Batlles J, Ramirez JF, Sole M. CT of pulmonary epithelioid hemangioendothelioma. J Comput Assist Tomogr. 1994;18:562–5.
18. Bagan P, Hassan M, Le Pimpec Barthes F, et al. Prognostic factors and surgical indications of pulmonary epithelioid hemangioendothelioma: a review of the literature. Ann Thorac Surg. 2006;82:2010–3.
19. Mukundan G, Urban BA, Askin FB, Fishman EK. Pulmonary epithelioid hemangioendothelioma: atypical radiologic findings of a rare tumor with pathologic correlation. J Comput Assist Tomogr. 2000;24:719–20.
20. Crotty EJ, McAdams HP, Erasmus JJ, Sporn TA, Roggli VL. Epithelioid hemangioendothelioma of the pleura: clinical and radiologic features. AJR Am J Roentgenol. 2000;175:1545–9.
21. Gillmore JD, Hawkins PN. Amyloidosis and the respiratory tract. Thorax. 1999;54:444–51.
22. Urban BA, Fishman EK, Goldman SM, et al. CT evaluation of amyloidosis: spectrum of disease. Radiographics. 1993;13:1295–308.
23. Travis WD, Hoffman GS, Leavitt RY, Pass HI, Fauci AS. Surgical pathology of the lung in Wegener's granulomatosis. Review of 87 open lung biopsies from 67 patients. Am J Surg Pathol. 1991;15:315–33.
24. Lee KS, Kim TS, Fujimoto K, et al. Thoracic manifestation of Wegener's granulomatosis: CT findings in 30 patients. Eur Radiol. 2003;13:43–51.
25. Mukhtyar C, Flossmann O, Hellmich B, et al. Outcomes from studies of antineutrophil cytoplasm antibody associated vasculitis: a systematic review by the European league against rheumatism systemic vasculitis task force. Ann Rheum Dis. 2008;67:1004–10.

# 20 Ground-Glass Opacity with Reticulation

## Ground-Glass Opacity with Reticulation and Fibrosis

### Definition

Ground-glass opacity (GGO) appears at thin-section CT (TSCT) as hazy increased opacity of the lung, with the preservation of bronchial and vascular margins. It is caused by partial filling of airspaces; interstitial thickening due to fluid, cells, or fibrosis; partial collapse of alveoli; increased capillary blood volume; or combination of these, the common factor being the partial displacement of air [1]. The GGO is less opaque than consolidation, in which bronchovascular margins are obscured (Fig. 20.1).

Reticulation at TSCT includes interlobular septal thickening, intralobular lines, or the cyst walls of honeycombing (HC) [2]. When GGO lesions were admixed with reticulation, traction bronchiectasis, and architectural distortion, the lesions represent histologically the area of pulmonary fibrosis.

### Diseases Causing the Pattern

*Usual interstitial pneumonia* (*UIP*) (Fig. 20.2) and fibrotic or mixed fibrotic and cellular *nonspecific interstitial pneumonia* (*NSIP*) (Figs. 20.3 and 20.4) are the two most common diseases that show GGO mixed with reticulation with or without honeycombing.

### Distribution

Subpleural and basal predominance is one of the four major prerequisites (subpleural and basal predominance, reticular abnormality, HC with or without traction bronchiectasis, and absence of features listed as inconsistent with UIP pattern) to be called UIP pattern at TSCT [3]. The TSCT features that help differentiate best NSIP from UIP or chronic hypersensitivity pneumonitis are relative subpleural sparing of GGO and reticulation [4] (Fig. 20.3). NSIP may also demonstrate bronchovascular distribution of lung lesions and subpleural distribution as well (Fig. 20.4).

### Clinical Considerations

Patients with UIP or fibrotic NSIP who have a high fibrotic score (the extent of reticulation plus HC) at TSCT and a low DLco level appear to have a high death risk [5]. Even in cases of UIP and fibrotic NSIP with little HC, serial CT discloses an increase in the extent of HC and reticulation and a decrease in the extent of GGO. Overall extent of lung fibrosis (reticulation and HC) at the baseline CT examination appears predictive of survival in UIP and fibrotic NSIP with little HC [6].

Honeycombing with Subpleural or Basal Predominance
Chap. 17.

**Key Points for Differential Diagnosis**

| | Distribution | | | | | | | | Clinical presentations | | | |
|---|---|---|---|---|---|---|---|---|---|---|---|---|
| | Zones | | | | | | | | | | | |
| Diseases | U | M | L | SP | C | R | BV | R | Acute | Subacute | Chronic | Others |
| IPF/UIP | | + | + | + | | | | + | | | + | |
| NSIP | | + | + | + | + | | + | + | | + | + | Female predominance; subpleural sparing and along BV bundles |

*Note*: *IPF* idiopathic pulmonary fibrosis, *UIP* usual interstitial pneumonia, *NSIP* nonspecific interstitial pneumonia, *U* upper, *M* middle, *L* lower, *R* random, *SP* subpleural, *C* central, *BV* bronchovascular

K.S. Lee et al., *Radiology Illustrated: Chest Radiology*, Radiology Illustrated,
DOI 10.1007/978-3-642-37096-0_20, © Springer-Verlag Berlin Heidelberg 2014

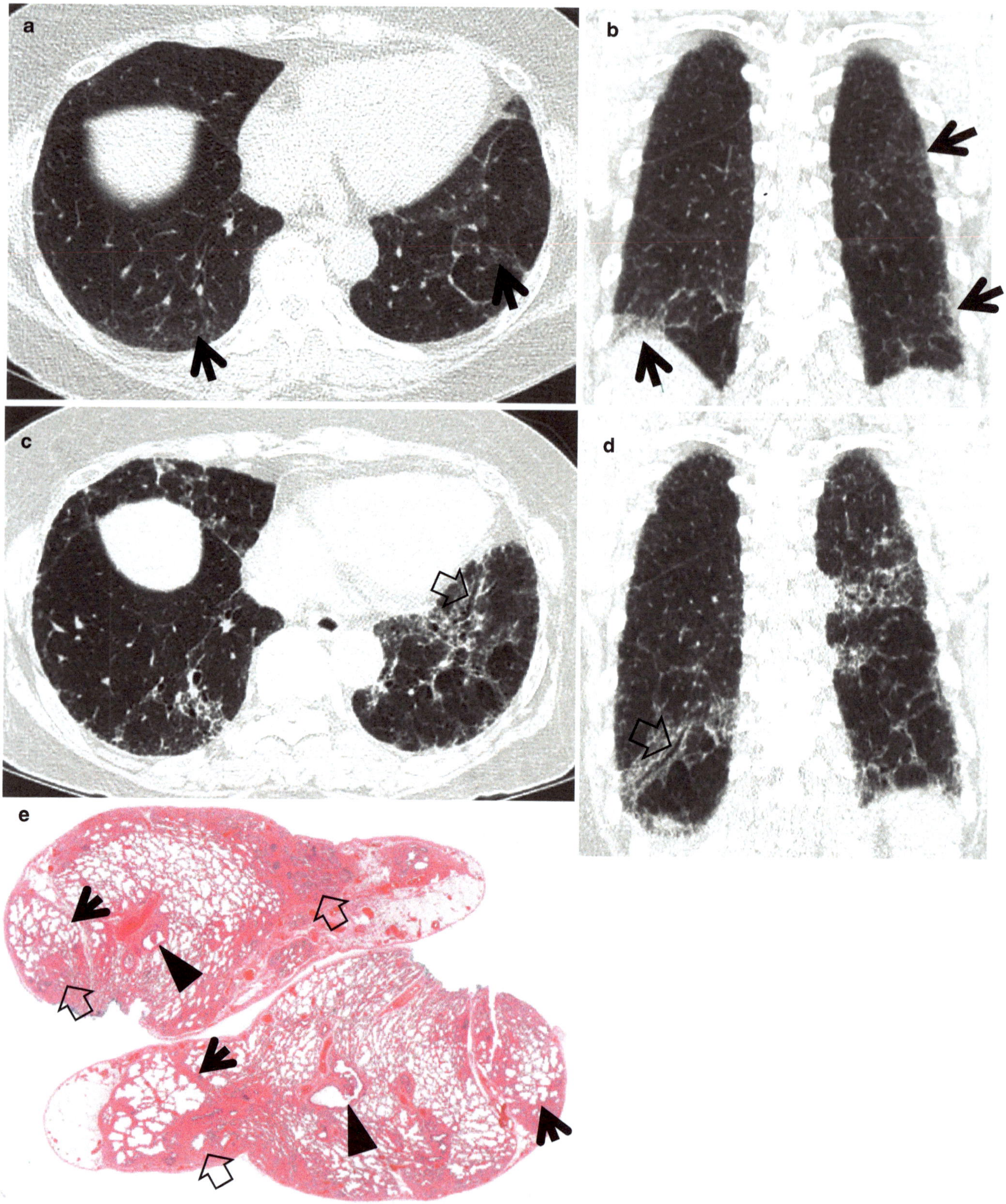


**Fig. 20.1** Usual interstitial pneumonia manifesting as subpleural patchy areas of reticulation and ground-glass opacity without honeycombing cyst in a 73-year-old man. (**a**) Lung window image of thin-section (1.0-mm section thickness) CT scan obtained at level of liver dome shows patchy areas of reticulation and ground-glass opacity (*arrows*) in bilateral lower lung zones. (**b**) Coronal reformatted image (2.0-mm section thickness) also shows patchy areas of reticulation and ground-glass opacity (*arrows*) in lower lung zones. (**c**) Three-year follow-up CT demonstrates increased extent of reticulation and ground-glass opacity in both lungs. Also note traction bronchiectasis (*open arrow*). (**d**) Coronal reformatted image (2.0-mm section thickness) also shows increased extent of reticulation and ground-glass opacity in both lungs. Also note traction bronchiectasis (*open arrow*). (**e**) Low-magnification (×10) photomicrograph of surgical biopsy specimen obtained from right lower lobe and at follow-up CT acquisition time discloses heterogeneous areas of inflammation (*arrows*) and fibrosis (*open arrows*) in alveolar walls in terms of time and region. Also note airway wall thickening and dilatation (*arrowheads*)

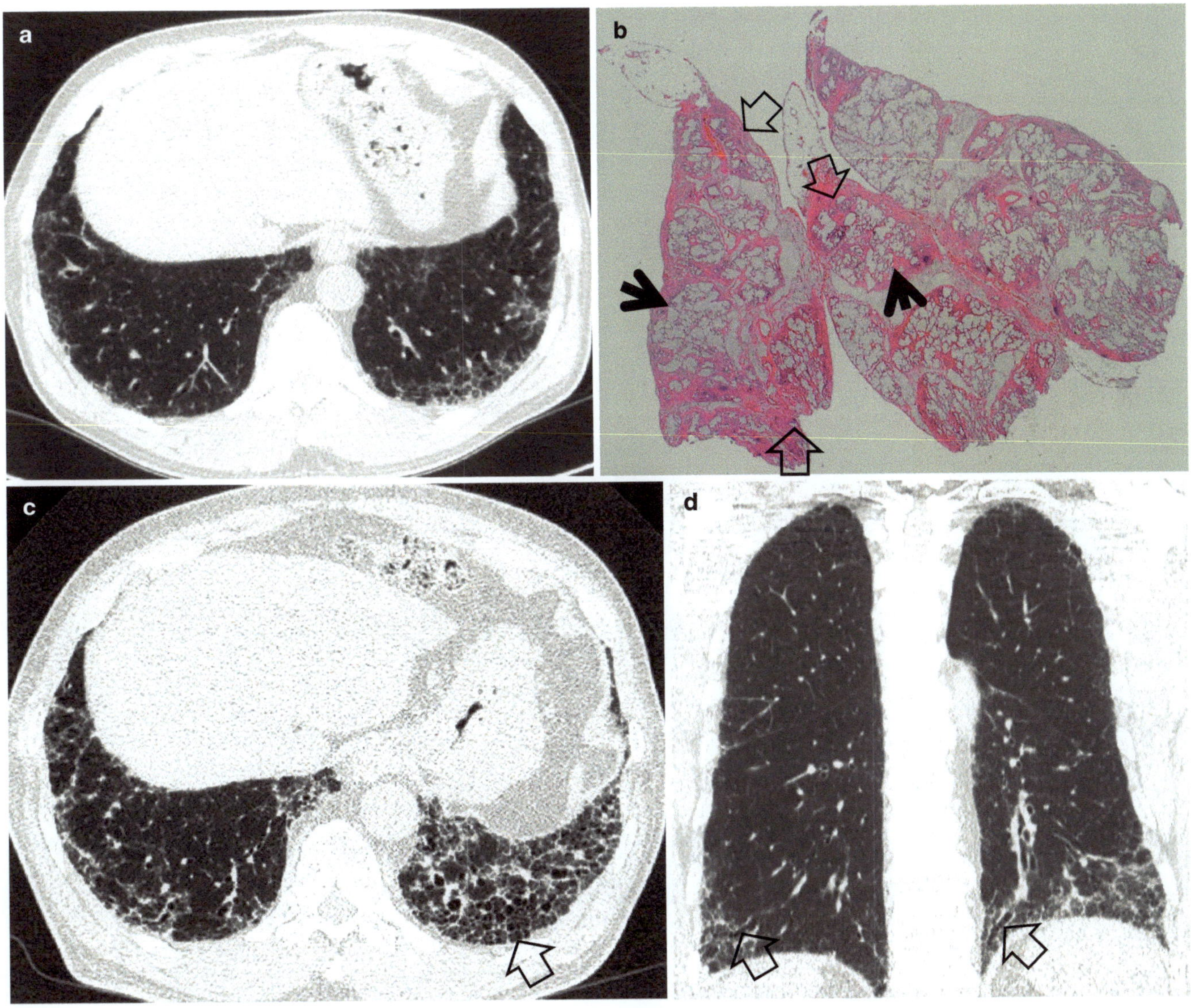


**Fig. 20.2** Usual interstitial pneumonia manifesting as subpleural patchy areas of reticulation and ground-glass opacity without honeycombing cyst in a 62-year-old man. (**a**) Lung window image of thin-section (1.5-mm section thickness) CT scan obtained at level of liver dome shows patchy areas of reticulation and ground-glass opacity in bilateral lower lung zones. (**b**) Low-magnification (×4) photomicrograph of surgical biopsy specimen obtained from left lower lobe discloses heterogeneous areas of inflammation (*arrows*) and fibrosis (*open arrows*) in alveolar walls in terms of time and region. (**c**) Seven-year follow-up CT demonstrates increased extent of reticulation in both lungs. Also note new area of honeycombing (*open arrow*). (**d**) Follow-up CT in coronal reformatted view depicts reticulation predominant abnormalities with lower lung zone predominance. Also note traction bronchiectasis (*open arrows*)

## Ground-Glass Opacity with Reticulation, but without Fibrosis (Crazy-Paving Appearance)

### Definition

The crazy-paving appearance consists of a network of a smooth linear pattern superimposed on the area of ground-glass opacity (GGO) on high-resolution CT scans (Fig. 20.5). Once thought as specific finding for pulmonary alveolar proteinosis (PAP), currently the crazy-paving appearance is a nonspecific finding seen in a variety of interstitial and airspace lung diseases [7].

### Diseases Causing the Pattern

The diseases causing crazy-paving pattern include acute bacterial, viral, or *Pneumocystis* pneumonia (Fig. 20.6), acute interstitial pneumonia (AIP) or adult respiratory distress syndrome (ARDS), diffuse alveolar damage superimposed on usual interstitial pneumonia (UIP), diffuse alveolar hemorrhage (DAH) (Fig. 20.5), pulmonary interstitial edema, *pulmonary alveolar proteinosis* (PAP) (Fig. 20.7), nonspecific interstitial pneumonia (NSIP), subacute hypersensitivity pneumonitis (HP), organizing pneumonia, sarcoidosis, *lipoid pneumonia* (Fig. 20.8), and *diffuse form of mucinous or nonmucinous*

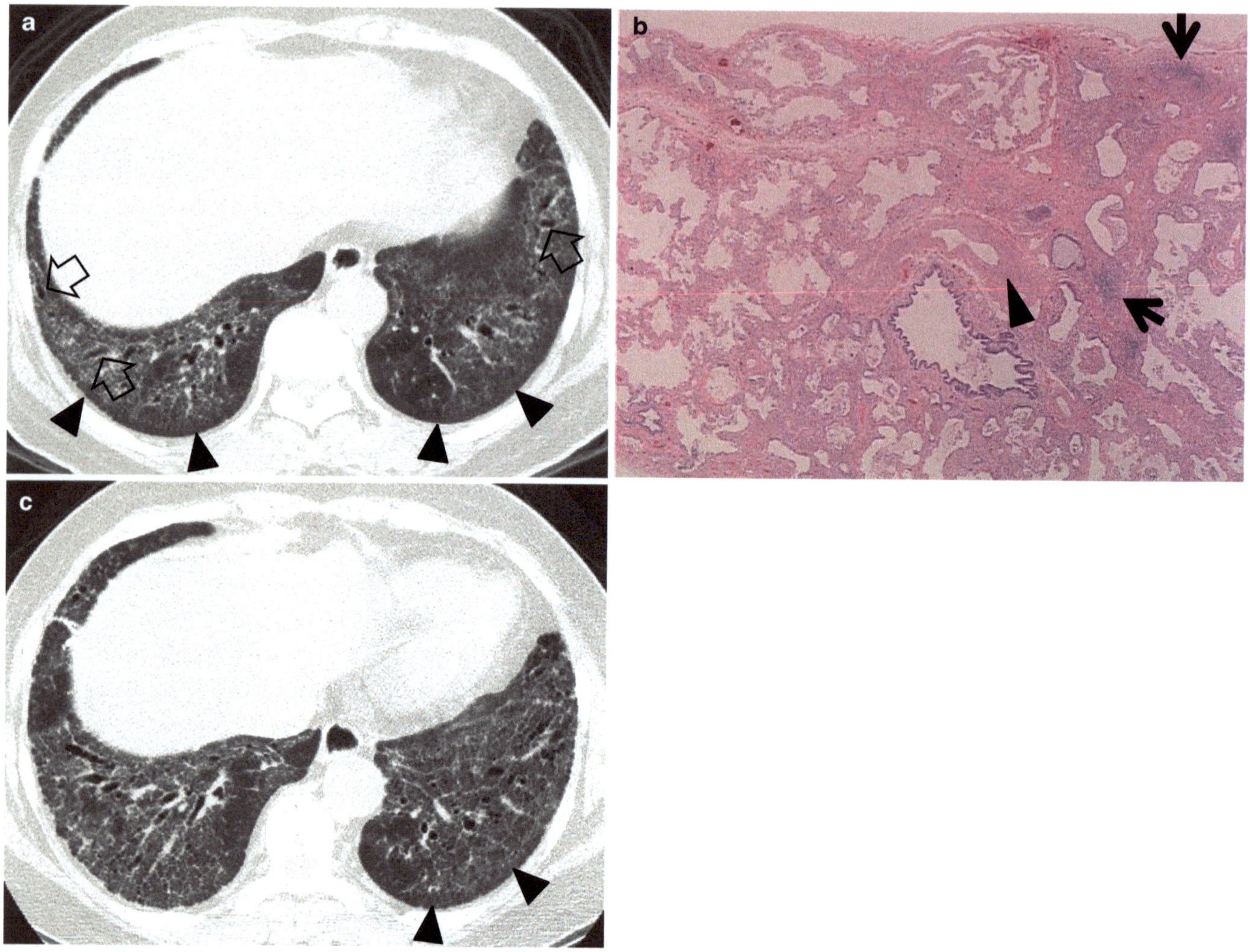


**Fig. 20.3** Fibrotic nonspecific interstitial pneumonia in a 50-year-old woman. (**a**) Lung window image of thin-section (1.0-mm section thickness) CT scan obtained at level of liver dome shows patchy areas of reticulation and ground-glass opacity in bilateral lower lung zones. Subpleural sparing (*arrowheads*), one of important signs that help differentiate usual interstitial pneumonia from this disease on CT, is clearly seen. Also note traction bronchiectasis (*open arrows*). (**b**) Low-magnification (×40) photomicrograph of surgical biopsy specimen obtained from right lower lobe discloses clearly temporal and regional homogeneity; namely, whole alveolar wall shows fibrotic changes with little lymphocytic infiltration. Also note few areas (*arrows*) of lymphocytic infiltration and thickened vessel walls (*arrowhead*). (**c**) Four-year follow-up CT demonstrates slightly increased extent of reticulation in both lungs. Still subpleural sparing (*arrowheads*) is overt particularly in left lung

*adenocarcinoma* (AIS, former bronchioloalveolar carcinoma [BAC]) or lung adenocarcinoma [7, 8] (Fig. 20.9).

## Distribution

In most diseases, lung abnormalities show random and patchy and extensive distribution. In NSIP and organizing pneumonia, the abnormalities usually demonstrate subpleural and lower lung zone predominance. In lipoid pneumonia, the crazy-paving appearance is usually located in the right middle lobe, lingular division of the left upper lobe, or in both the lower lobes.

## Clinical Considerations

The speed of disease development may help distinguish among various diseases. For example, acute disease process suggest the diagnosis of *Pneumocystis* or other infectious pneumonia, ARDS, AIP or acute exacerbation of

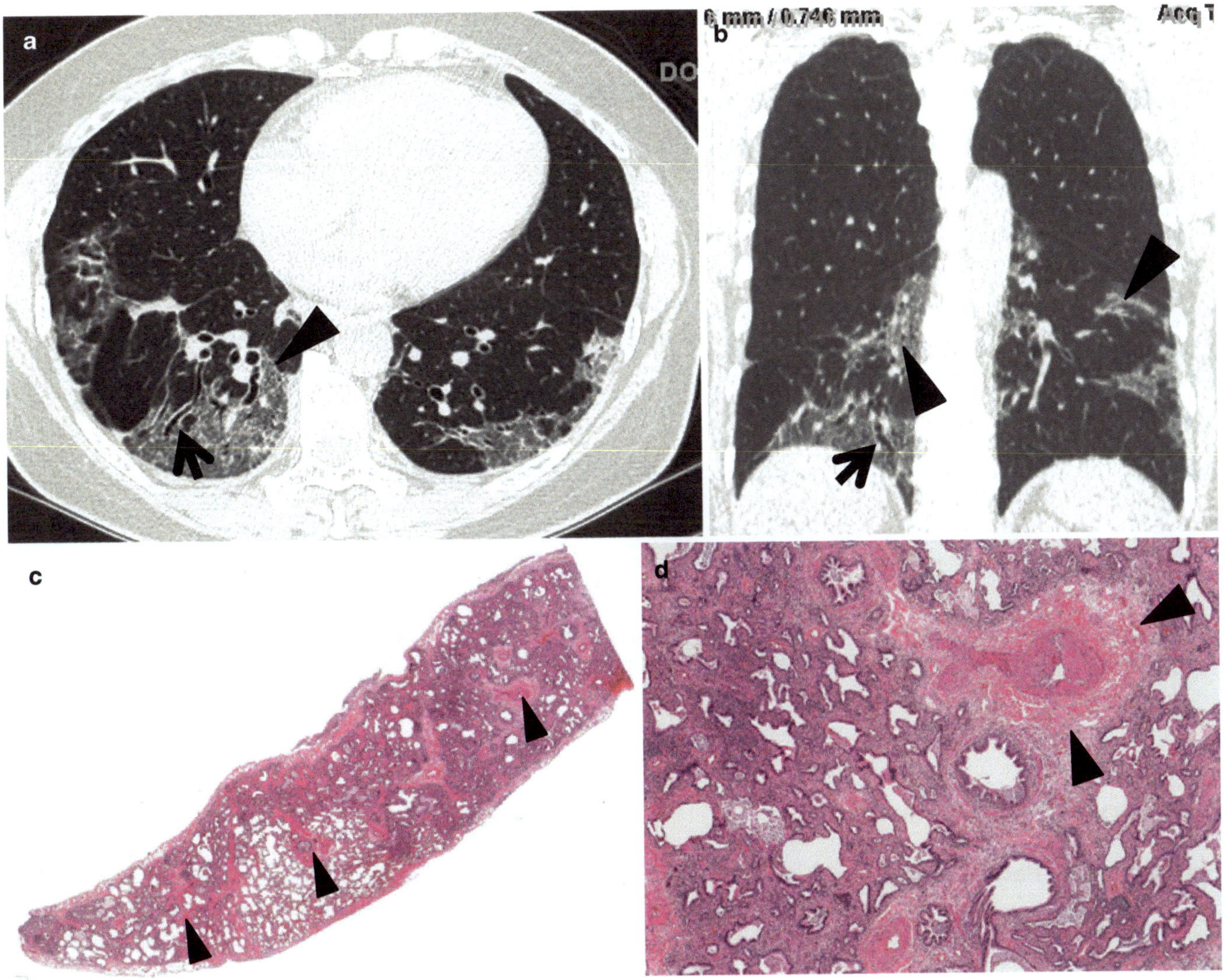


Fig. 20.4 Fibrotic nonspecific interstitial pneumonia in a 60-year-old woman. (**a**) Lung window image of thin-section (1.0-mm section thickness) CT scan obtained at level of cardiac ventricle shows patchy areas of ground-glass opacity and reticulation. Please note involvement of central portion (*arrowhead*) of lung as well as subpleural lungs, which is somewhat more peculiar to nonspecific interstitial pneumonia than usual interstitial pneumonia. Also note traction bronchiectasis (*arrow*). (**b**) Coronal reformatted imaged demonstrates central involvement (*arrowheads*) involvement of lung lesions along bronchovascular bundles, not to mention of subpleural lung involvement. Also note traction bronchiectasis (*arrow*). (**c**) Low-magnification (×4) photomicrograph of surgical biopsy specimen obtained from right lower lobe exhibits uniform interstitial expansion with fibrosis and little lymphocytic infiltration. Also note thickened vessel walls (*arrowheads*). (**d**) Somewhat closer look (×40) of surgical biopsy specimen discloses clearly temporal and regional homogeneity, namely, uniform interstitial expansion due to fibrosis. Also thickened vessel wall, which is postinflammatory changes (*arrowheads*)

UIP, DAH, and interstitial edema, whereas chronic indolent course may indicate the presence of PAP, lipoid pneumonia, and diffuse form of lung adenocarcinoma or mucinous adenocarcinoma in situ (AIS). Other patient history and clinical presentation may also be useful for helping make a specific diagnosis.

**Key Points for Differential Diagnosis**

| | Distribution | | | | | | | | | | | |
|---|---|---|---|---|---|---|---|---|---|---|---|---|
| | Zones | | | | | | | | Clinical presentations | | | |
| Diseases | U | M | L | SP | C | R | BV | R | Acute | Subacute | Chronic | Others |
| *Pneumocystis* pneumonia | + | + | + | | | + | | + | + | | | |
| AIP or ARDS | + | + | + | | | + | | + | + | | | |
| DAD superimposed on UIP | | + | + | + | | | | | + | | | Acute exacerbation of UIP |
| DAH | + | + | + | | | + | | + | + | | | Subpleural (apical and costophrenic angle) sparing |
| PE | | + | + | | | + | | + | + | | | |
| PAP | + | + | + | | | + | | + | | + | | |
| NSIP | | + | + | + | + | | + | + | | + | | |
| Subacute HP | + | + | | | | + | | + | | + | | |
| OP | | + | + | + | | | + | | | + | | |
| Sarcoidosis | + | + | | | | + | + | | | | + | |
| LP | | + | + | | | + | | + | | | + | |
| Mucinous AD | + | + | + | | | + | | + | | | + | |

*Note*: *AIP* acute interstitial pneumonia, *ARDS* adult respiratory distress syndrome, *DAD* diffuse alveolar damage, *UIP* usual interstitial pneumonia, *DAH* diffuse alveolar hemorrhage, *PE* pulmonary edema, *PAP* pulmonary alveolar proteinosis, *NSIP* nonspecific interstitial pneumonia, *HP* hypersensitivity pneumonitis, *OP* organizing pneumonia, *LP* lipoid pneumonia, *AD* adenocarcinoma, *U* upper, *M* middle, *L* lower, *SP* subpleural, *C* central, *R* random, *BV* bronchovascular

## *Pneumocystis jirovecii* Pneumonia

### Pathology and Pathogenesis

The alveoli are filled by a foamy, pale, and eosinophilic exudate (Fig. 20.6). The fungus is unstained in Hematoxylin and Eosin preparations but with silver stain the alveoli are seen to contain numerous round cysts that measure about 5 μm across. Crescent-shaped forms represent collapsed cysts. Other helpful feature is a dot, generally seen on the edge of the cyst. In bronchoalveolar lavage fluids, frothy exudate is frequently seen and it may be a diagnostic tool if a biopsy cannot be studied [9].

### Symptoms and Signs

*Pneumocystis jirovecii* pneumonia can occur in immunocompromised individuals, especially hematopoietic stem and solid organ transplants, those receiving high-dose corticosteroid therapy, and persons with advanced HIV infection [10]. A slow indolent time course with symptoms of pneumonia progressing over weeks to months is characteristic in HIV-infected patients. Fulminant respiratory failure associated with fever and dry cough is typical in non-HIV-infected patients.

### CT Findings

Thin-section CT (TSCT) typically shows bilateral areas of GGO [11] (Fig. 20.6). The areas of GGO may be patchy, have a geographic appearance, be diffuse, or involve mainly the perihilar regions or upper lobes. Reticulation or interlobular septal thickening is seen in approximately 20 % of patients forming "crazy-paving appearance" (Fig. 20.6). Cyst formation is seen in about 30 % of patients. The cysts are variable in appearance, but most measure 5–30 mm in diameter, are thin walled, and are located in the upper lobes. Unusual manifestations include nodules and a miliary pattern [12].

### CT–Pathology Comparisons

The GGO reflects thickening of alveolar wall by edema or interstitial pneumonitis and foamy nature of alveolar exudates, whereas the reticulation reflects the organization of intra-alveolar materials or fibrosis [8].

### Patient Prognosis

The first-line drug for treatment and prevention is trimethoprim–sulfamethoxazole. To reduce the incidence of

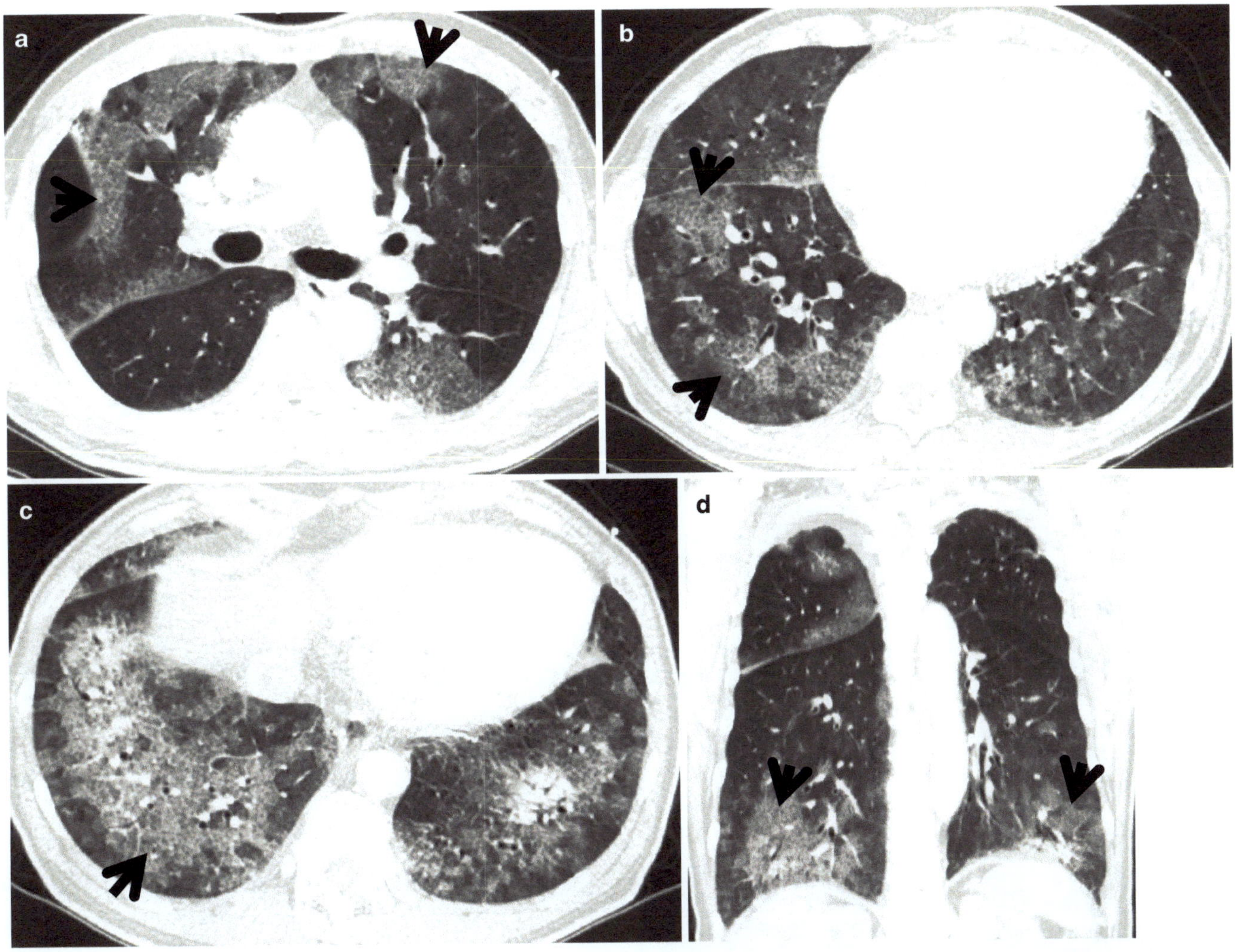


**Fig. 20.5** Diffuse alveolar hemorrhage manifesting as crazy-paving appearance at thin-section CT in a 60-year-old man who had ischemic cardiomyopathy and received heparin and warfarin therapy. (**a–c**) Lung window images of CT scans (2.5-mm section thickness) obtained at levels of main bronchi (**a**), cardiac ventricle (**b**), and liver dome (**c**), respectively, show patchy and extensive areas of ground-glass opacity containing internal reticulation (crazy-paving appearance, *arrows*) in both lungs. Subpleural sparing is overt in all lung zones. (**d**) Coronal reformatted image (2.0-mm section thickness) also demonstrates crazy-paving appearance (*arrows*) in both lungs with subpleural sparing

respiratory failure due to a severe inflammation caused by microbial degradation after antimicrobial therapy, the addition of corticosteroids is indicated for all patients with HIV infection and confirmed cases [10].

## Lipoid Pneumonia

### Pathology and Pathogenesis

There are two types of lipoid pneumonia: exogenous lipoid pneumonia and endogenous one (also called cholesterol pneumonia or golden pneumonia). Exogenous lipoid pneumonia is caused by repeated episodes of aspiration or inhalation of fat or oils, resulting in their accumulation within alveolar macrophages that are incapable of metabolizing the fatty substances. Therefore, oil is repeatedly released into the alveoli, eliciting a foreign-body reaction. Mineral oil is the most common irritant.

Histologically, multiple round to oval cystic spaces (lipid vacuoles that are washed out during processing) surrounded by varying amounts of histiocytes and multinucleated foreign-body giant cells are found (Fig. 20.8). Endogenous lipoid pneumonia is usually associated with bronchial obstruction, thus resulting in the accumulation of cellular breakdown products including cholesterol and its esters from destroyed alveolar cell walls. These lipids are phagocytized by macrophages, which then accumulate within the alveolar spaces. Histologically, there are intra-alveolar accumulation of foamy macrophages containing

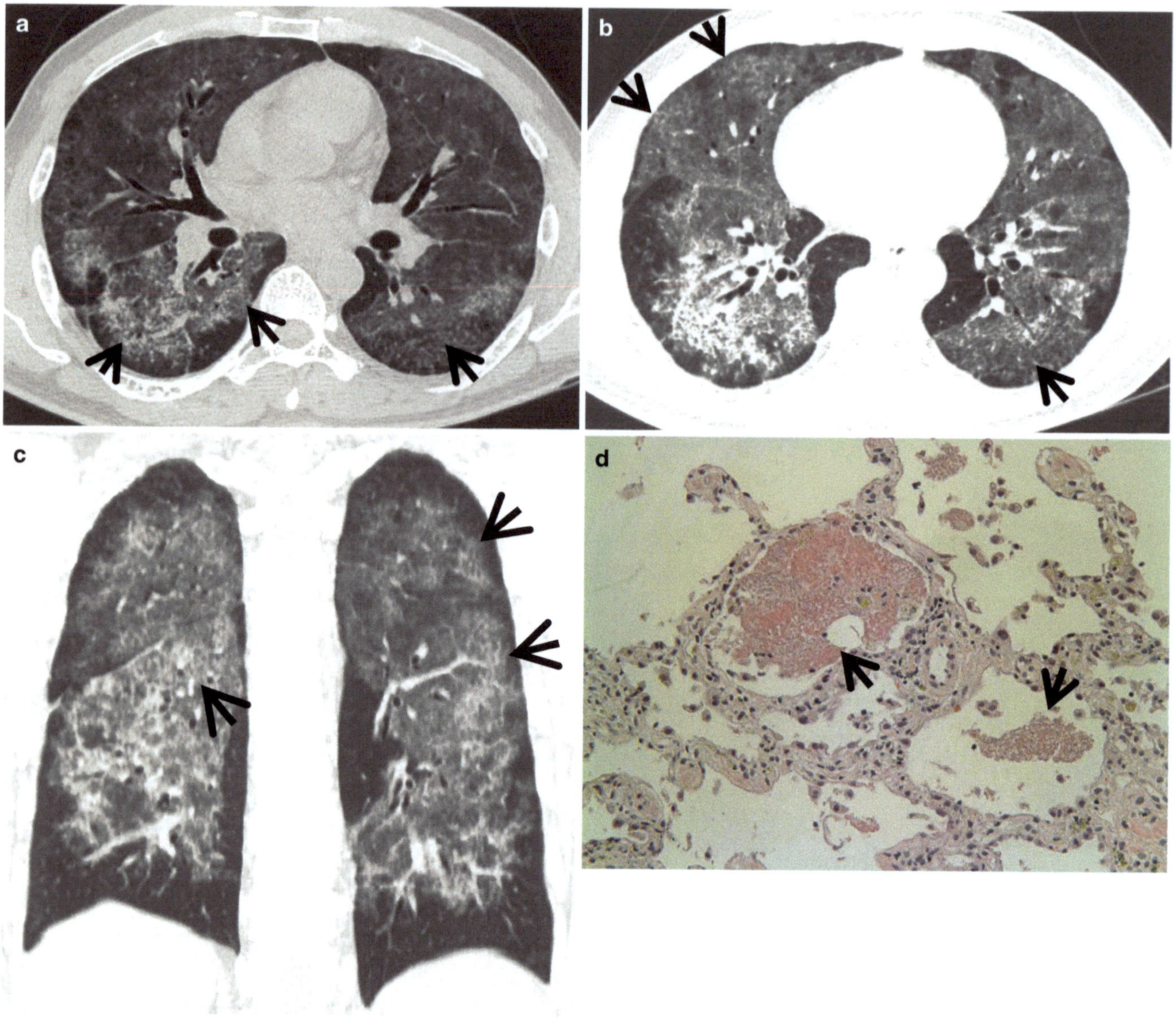


**Fig. 20.6** *Pneumocystis jirovecii* pneumonia in a 48-year-old man with asthma who received corticosteroid therapy. (**a**, **b**) Lung window images of CT scans (2.5-mm section thickness) obtained at levels of right middle lobar bronchus (**a**) and right inferior pulmonary vein (**b**), respectively, show diffuse ground-glass opacity harboring internal reticulation (crazy-paving appearance, *arrows*) in both lungs. Subpleural sparing is seen in all lung zones. (**c**) Coronal reformatted image (2.0-mm section thickness) also demonstrates crazy-paving appearance (*arrows*) in both lungs with subpleural sparing. (**d**) High-magnification (×200) photomicrograph of transbronchial lung biopsy specimen obtained from right lower lobe discloses intra-alveolar foamy exudate (*arrows*) and mild interstitial inflammation and fibrosis suggesting *Pneumocystis* pneumonia and acute lung injury

fine lipid vacuoles (less than 1 μm) and eosinophilic proteinaceous materials derived from degenerating cells, including surfactant from type II pneumocytes, in the alveoli distal to the bronchial obstruction [13].

## Symptoms and Signs

Symptoms can vary significantly among affected patients, ranging from asymptomatic to severe life-threatening disease [14]. However, symptoms are usually mild. Chronic cough and dyspnea are the most common symptoms.

## CT Findings

The most common CT findings of acute or chronic lipoid pneumonia are low attenuation areas of consolidation and a crazy-paving pattern (Fig. 20.8). The consolidation is most commonly seen within the dependent portions of the lungs.

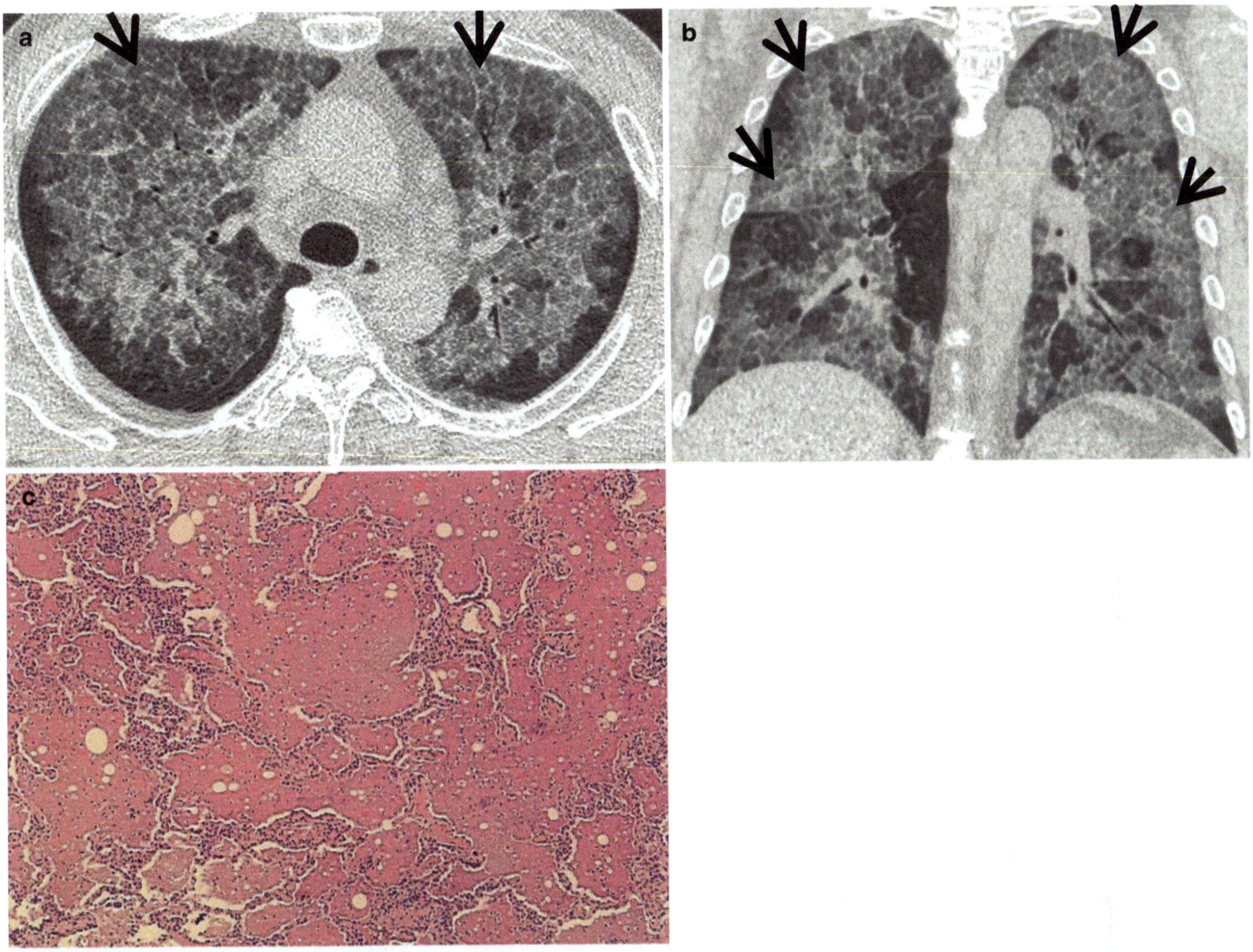


Fig. 20.7 Pulmonary alveolar proteinosis in a 52-year-old man. (**a**) Lung window image of CT scan (1.5-mm section thickness) obtained at level of azygos arch shows diffuse ground-glass opacity containing internal reticulation (crazy-paving appearance, *arrows*) in both lungs. Subpleural sparing is seen. (**b**) Coronal reformatted image (2.0-mm section thickness) also demonstrates crazy-paving appearance (*arrows*) in both lungs. (**c**) High-magnification (×200) photomicrograph of surgical biopsy specimen obtained from right lower lobe discloses filling of alveolar airspaces with finely granular eosinophilic material. Also note normal alveolar walls

Chronic lipoid pneumonia most commonly results in a focal, mass-like area of consolidation [15, 16].

## CT–Pathology Comparisons

The crazy-paving pattern reflects intra-alveolar and interstitial accumulation of lipid-laden macrophages and hyperplasia of type II pneumocytes in the alveolar lining [17].

## Patient Prognosis

The key in the management is identification and discontinuation of the exposure to the offending agent. Treatment is primarily supportive and generally conservative. Acute, sometimes fatal, cases can occur, but the disease is usually indolent.

# Pulmonary Alveolar Proteinosis

## Pathology and Pathogenesis

Pulmonary alveolar proteinosis (PAP) is characterized by an intra-alveolar accumulation of lipid-rich eosinophilic material (Fig. 20.7). In primary PAP, it occurs as a result of impaired clearance of surfactant by alveolar macrophages due to the effects of an autoantibody directed against granulocyte-macrophage colony-stimulating factor (GM-CSF). The gross lung shows firm yellow-white nodules, some as large as 2 cm in diameter. Microscopically,

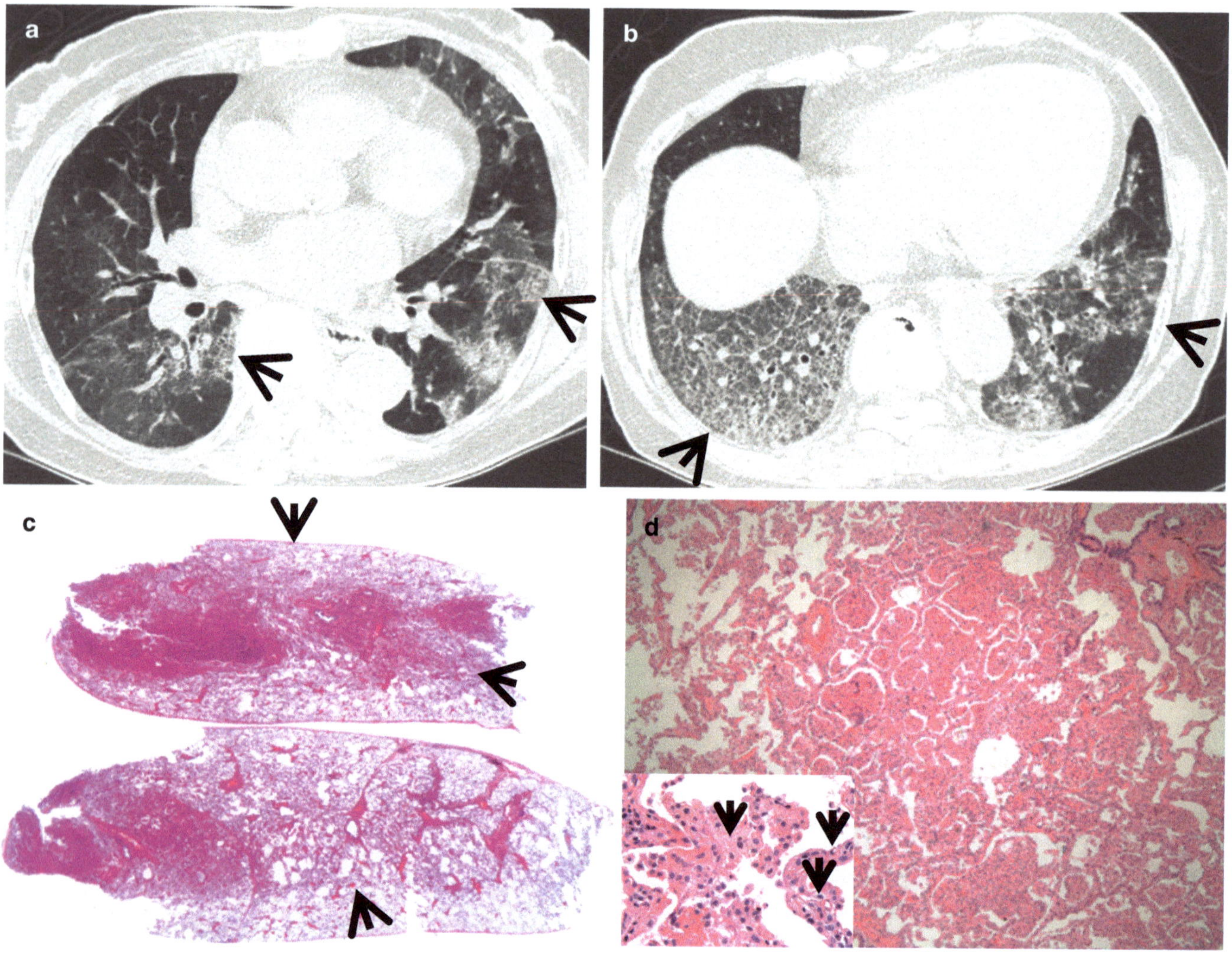


Fig. 20.8 Lipoid pneumonia (squalene aspiration pneumonia) in a 73-year-old man. (**a**, **b**) Lung window images of CT scans (2.5-mm section thickness) obtained at levels of right middle lobar bronchus (**a**) and liver dome (**b**), respectively, show patchy and extensive areas of ground-glass opacity harboring internal reticulation (crazy-paving appearance, *arrows*) in both lungs. (**c**) Low-magnification (×10) photomicrograph of surgical biopsy specimen obtained from right lower lobe demonstrates consolidative lesions filled with inflammatory cells as well as areas (*arrows*) of interstitial thickening with loose fibrosis and inflammation. (**d**) High-magnification (×100) photomicrograph discloses alveolar filling with lipid-laden macrophages, other inflammatory cells, and fibrin. *Inset*: lipid-laden macrophages (*arrows*)

pink granular material fills the air spaces, sometimes with a rim of retraction that separates the alveolar wall slightly from the exudates. Closer inspection of this material shows embedded clumps of dense globular material and cholesterol clefts [18].

## Symptoms and Signs

Most patients with PAP present with progressive exertional dyspnea of insidious onset and cough [19]. Less commonly, fever, chest pain, or hemoptysis also occurs, especially if secondary infection is present. Almost one-third of patients are asymptomatic. The findings on physical examination can be unremarkable, but there are inspiratory crackles in 50 % of patients and cyanosis in 25 %.

## CT Findings

The characteristic TSCT finding is areas of GGO. The areas of GGO often have sharply defined margins, giving them a geographic appearance (Fig. 20.7). In most cases, intralobular interstitial and interlobular septal thickening can be seen, superimposed on the areas of GGO, forming the "crazy-paving appearance" [20, 21] (Fig. 20.7). The distribution of disease is variable: most commonly, it is random. Sometimes, areas of airspace consolidation may be present.

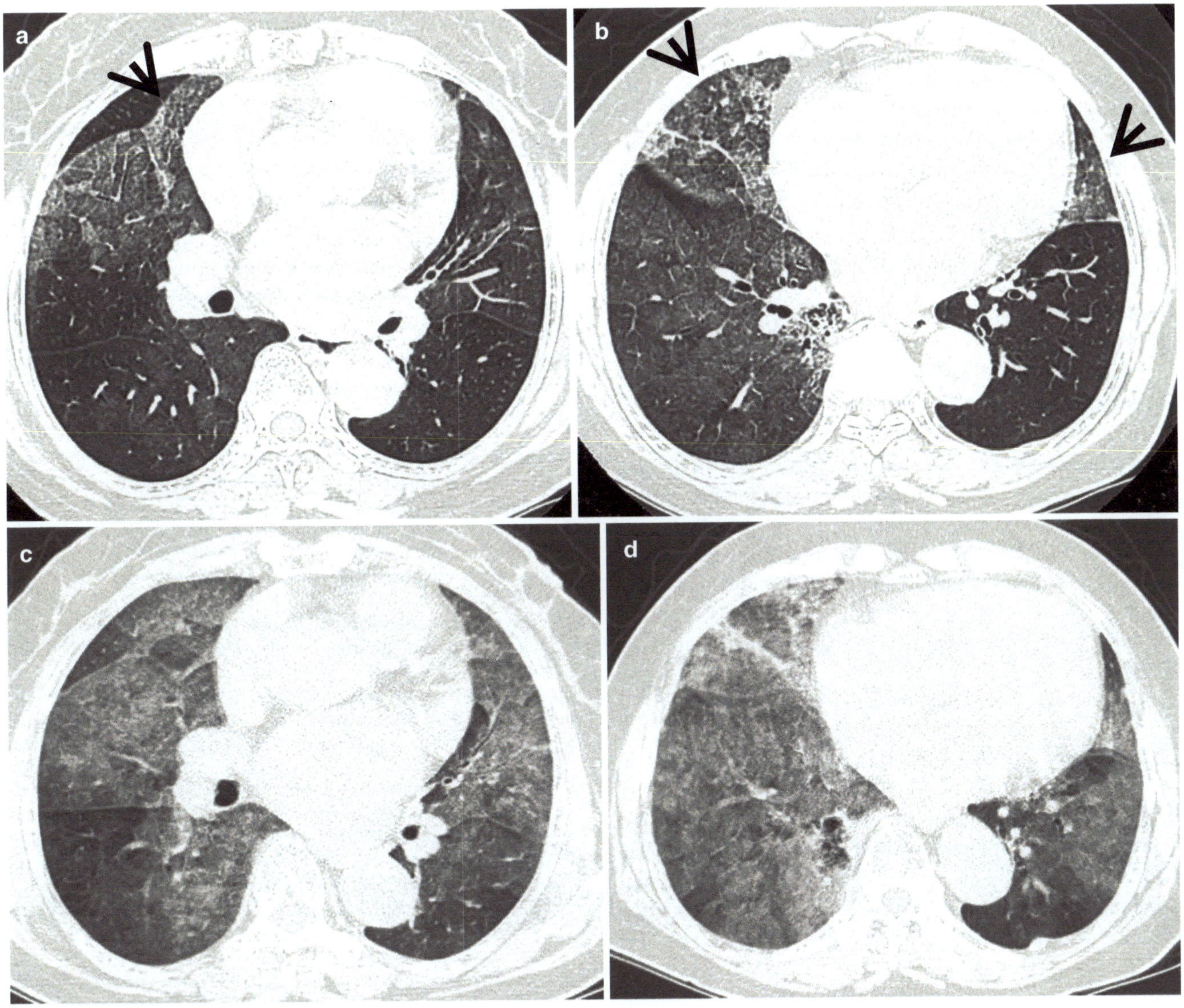


**Fig. 20.9** Diffuse nonmucinous adenocarcinoma in situ in a 70-year-old woman. (**a**, **b**) Lung window images of CT scans (2.5-mm section thickness) obtained at levels of right bronchus intermedius (**a**) and right inferior pulmonary vein (**b**), respectively, show patchy extensive areas of ground-glass opacity having internal reticulation (crazy-paving appearance, *arrows*) in both lungs. (**c**, **d**) Ten-month follow-up CT scans obtained at similar levels to **a** and **b**, respectively, demonstrate progressive disease with diffuse ground-glass opacity in both lungs

## CT–Pathology Comparisons

Areas of GGO represent alveolar filling with finely granular eosinophilic materials. Crazy-paving appearance results from septal edema or from accumulation of lipoproteins in the airspaces adjacent to normal interlobular septa [22].

## Patient Prognosis

From spontaneous remission to death, disease evolution is unpredictable. Acquired pulmonary alveolar proteinosis has been treated successfully since 1960s by whole lung lavage, and this procedure remains the standard of care. Novel therapy targeting alveolar macrophage with granulocyte-macrophage colony-stimulating factor is now considered an alternative to whole lung lavage.

# Mucinous Adenocarcinoma or Adenocarcinoma in Situ, Diffuse Form

## Pathology and Pathogenesis

Invasive mucinous adenocarcinoma (formerly mucinous BAC) has a distinctive histologic appearance with tumor cells having a goblet or columnar cell morphology with abundant intracytoplasmic mucin. Cytologic atypia is usually inconspicuous or absent. Alveolar spaces often contain mucin. When stromal invasion is seen, the malignant cells may show less cytoplasmic mucin and more atypia. These tumors differ from mucinous adenocarcinoma in situ and minimally invasive adenocarcinoma by one or more of the following criteria: size (>3 cm in diameter), amount of invasion (>0.5 cm in thickness), multiple nodules, or lack of a circumscribed border with military spread into adjacent lung parenchyma. There is a strong tendency for multicentric, multilobar, and bilateral lung involvement, which may reflect aerogenous spread [23].

## Symptoms and Signs

Most patients are asymptomatic. Cough and exertional dyspnea are the most common respiratory symptoms when it progresses diffusely to bilateral lung. Due to abundant mucin production of the cancer cells, patients with invasive mucinous adenocarcinoma can complain of copious amount of sputum, so-called bronchorrhea. Constitutional symptoms including anorexia, weight loss, and malaise may be present.

## CT Findings

Diffuse nonmucinous or mucinous adenocarcinoma or AIS may be seen as three predominant patterns: GGO (4 of 38, 10 %) (Fig. 20.9), consolidation (22 of 38, 58 %), and multiple nodules (12 of 38, 32 %) [24]. When reticular attenuation is superimposed on GGO lesions, the tumor may manifest crazy-paving pattern.

## CT–Pathology Comparisons

The GGO reflects the low-density intra-alveolar material (glycoprotein), whereas the superimposed reticular attenuation is due to infiltration of the interstitium by inflammatory or tumor cells [24, 25].

## Patient Prognosis

The overall prognosis for patients with invasive mucinous adenocarcinoma is worse than for those with the nonmucinous adenocarcinoma. Invasive mucinous adenocarcinoma has a strong tendency for multifocal, multilobar, and bilateral lung involvement, which may reflect aerogenous spread. Even if surgically resected in the localized stage, it frequently recurs in the remaining lung.

## References


1. Remy-Jardin M, Giraud F, Remy J, Copin MC, Gosselin B, Duhamel A. Importance of ground-glass attenuation in chronic diffuse infiltrative lung disease: pathologic-CT correlation. Radiology. 1993;189:693–8.
2. Hansell DM, Bankier AA, MacMahon H, McLoud TC, Muller NL, Remy J. Fleischner Society: glossary of terms for thoracic imaging. Radiology. 2008;246:697–722.
3. Raghu G, Collard HR, Egan JJ, et al. An official ATS/ERS/JRS/ALAT statement: idiopathic pulmonary fibrosis: evidence-based guidelines for diagnosis and management. Am J Respir Crit Care Med. 2011;183:788–824.
4. Silva CI, Muller NL, Lynch DA, et al. Chronic hypersensitivity pneumonitis: differentiation from idiopathic pulmonary fibrosis and nonspecific interstitial pneumonia by using thin-section CT. Radiology. 2008;246:288–97.
5. Shin KM, Lee KS, Chung MP, et al. Prognostic determinants among clinical, thin-section CT, and histopathologic findings for fibrotic idiopathic interstitial pneumonias: tertiary hospital study. Radiology. 2008;249:328–37.
6. Lee HY, Lee KS, Jeong YJ, et al. High-resolution CT findings in fibrotic idiopathic interstitial pneumonias with little honeycombing: serial changes and prognostic implications. AJR Am J Roentgenol. 2012;199:982–9.
7. Johkoh T, Itoh H, Muller NL, et al. Crazy-paving appearance at thin-section CT: spectrum of disease and pathologic findings. Radiology. 1999;211:155–60.
8. Rossi SE, Erasmus JJ, Volpacchio M, Franquet T, Castiglioni T, McAdams HP. "Crazy-paving" pattern at thin-section CT of the lungs: radiologic-pathologic overview. Radiographics. 2003;23:1509–19.
9. Watts JC, Chandler FW. Pneumocystis carinii pneumonitis. The nature and diagnostic significance of the methenamine silver-positive "intracystic bodies". Am J Surg Pathol. 1985;9:744–51.
10. Gilroy SA, Bennett NJ. Pneumocystis pneumonia. Semin Respir Crit Care Med. 2011;32:775–82.
11. Kuhlman JE, Kavuru M, Fishman EK, Siegelman SS. Pneumocystis carinii pneumonia: spectrum of parenchymal CT findings. Radiology. 1990;175:711–4.
12. Boiselle PM, Crans Jr CA, Kaplan MA. The changing face of Pneumocystis carinii pneumonia in AIDS patients. AJR Am J Roentgenol. 1999;172:1301–9.
13. Betancourt SL, Martinez-Jimenez S, Rossi SE, Truong MT, Carrillo J, Erasmus JJ. Lipoid pneumonia: spectrum of clinical and radiologic manifestations. AJR Am J Roentgenol. 2010;194:103–9.
14. Marchiori E, Zanetti G, Mano CM, Hochhegger B. Exogenous lipoid pneumonia. Clinical and radiological manifestations. Respir Med. 2011;105:659–66.
15. Lee KS, Muller NL, Hale V, Newell Jr JD, Lynch DA, Im JG. Lipoid pneumonia: CT findings. J Comput Assist Tomogr. 1995;19:48–51.
16. Yi MS, Kim KI, Jeong YJ, Park HK, Lee MK. CT findings in hydrocarbon pneumonitis after diesel fuel siphonage. AJR Am J Roentgenol. 2009;193:1118–21.
17. Franquet T, Gimenez A, Bordes R, Rodriguez-Arias JM, Castella J. The crazy-paving pattern in exogenous lipoid pneumonia: CT-pathologic correlation. AJR Am J Roentgenol. 1998;170:315–7.
18. Khan A, Agarwal R. Pulmonary alveolar proteinosis. Respir Care. 2011;56:1016–28.
19. Trapnell BC, Whitsett JA, Nakata K. Pulmonary alveolar proteinosis. N Engl J Med. 2003;349:2527–39.
20. Murch CR, Carr DH. Computed tomography appearances of pulmonary alveolar proteinosis. Clin Radiol. 1989;40:240–3.

21. Lee KN, Levin DL, Webb WR, Chen D, Storto ML, Golden JA. Pulmonary alveolar proteinosis: high-resolution CT, chest radiographic, and functional correlations. Chest. 1997;111:989–95.
22. Kang EY, Grenier P, Laurent F, Muller NL. Interlobular septal thickening: patterns at high-resolution computed tomography. J Thorac Imaging. 1996;11:260–4.
23. Travis WD, Brambilla E, Noguchi M, et al. International association for the study of lung cancer/American thoracic society/European respiratory society international multidisciplinary classification of lung adenocarcinoma. J Thorac Oncol. 2011;6:244–85.
24. Akira M, Atagi S, Kawahara M, Iuchi K, Johkoh T. High-resolution CT findings of diffuse bronchioloalveolar carcinoma in 38 patients. AJR Am J Roentgenol. 1999;173:1623–9.
25. Tan RT, Kuzo RS. High-resolution CT findings of mucinous bronchioloalveolar carcinoma: a case of pseudopulmonary alveolar proteinosis. AJR Am J Roentgenol. 1997;168:99–100.

# Ground-Glass Opacity without Reticulation

# 21

## Ground-Glass Opacity without Reticulation, Subpleural and Patchy Distribution

### Definition

Ground-glass opacity (GGO) is caused by partial displacement of air in lung parenchyma. The opacity is caused by partial filling of airspaces, interstitial thickening (due to fluid, cells, or fibrosis) (Figs. 21.1 and 21.2), partial collapse of alveoli, and increased capillary blood volume. Without reticulation, the GGO areas usually represent active inflammatory or reversible disease state.

### Diseases Causing the Pattern

*Cellular nonspecific interstitial pneumonia (NSIP)* (Fig. 21.1), *desquamative interstitial pneumonia (DIP)* (Fig. 21.2), cryptogenic organizing pneumonia (COP), and eosinophilic pneumonia (allergic lung disease) depict GGO lesions without reticulation on thin-section CT (TSCT).

### Distribution

The distribution of GGO lesions in cellular NSIP is subpleural, usually without obvious upper–lower lung zone gradient (this gradient, overt in usual interstitial pneumonia with lower lung zone predominance) [1]. In DIP, the opacity had subpleural and lower lung zone predominance [1]. In two-thirds of patients, the opacity lesions in COP are distributed along the bronchovascular bundles or subpleural lungs [2]. In chronic eosinophilic pneumonia, CT shows subpleural opacity with slight upper lung zone predominance [3].

### Clinical Considerations

The presence of asthma history suggests the diagnosis of eosinophilic lung disease (approximately 40 % of patients with chronic eosinophilic lung disease have asthma) [3]. In drug-induced lung disease and lung involvements of collagen vascular diseases, lung abnormalities can be assessed with pattern approach, namely NSIP, DIP, COP, and eosinophilic lung disease-like patterns [4, 5].

**Key Points for Differential Diagnosis**

| | Distribution | | | | | | | | Clinical presentations | | | |
|---|---|---|---|---|---|---|---|---|---|---|---|---|
| | Zones | | | | | | | | | | | |
| Diseases | U | M | L | SP | C | R | BV | R | Acute | Subacute | Chronic | Others |
| Cellular NSIP | | + | + | + | + | | + | + | | | + | |
| DIP | | + | + | + | | | | + | | + | + | Smokers' lung disease |
| COP | | + | + | + | | | + | | | + | + | Consolidation predominant |
| CEP | + | + | | + | | | | + | | + | + | Consolidation predominant; asthma in 40 % of patients |

*Note*: *NSIP* nonspecific interstitial pneumonia, *DIP* desquamative interstitial pneumonia, *COP* cryptogenic organizing pneumonia, *CEP* chronic eosinophilic pneumonia, *U* upper, *M* middle, *L* lower, *R* random, *SP* subpleural, *C* central, *BV* bronchovascular

K.S. Lee et al., *Radiology Illustrated: Chest Radiology*, Radiology Illustrated,
DOI 10.1007/978-3-642-37096-0_21, © Springer-Verlag Berlin Heidelberg 2014

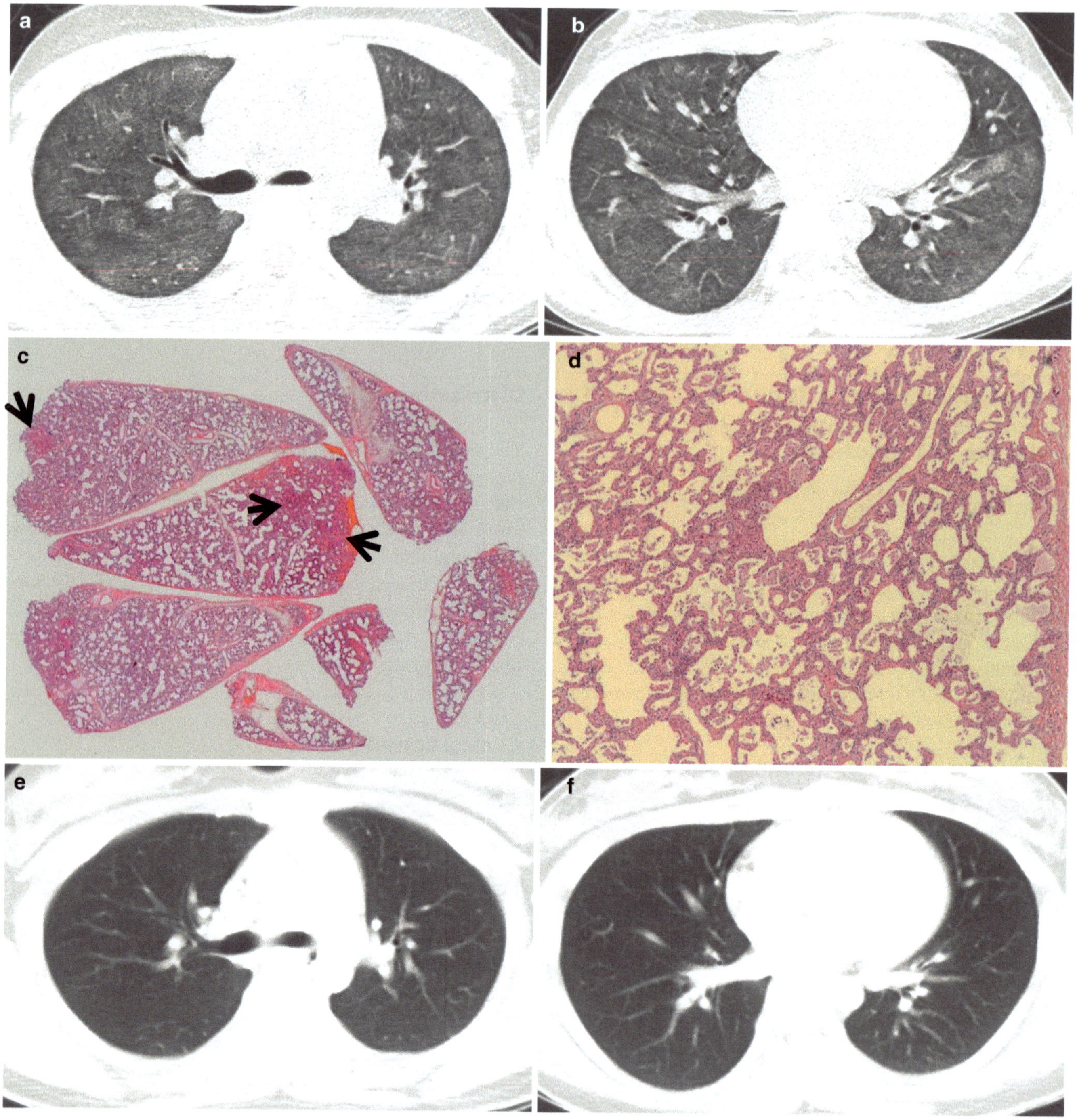


Fig. 21.1 Cellular nonspecific interstitial pneumonia manifesting as diffuse ground-glass opacity without reticulation in a 10-year-old girl. (**a**, **b**) Lung window images of CT scans (2.5-mm section thickness) obtained at levels of right upper lobar bronchus (**a**) and inferior pulmonary veins (**b**), respectively, show diffuse ground-glass opacity in both lungs. (**c**) Low-magnification (×40) photomicrograph of surgical lung biopsy specimen obtained from right lower lobe demonstrates diffuse alveolar wall thickening with inflammatory cell infiltration. Lesions are temporally homogeneous and uniform in alveolar wall thickening. Areas of focal organizing pneumonia (*arrows*) are associated. (**d**) High-magnification (×200) photomicrograph discloses alveolar wall thickening with chronic inflammatory cell infiltration and mild alveolar pneumocytes hyperplasia and many intra-alveolar macrophage aggregation. (**e**, **f**) Two-year follow-up CT scans obtained at similar levels to **a** and **b**, respectively, exhibit complete disappearance of ground-glass opacity in both lungs. Patient received corticosteroid therapy

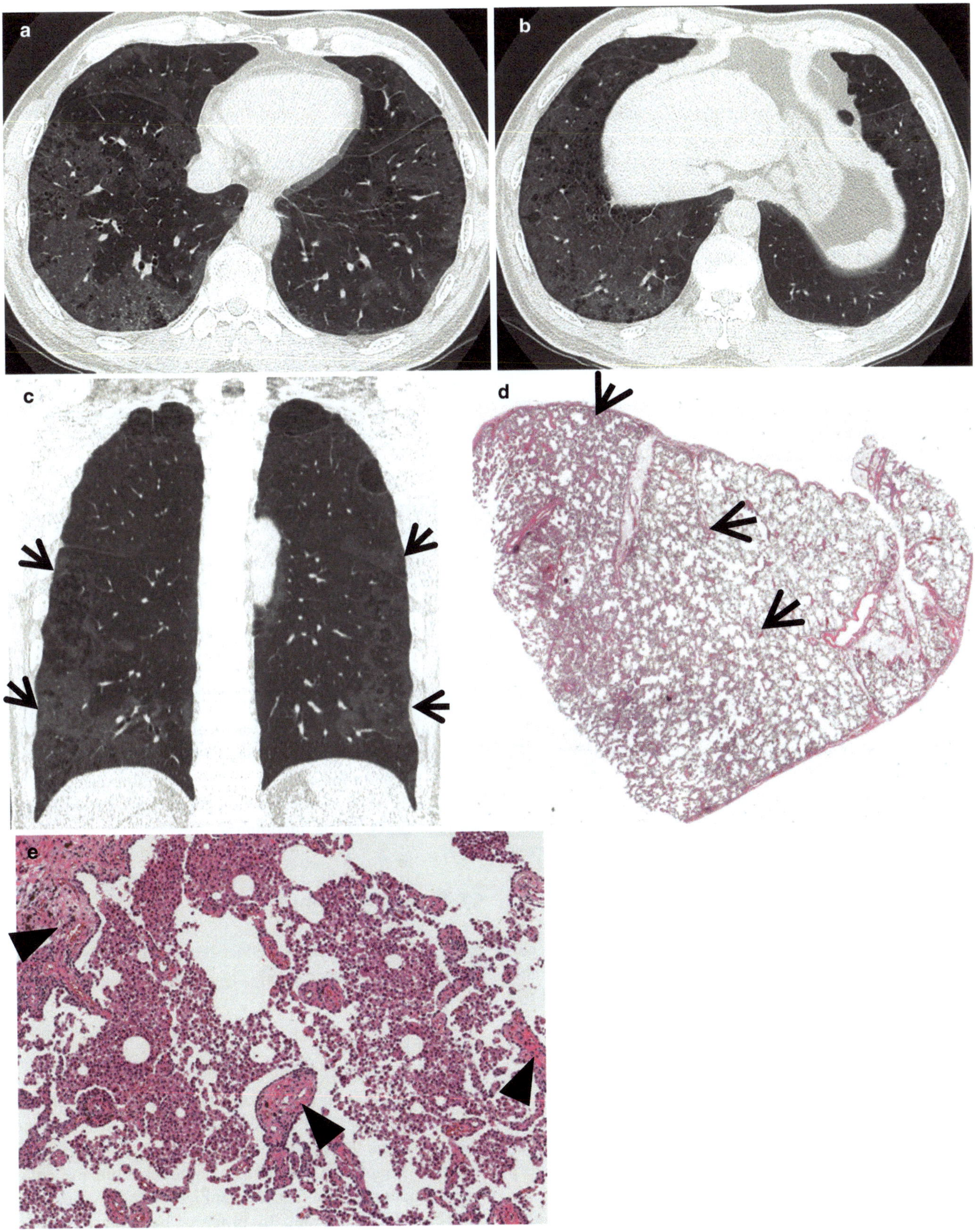


**Fig. 21.2** Desquamative interstitial pneumonia presenting as patchy areas of ground-glass opacity without reticulation in a 51-year-old smoker man. (**a, b**) Lung window images of CT scans (1.5-mm section thickness) obtained at levels of suprahepatic inferior vena cava (**a**) and liver dome (**b**), respectively, show patchy and extensive but subpleural areas of ground-glass opacity in both lungs. (**c**) Coronal reformatted CT image (2.0-mm section thickness) demonstrates subpleural patchy areas of ground-glass opacity (*arrows*) in both lungs. Also note bullae in upper lung zones. (**d**) Low-magnification (×40) photomicrograph of surgical lung biopsy specimen obtained from right lower lobe exhibits areas of uniform accumulation of inflammatory cells in intra-alveolar spaces and mildly in interstitium (alveolar walls) (*arrows*). (**e**) High-magnification (×200) photomicrograph discloses intra-alveolar macrophage accumulation and mild interstitial fibrosis (*arrowheads*)

## Cellular Nonspecific Interstitial Pneumonia

### Pathology and Pathogenesis

The inflammatory process in cellular NSIP is diffuse and uniform, mainly involving the alveolar walls and variably affecting the bronchovascular sheaths and pleura (Fig. 21.1). When air space organization (the organizing pneumonia pattern) is present, it is not uniformly distributed as might occur in organizing infectious pneumonia. When fibrosis occurs in NSIP, it is usually mild and preserves lung structure. Peribronchiolar metaplasia of variable extent may be seen, but microscopic honeycombing (HC) is characteristically absent [6].

### Symptoms and Signs

The typical clinical presentation of NSIP is breathlessness and cough of approximately 6–7 months' duration, predominantly in women, in never-smokers, and in the sixth decade of life [7]. Chest examination reveals bilateral inspiratory crackles in most patients. Digital clubbing is rarely seen in cellular nonspecific interstitial pneumonia. Systemic symptoms, including fever and arthralgia, are frequently observed.

### CT Findings

Cellular NSIP is often characterized by the absence of severe fibrotic changes or HC. The most common CT findings of NSIP are GGO (Fig. 21.1) and fine reticular abnormality [8]. Traction bronchiectasis may be present or absent. All these findings have a symmetric lower lung zone distribution. Consolidation sometimes is seen, but is not the primary abnormality of NSIP. If rapidly developing airspace consolidation or GGO is seen in a patient with NSIP, one should consider the possibility of an acute exacerbation or infection [9]. Although cellular NSIP is characterized by the absence of severe fibrotic changes, imaging features of cellular and fibrotic NSIP often overlap and there is no reliable way to differentiate between cellular and fibrotic NSIP [10].

### CT–Pathology Comparisons

Cellular NSIP demonstrates prominent inflammation without significant fibrosis. Areas of GGO correspond histologically to the areas of interstitial thickening by inflammatory cells and fibrous tissue (Fig. 21.1), whereas the areas of consolidation are related to areas of cryptogenic organizing pneumonia [11].

### Patient Prognosis

Prognosis of cellular NSIP is excellent, with a 10-year survival up to 100 %. Corticosteroids are the main drugs for the treatment.

## Desquamative Interstitial Pneumonia

### Pathology and Pathogenesis

On scanning magnification, the DIP has an eosinophilic appearance due to the presence of eosinophilic macrophages uniformly filling air spaces (Fig. 21.2). Mild interstitial thickening by fibrous tissue is the rule and is uniform in appearance. When chronic inflammation is evident at scanning magnification, it is centrilobular and associated with respiratory bronchioles [12].

### Symptoms and Signs

The clinical presentation of patients with DIP is nonspecific. It consists of chronic cough and dyspnea [13]. Physical examination reveals inspiratory crackles in approximately 60 % and digital clubbing in 25–50 % of patients.

### CT Findings

The predominant TSCT finding of DIP is bilateral areas of GGO with subpleural and basal predominance [14] (Fig. 21.2). Although reticular opacity may be associated with the GGO, HC is uncommon.

### CT–Pathology Comparisons

Areas of GGO on TSCT reflect the filling of alveolar airspaces by macrophages [15] (Fig. 21.2).

### Patient Prognosis

Smoking cessation is the first and most important therapeutic intervention for individuals with DIP who smoke. Pharmacologic therapy with corticosteroids is often used in patients with marked symptoms or significant impairment of lung function. Spontaneous remission has also been described. DIP can gradually progress, particularly in those who continue to smoke.

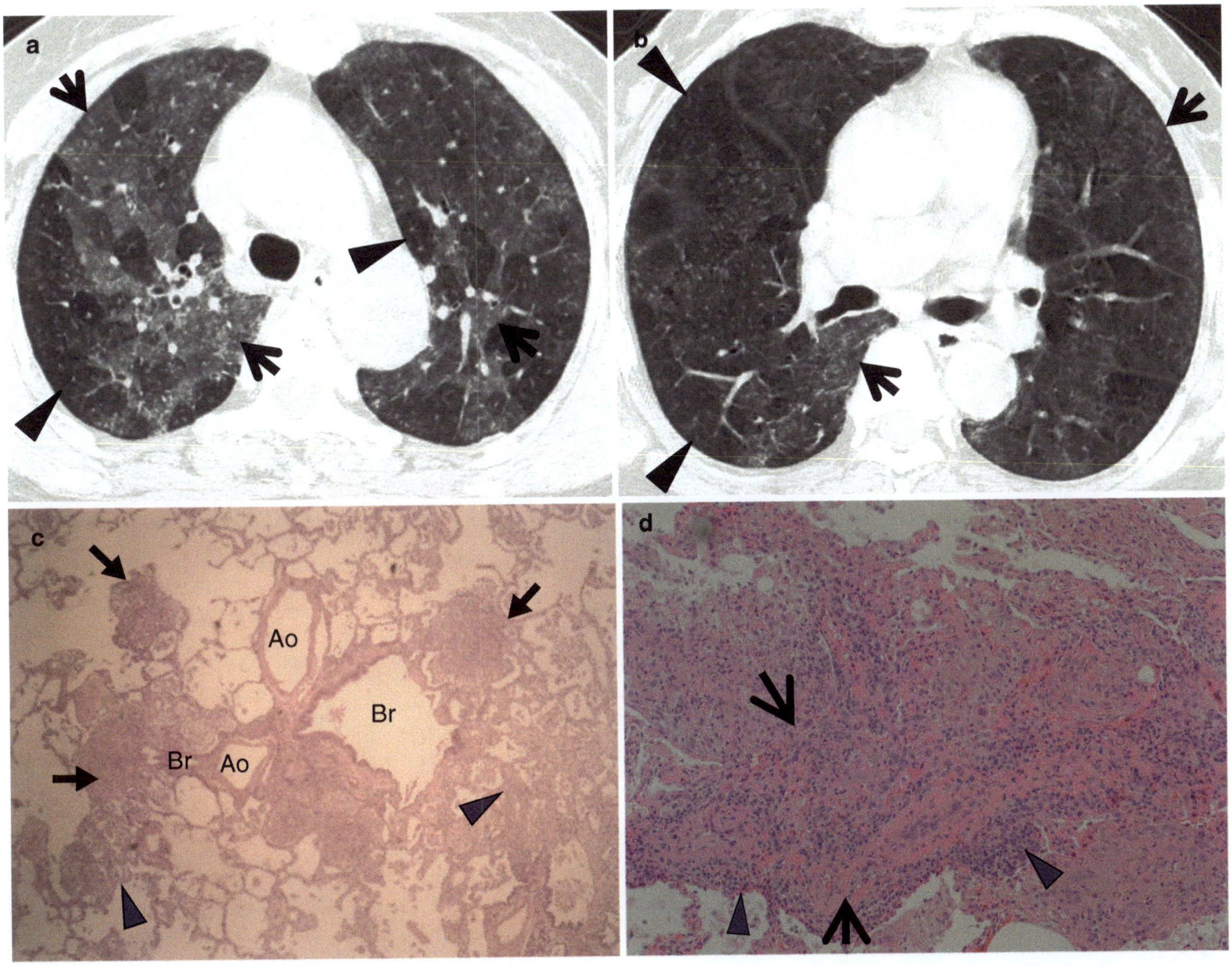


**Fig. 21.3** Subacute hypersensitivity pneumonitis in a 66-year-old woman. (**a**, **b**) Lung window images of thin-section (1.0-mm section thickness) CT scans obtained at levels of azygos arch (**a**) and distal bronchus intermedius (**b**), respectively, show the so-called head cheese sign with mixed infiltrative (ground-glass opacity, *arrows*) and obstructive (mosaic attenuation, *arrowheads*) abnormalities. Ground-glass opacity is caused by lung infiltration, whereas mosaic perfusion with decreased vessel sign is usually caused by small airway disease. (**c**) High-magnification (×100) photomicrograph of surgical biopsy specimen obtained from right upper lobe demonstrates bronchiolocentric granulomas (*arrows*) along with lymphocyte infiltration (*arrowheads*) in peribronchiolar interstitium (alveolar walls). *Ao* arteriole, *Br* bronchiole. (**d**) High-magnification photomicrograph (×200) discloses loosely formed granuloma (*arrows*) comprising epithelioid histiocytes and giant cells and surrounding lymphocyte cuff (*arrowheads*)

## Ground-Glass Opacity without Reticulation, with Small Nodules

### Definition

Ground-glass opacity (GGO) is caused by partial displacement of air in lung parenchyma. The opacity is caused by partial filling of airspaces, interstitial thickening (due to fluid, cells, or fibrosis), partial collapse of alveoli, or increased capillary blood volume. Without reticulation, the GGO areas usually represent active inflammatory or reversible disease state (repetition see section "Ground-Glass Opacity without Reticulation, Subpleural and Patchy Distribution"). In several diseases, the diffuse areas of GGO may contain small identifiable poorly defined (GGO) nodules within the lesions or be associated with the nodules (Figs. 21.3, 21.4, and 21.5).

### Diseases Causing the Pattern

*Subacute hypersensitivity pneumonitis* (*HP*) (Fig. 21.3), *cytomegalovirus pneumonia* (*CMV pneumonia*) (Fig. 21.4),

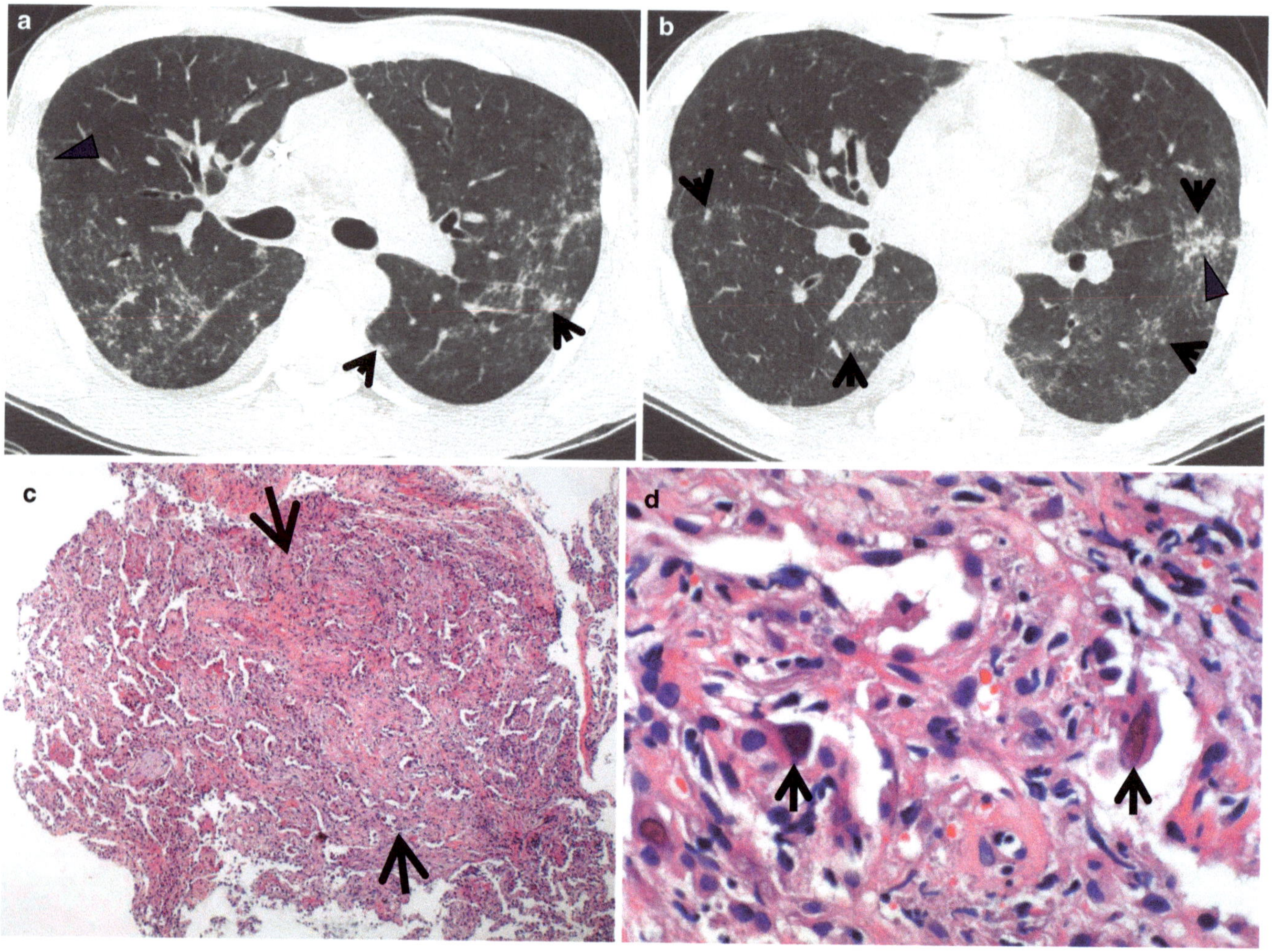


**Fig. 21.4** Cytomegalovirus pneumonia in a 28-year-old man with acute myeloid leukemia. (**a**, **b**) Lung window images of thin-section (1.0-mm section thickness) CT scans obtained at levels of main bronchi (**a**) and basal trunk (**b**), respectively, show patchy areas of ground-glass opacity in both lungs associated with branching small nodular structures (tree-in-bud sign, *arrowheads*) and somewhat larger nodules (*arrows*) of acinus size. (**c**) High-magnification (×100) photomicrograph of surgical lung biopsy specimen obtained from left lower lobe demonstrates organizing pneumonia (*arrows*) pattern with viral inclusion in epithelial cells consistent with cytomegalovirus pneumonia. (**d**) High-magnification (×200) photomicrograph discloses viral inclusion bodies (*arrows*) in epithelial cells

and *diffuse alveolar hemorrhage (DAH) particularly associated with pulmonary vasculitis* (Fig. 21.5) may exhibit diffuse or extensive areas of GGO containing small poorly formed nodular (mainly GGO nodules) lesions [16].

## Distribution

The areas of GGO in subacute HP are usually extensive, bilateral, and symmetric [17]. In some patients, they are patchy or asymmetric. Also in cytomegalovirus pneumonia, the GGO lesions show diffuse or patchy distribution without zonal predominance [18, 19]. The lesions in DAH are diffuse in the upper and lower lobes in approximately 75 % of patients or are localized in the lower part of the lungs in 25 % of patients. In both the cases, the apices and costophrenic angles are usually spared [20].

## Clinical Considerations

Bird fancier's lung and farmer's lung are the two most leading cause of hypersensitivity pneumonitis [21]. CMV pneumonia is a common life-threatening complication seen in immunocompromised patients. It occurs most commonly after bone marrow and solid organ transplantation and in patients with AIDS [19]. The clinical syndrome in DAH includes hemoptysis, anemia, diffuse radiologic pulmonary opacity, and hypoxemic respiratory failure. The most common underlying histology of DAH is of a small vessel vasculitis known as pulmonary capillaritis, usually seen with seropositive systemic vasculitis, or a connective tissue disorder (bland pulmonary hemorrhage), and diffuse alveolar damage due to a number of injuries including, drugs, coagulation disorders, and infection [22] .

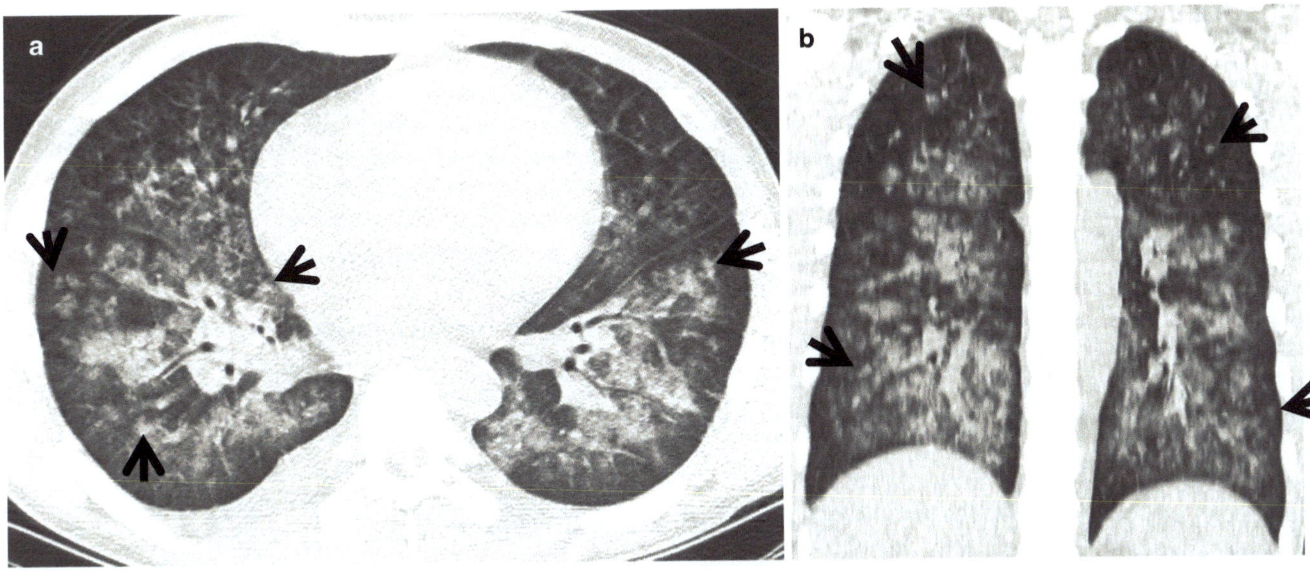


**Fig. 21.5** Diffuse alveolar hemorrhage in a 15-year-old boy with IgA nephropathy and pulmonary capillaritis. (**a**, **b**) Lung window image of CT (2.5-mm section thickness) scan obtained at level of inferior pulmonary veins shows patchy and extensive parenchymal opacity in both lungs. Please also note small poorly formed centrilobular nodules (*arrows*) in both lungs

**Key Points for Differential Diagnosis**

| | Distribution | | | | | | | | Clinical presentations | | | |
|---|---|---|---|---|---|---|---|---|---|---|---|---|
| | Zones | | | | | | | | | | | |
| Diseases | U | M | L | SP | C | R | BV | R | Acute | Subacute | Chronic | Others |
| Subacute HP | + | + | + | | | + | | + | | + | | Bird fanciers, farmers |
| CMV pneumonia | + | + | + | | | + | | + | + | | | Immunocompromised patients |
| DAH | + | + | + | | | + | | + | + | | | Hemoptysis, anemia, pulmonary vasculitis |
| | | | | | | | | | | | | Interlobular septal thickening |

*Note*: *HP* hypersensitivity pneumonitis, *CMV* cytomegalovirus, *DAH* diffuse alveolar hemorrhage, *U* upper, *M* middle, *L* lower, *SP* subpleural, *C* central, *R* random, *BV* bronchovascular

## Subacute Hypersensitivity Pneumonitis

### Pathology and Pathogenesis

The histopathologic features of subacute HP are a subacute or chronic inflammatory interstitial pneumonia associated with bronchiolitis and small, indistinct, non-necrotizing interstitial granulomas. The histopathology of HP raises a differential diagnosis that includes other cellular interstitial pneumonias, such as NSIP. At low magnification, the surgical lung biopsy shows a moderately dense interstitial infiltrate, composed of plasma cells and small lymphocytes, causing slight widening of the alveolar walls. A bronchiolocentric distribution may be evident (Fig. 21.3) and thus is called a granulomatous interstitial bronchiolocentric pneumonitis. Typically, the granulomas are small, non-necrotizing, poorly formed, and loosely arranged [23].

### Symptoms and Signs

Subacute form of HP is characterized by gradual development of cough and dyspnea over several days and weeks [24]. Some patients present with fever, fatigue, anorexia, and weight loss. Physical examination reveals tachypnea and bibasilar inspiratory crackles.

### CT Findings

The most characteristic features of subacute HP on thin-section CT are bilateral patchy areas of GGO, poorly defined small centrilobular nodules, and lobular areas of mosaic attenuation on inspiratory images and of air trapping on expiratory CT images [17, 25] (Fig. 21.3). Sometimes, thin-walled cysts can be seen in a small percentage of patients [26].

## CT–Pathology Comparisons

At histologic examination, centrilobular small nodules correspond to cellular bronchiolitis, non-caseating granulomas, and bronchiolocentric interstitial pneumonitis [27] (Fig. 21.3). The lobular areas of mosaic attenuation and air trapping are presumed to be secondary to small airway obstruction due to cellular bronchiolitis or, less commonly, constrictive bronchiolitis. Thin-walled cysts are presumed to result from bronchiolitis and bronchiolar obstruction.

## Patient Prognosis

Early diagnosis and avoidance of antigen exposure are crucial in the management. Corticosteroids are recommended in severe respiratory impairment with hypoxemia. If the diagnosis is correctly and timely done, outcome is usually good.

# Cytomegalovirus Pneumonia

## Pathology and Pathogenesis

CMV pneumonia shows features of interstitial pneumonitis, and some of the alveolar epithelial cells are enlarged and contain characteristic inclusions. These measure up to as much as 10 μm in diameter and are surrounded by a clear zone inside the nuclear membrane. These Cowdry type A intranuclear inclusions have been likened to an owl's eyes. The inclusions represent clumped chromatin and the clear zone the virus. Cytoplasmic inclusions up to 2 μm in diameter are often also present. Severe cases may show a necrotizing pneumonia or tracheobronchitis. Immunocytochemistry or in situ hybridization may be useful in cases that the inclusions being well not developed. Diffuse alveolar damage is a further pattern of disease that is occasionally seen in CMV pneumonia [28] (Fig. 21.4).

## Symptoms and Signs

Clinical manifestations of CMV pneumonia may range from mild dyspnea to severe respiratory insufficiency [29]. Most patients present with fever, cough, hypoxia, and dyspnea.

## CT Findings

On high-resolution CT, bilateral parenchymal abnormalities consisting of consolidation, GGO, and nodules less than 10 mm in size are the most common findings [19] (Fig. 21.4). GGO have patchy or diffuse distribution without zonal predominance. Nodules tend to be bilateral and symmetric and to have a centrilobular distribution and are sometimes associated with a halo of GGO [18] (Fig. 21.4). Airspace consolidation usually has a lobular or subsegmental distribution. Other findings include thickening of bronchovascular bundles and tree-in-bud patterns.

## CT–Pathology Comparisons

Patchy or diffuse areas of GGO histopathologically correspond to areas of diffuse alveolar damage. Poorly defined nodules or nodules with an associated halo represent focal areas of inflammation or hemorrhage [19] (Fig. 21.4).

## Patient Prognosis

Antiviral therapy with ganciclovir with or without hyperimmune globulin enriched for CMV antibodies or foscarnet is effective, but it has a high mortality especially in bone marrow transplantation recipients.

# Diffuse Alveolar Hemorrhage

## Pathology and Pathogenesis

Whatever the etiology, biopsy shows a combination of alveolar hemorrhage and hemosiderosis. The cause of the hemorrhage is often not evident histologically but there may be intense neutrophil infiltration of the alveolar walls representing capillaritis and rare cases show diffuse alveolar damage [30].

## Symptoms and Signs

Patients with DAH present with cough, dyspnea, and hemoptysis [22]. In fact, one-third of patients will not have hemoptysis, despite active intra-alveolar bleeding. Fever and other systemic symptoms may be present, depending on the etiology of the diffuse alveolar hemorrhage. Careful attention should be given to the nasal and oropharyngeal examination to exclude clues to a vasculitis.

## CT Findings

The most common CT features of DAH are bilateral GGO and consolidation [20]. The lesions are diffuse in the upper and lower lobes in approximately three-fourths of patients or are localized in the lower part of the lungs in 25 % of patients. Typically, the halo sign may be seen with parenchymal nodules or masses and consolidation on CT scans (Fig. 21.5).

Smooth interlobular septal thickening becomes superimposed on areas of GGO (a crazy-paving appearance) within 2–3 days. These findings may show improvement in the course of hemorrhage resorption. Ill-defined centrilobular small nodules have been reported to be uniform in size (1–3 mm in diameter) and are diffusely distributed with no zonal predominance.

### CT–Pathology Comparisons

Areas of GGO and consolidation histopathologically correlate with pulmonary hemorrhage, both with or without capillaritis [31]. Ill-defined centrilobular small nodules reflect intra-alveolar accumulation of pulmonary macrophages [32].

### Patient Prognosis

The treatment of DAH depends on the underlying cause of hemorrhage. Corticosteroids are a mainstay of therapy in most cases. Cyclophosphamide or azathioprine may be added. Plasmapheresis may be tried in the cases of the immune etiology. Mortality is considerable especially in small vessel vasculitis.

## Ground-Glass Opacity without Reticulation, Diffuse Distribution

### Definition

Ground-glass opacity (GGO) is caused by partial displacement of air in lung parenchyma. The opacity is caused by partial filling of airspaces, interstitial thickening (due to fluid, cells, or fibrosis), partial collapse of alveoli, or increased capillary blood volume. Without reticulation, the GGO areas usually represent active inflammatory or reversible disease state (repetition see section "Ground-Glass Opacity without Reticulation, Subpleural and Patchy Distribution") (Figs. 21.6, 21.7, and 21.8).

### Diseases Causing the Pattern

Diffuse GGO lesions may be observed in *acute hypersensitivity pneumonitis* (*HP*) (Fig. 21.6), *Pneumocystis jiroveci* pneumonia (PJP), cytomegalovirus pneumonia (CMV pneumonia), pulmonary edema, diffuse alveolar hemorrhage (DAH), acute interstitial pneumonia (AIP), and *acute eosinophilic pneumonia* (*AEP*) (Figs. 21.7 and 21.8).

### Distribution

Although diffuse in distribution, subpleural lungs including apices and costophrenic angles may be spared in pulmonary edema and DAH. In PJP, the parenchymal lesions may commence in the infrahilar regions and extend to the peripheral lungs.

### Clinical Considerations

In the acute stage ± of HP after direct exposure to the antigen, there is fever, chills, nonproductive cough, dyspnea, malaise, and myalgia, all resembling influenza. Exposure to known offending allergens lead to acute symptoms within 4–8 h after the exposure and positive precipitating antibodies to the offending antigen [33]. PJP is the most

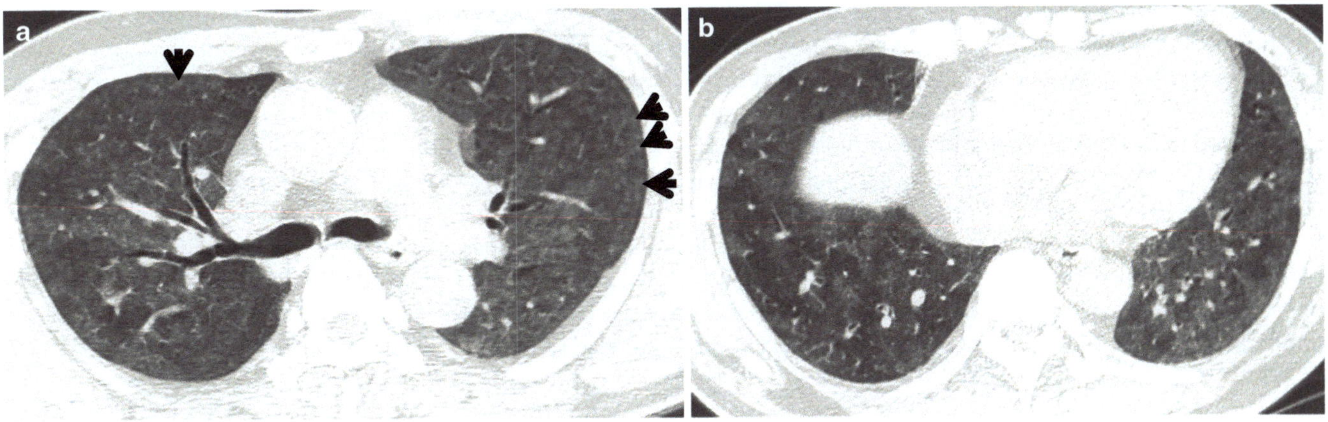


**Fig. 21.6** Acute hypersensitivity pneumonitis in a 53-year-old farmer man. (**a**, **b**) Lung window images of CT scans (1.5-mm section thickness) obtained at levels of right upper lobar bronchus (**a**) and liver dome (**b**), respectively, show diffuse ground-glass opacity in both lungs. Also note poorly formed centrilobular nodules (*arrows*)

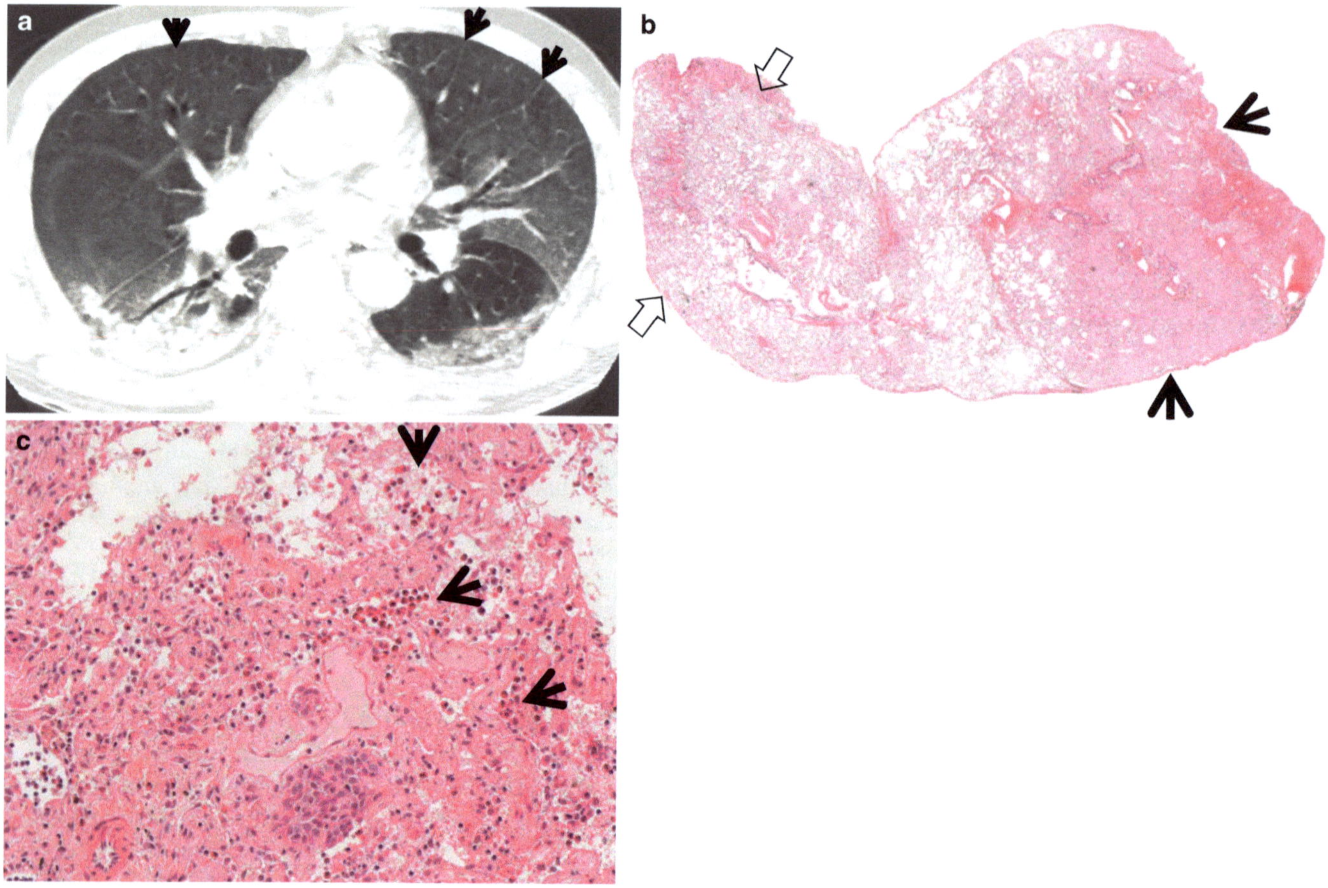


**Fig. 21.7** Acute eosinophilic pneumonia in a 45-year-old man. Patient complains of fever, cough, and dyspnea. (**a**) Lung window of CT scan (5.0-mm section thickness) obtained at level of bronchus intermedius shows diffuse ground-glass opacity in both lungs. Some areas of consolidation are seen in dependent portion of lungs. Also note smooth interlobular septal thickening (*arrows*). (**b**) Low-magnification (×40) photomicrograph demonstrates areas of acute eosinophilic pneumonia and associated diffuse alveolar damage of proliferative stage and organizing pneumonia pattern (*arrows*). Please note other area (*open arrows*) of different stage of diffuse alveolar damage (*open arrows*, early exudative stage). (**c**) High-magnification (×200) photomicrograph discloses characteristic eosinophilic aggregates (*arrows*) in alveolar spaces along with interstitial fibroblastic thickening due to acute lung damage

common opportunistic infection among persons with AIDS in the United States. The incidence of PJP in solid organ and hematopoietic stem cell transplant recipients remains low because of widespread chemoprophylaxis. Most transplant-related PJP infections occur in the early posttransplant period [34]. CMV pneumonia occurs most commonly after bone marrow and solid organ transplantation and in patients with AIDS [19]. The most common underlying histology of DAH is of a small vessel vasculitis known as pulmonary capillaritis, usually seen with seropositive systemic vasculitides, or a connective tissue disorder (bland pulmonary hemorrhage), and diffuse alveolar damage due to a number of injuries including, drugs, coagulation disorders, and infection [22]. AIP is a fulminant disease of unknown etiology that usually occurs in a previously healthy person and produces histologic findings of diffuse alveolar damage. The patients present with symptoms of acute respiratory failure and require mechanical ventilation within 1–2 weeks of symptom onset. AEP is characterized clinically by acute febrile illness, severe hypoxemia, diffuse pulmonary opacity, increased eosinophil counts in bronchoalveolar lavage fluid, no infectious or atopic illness, rapid improvement with steroid therapy, and no relapse [35, 36].

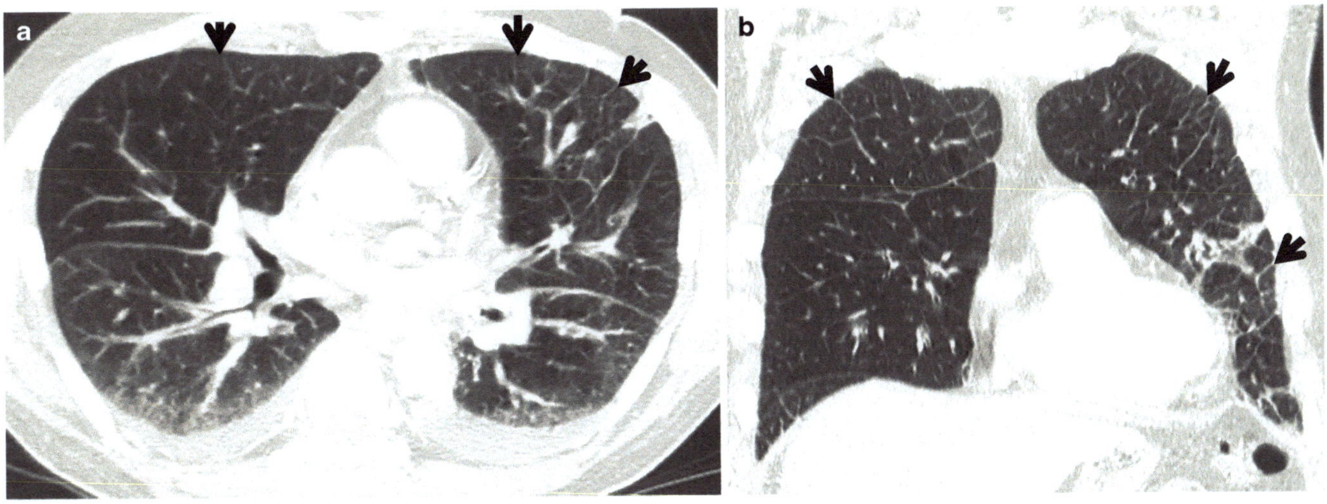


**Fig. 21.8** Acute eosinophilic pneumonia in a 57-year-old man. Patient complains of cough and sputum. (**a**) Lung window of CT scan (5.0-mm section thickness) obtained at level of right middle lobar bronchus shows subpleural areas of ground-glass opacity particularly in posterior aspects. Also note smooth interlobular septal thickening (*arrows*). (**b**) Coronal reformatted image (2.0-mm section thickness) demonstrates patchy area of parenchymal opacity and smooth interlobular septal thickening (*arrows*)

**Key Points for Differential Diagnosis**

| | Distribution | | | | | | | | Clinical presentations | | | |
|---|---|---|---|---|---|---|---|---|---|---|---|---|
| | Zones | | | | | | | | | | | |
| Diseases | U | M | L | SP | C | R | BV | R | Acute | Subacute | Chronic | Others |
| Acute HP | + | + | + | | | + | | + | + | | | Unknown causes, immediately after heavy smoking |
| *Pneumocystis* pneumonia | + | + | + | | | + | | + | + | | | AIDS, transplanted patients |
| CMV pneumonia | + | + | + | | | + | | + | + | | | Immunocompromised patients |
| Pulmonary edema | + | + | + | | | + | | + | + | | | With smooth interlobular septal thickening |
| DAH | + | + | + | | | + | | + | + | | | Hemoptysis, anemia, pulmonary vasculitis |
| | | | | | | | | | | | | Interlobular septal thickening |
| AIP | + | + | + | | | + | | + | + | | | Idiopathic diffuse alveolar damage |
| AEP | + | + | + | | | + | | + | + | | | With smooth interlobular septal thickening or cardiomegaly |

*Note*: *HP* hypersensitivity pneumonitis, *CMV* cytomegalovirus, *DAH* diffuse alveolar hemorrhage, *AIP* acute interstitial pneumonia, *AEP* acute eosinophilic pneumonia, *U* upper, *M* middle, *L* lower, *SP* subpleural, *C* central, *R* random, *BV* bronchovascular, *AIDS* acquired immune deficiency syndrome

## Acute Hypersensitivity Pneumonitis

### Pathology and Pathogenesis

The current classification of HP in acute, subacute, and chronic phases is now challenged. Cellular nonspecific interstitial pneumonitis and cryptogenic organizing pneumonia patterns may be the sole histologic expression of the disease [37].

### Symptoms and Signs

Symptoms of acute HP occur abruptly, a few hours after exposure to the provoking antigen [24]. It consists of a flu-like syndrome characterized by fever, chills, headache, and malaise. Patients may present with severe dyspnea, chest tightness, and nonproductive cough. The episodes subside within 24–48 h once the patient is removed from the antigen exposure, but recur after the next antigen contact. Tachypnea and diffuse fine crackles are observed on physical examination.

### CT Findings

The most common HRCT findings of acute HP consist of diffuse GGO and consolidation [38]. Centrilobular nodules also may be seen (Fig. 21.6).

### CT–Pathology Comparisons

Diffuse GGO and consolidation may be due to cellular interstitial pneumonia or acute organizing pneumonia [27, 37].

### Patient Prognosis

Early diagnosis and avoidance of antigen exposure are crucial in the management. Corticosteroids are recommended in severe respiratory impairment with hypoxemia. If the diagnosis is correctly and timely done, outcome is usually good.

## Acute Eosinophilic Pneumonia

### Pathology and Pathogenesis

AEP shows the features of diffuse alveolar damage in its exudative or organizing phases, coupled with a heavy interstitial infiltrate. In its exudative phase, diffuse alveolar damage is characterized by hyaline membranes and in its organizing phase by interstitial fibroblast proliferation, prominent alveolar epithelial regeneration, and organizing alveolar exudates [39].

### Symptoms and Signs

Patients present with rapid onset of cough, tachypnea, and dyspnea of usually less than 7 days duration. Patients can progress from mild dyspnea to life-threatening respiratory failure in only a few hours. Fever is invariably present. Pleuritic chest pain and myalgia are common. Crackles are present in 80 % of patients. The disease is frequently misdiagnosed as severe community-acquired pneumonia [40].

### CT Findings

The predominant patterns of parenchymal abnormality seen at HRCT are bilateral patchy areas of GGO, frequently accompanied by interlobular septal thickening and sometimes by consolidation or poorly defined small nodules [36, 41] (Figs. 21.7 and 21.8).

### CT–Pathology Comparisons

Bilateral areas of GGO on HRCT correspond histopathologically to diffuse alveolar damage associated with interstitial and alveolar eosinophilia [42].

### Patient Prognosis

Approximately two-thirds of patients require mechanical ventilation, but they respond rapidly and completely to corticosteroids. Most patients have complete recovery with no long-term pulmonary symptoms [43].

## References


1. Mueller-Mang C, Grosse C, Schmid K, Stiebellehner L, Bankier AA. What every radiologist should know about idiopathic interstitial pneumonias. Radiographics. 2007;27:595–615.
2. Lee KS, Kullnig P, Hartman TE, Muller NL. Cryptogenic organizing pneumonia: CT findings in 43 patients. AJR Am J Roentgenol. 1994;162:543–6.
3. Kim Y, Lee KS, Choi DC, Primack SL, Im JG. The spectrum of eosinophilic lung disease: radiologic findings. J Comput Assist Tomogr. 1997;21:920–30.
4. Min JH, Lee HY, Lim H, et al. Drug-induced interstitial lung disease in tyrosine kinase inhibitor therapy for non-small cell lung cancer: a review on current insight. Cancer Chemother Pharmacol. 2011;68:1099–109.
5. Kim EA, Lee KS, Johkoh T, et al. Interstitial lung diseases associated with collagen vascular diseases: radiologic and histopathologic findings. Radiographics. 2002;22 Spec No:S151–65.
6. Katzenstein AL, Fiorelli RF. Nonspecific interstitial pneumonia/fibrosis. Histologic features and clinical significance. Am J Surg Pathol. 1994;18:136–47.
7. Travis WD, Hunninghake G, King Jr TE, et al. Idiopathic nonspecific interstitial pneumonia: report of an American Thoracic Society Project. Am J Respir Crit Care Med. 2008;177:1338–47.
8. Kligerman SJ, Groshong S, Brown KK, Lynch DA. Nonspecific interstitial pneumonia: radiologic, clinical, and pathologic considerations. Radiographics. 2009;29:73–87.
9. Park IN, Kim DS, Shim TS, et al. Acute exacerbation of interstitial pneumonia other than idiopathic pulmonary fibrosis. Chest. 2007;132:214–20.
10. Tsubamoto M, Muller NL, Johkoh T, et al. Pathologic subgroups of nonspecific interstitial pneumonia: differential diagnosis from other idiopathic interstitial pneumonias on high-resolution computed tomography. J Comput Assist Tomogr. 2005;29:793–800.
11. Kim TS, Lee KS, Chung MP, et al. Nonspecific interstitial pneumonia with fibrosis: high-resolution CT and pathologic findings. AJR Am J Roentgenol. 1998;171:1645–50.
12. Yousem SA, Colby TV, Gaensler EA. Respiratory bronchiolitis-associated interstitial lung disease and its relationship to desquamative interstitial pneumonia. Mayo Clin Proc. 1989;64:1373–80.
13. Vassallo R. Diffuse lung diseases in cigarette smokers. Semin Respir Crit Care Med. 2012;33:533–42.

14. Hartman TE, Primack SL, Swensen SJ, Hansell D, McGuinness G, Muller NL. Desquamative interstitial pneumonia: thin-section CT findings in 22 patients. Radiology. 1993;187:787–90.
15. Hidalgo A, Franquet T, Gimenez A, Bordes R, Pineda R, Madrid M. Smoking-related interstitial lung diseases: radiologic-pathologic correlation. Eur Radiol. 2006;16:2463–70.
16. Okada F, Ando Y, Yoshitake S, et al. Clinical/pathologic correlations in 553 patients with primary centrilobular findings on high-resolution CT scan of the thorax. Chest. 2007;132:1939–48.
17. Hansell DM, Wells AU, Padley SP, Muller NL. Hypersensitivity pneumonitis: correlation of individual CT patterns with functional abnormalities. Radiology. 1996;199:123–8.
18. Moon JH, Kim EA, Lee KS, Kim TS, Jung KJ, Song JH. Cytomegalovirus pneumonia: high-resolution CT findings in ten non-AIDS immunocompromised patients. Korean J Radiol. 2000;1:73–8.
19. Franquet T, Lee KS, Muller NL. Thin-section CT findings in 32 immunocompromised patients with cytomegalovirus pneumonia who do not have AIDS. AJR Am J Roentgenol. 2003;181:1059–63.
20. Chung MP, Yi CA, Lee HY, Han J, Lee KS. Imaging of pulmonary vasculitis. Radiology. 2010;255:322–41.
21. Morell F, Roger A, Reyes L, Cruz MJ, Murio C, Munoz X. Bird fancier's lung: a series of 86 patients. Medicine (Baltimore). 2008;87:110–30.
22. Lara AR, Schwarz MI. Diffuse alveolar hemorrhage. Chest. 2010;137:1164–71.
23. Selman M, Pardo A, King Jr TE. Hypersensitivity pneumonitis: insights in diagnosis and pathobiology. Am J Respir Crit Care Med. 2012;186:314–24.
24. Selman M, Buendia-Roldan I. Immunopathology, diagnosis, and management of hypersensitivity pneumonitis. Semin Respir Crit Care Med. 2012;33:543–54.
25. Small JH, Flower CD, Traill ZC, Gleeson FV. Air-trapping in extrinsic allergic alveolitis on computed tomography. Clin Radiol. 1996;51:684–8.
26. Franquet T, Hansell DM, Senbanjo T, Remy-Jardin M, Muller NL. Lung cysts in subacute hypersensitivity pneumonitis. J Comput Assist Tomogr. 2003;27:475–8.
27. Silva CI, Churg A, Muller NL. Hypersensitivity pneumonitis: spectrum of high-resolution CT and pathologic findings. AJR Am J Roentgenol. 2007;188:334–44.
28. Wallace JM, Hannah J. Cytomegalovirus pneumonitis in patients with AIDS. Findings in an autopsy series. Chest. 1987;92:198–203.
29. de Maar EF, Verschuuren EA, Harmsen MC, The TH, van Son WJ. Pulmonary involvement during cytomegalovirus infection in immunosuppressed patients. Transpl Infect Dis. 2003;5:112–20.
30. Lombard CM, Colby TV, Elliott CG. Surgical pathology of the lung in anti-basement membrane antibody-associated Goodpasture's syndrome. Hum Pathol. 1989;20:445–51.
31. Primack SL, Miller RR, Muller NL. Diffuse pulmonary hemorrhage: clinical, pathologic, and imaging features. AJR Am J Roentgenol. 1995;164:295–300.
32. Cheah FK, Sheppard MN, Hansell DM. Computed tomography of diffuse pulmonary haemorrhage with pathological correlation. Clin Radiol. 1993;48:89–93.
33. Blatman KH, Grammer LC. Chapter 19: Hypersensitivity pneumonitis. Allergy Asthma Proc. 2012;33 Suppl 1:S64–6.
34. Catherinot E, Lanternier F, Bougnoux ME, Lecuit M, Couderc LJ, Lortholary O. Pneumocystis jirovecii pneumonia. Infect Dis Clin North Am. 2010;24:107–38.
35. Allen JN, Pacht ER, Gadek JE, Davis WB. Acute eosinophilic pneumonia as a reversible cause of noninfectious respiratory failure. N Engl J Med. 1989;321:569–74.
36. Cheon JE, Lee KS, Jung GS, Chung MH, Cho YD. Acute eosinophilic pneumonia: radiographic and CT findings in six patients. AJR Am J Roentgenol. 1996;167:1195–9.
37. Lacasse Y, Girard M, Cormier Y. Recent advances in hypersensitivity pneumonitis. Chest. 2012;142:208–17.
38. Silver SF, Muller NL, Miller RR, Lefcoe MS. Hypersensitivity pneumonitis: evaluation with CT. Radiology. 1989;173:441–5.
39. Tazelaar HD, Linz LJ, Colby TV, Myers JL, Limper AH. Acute eosinophilic pneumonia: histopathologic findings in nine patients. Am J Respir Crit Care Med. 1997;155:296–302.
40. Rhee CK, Min KH, Yim NY, et al. Clinical characteristics and corticosteroid treatment of acute eosinophilic pneumonia. Eur Respir J. 2013;41:402–9.
41. King MA, Pope-Harman AL, Allen JN, Christoforidis GA, Christoforidis AJ. Acute eosinophilic pneumonia: radiologic and clinical features. Radiology. 1997;203:715–9.
42. Jeong YJ, Kim KI, Seo IJ, et al. Eosinophilic lung diseases: a clinical, radiologic, and pathologic overview. Radiographics. 2007;27:617–37; discussion 637–9.
43. Allen J. Acute eosinophilic pneumonia. Semin Respir Crit Care Med. 2006;27:142–7.

# Consolidation

# 22

## Consolidation with Subpleural or Patchy Distribution

### Definition

Consolidation refers to an area of homogeneous increase in lung parenchymal attenuation that obscures the margins of vessels and airway walls [1]. Air bronchograms may be present with consolidative area. Pathologically, consolidation represents an exudate or other product of disease that replaces alveolar air, rendering the lung solid [2, 3].

### Diseases Causing the Pattern

*Cryptogenic organizing pneumonia* (*COP*) (Fig. 22.1), *chronic eosinophilic pneumonia* (*CEP*) (Fig. 22.2), *Churg–Strauss syndrome* (*CSS*) (Fig. 22.3), and *radiation pneumonitis* (Fig. 22.4) usually depict subpleural or patchy areas of consolidation in both lungs.

### Distribution

Consolidation in COP is present alone or as part of a mixed pattern and has a predominantly subpleural or peribronchovascular distribution [4]. The consolidation usually involves both lungs and shows middle and lower lung zone predominance [5, 6]. In CEP, CT scans show subpleural consolidation with upper and middle lung zone predominance [7]. Consolidation in CSS is present, usually mixed with other patterns of abnormalities including small nodules and ground-glass opacity (GGO), and shows random distribution [8]. Consolidation in radiation pneumonitis involves uniformly the irradiated lung portion, but not necessarily conforming to the shape of the irradiation portal [9]. The consolidation may show patchy and extensive distribution.

### Clinical Considerations

The presence of asthma history suggests the diagnosis of chronic eosinophilic lung disease (almost all patients in CSS and approximately 40 % of patients with CEP) [10]. COP or COP-like lung lesion may be seen in collagen vascular disease, occupational lung disease, or drug-induced lung disease. Abnormal lung lesions like consolidation occur equally in irradiated and unirradiated lung in radiation pneumonitis. This fact, along with prompt improvement of the lesions after corticosteroid therapy, suggests an immunologically mediated mechanism such as a hypersensitivity pneumonitis [11].

**Key Points for Differential Diagnosis**

| | Distribution | | | | | | | | Clinical presentations | | | |
|---|---|---|---|---|---|---|---|---|---|---|---|---|
| | Zones | | | | | | | | | | | |
| Diseases | U | M | L | SP | C | R | BV | R | Acute | Subacute | Chronic | Others |
| COP | | + | + | + | | | + | | | + | + | Nodules, reversed halo sign |
| CEP | + | + | | + | | | | + | | + | + | Asthma in 40 % of patients |
| CSS | + | + | + | | | + | | + | | + | + | Asthma in all patients, airway disease components |
| Radiation pneumonitis | + | + | + | | | + | | + | | + | + | Usually irradiated region; consolidation beyond irradiated field, hypersensitivity pneumonitis? |

*Note*: *COP* cryptogenic organizing pneumonia, *CEP* chronic eosinophilic pneumonia, *CSS* Churg–Strauss syndrome, *U* upper, *M* middle, *L* lower, *SP* subpleural, *C* central, *R* random, *BV* bronchovascular

K.S. Lee et al., *Radiology Illustrated: Chest Radiology*, Radiology Illustrated,
DOI 10.1007/978-3-642-37096-0_22, © Springer-Verlag Berlin Heidelberg 2014

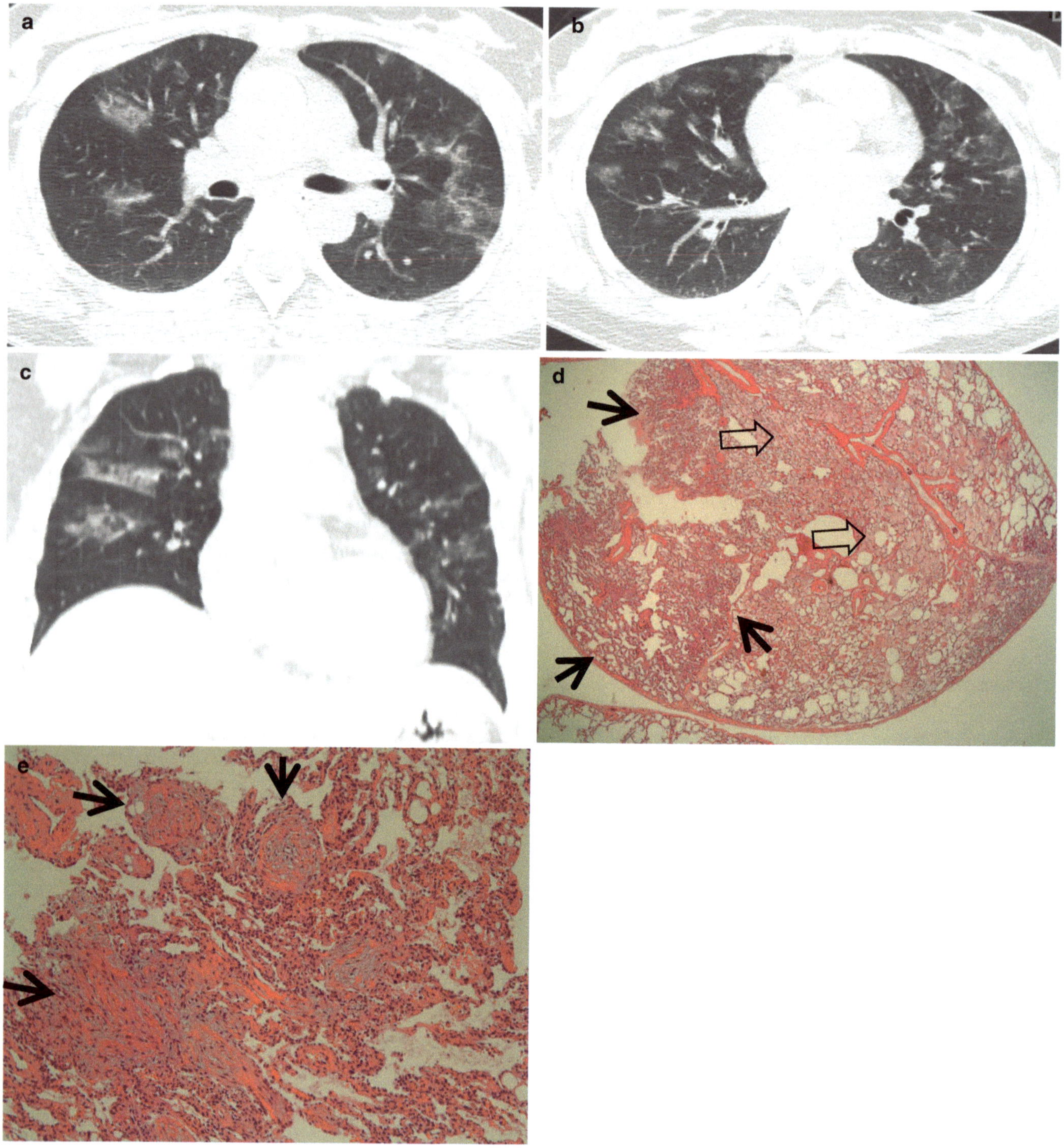

**Fig. 22.1** Cryptogenic organizing pneumonia in a 44-year-old woman. (**a**, **b**) Lung window images of CT scans (2.5-mm section thickness) obtained at levels of distal main bronchi (**a**) and inferior pulmonary veins (**b**), respectively, show patchy areas of consolidation, ground-glass opacity, or ground-glass opacity nodules in both lungs. Lung lesions show typically peribronchovascular or subpleural distribution. (**c**) Coronal reformatted image (2.0-mm section thickness) also demonstrates same pattern of lung abnormalities distributed along bronchovascular bundles. (**d**) Low-magnification (×40) photomicrograph of surgical lung biopsy specimen obtained from right middle lobe shows alveolar-filling process with inflammation (*arrows*) and fibrinous exudate (*open arrows*). (**e**) High-magnification (×100) photomicrograph discloses granulation plugs (*arrows*) filling alveolar spaces and alveolar ducts. Patient also has histopathologically some component of capillaritis and alveolar hemorrhage

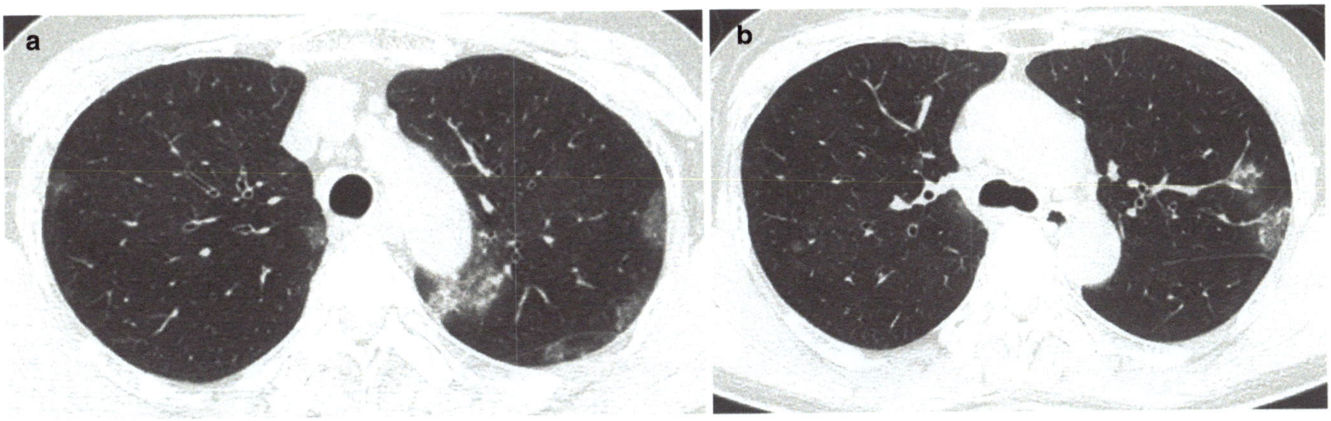


Fig. 22.2 Chronic eosinophilic pneumonia in a 55-year-old asthmatic woman. (**a**, **b**) Lung window images of CT scans (1.5-mm section thickness) obtained at levels of aortic (**a**) and azygos (**b**) arches, respectively, show patchy areas of consolidation and ground-glass opacity in both lungs

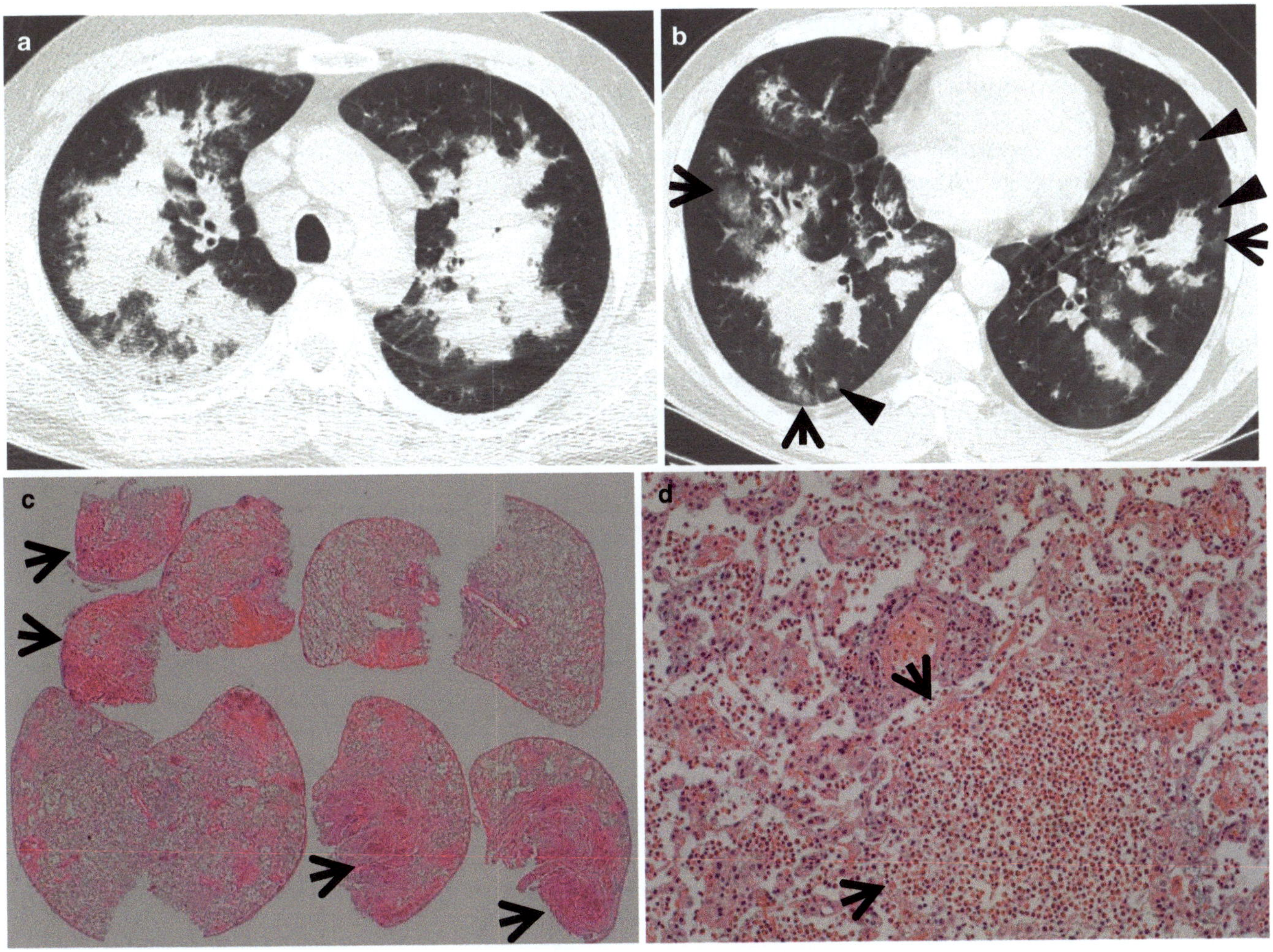


Fig. 22.3 Churg–Strauss syndrome in a 39-year-old asthmatic man. (**a**, **b**) Lung window images of CT scans (2.5-mm section thickness) obtained at levels of aortic arch (**a**) and cardiac ventricle (**b**), respectively, show patchy and extensive areas of consolidation in both lungs. Also note some areas of ground-glass opacity (*arrows*) and poorly defined nodules (*arrowheads*). (**c**) Low-magnification (×40) photomicrograph of surgical lung biopsy specimen obtained from right upper lobe demonstrates alveolar-filling process with eosinophils (*arrows*). (**d**) High-magnification (×100) photomicrograph discloses alveolar spaces filled with eosinophils (eosinophilic pneumonia) (*arrows*). In other areas, small extravascular granulomas and few areas of capillaritis were seen (not shown here)

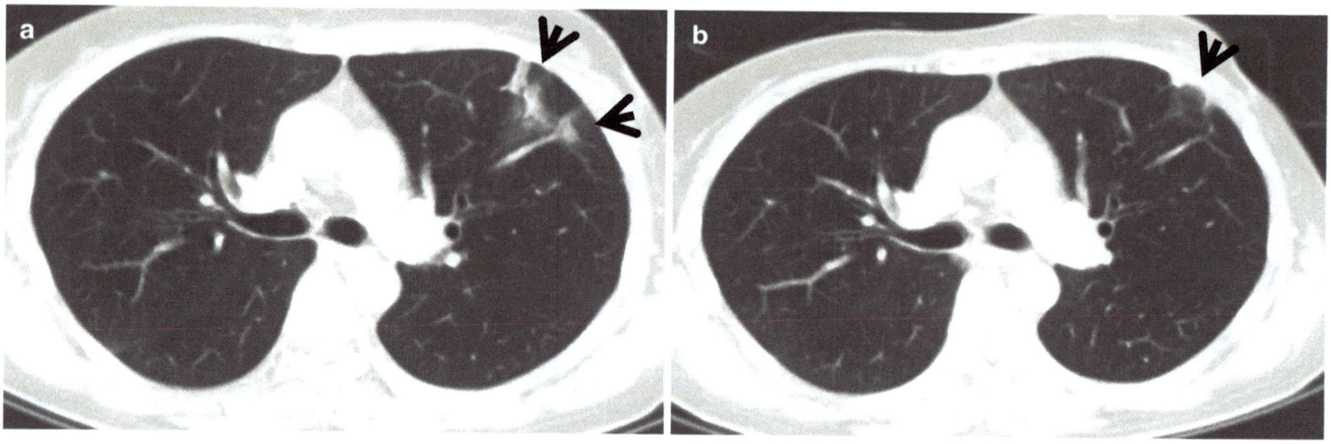


Fig. 22.4 Radiation pneumonitis in a 44-year-old woman with left breast cancer. (**a**, **b**) Lung window images of consecutive CT scans (2.5-mm section thickness) obtained at level of right upper lobar bronchus show focal parenchymal consolidation (*arrows*) in anterior segment of left upper lobe. Patient received conformational irradiation after partial left mastectomy

## Cryptogenic Organizing Pneumonia

### Pathology and Pathogenesis

COP is characterized by variably dense airspace aggregates of fibroblasts in immature collagen matrix. This alveolar-filling process can be seen to extend into or from terminal bronchioles. Typically, the lung architecture is preserved in COP, and lymphocytes, plasma cells, and histiocytes are present in variable numbers within the interstitium (Fig. 22.1). Fibrin may be seen focally in association with airspace organization. Alveolar macrophage accumulation may be present, attesting to some degree of airway obstruction. Interstitial fibrosis and honeycomb lung remodeling are not components of the cryptogenic (idiopathic) form of organizing pneumonia [12].

### Symptoms and Signs

The initial manifestations are nonspecific, with a flu-like illness of fever, malaise, and cough [13]. It is followed by progressive and usually mild dyspnea. Dyspnea may occasionally be severe. In most cases, the duration of onset is less than 3 months. The disease is frequently misdiagnosed as infectious pneumonia. Hemoptysis, chest pain, and night sweating are rare. Finger clubbing is absent. Bibasilar inspiratory crackles are observed at auscultation.

### CT Findings

The characteristic HRCT finding of COP consists of unilateral or bilateral areas of airspace consolidation with subpleural or peribronchial distribution [4, 14] (Fig. 22.1). An air bronchogram with bronchial dilatation may be seen in patients who have extensive consolidation, and air bronchograms are usually restricted to these consolidative areas. GGOs are commonly present in association with the areas of consolidation. Curvilinear opacity with an arcade-like appearance (perilobular pattern) is seen in more than half of the patients [15]. Small, ill-defined nodules, often in a centrilobular distribution, are seen in 30–50 % of cases. Occasionally, the disease is manifested as a large nodule or mass-like area of consolidation. Sometimes, COP shows a reversed halo sign, which is defined as central GGO surrounded by more dense airspace consolidation with crescent and ring shapes [5].

### CT–Pathology Comparisons

The areas of consolidation correspond histologically to the regions of lung parenchyma that show organizing pneumonia: granulation plugs lying within small airways, alveolar ducts, and alveoli [16] (Fig. 22.1). The GGO correlates with areas of alveolar septal inflammation and minimal airspace fibrosis. The small nodules are related to foci of organizing pneumonia limited to the peribronchial region or to fibroblastic tissue plugs within the bronchiolar lumen. Perilobular pattern pathologically reflects the area of organizing exudate accumulation in the perilobular alveoli, with or without interlobular septal thickening [15]. Reversed halo sign correspond to central area of alveolar septal inflammation and peripheral area of organizing pneumonia within the alveolar ducts [5].

### Patient Prognosis

COP responds well to corticosteroids. Corticosteroids result in dramatic clinical improvement, with regression of symptoms within days. The overall prognosis is excellent.

Spontaneous improvement over 3–6 months has been reported. Relapse occurs in 13–58 % of patients on decreasing or after stopping corticosteroid therapy.

## Chronic Eosinophilic Pneumonia

### Pathology and Pathogenesis

Microscopically, eosinophils fill the alveoli and infiltrate the interstitium (Fig. 22.2). The alveoli also contain a variable number of macrophages. The eosinophil infiltrate may involve small blood vessels but necrotizing vasculitis is not encountered: its presence would suggest Churg–Strauss allergic granulomatosis [17].

### Symptoms and Signs

Cough and dyspnea are invariably present [18]. The severity of dyspnea is highly variable from one case to another. Wheezing occurs in about half of the case. Chest pain and hemoptysis are rare. The symptoms are most often present for at least 1 month before diagnosis is made. Weight loss, night sweating, and fever are frequent. The most common extrathoracic manifestations are cardiac, including chest pain with ST segment changes or associated pericarditis.

### CT Findings

The characteristic CT finding of CEP is non-segmental areas of airspace consolidation and GGO with peripheral predominance [19, 20] (Fig. 22.2). The consolidation and GGO usually have upper lobe predominance. Less common findings include crazy-paving pattern, nodules, and reticulation. These less common findings predominate in the later stages of CEP. CT performed more than 2 months after the onset of symptoms shows linear band-like areas of parenchymal opacity parallel to the pleural surface. Pleural effusion is observed in less than 10 % of cases.

### CT–Pathology Comparisons

Areas of consolidation on HRCT correspond histologically to accumulations of eosinophils and lymphocytes in the alveoli and interstitium and interstitial fibrosis (Fig.22.2).

### Patient Prognosis

All the reports have confirmed the dramatic response to corticosteroids. Symptoms and pulmonary infiltrates on imaging improve within a few days of initiation of corticosteroid therapy. However, relapses are observed in up to 50 % of patients while tapering or after stopping the doses of corticosteroids. Long-term corticosteroid therapy is required in more than 50 % of the cases.

## Churg–Strauss Syndrome

### Pathology and Pathogenesis

The findings on lung biopsy depend on the stage of the disease during which the biopsy is obtained and whether or not the patient has received therapy, particularly steroids. Lung biopsies from CSS patients in the full blown vasculitic phase may show asthmatic bronchitis, eosinophilic pneumonia, extravascular stellate granulomas, and vasculitis (Fig. 22.3). Vasculitis can affect arteries, veins, or capillaries. Diffuse pulmonary hemorrhage and capillaritis can be seen [21].

### Symptoms and Signs

Mean age of onset is 38 years. Asthma is essentially universal in CSS [22]. Virtually all patients have eosinophilia. Cardiac involvement is relatively common and is a major cause of mortality. Compared with ANCA-associated granulomatous vasculitis and microscopic polyangiitis, peripheral nerve involvement is more common while pulmonary hemorrhage and glomerulonephritis are much less common.

### CT Findings

The most common HRCT findings consist of small centrilobular nodules, GGO, consolidation in a patchy or a predominantly subpleural distribution, bronchial wall thickening and dilatation, interlobular septal thickening, and a mosaic perfusion pattern [8] (Fig. 22.3). Unilateral or bilateral pleural effusion is seen in up to 50 % of patients.

### CT–Pathology Comparisons

Small nodules histopathologically correlate with areas of dense eosinophilic and lymphocytic infiltration in the bronchiolar walls and patchy areas of capillaritis in alveolar walls. The areas of consolidation correspond histopathologically to the area of eosinophilic or granulomatous inflammation predominantly in the alveoli and alveolar walls. Interlobular septal thickening may be caused by septal edema, eosinophilic infiltration, and mild fibrosis [8, 23].

### Patient Prognosis

Systemic corticosteroids remain the mainstay of therapy. Cyclophosphamide can be used in combination with corticosteroids in cases with severe disease. The mortality rates attributable to CSS or complications of therapy are less than 10–20 %. Older age, azotemia, and cardiac involvement are poor prognostic factors.

## Radiation Pneumonitis

### Pathology and Pathogenesis

Microscopic findings may include diffuse alveolar damage, acute interstitial pneumonia, and interstitial lymphocytic infiltration in the early phase. There may be variable interstitial, alveolar, and replacement fibrosis in the late phase. Vascular intimal fibrosis with foamy macrophages can be seen [24].

### Symptoms and Signs

Symptoms of radiation pneumonitis, including low-grade fever, dry cough, pleuritic chest discomfort, sensation of chest fullness, and dyspnea, usually develop 1–3 months after completion of radiation therapy [25]. In severe cases, patients may present with respiratory failure. Hemoptysis is rare.

### CT Findings

The hallmark of radiation pneumonitis on CT is the presence of increased lung attenuation corresponding closely to the location of irradiation ports (Fig. 22.4). Increased lung attenuations include homogeneous GGO that uniformly involves the irradiated portions, patchy consolidation that is contained within the irradiated lung, or discrete consolidation that conforms to the shape of the radiation ports [9, 26]. Subtle GGO or patchy consolidation can be detected outside of the radiation portal in 10–20 % of cases and is less severe than those seen within the radiation ports [9].

### CT–Pathology Comparisons

Areas of GGO correspond histologically to airspace and interstitial edema and those of consolidation to diffuse alveolar damage.

### Patient Prognosis

Corticosteroids are the mainstay of therapy. It has been shown to improve symptoms and lung function. Signs and symptoms may recur after the cessation of the therapy. Supplemental oxygen may be necessary. Late pulmonary adverse effects include pulmonary fibrosis, which is permanent and associated with marked dyspnea.

## Consolidation with Diffuse Distribution

### Definition

Consolidation refers to an area of homogeneous increase in lung parenchymal attenuation that obscures the margins of vessels and airway walls [1]. Air bronchograms may be present with consolidative area (Repetition section "Ground-Glass Opacity without Reticulation, Subpleural and Patchy Distribution" in Chap. 21). In certain diseases, the areas of consolidation are widely spread or scattered (diffuse) throughout the lungs.

### Diseases Causing the Pattern

*Extensive acute pneumonias including viral* (Fig. 22.5) and *Pneumocystis* pneumonia, *acute interstitial pneumonia* (*AIP*) (Figs. 22.6 and 22.7) or adult respiratory distress syndrome (ARDS), pulmonary edema, *diffuse alveolar hemorrhage* (*DAH*) (Fig. 22.8) show diffuse areas of consolidation in both lungs.

### Distribution

Although diffuse in distribution, subpleural lungs including apices and costophrenic angles may be spared in pulmonary edema and DAH. In *Pneumocystis* pneumonia, the parenchymal lesions may commence in the infrahilar regions and extend to the peripheral lungs. Parenchymal lesions in half of patients with AIP equally involve all three lung zones and those in 39 % of patients have lower lung zone predominance.

### Clinical Considerations

Viral pneumonia in adults can be classified into two clinical groups: so-called atypical pneumonia in otherwise healthy hosts and viral pneumonia in immunocompromised hosts.

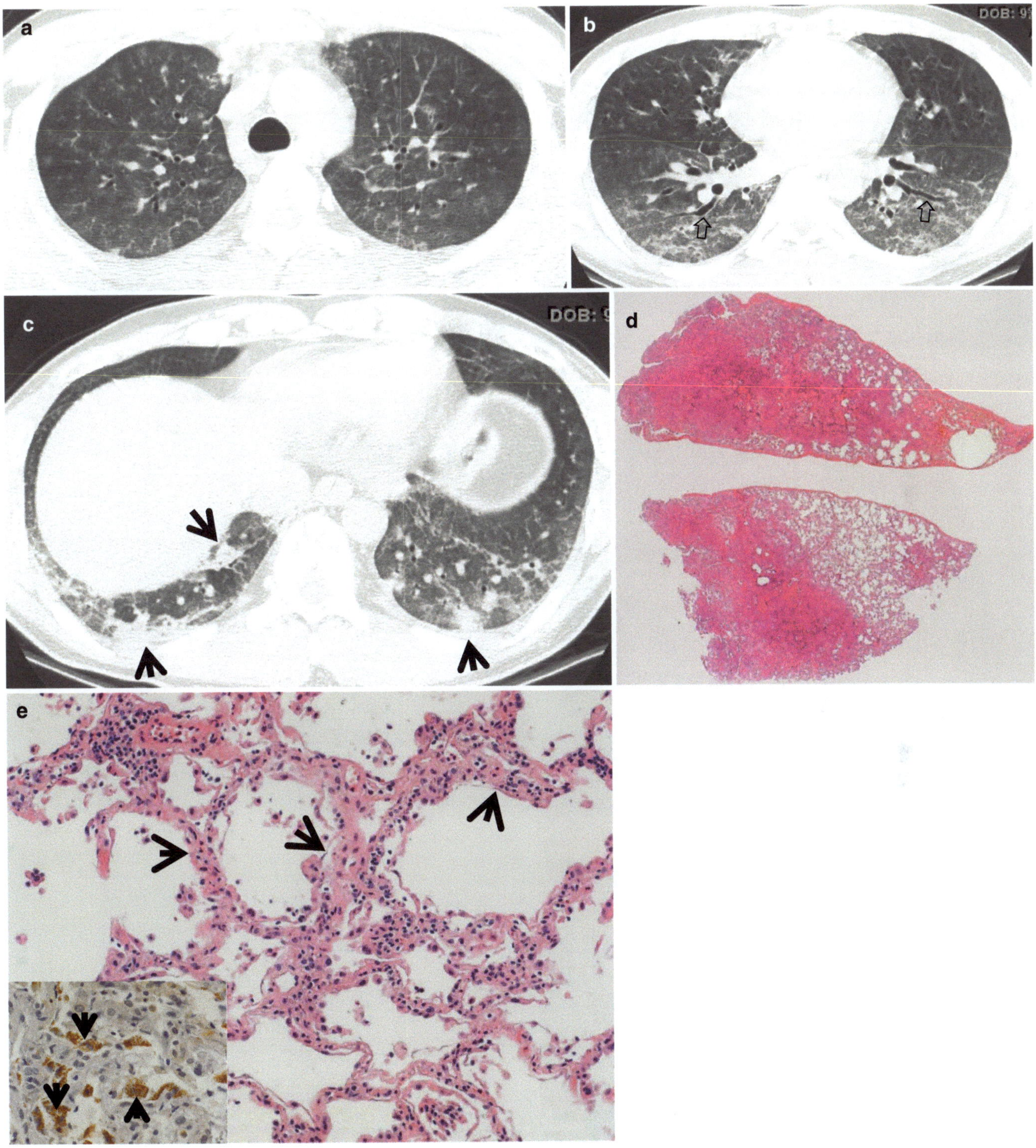

**Fig. 22.5** Viral pneumonia presenting as diffuse alveolar damage in a 28-year-old man. Patient has no underlying illness. (a–c) Lung window images of CT scans (2.5-mm section thickness) obtained at levels of azygos arch (**a**), inferior pulmonary veins (**b**), and liver dome (**c**), respectively, show diffuse ground-glass opacity in both lungs and patchy areas of consolidation (*arrows*) in lower lung zones. Also note bronchial dilatation (*open arrows*) in lower lung zones. (**d**) Low-magnification (×10) photomicrograph of surgical biopsy specimen obtained from right upper lobe demonstrates alveolar filling with fibromyxoid tissue admixed with some inflammatory cells. (**e**) High-magnification (×200) photomicrograph focused on interstitial disease process discloses alveolar wall thickening with mononuclear cell and fibroblastic proliferation (*arrows*). *Inset*: immune staining showing many positive particles (*arrows*) in nucleus of pneumocytes

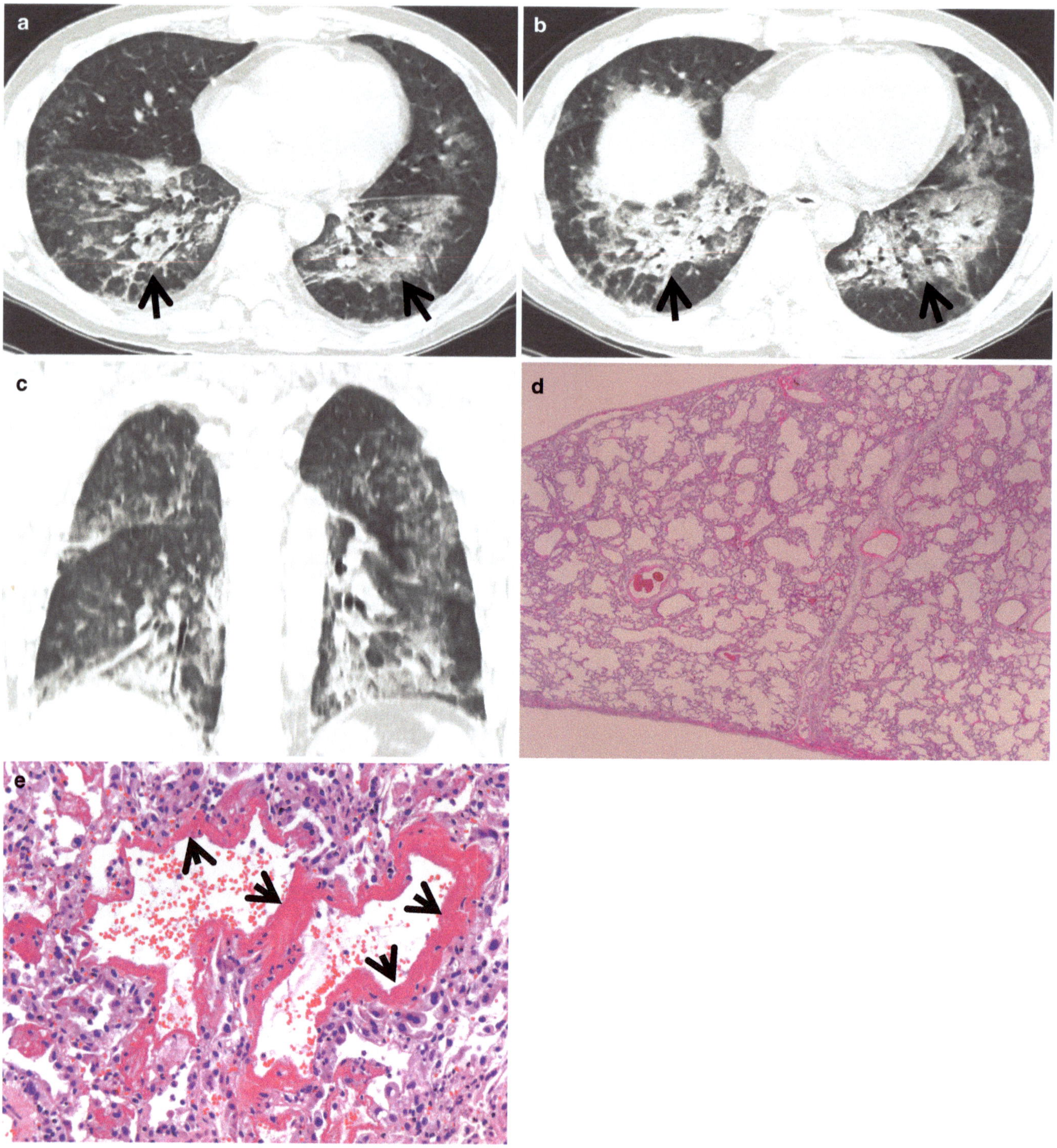


**Fig. 22.6** Acute interstitial pneumonia in a 27-year-old man. (**a**, **b**) Lung window images of CT scans (2.5-mm section thickness) obtained at levels of cardiac ventricle (**a**) and liver dome (**b**), respectively, show patchy areas of consolidation and ground-glass opacity in both lungs (*arrows*). (**c**) Coronal reformatted image (2.0-mm section thickness) demonstrates diffuse areas of parenchymal opacity in both lungs. (**d**) Low-magnification (×10) photomicrograph of surgical biopsy specimen obtained from right lower lobe demonstrates diffuse interstitial thickening with edema, fibroblastic proliferation, and mononuclear cell infiltration. (**e**) High-magnification (×200) photomicrograph discloses interstitial fibroblastic proliferation and mononuclear cell (lymphocyte) infiltration. Also note hyaline membranes (*arrows*) lining alveolar walls

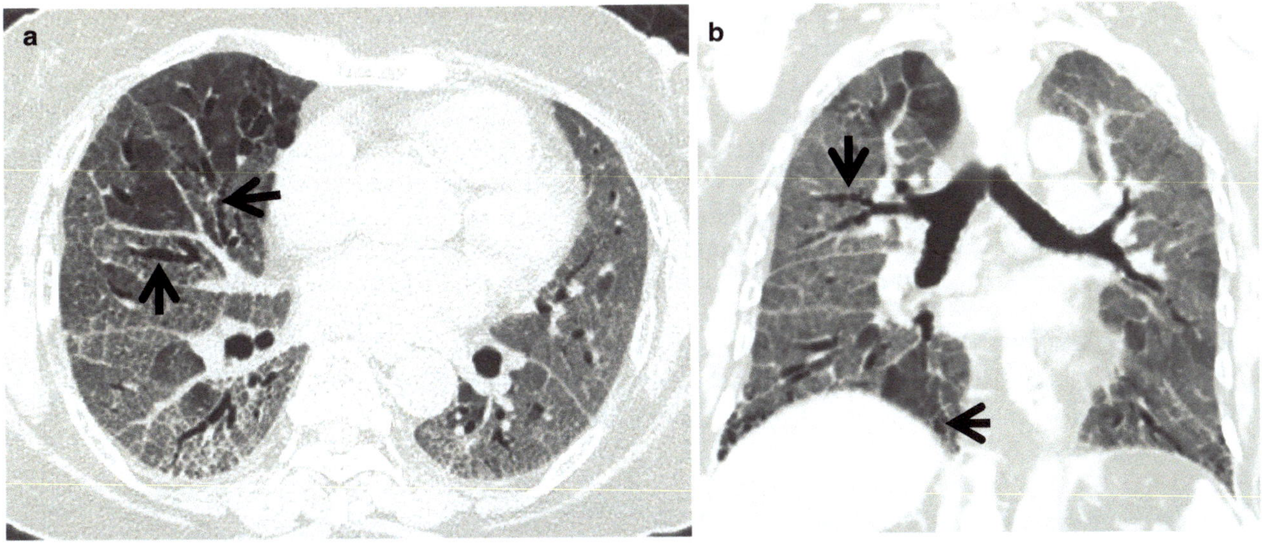


**Fig. 22.7** Acute interstitial pneumonia in proliferative phase in a 69-year-old woman. (**a**) Lung window image of CT scans (2.5-mm section thickness) obtained at level of basal trunks shows extensive areas of ground-glass opacity with crazy-paving appearance. Also note traction bronchiectasis (*arrows*) within ground-glass opacity lesions. (**b**) Coronal reformatted image (2.0-mm section thickness) demonstrates diffuse areas of ground-glass opacity and crazy-paving lesions. Also note traction bronchiectasis (*arrows*)

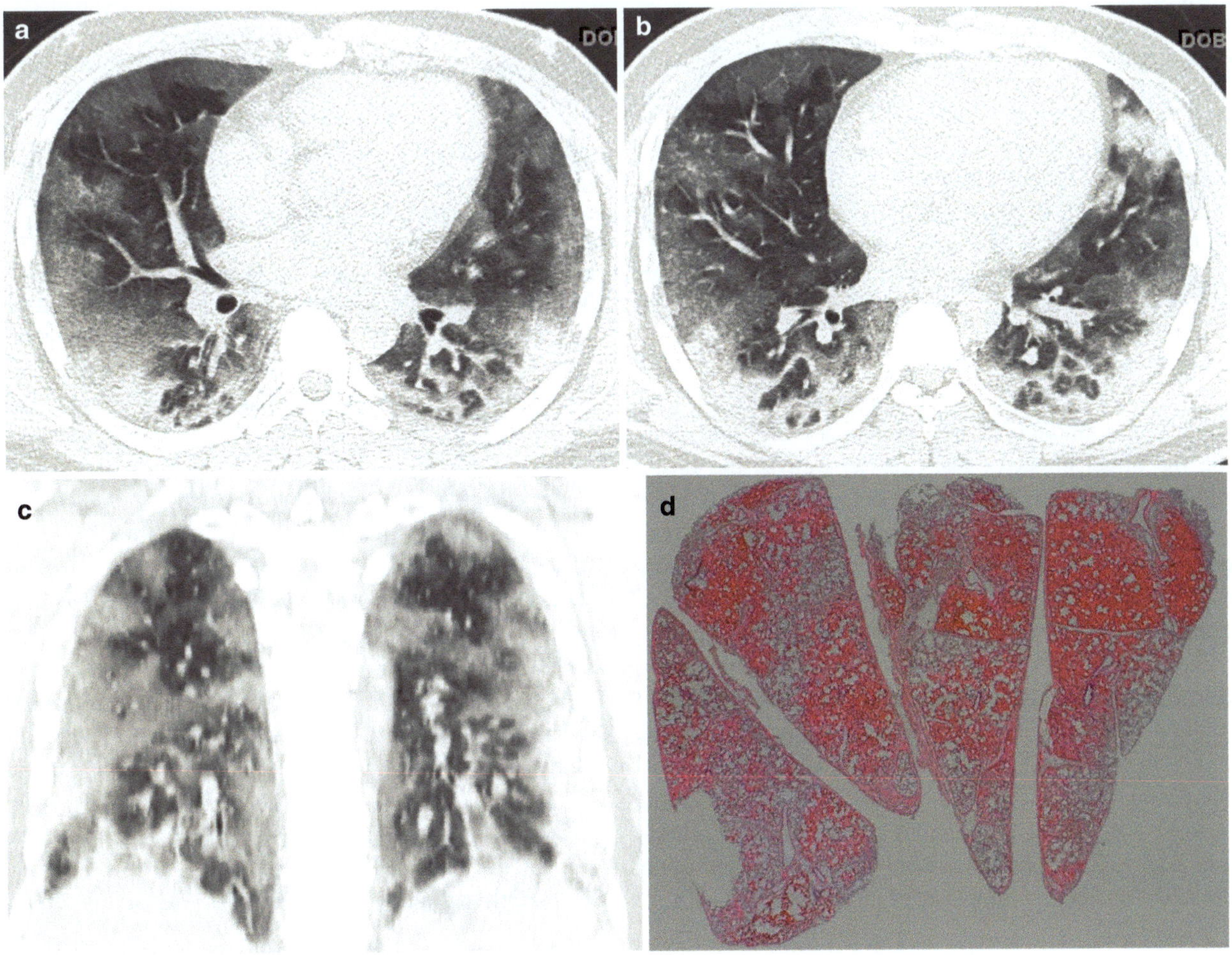


**Fig. 22.8** Diffuse alveolar hemorrhage in a 27-year-old man without specific underlying disease identified. (**a, b**) Lung window images of CT scans (2.5-mm section thickness) obtained at levels of right middle lobar bronchus (**a**) and segmental bronchi (**b**), respectively, show diffuse areas of parenchymal opacity (consolidation and ground-glass opacity) in both lungs. (**c**) Coronal reformatted image (2.0-mm section thickness) demonstrates diffuse areas of parenchymal opacity in both lungs. (**d**) Low-magnification (×10) photomicrograph of surgical biopsy specimen obtained from right lower lobe exhibits alveolar filling with diffuse intra-alveolar hemorrhage. Specific cause of diffuse alveolar hemorrhage was not elucidated with additional histopathologic studies

Influenza virus types A and B cause most cases of viral pneumonia in immunocompetent adults. Immunocompromised hosts are susceptible to pneumonias caused by cytomegalovirus, herpes virus, measles virus, and adenovirus [27]. AIP is a fulminant disease of unknown etiology, usually occurring in a previously healthy person and producing histologic findings of diffuse alveolar damage (DAD) [28]. CT assessment is potentially helpful in predicting patient prognosis in AIP regardless of physiologic abnormality; namely in survivors, the extent of ground-glass opacity (GGO) or consolidation associated with traction bronchiolectasis or bronchiectasis was less and architectural distortion was also less frequent [29]. ARDS, also called acute respiratory distress syndrome, is a type of lung failure that may result from any disease that causes large amounts of fluid to collect in the lungs (DAD as in AIP). ARDS is not itself a specific disease, but a syndrome, a group of symptoms and signs that make up one of the most important forms of *respiratory failure*. As mentioned in a previous chapter, the most common underlying histology of DAH is of a small vessel vasculitis known as pulmonary capillaritis, usually seen with seropositive systemic vasculitides, or a connective tissue disorder (bland pulmonary hemorrhage), and DAD due to a number of injuries including, drugs, coagulation disorders and infection [30].

**Key Points for Differential Diagnosis**

| | Distribution | | | | | | | | | | | |
|---|---|---|---|---|---|---|---|---|---|---|---|---|
| | Zones | | | | | | | | Clinical presentations | | | |
| Diseases | U | M | L | SP | C | R | BV | R | Acute | Subacute | Chronic | Others |
| Extensive pneumonia, especially viral pneumonias | + | + | + | | | + | | + | + | | | Mixed with small poorly defined nodules and GGO lesions |
| AIP or ARDS | + | + | + | | | + | | + | + | | | Subpleural lungs are usually involved; CT air-bronchogram sign |
| Pulmonary edema | + | + | + | | | + | | + | + | | | Renal edema; apices and costophrenic angles, spared |
| DAH | + | + | + | | | + | | + | + | | | Apices and costophrenic angles, spared |

*Note*: *AIP* acute interstitial pneumonia, *ARDS* adult (acute) respiratory distress syndrome, *DAH* diffuse alveolar hemorrhage, *U* upper, *M* middle, *L* lower, *SP* subpleural, *C* central, *R* random, *BV* bronchovascular, *GGO* ground-glass opacity

## Viral Pneumonias

### Pathology and Pathogenesis

The microscopic findings in most pulmonary viral infections include the direct effect of the virus as well as the host's inflammatory response. The clinical outcome depends upon the virulence of the organism and the nature of the host response; and, consequent pathology includes DAD (Fig. 22.5), diffuse or patchy bronchiolitis and interstitial pneumonitis, giant cell reactions, or even minimal change. The histopathologic diagnosis of viral infection is impossible without the identification of the characteristic cytopathic effect (CPE). DAD, often with bronchiolitis, is the most typical pattern of viral lung injury. However, DAD also occurs in bacterial, mycobacterial, and fungal pneumonias; therefore, a careful search for specific viral CPE becomes important. For the surgical pathologist, CPE manifests mainly as the viral inclusion present in the nucleus or cytoplasm of an infected cell [31].

### Symptoms and Signs

In general, clinical manifestations of viral pneumonia are similar to those of bacterial pneumonia. However, wheezing and rhinorrhea are more common while viral pneumonia is less frequently febrile [32]. Mixed or superimposed infection of bacterial agents is common. Acute severe pneumonia progressing to ARDS in viral pneumonia has been increasingly reported.

### CT Findings

On CT, viral pneumonia manifests as poorly defined centrilobular small nodules, GGO with a lobular distribution, and segmental consolidation. Because of the presence of associated cellular bronchiolitis, hyperinflation is commonly seen. With progression, the rapid confluence of consolidation leads to DAD (Fig. 22.5), consisting of homogeneous or patchy unilateral or bilateral airspace consolidation and GGO or poorly defined centrilobular nodules [27].

### CT–Pathology Comparisons

CT findings of viral pneumonia reflect the variable extents of DAD (intra-alveolar edema, fibrin, and variable cellular infiltrates with a hyaline membrane), intra-alveolar hemorrhage, and interstitial (intrapulmonary or airway) inflammatory cell infiltration (Fig. 22.5).

### Patient Prognosis

While therapy for most of viral pneumonia has not been fully clarified, it is reasonable to assume antiviral agents may work if introduced early enough in the course of infection. Viral pneumonia presenting with ARDS requires mechanical ventilation and shows a mortality of 20–25 %.

## Acute Interstitial Pneumonia

### Pathology and Pathogenesis

Because AIP is idiopathic, other specific causes of acute lung injury must be excluded before making this diagnosis. Considerations in the differential diagnosis include infection, collagen vascular disease, acute exacerbation of idiopathic pulmonary fibrosis (IPF), drug effect, and other causes of DAD. Most cases of DAD are not AIP, and detailed clinical information, radiologic findings, serologic data, and microbiologic results will often point to or rule out a specific etiologic condition. Use of special stains applied to tissue sections or cytologic preparations also is essential to rule out infectious organisms in this setting. AIP is characterized by the histologic pattern of DAD (Fig. 22.6). AIP cannot be distinguished from DAD on histology alone [33].

### Symptoms and Signs

AIP can affect patients of any age and sex. The disease if often preceded by a viral-like or flu-like prodromal illness or upper respiratory tract infection characterized by fatigue and myalgia, followed by acute onset of dyspnea, fever and hypoxemia [34]. The duration of symptoms is usually less than 4–8 weeks. The patients have been previously healthy.

### CT Findings

The early HRCT findings of AIP consist of patchy or diffuse bilateral GGO and airspace consolidation with interlobular septal and intralobular interstitial thickening [28, 35] (Fig. 22.6). Half of patients have no zonal predominance and 39 % of patients have lower lung zone predominance. With disease progression of disease, the GGO become diffuse, the areas of consolidation become more extensive, and architectural distortion and traction bronchiectasis become evident (Fig. 22.7). Honeycombing is seen in a small percentage of patients.

### CT–Pathology Comparisons

Areas of GGO and consolidation without traction bronchiectasis occur in the exudative or early proliferative phase of AIP, whereas traction bronchiectasis is seen in the late proliferative and fibrotic phases of AIP [36]. Honeycombing correlates with the presence of dense interstitial fibrosis and restructuring of distal airspaces.

### Patient Prognosis

There is no proven effective therapy. Virtually all patients require mechanical ventilation and supportive care. Many patients are treated with high-dose corticosteroids. The prognosis is poor. Overall, approximately half of patients die within 2 months. However, variable numbers of survivors have been reported [37].

## Diffuse Alveolar Hemorrhage

### Pathology and Pathogenesis

The histopathology of DAH is stereotypical (Fig. 22.8), regardless of etiology and a specific diagnosis requires clinical and serologic data. Most causes of DAH are immunologically mediated. Some of these diseases have specific patterns of immunoglobulin deposition that can be visualized in tissue sections by using immunofluorescence staining of a specially prepared portion of the surgical lung biopsy. In practice today, immunofluorescence staining is rarely necessary for diagnosis because serologic studies are widely available and reasonably specific for the subtypes of DAH [38].

### Symptoms and Signs

Patients with DAH present with cough, dyspnea, and hemoptysis [30]. In fact, one-third of patients will not have hemoptysis, despite active intra-alveolar bleeding. Fever and other systemic symptoms may be present, depending on the etiology of the diffuse alveolar hemorrhage. Careful attention should be given to the nasal and oropharyngeal examination to exclude clues to a vasculitis.

### CT Findings

The most common CT features of DAH are bilateral GGOs and consolidation (Fig. 22.8). The lesions are diffuse in the upper and lower lobes in approximately three-fourths of patients or are localized in the lower part of the lungs in 25 % of patients. Typically, the halo sign may be seen with parenchymal nodules or masses and consolidation on CT scans, representing the hemorrhagic nature of these parenchymal lesions. Smooth interlobular septal thickening becomes superimposed on areas of GGO (a crazy-paving appearance) within 2–3 days. These findings may show improvement in the course of hemorrhage resorption.

Additionally, ill-defined centrilobular nodules may be present, reflecting intra-alveolar accumulation of pulmonary macrophages. Nodules have been reported to be uniform in size (1–3 mm in diameter) and are diffusely distributed with no zonal predominance [39].

## CT–Pathology Comparisons

The airspace lesions histopathologically correlate with pulmonary hemorrhage, both with or without capillaritis [40] (Fig. 22.8).

## Patient Prognosis

The treatment of DAH depends on the underlying cause of hemorrhage. Corticosteroids are a mainstay of therapy in most cases. Cyclophosmide or azathioprine may be added. Plasmapheresis may be tried in the cases of the immune etiology. Mortality is considerable especially in small vessel vasculitis.

## References


1. Leung AN, Miller RR, Muller NL. Parenchymal opacification in chronic infiltrative lung diseases: CT-pathologic correlation. Radiology. 1993;188:209–14.
2. Lee KS, Kim EA. High-resolution CT of alveolar filling disorders. Radiol Clin North Am. 2001;39:1211–30.
3. Hansell DM, Bankier AA, MacMahon H, McLoud TC, Muller NL, Remy J. Fleischner Society: glossary of terms for thoracic imaging. Radiology. 2008;246:697–722.
4. Lee KS, Kullnig P, Hartman TE, Muller NL. Cryptogenic organizing pneumonia: CT findings in 43 patients. AJR Am J Roentgenol. 1994;162:543–6.
5. Kim SJ, Lee KS, Ryu YH, et al. Reversed halo sign on high-resolution CT of cryptogenic organizing pneumonia: diagnostic implications. AJR Am J Roentgenol. 2003;180:1251–4.
6. Lee JW, Lee KS, Lee HY, et al. Cryptogenic organizing pneumonia: serial high-resolution CT findings in 22 patients. AJR Am J Roentgenol. 2010;195:916–22.
7. Mayo JR, Muller NL, Road J, Sisler J, Lillington G. Chronic eosinophilic pneumonia: CT findings in six cases. AJR Am J Roentgenol. 1989;153:727–30.
8. Kim YK, Lee KS, Chung MP, et al. Pulmonary involvement in Churg-Strauss syndrome: an analysis of CT, clinical, and pathologic findings. Eur Radiol. 2007;17:3157–65.
9. Libshitz HI, Shuman LS. Radiation-induced pulmonary change: CT findings. J Comput Assist Tomogr. 1984;8:15–9.
10. Kim Y, Lee KS, Choi DC, Primack SL, Im JG. The spectrum of eosinophilic lung disease: radiologic findings. J Comput Assist Tomogr. 1997;21:920–30.
11. Gibson PG, Bryant DH, Morgan GW, et al. Radiation-induced lung injury: a hypersensitivity pneumonitis? Ann Intern Med. 1988;109: 288–91.
12. Colby TV. Pathologic aspects of bronchiolitis obliterans organizing pneumonia. Chest. 1992;102:38S–43.
13. Cottin V, Cordier JF. Cryptogenic organizing pneumonia. Semin Respir Crit Care Med. 2012;33:462–75.
14. Muller NL, Staples CA, Miller RR. Bronchiolitis obliterans organizing pneumonia: CT features in 14 patients. AJR Am J Roentgenol. 1990;154:983–7.
15. Ujita M, Renzoni EA, Veeraraghavan S, Wells AU, Hansell DM. Organizing pneumonia: perilobular pattern at thin-section CT. Radiology. 2004;232:757–61.
16. Nishimura K, Itoh H. High-resolution computed tomographic features of bronchiolitis obliterans organizing pneumonia. Chest. 1992;102:26S–31.
17. Allen JN, Davis WB. Eosinophilic lung diseases. Am J Respir Crit Care Med. 1994;150:1423–38.
18. Marchand E, Cordier JF. Idiopathic chronic eosinophilic pneumonia. Semin Respir Crit Care Med. 2006;27:134–41.
19. Johkoh T, Muller NL, Akira M, et al. Eosinophilic lung diseases: diagnostic accuracy of thin-section CT in 111 patients. Radiology. 2000;216:773–80.
20. Jeong YJ, Kim KI, Seo IJ, et al. Eosinophilic lung diseases: a clinical, radiologic, and pathologic overview. Radiographics. 2007;27:617–37; discussion 637–9.
21. Koss MN, Antonovych T, Hochholzer L. Allergic granulomatosis (Churg-Strauss syndrome): pulmonary and renal morphologic findings. Am J Surg Pathol. 1981;5:21–8.
22. Keogh KA, Specks U. Churg-Strauss syndrome. Semin Respir Crit Care Med. 2006;27:148–57.
23. Silva CI, Muller NL, Fujimoto K, Johkoh T, Ajzen SA, Churg A. Churg-Strauss syndrome: high resolution CT and pathologic findings. J Thorac Imaging. 2005;20:74–80.
24. Fajardo LF, Berthrong M. Radiation injury in surgical pathology. Part I Am J Surg Pathol. 1978;2:159–99.
25. Graves PR, Siddiqui F, Anscher MS, Movsas B. Radiation pulmonary toxicity: from mechanisms to management. Semin Radiat Oncol. 2010;20:201–7.
26. Ikezoe J, Takashima S, Morimoto S, et al. CT appearance of acute radiation-induced injury in the lung. AJR Am J Roentgenol. 1988; 150:765–70.
27. Kim EA, Lee KS, Primack SL, et al. Viral pneumonias in adults: radiologic and pathologic findings. Radiographics. 2002;22 (Spec No):S137–49.
28. Johkoh T, Muller NL, Taniguchi H, et al. Acute interstitial pneumonia: thin-section CT findings in 36 patients. Radiology. 1999;211: 859–63.
29. Ichikado K, Suga M, Muller NL, et al. Acute interstitial pneumonia: comparison of high-resolution computed tomography findings between survivors and nonsurvivors. Am J Respir Crit Care Med. 2002;165:1551–6.
30. Lara AR, Schwarz MI. Diffuse alveolar hemorrhage. Chest. 2010;137:1164–71.
31. Mizgerd JP. Acute lower respiratory tract infection. N Engl J Med. 2008;358:716–27.
32. Cesario TC. Viruses associated with pneumonia in adults. Clin Infect Dis. 2012;55:107–13.
33. Katzenstein AL, Myers JL, Mazur MT. Acute interstitial pneumonia. A clinicopathologic, ultrastructural, and cell kinetic study. Am J Surg Pathol. 1986;10:256–67.
34. Swigris JJ, Brown KK. Acute interstitial pneumonia and acute exacerbations of idiopathic pulmonary fibrosis. Semin Respir Crit Care Med. 2006;27:659–67.
35. Primack SL, Hartman TE, Ikezoe J, Akira M, Sakatani M, Muller NL. Acute interstitial pneumonia: radiographic and CT findings in nine patients. Radiology. 1993;188:817–20.
36. Ichikado K, Johkoh T, Ikezoe J, et al. Acute interstitial pneumonia: high-resolution CT findings correlated with pathology. AJR Am J Roentgenol. 1997;168:333–8.

37. Suh GY, Kang EH, Chung MP, et al. Early intervention can improve clinical outcome of acute interstitial pneumonia. Chest. 2006;129:753–61.
38. Travis WD, Colby TV, Lombard C, Carpenter HA. A clinicopathologic study of 34 cases of diffuse pulmonary hemorrhage with lung biopsy confirmation. Am J Surg Pathol. 1990;14:1112–25.
39. Chung MP, Yi CA, Lee HY, Han J, Lee KS. Imaging of pulmonary vasculitis. Radiology. 2010;255:322–41.
40. Primack SL, Miller RR, Muller NL. Diffuse pulmonary hemorrhage: clinical, pathologic, and imaging features. AJR Am J Roentgenol. 1995;164:295–300.

# 23 Decreased Opacity with Cystic Walls

## Cavities

### Definition

Please refer to section "Cavity" in Chap. 12.

### Diseases Causing Cavities

In patients with diffuse lung diseases, multiple cavities are seen in patients with Langerhans cell histiocytosis, fungal infection, and sarcoidosis. Cavitary nodules are also seen in patients with *rheumatoid lung disease* (Fig. 23.1), antineutrophil cytoplasmic antibody (ANCA)-associated granulomatous vasculitis (former Wegener's granulomatosis), septic embolism, and *metastatic tumors* (*squamous cell carcinoma of head and neck and the uterine cervix*) (Fig. 23.2).

### Distribution

In Langerhans cell histiocytosis, the cavitating nodules are associated with noncavitating nodules and are distributed mainly in the upper and middle lung zones, sparing the lower lung zones [1]. Cavitary nodules in patients with (ANCA)-associated granulomatous vasculitis have no predilection for any lung zones [2]. Rheumatoid lung nodules, metastatic tumors, fungal infection, and septic embolism nodules tend to predominate in the lung periphery [3–5].

### Clinical Considerations

Cigarette smoking is highly related to pulmonary Langerhans cell histiocytosis, and the cavitating nodules in the disease are reversible with corticosteroid or cytotoxic drug therapy [6]. Immunocompromised patients and patients with underlying lung disease are at increased risk of fungal infection. Rheumatoid lung nodules are typically seen in patients with subcutaneous nodules and tend to wax and wane in proportion to the activity of the arthritis [3]. Septic embolism occurs most commonly in intravenous drug users and in immunocompromised patients with central venous lines. The site of the primary neoplasm with cavitation is most frequently in the head and neck in men and the uterine cervix in women [7]. Cavitation also may occur in metastatic adenocarcinomas, particularly in lesions originating from the large bowel, and in metastatic sarcoma, particularly osteogenic.

K.S. Lee et al., *Radiology Illustrated: Chest Radiology*, Radiology Illustrated,
DOI 10.1007/978-3-642-37096-0_23, © Springer-Verlag Berlin Heidelberg 2014

## Key Points for Differential Diagnosis

| Diseases | Distribution | | | | | | | | Clinical presentations | | | Others |
|---|---|---|---|---|---|---|---|---|---|---|---|---|
| | Zones | | | | | | | | | | | |
| | U | M | L | SP | C | R | BV | R | Acute | Subacute | Chronic | |
| LCH | + | + | | | | + | | + | | | + | Associated with irregular cysts or nodules, spare CPA |
| Fungal infection | + | + | + | + | | + | | + | + | | | With GGO halo |
| Sarcoidosis | + | + | | | | + | + | | | | + | Mediastinal or hilar LN enlargement, female predominance, African Americans |
| Rheumatoid nodules | + | + | | + | | + | | + | | | + | Variable in size, unpredictable natural course |
| ANCA-associated granulomatous vasculitis | + | + | + | + | | | + | | | + | + | Large necrotic area on enhanced scans |
| Septic lung | + | + | + | + | | + | | + | | | | Feeding vessel sign |
| Pulmonary metastasis | | + | + | + | | + | | + | | | + | Variable-sized nodules |

*Note*: *LCH* Langerhans cell histiocytosis, *ANCA* antineutrophil cytoplasmic antibody, *U* upper, *M* middle, *L* lower, *SP* subpleural, *C* central, *R* random, *BV* bronchovascular, *CPA* costophrenic angle, *GGO* ground-glass opacity, *LN* lymph node

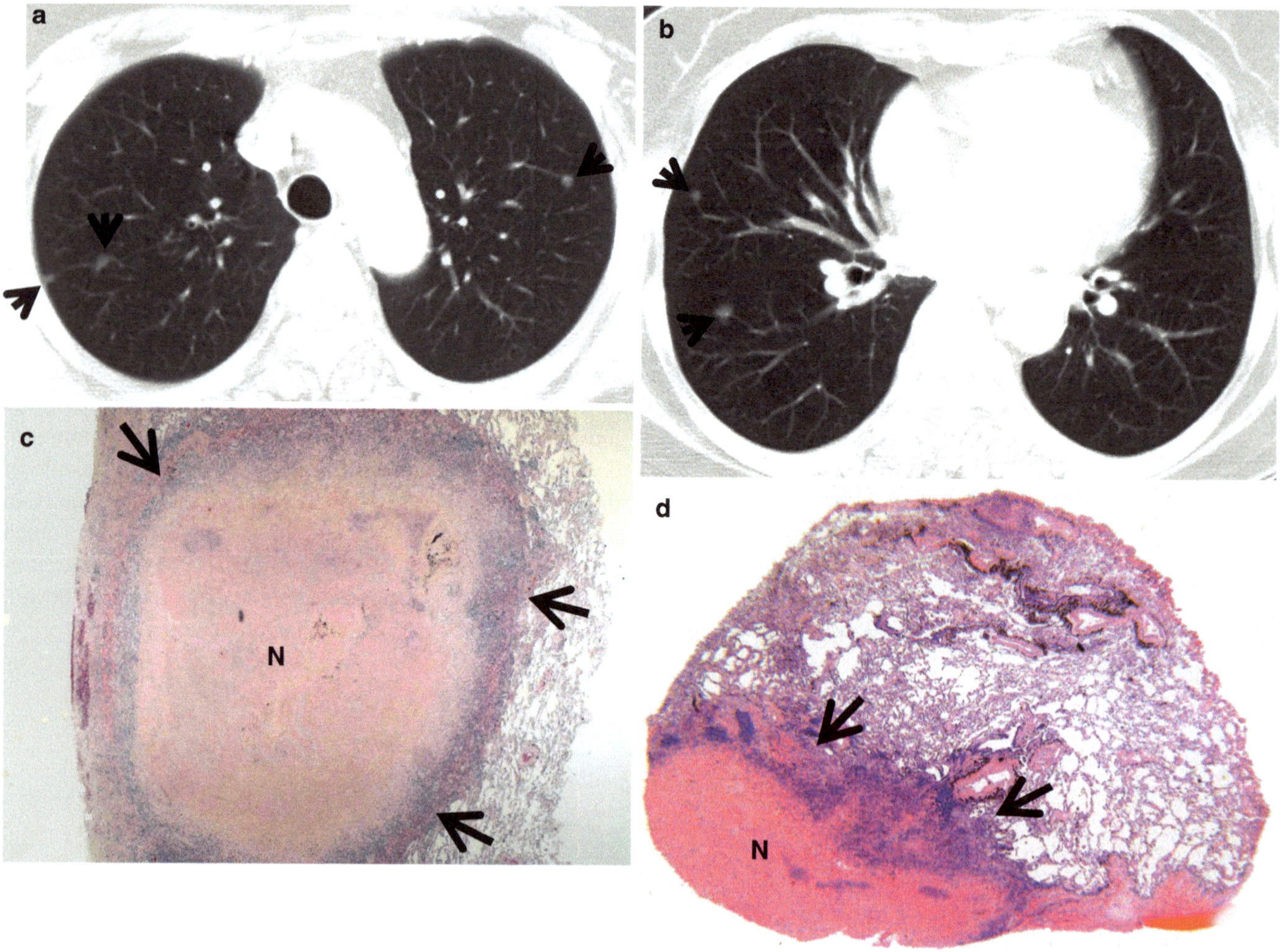


**Fig. 23.1** Rheumatoid nodules in a 70-year-old woman who has suffered from rheumatoid arthritis for 10 years. (**a**, **b**) Lung window images of CT scans (5.0-mm section thickness) obtained at levels of aortic arch (**a**) and basal trunks (**b**), respectively, show multiple small nodules (*arrows*) in both lungs. Mediastinal window images exhibit necrosis in central portion of nodules. (**c**) Low-magnification (×4) photomicrograph of surgical biopsy specimen obtained from right lower lobe demonstrates a nodule containing necrotic portion (*N*) and surrounding rim (*arrows*) of epithelioid histiocytes and fibrotic tissue. (**d**) Another low-magnification (×10) photomicrograph discloses necrotic portion (*N*), a rim of epithelioid histiocytes and fibrotic tissue (*arrows*), and normal lung

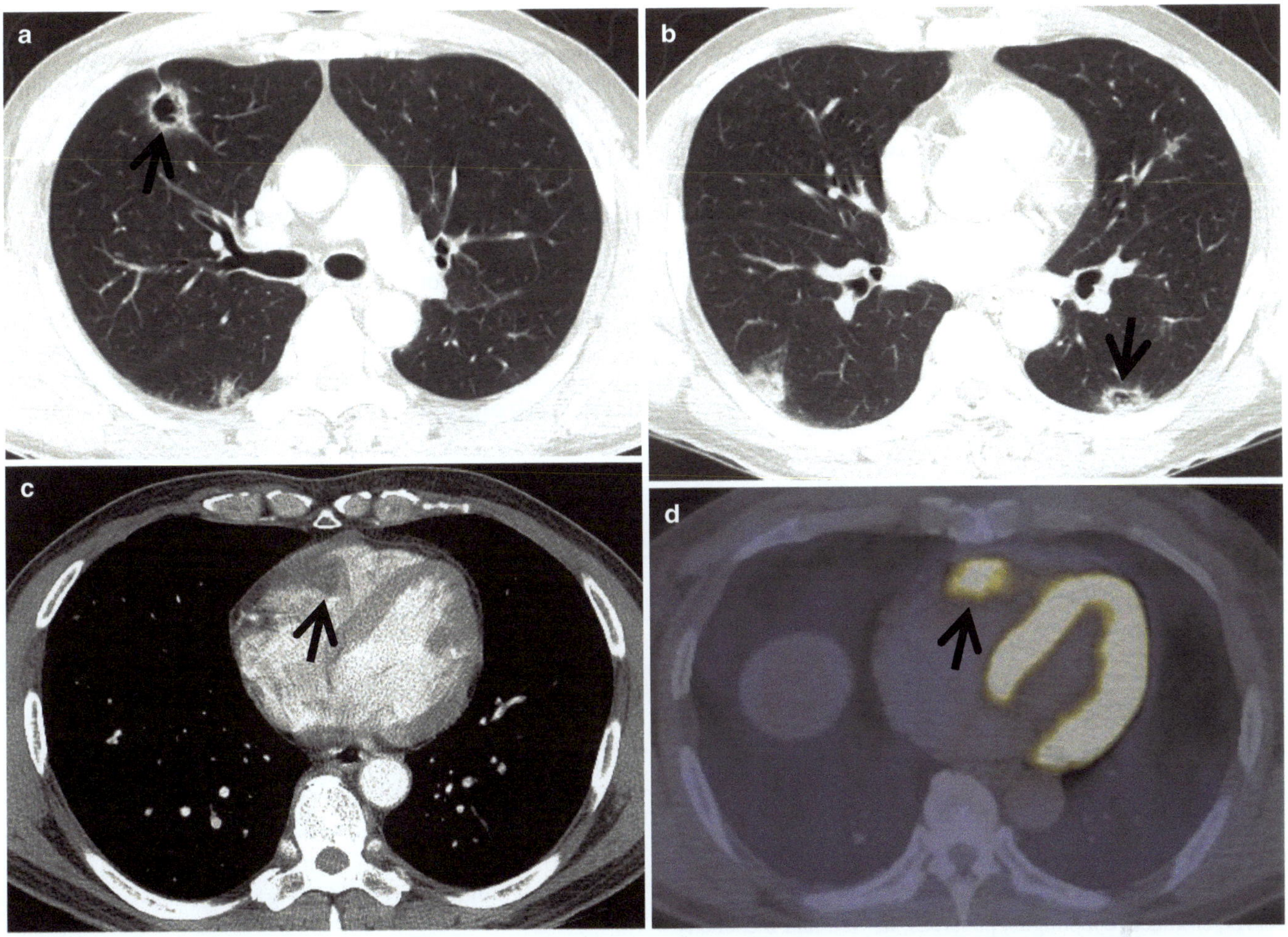


**Fig. 23.2** Cavitary lung nodules representing pulmonary metastatic nodules in a 50-year-old man with renal cell carcinoma. (**a, b**) Lung window images of CT scans (5.0-mm section thickness) obtained at levels of right upper lobar bronchus (**a**) and basal trunks (**b**), respectively, show multiple cavitating (*arrows*) and noncavitating nodules in both lungs. (**c**) Enhanced CT scan obtained at level of cardiac ventricle shows a low-attenuation nodule (*arrow*) in right ventricle abutting lateral wall of the chamber. (**d**) Fluorodeoxyglucose positron emission tomography displays high uptake of glucose (*arrow*) at right ventricular nodule. *Arrows* in (**c**) and (**d**) indicate metastatic nodules in right cardiac ventricle

## Rheumatoid Lung Nodules

### Pathology and Pathogenesis

The rheumatoid lung nodules have a necrotic center of finely granular eosinophilic debris surrounded by a capsule of chronic inflammatory granulation tissue. The boundary between dead and viable tissue is marked by a characteristic palisade of radially oriented macrophages (Fig. 23.1). The inflammatory cells include a small number of giant cells as well as plentiful lymphocytes and plasma cells [8].

### Symptoms and Signs

Most patients with rheumatoid lung nodules are asymptomatic. Occasionally, cavitation may lead to hemoptysis [9]. Due to their typical subpleural distribution, complications, including pneumothorax, empyema, pleural effusions, and bronchopleural fistula, may occur.

### CT Findings

Rheumatoid nodules have a maximum diameter of 0.5–5.0 cm and are usually located in peripheral zones of the upper and middle lung regions [10] (Fig. 23.1). Pulmonary nodules may increase in size or resolve spontaneously. Cavitation of nodules is common and is rarely associated with rupturing into the pleural space, producing bronchopleural fistula, pneumothorax, pleural effusion, or empyema [11]. Calcification of rheumatoid pulmonary nodules is not a frequent finding but may be seen in some patients with Caplan syndrome.

### CT–Pathology Comparisons

Rheumatoid pulmonary nodule is pathologically identical to subcutaneous rheumatoid nodule. They contain three histologically distinct zones: central fibrinoid necrosis, surrounding palisading epithelioid cells, and an outer zone of lymphocytes, plasma cells, and fibroblasts [12]. The necrotic central zone becomes cavitary or cystic, likely with the resolution of necrosis and subsequent inflation resulting from airflow in the lumen. Therefore, patients exhibit rheumatoid pulmonary nodules in various stages from new nodules with central necrosis to older nodules with cavitary or cystic changes.

### Patient Prognosis

Rheumatoid lung nodules may remain stable, regress spontaneously, or enlarge. Depending on the clinical circumstances, serial radiographic follow-up or surgical resection may be required.

## Cavitary Metastasis

### Pathology and Pathogenesis

Cavitation in pulmonary metastases is thought to be uncommon. The primary sites were the large intestine, opposite lung, cervix, stomach, esophagus, pancreas, larynx, and mesenchymal tumors. It seems that the principal cause of necrosis and subsequent cavitation in metastatic tumors of the lung is interference with their blood supply by vascular involvement [13].

### Symptoms and Signs

Significant number of patients with cavitary lung metastasis is asymptomatic. Hemoptysis can occur. Nonspecific symptoms including cough, vague chest discomfort, and dyspnea can result from a very large tumor burden. Constitutional symptoms such as weight loss, anorexia, and generalized weakness may be accompanied.

### CT Findings

CT finding of cavitary metastasis consists of multiple nodules with or without cavitation (Fig. 23.2). The size of nodules range from a few millimeters to several centimeters in diameter, and nodules are usually of varying size. They tend to be most numerous in the outer third of lungs, particularly the subpleural regions of the lower zones, and have a random distribution within the secondary pulmonary lobules [14, 15]. Most nodules are round and have smooth margins. They may be lobulated, however, and have irregular margins. The wall of cavitary metastatic nodule is generally thick and irregular, although thin-walled cavities can be found with metastases from sarcomas and adenocarcinomas [7].

### CT–Pathology Comparisons

Please note section “Cavity” in Chap. 12 and section “Pulmonary Metastasis” in Chap. 19.

### Patient Prognosis

Prognosis of the patients with cavitary lung metastasis is poor since the primary tumor is not highly responsive to anticancer chemotherapy.

## Cysts

### Definition

A cyst is a round parenchymal lucency or low-attenuating area with a well-defined interface with normal lung. Cysts have variable wall thickness but are usually thin walled (<2 mm). The cysts usually contain air but occasionally contain fluid or solid material [16] (Fig. 23.3).

### Diseases Causing Multiple Cysts

Many diffuse lung diseases may manifest cysts as the primary abnormality [17, 18]. *Lymphangioleiomyomatosis* (*LAM*) (Fig. 23.3) and Langerhans cell histiocytosis (LCH) are the most common to present with diffuse lung cysts. Other interstitial lung diseases that may cause multiple cysts include *lymphocytic interstitial pneumonia* (*LIP*) (Fig. 23.4), desquamative interstitial pneumonia (DIP), subacute hypersensitivity pneumonitis, and amyloidosis. *Cystic pulmonary metastasis* (*angiosarcoma*) (Figs. 23.5 and 23.6) and Birt–Hogg–Dube syndrome also cause multiple pulmonary cysts. Honeycombing cysts in various interstitial lung diseases (usual interstitial pneumonia, nonspecific interstitial pneumonia, asbestosis, chronic hypersensitivity pneumonitis, advanced fibrotic sarcoidosis) also appear as multiple pulmonary cysts (please note section “Cyst” in Chap. 12 and section “Honeycombing with Subpleural or Basal Predominance” in Chap. 17).

### Distribution

Please note section “Cyst” in Chap. 12 and section “Honeycombing with Subpleural or Basal Predominance” in Chap. 17.

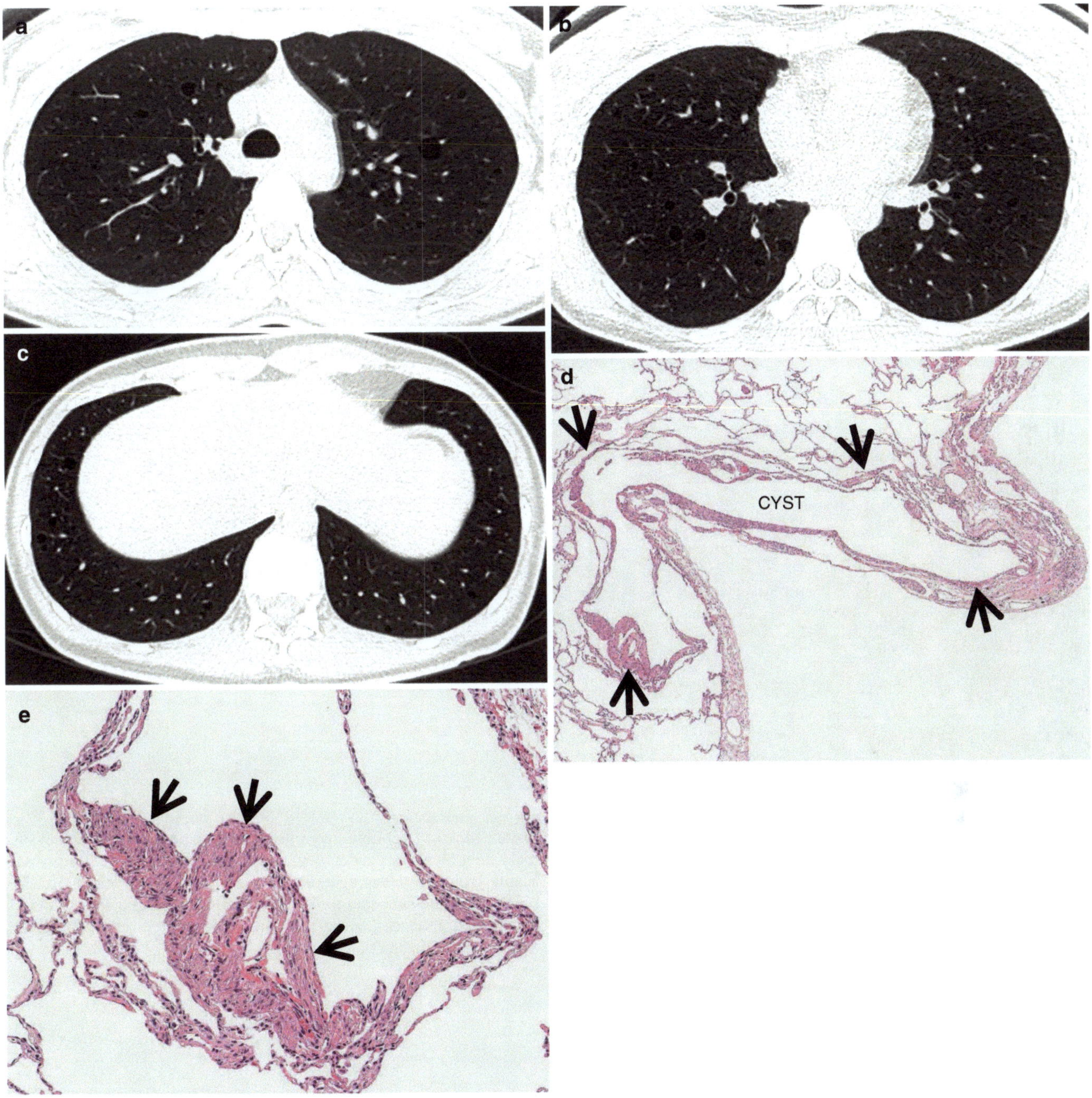


**Fig. 23.3** Lymphangioleiomyomatosis in a 37-year-old woman. (**a–c**) Lung window images of thin-section (1.5-mm section thickness) CT scans obtained at levels of aortic arch (**a**), inferior pulmonary veins (**b**), and liver dome (**c**), respectively, show multiple variable-sized air-filled cysts in both lungs. Please note involvement of lung bases that are spared in Langerhans cell histiocytosis. (**d**) Low-magnification (×40) photomicrograph of surgical lung biopsy specimen depicts a cystic lesion (*CYST*) and its wall composed of spindle or ovoid smooth muscle cells (*arrows*). (**e**) High-magnification (×100) photomicrograph discloses clearly cystic wall composed of spindle or ovoid smooth muscle cells (*arrows*)

## Clinical Considerations

Please note section "Cyst" in Chap. 12. LAM is associated with tuberous sclerosis (seizure, skin lesions) and is more common than sporadic or lone LAM [19]. Cystic pulmonary metastases occur most frequently in tumors of epithelial origin and less frequently in tumors of mesenchymal (angiosarcoma, leiomyosarcoma, synovial cell sarcoma, epithelioid cell sarcoma, and endometrial stromal sarcoma) origins [20].

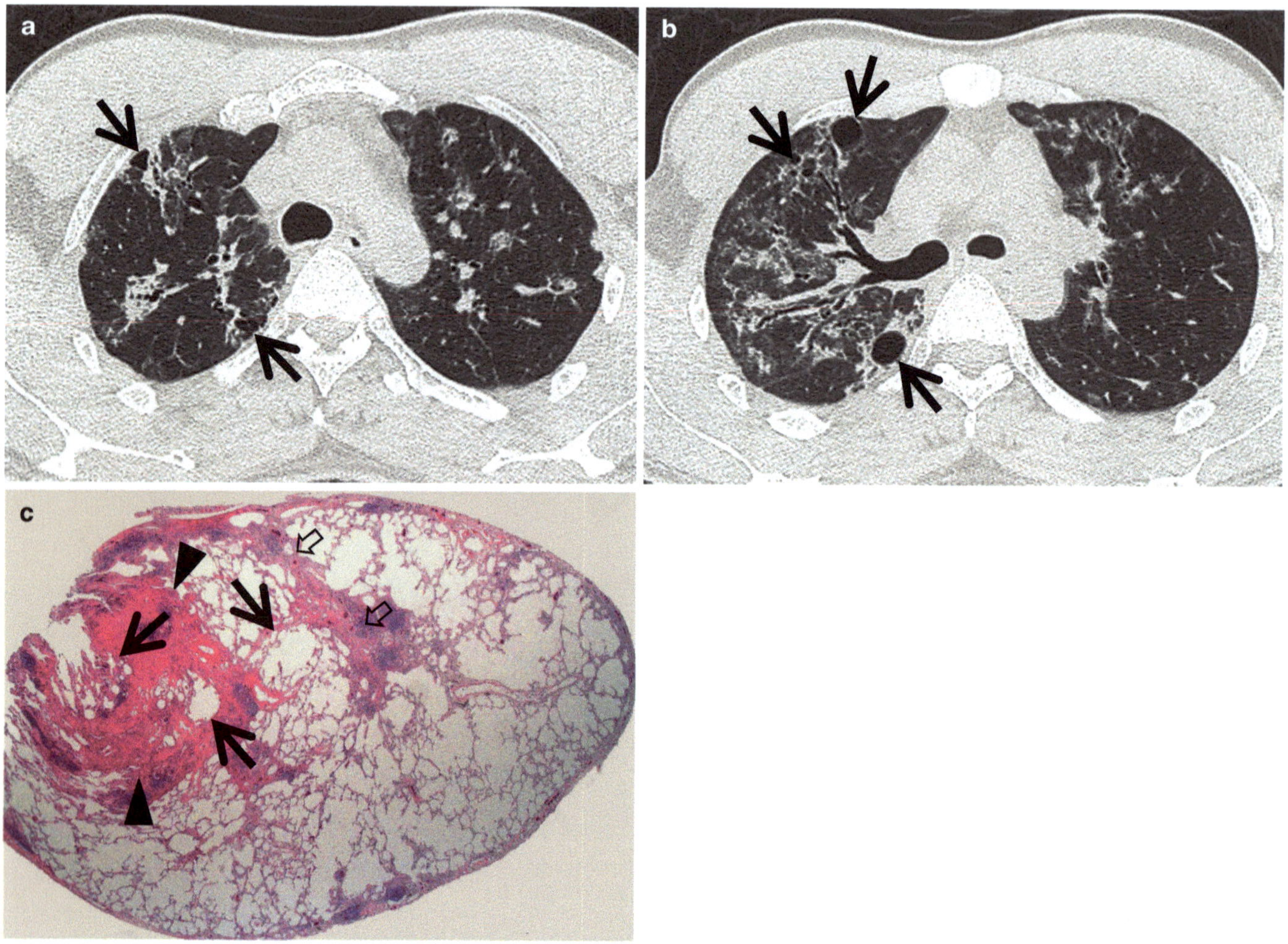


**Fig. 23.4** Lymphocytic interstitial pneumonia in a 37-year-old man with Sjögren's syndrome. (**a**, **b**) Lung window images of thin-section (1.5-mm section thickness) CT scans obtained at levels of aortic arch (**a**) and right upper lobar bronchus (**b**), respectively, show ground-glass opacity nodules or ground-glass opacity in both lungs along bronchovascular bundles or along subpleural lungs. Also note cystic lung lesions (*arrows*). (**c**) Low-magnification (×40) photomicrograph of surgical lung biopsy specimen depicts peribronchiolar dense fibrosis and scanty lymphocyte aggregations (*arrowheads*). Such changes are also seen in interlobular septa (*open arrows*) and subpleural region. Please note cystic changes (*arrows*) of alveoli associated with bronchiolar fibrosis and inflammation

### Key Points for Differential Diagnosis

| | Distribution | | | | | | | | | | | |
|---|---|---|---|---|---|---|---|---|---|---|---|---|
| | Zones | | | | | | | | Clinical presentations | | | |
| Diseases | U | M | L | SP | C | R | BV | R | Acute | Subacute | Chronic | Others |
| LAM | + | + | + | | | + | | + | | | + | Round or oval cysts, involve CPA |
| LCH | + | + | | | | + | | + | | | + | Irregular cysts, cysts with nodules, spare CPA |
| LIP | | | + | | | | + | | | + | + | With GGO and poorly defined centrilobular nodules |
| DIP | | | + | + | | | | | | + | + | A combination of lack of a perceptible cyst wall and areas of GGO around cysts |
| Cystic pulmonary metastasis | + | + | + | + | | + | | + | | + | + | Angiosarcoma, characteristic |
| Birt–Hogg–Dube syndrome | | | + | + | | | | | | | + | Large dominant cysts tend to be located in the lung bases and may be multiseptated |

*Note*: *LAM* lymphangioleiomyomatosis, *LCH* Langerhans cell histiocytosis, *LIP* lymphocytic interstitial pneumonia, *DIP* desquamative interstitial pneumonia, *U* upper, *M* middle, *L* lower, *SP* subpleural, *C* central, *R* random, *BV* bronchovascular, *CPA* costophrenic angle, *GGO* ground-glass opacity

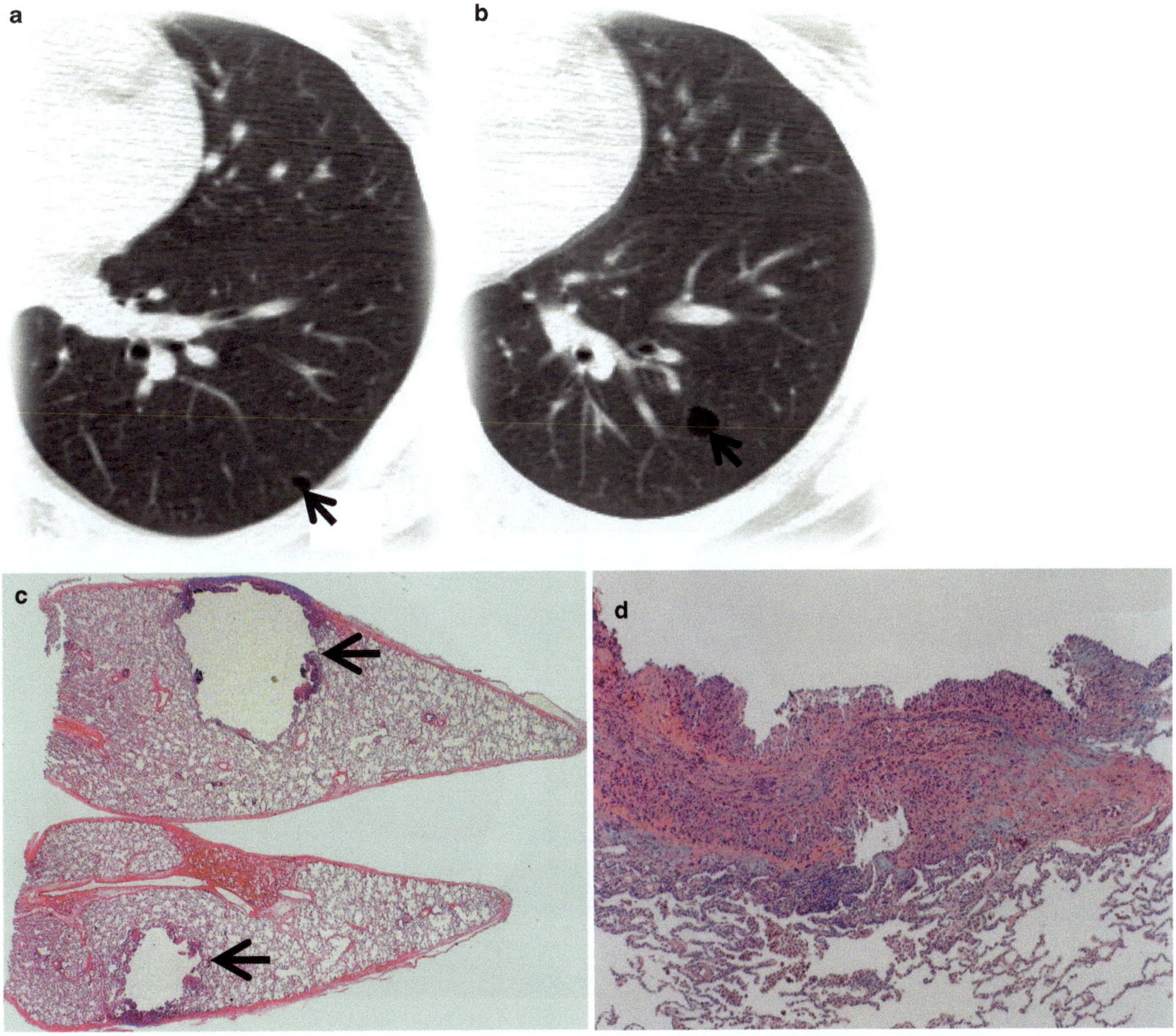


**Fig. 23.5** Cystic metastasis in a 20-year-old man with osteogenic sarcoma in right thigh. (**a**, **b**) Lung window images of CT scan (5.0-mm section thickness) obtained at levels of left inferior pulmonary vein (**a**) and basal segmental bronchi (**b**), respectively, show cystic lung lesions (*arrows*). (**c**) Low-magnification (×4) photomicrograph of surgical biopsy specimen depicts a unilocular cyst with thin wall (*arrows*) which is composed of metastatic tumor cells. (**d**) High-magnification (×100) photomicrograph discloses cyst wall composed of spindle-shaped pleomorphic tumor cells permeating bronchiolar wall

## Lymphangioleiomyomatosis

### Pathology and Pathogenesis

The essential pathologic feature is a proliferation of unusual smooth muscle cells that involves all parts of the lungs (Fig. 23.3). They are generally plump and spindle-shaped with pale eosinophilic cytoplasm but the cytoplasm may be clear and the cells are polygonal in outline so that they appear epithelioid. The alveolar walls are infiltrated by the unusual smooth muscle cells and consequently thickened, often in nodular fashion. Narrow lymphatic channels are often evident within these cell collections. Consequent breakdown of the alveolar walls leads to focal cystic change, which ultimately culminates in gross "honeycombing" throughout the lungs. Airway collapse consequent upon this cystic change is the principal mechanism contributing to airflow limitation. Rupture of the cysts explains the frequent pneumothoraces which are one of the distinctive complications of this disease [21].

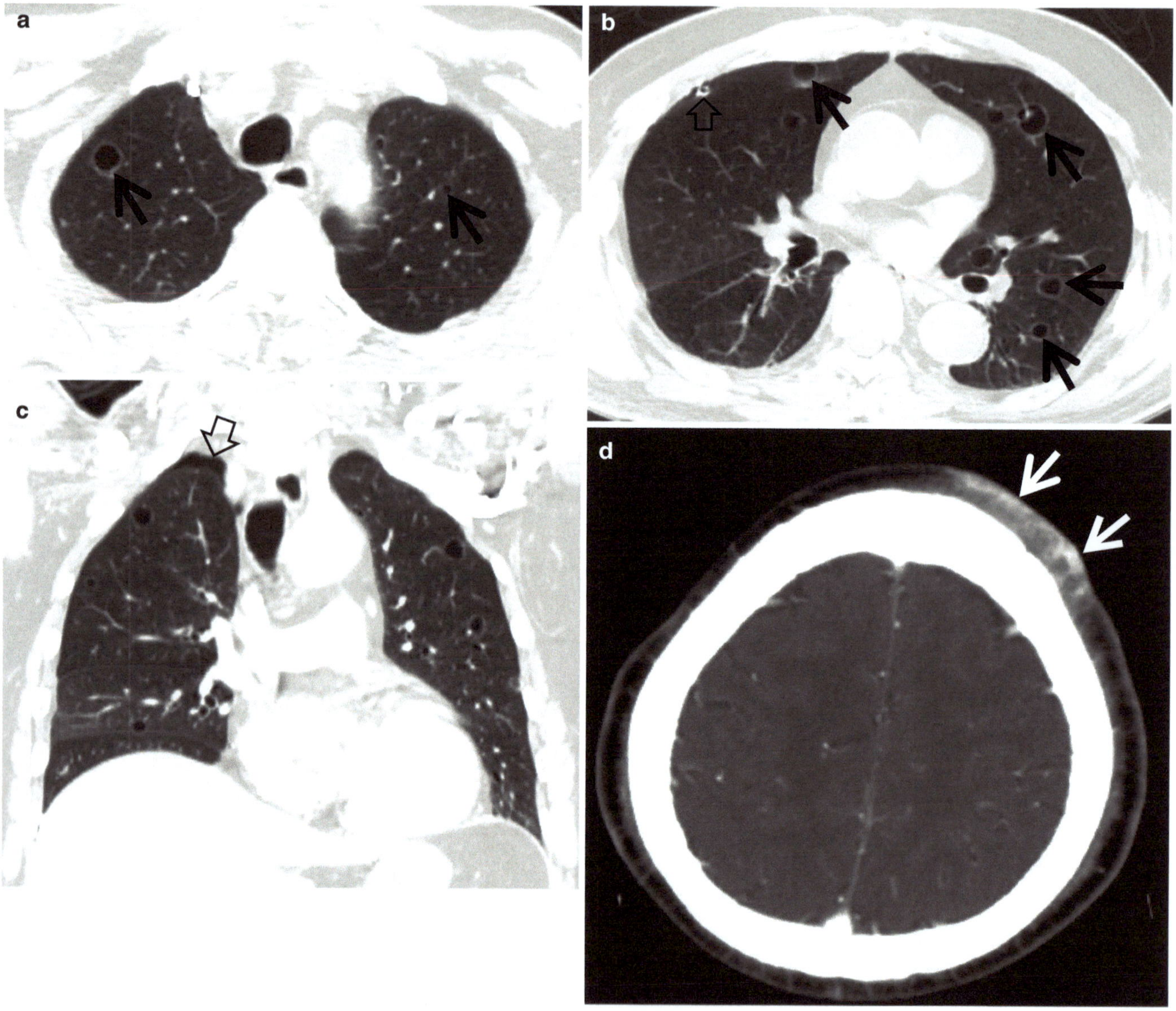


**Fig. 23.6** Cystic metastasis in an 82-year-old man with angiosarcoma in his scalp. (**a**, **b**) Lung window images of CT scan (5.0-mm section thickness) obtained at levels of aortic arch (**a**) and arising portion of right middle lobar bronchus (**b**), respectively, show cystic lung lesions (*arrows*) in both lungs. A pigtail catheter (*open arrow*) was inserted in right pleural space in order to evacuate pneumothorax caused by rupture of cystic lung lesions. (**c**) Coronal reformatted image (2.0-mm section thickness) also demonstrates multiple cystic lung lesions. Also note pneumothorax (*open arrow*) in right apex. (**d**) Enhanced CT (5.0-mm section thickness) scan of brain depicts a band-like highly enhancing soft tissue tumor (*arrows*) in left scalp, anteriorly, which turned out to be an angiosarcoma

## Symptoms and Signs

Patients with LAM usually develop progressive dyspnea and recurrent pneumothorax, chylous effusions, and occasional hemoptysis [22]. Extrapulmonary lymphadenopathy and cystic masses of the axial lymphatics can be found in abdomen or pelvis. In patients with tuberous sclerosis, LAM is often associated with angiomyolipoma in the kidneys and liver. Meningioma is also frequently found.

## CT Findings

Characteristic HRCT findings of LAM are diffuse thin-walled cysts surrounded by normal lung without regional sparing [18, 23] (Fig. 23.3). Cysts are usually 2–5 mm but can be as large as 25–30 mm. Cysts are typically round or ovoid, but they may become polygonal with severe parenchymal involvement. Other findings include thickening of interlobular septa, small centrilobular nodules, and focal areas of ground-glass opacity (GGO).

### CT–Pathology Comparisons

The pathogenesis of cyst development is unclear, but it may arise from air trapping caused by peribronchiolar smooth muscle proliferation [18]. Small centrilobular nodules correspond to hyperplastic muscle or pneumocyte hyperplasia, and focal areas of GGO may be due to smooth muscle proliferation, hemosiderosis, or pulmonary hemorrhage. Interlobular septal thickening represents edema caused by obstruction of pulmonary lymphatics.

### Patient Prognosis

The management of LAM is basically supportive, including care for recurrent pneumothorax and oxygen for dyspnea. Lung transplantation is the last treatment option. Sirolimus, as an mTOR inhibitor, can be the promising medical therapy [24]. Predicting the prognosis of individual patient is difficult. More advance disease at the time of diagnosis and rapid decline in lung function are the poor prognostic factors.

## Lymphocytic Interstitial Pneumonia

### Pathology and Pathogenesis

The definition of LIP by American Thoracic Society/European Respiratory Society 02 consensus classification is limited to the diseases with extensive alveolar septal infiltration of lymphoid cells based on the concept that LIP is one of the interstitial pneumonias [25]. The definition also excluded many of the previously diagnosed LIPs with predominant involvement of interstitium other than alveolar septa such as bronchovascular bundles and interlobular septa, which should be called diffuse lymphoid hyperplasia (Fig. 23.4).

### Symptoms and Signs

The majority of patients with LIP are women. The onset of symptoms typically occurs between the ages of 40 and 70 years [26]. Patients present with respiratory symptoms including cough and slowly progressive dyspnea, sometimes associated with pleuritic chest pain. Systemic symptoms such as weight loss, fever, fatigue, arthralgia, and night sweating are less common. In those patients with Sjögren's syndrome, dry mouth or dry eye may be observed.

### CT Findings

HRCT findings of LIP include areas of GGO, poorly defined centrilobular nodules, and thin-walled cysts with a basal predominance [27] (Fig. 23.4). Although the cysts may vary in size (1–30 mm), they are usually smaller than 30 mm. The cysts are typically less numerous than LAM or Langerhans cell histiocytosis. Other HRCT findings include peribronchovascular thickening, interlobular septal thickening, subpleural nodules, lymphadenopathy, and areas of consolidation.

### CT–Pathology Comparisons

The cysts in LIP may result from overdistension of airspaces distal to bronchioles that are partly obstructed by the lymphocytic infiltration [28]. Thickening of bronchovascular bundles, poorly defined centrilobular nodules, and interlobular septal thickening reflect the involvement of perilymphatic interstitium.

### Patient Prognosis

Corticosteroids are commonly employed and provide improvement in 50–60 % of patients. Up to one-third of patients may die within several years of diagnosis from progression of disease or infectious complications related to immunosuppressive therapy. Malignant transformation to lymphoma has been described.

## Cystic Pulmonary Metastasis, Particularly Angiosarcoma

### Pathology and Pathogenesis

Pulmonary metastasis of angiosarcomas commonly appears as extensive solid nodules; but, cystic or cavitary pulmonary lesions have also been reported. The cystic wall is composed of alveolar wall structures containing infiltrating spindle cell tumor. The spindle cell tumor comprises slit-like blood vessels harboring internal red blood cells. The tumor cells show strongly positive staining for CD31 and CD34 [29].

### Symptoms and Signs

Pulmonary metastasis of angiosarcoma is most frequently from the heart and the pulmonary artery trunk. Hemoptysis is the most frequent symptom even with diffuse pulmonary hemorrhage [30]. Other presenting symptoms include cough, dyspnea, chest pain, hemothorax, and pneumothorax, or pneumomediastinum.

### CT Findings

Pulmonary metastases of angiosarcoma commonly take the form of solid nodules with or without a GGO halo, but relatively few cases appear as cysts. A cystic pulmonary metastasis is a thin-walled, bulla-like lesion with or without accompanying nodules (Fig. 23.6). Pneumothorax or pneumomediastinum due to the rupture of cysts may occur [31].

### CT–Pathology Comparisons

Cystic metastases may be caused by excavation of a nodular tumor through discharge of the necrotic material inside, or by infiltration of malignant cells into the walls of a preexisting benign pulmonary bulla, or by infiltration of malignant cells into the walls of air sacs formed by cystic distension of small airways through the ball-valve effect of the tumor [31].

### Patient Prognosis

The prognosis of pulmonary metastasis of angiosarcoma is poor, with a median survival of 9 months after diagnosis.

## Emphysema

### Definition

Emphysema is characterized by permanently enlarged airspaces distal to the terminal bronchiole with destruction of alveolar walls [32]. The CT appearance of emphysema consists of focal areas or regions of low attenuation, usually without visible walls [16, 33] (Fig. 23.7).

Emphysema is usually classified in terms of the part of the acinus predominantly affected: proximal (centrilobular emphysema) (Fig. 23.7), distal (paraseptal emphysema) (Fig. 23.8), or whole acinus (panacinar or panlobular emphysema) (Fig. 23.9). The term *bullous emphysema* is bullous destruction of the lung parenchyma, usually on a background of paraseptal or panacinar emphysema. *Paracicatricial emphysema* is an irregular airspace enlargement occurring in patients with pulmonary fibrosis.

### Distribution

Centrilobular and paraseptal emphysema usually predominate in the upper lobes, whereas panlobular emphysema, associated with α1-antitrypsin deficiency, predominates in the lower lobes. Centrilobular emphysema affects the lobules around the central respiratory bronchioles, whereas panlobular emphysema uniformly affects the entire secondary lobule.

### Clinical Considerations

The term chronic obstructive pulmonary disease (COPD) is often used to describe patients who have chronic and irreversible airways obstruction, most commonly associated with combination of emphysema and chronic bronchitis. Centrilobular emphysema is the most common form of emphysema in cigarette smokers. Panlobular emphysema is the form of emphysema associated with α1-antitrypsin deficiency. Paraseptal emphysema can be an isolated phenomenon in young adults, often associated with spontaneous pneumothorax, or can be seen in older patients with centrilobular emphysema.

**Key Points for Differential Diagnosis**

1. Differentiation of paraseptal emphysema and honeycombing

   Areas of paraseptal emphysema usually occur in a single layer at the pleural surface, predominantly in the upper lobes, and may be associated with other findings of emphysema such as large bullae, but are typically unassociated with significant fibrosis. However, honeycombing cysts are usually smaller, occur in several layers in the subpleural lung, tend to predominate at the lung bases, and are associated with disruption of lobular architecture and other findings of fibrosis such as traction bronchiectasis.
2. Differentiation of centrilobular emphysema and lung cysts

   In patients with centrilobular emphysema, the focal areas of lucency lack visible walls; lung cysts, on the other hand, have walls recognizable on HRCT. However, in some patients with centrilobular emphysema, areas of lung destruction show very thin and less defined walls on HRCT, which reflect the presence of minimal lung fibrosis or compressed adjacent lung parenchyma. In patients with centrilobular emphysema, lucency can be seen involving only on part of a secondary pulmonary lobule. Lung cysts often appear larger than areas of centrilobular emphysema, which usually range from several millimeters to 10 mm.
3. The extent of emphysema is generally assessed by using CT densitometry parameters such as the relative low-attenuation area and the percentile of the frequency-attenuation distribution. Although several threshold values have been reported, a threshold

value of −960 to −970 HU has been shown to be suitable for quantifying emphysema in continuous volume data sets obtained with multidetector CT [34].

4. Numerous studies have demonstrated a significant correlation between the CT emphysema index (the proportion of the lung affected by emphysema) and pulmonary function test results [35]. However, airflow limitation in COPD is a complicated phenomenon that is related only in part to emphysematous lung destruction; therefore, the extent of emphysema does not always correlate with the severity of airflow limitation [36].
5. Although CT densitometry parameters may be used as rough indicators of the extent of emphysema, they provide no information about the distribution or size of low-attenuation clusters. Therefore, the anatomic distribution of emphysema should be taken into account in quantitative CT analysis of low-attenuation clusters (the size and number of clusters are calculated by grouping adjacent low-attenuation voxels together) [34].
6. Texture-based quantification of emphysema using an automated system shows better correlation with the lung function test results than densitometry-based quantification [37].
7. Quantitative CT analyses can help differentiate COPD phenotypes (emphysema predominant, airway predominant, and mixed) [38, 39].

## Centrilobular Emphysema

### Pathology and Pathogenesis

Centrilobular emphysema is characterized by destroyed centrilobular alveolar walls and enlargement of respiratory bronchioles and associated alveoli (Fig. 23.7). This is the most common form of emphysema in cigarette smokers [40].

### Symptoms and Signs

Depending on the extent of emphysema, clinical manifestations of the patients with centrilobular emphysema are variable. They may be asymptomatic or severely dyspneic even at rest. Tachypnea and barrel chest can be observed in severely dyspneic patients. Cyanosis is rare.

### CT Findings

Centrilobular emphysema is characterized by destroyed centrilobular alveolar walls and enlargement of respiratory bronchioles and associated alveoli. CT findings of centrilobular emphysema are centrilobular areas of decreased attenuation, usually without visible walls, of nonuniform distribution and are predominantly located in the upper lung zones [41] (Fig. 23.7). Areas of lucency often appear to be grouped near the centers of secondary pulmonary lobules, surrounding the centrilobular artery branches. With more severe centrilobular emphysema, areas of destruction can become confluent (Fig. 23.7).

### Patient Prognosis

Smoking cessation is the essential part of lung care. Prognosis is usually dependent on the lung function at the time of diagnosis. Bronchodilator therapy is often ineffective.

## Paraseptal Emphysema

### Pathology and Pathogenesis

Paraseptal emphysema is characterized by predominant involvement of the distal alveoli and their ducts and sacs. It is characteristically bounded by any pleural surface and the interlobular septa [32] (Fig. 23.8).

### Symptoms and Signs

Most patients are asymptomatic. Pulmonary function is normal or nearly normal. Sudden chest pain with dyspnea can occur in the cases of pneumothorax.

### CT Findings

Paraseptal emphysema is characterized by predominant involvement of the distal alveoli and their ducts and sacs. On CT it is characterized by subpleural and peribronchovascular regions of low attenuation separated by intact interlobular septa (Fig. 23.8).

### Patient Prognosis

Unless patients smoke, prognosis is excellent since pulmonary function is normal.

## Panacinar Emphysema Associated with α1-Antitrypsin Deficiency

### Pathology and Pathogenesis

Panacinar emphysema involves all portions of the acinus and secondary pulmonary lobule more or less uniformly. It predominates in the lower lobes and is the form of emphysema associated with α1-antitrypsin deficiency [40].

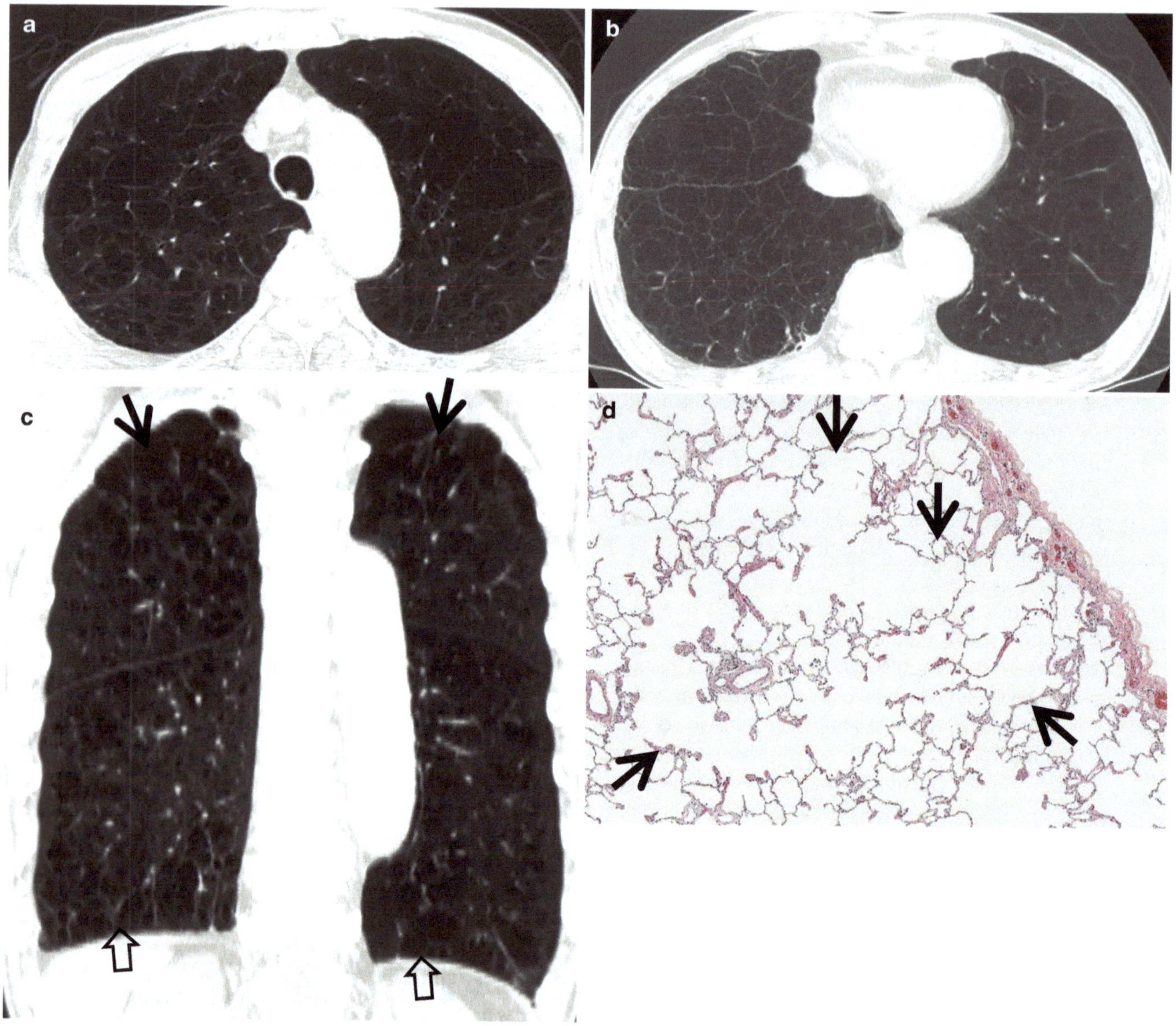


**Fig. 23.7** Centrilobular emphysema in a 65-year-old smoker man. (**a**, **b**) Lung window images of thin-section (1.0-mm section thickness) CT scans obtained at levels of aortic arch (**a**) and suprahepatic inferior vena cava (**b**), respectively, show extensive emphysema involving whole lungs. Emphysema is variable in their size and involves both upper and lower lung zones, suggesting extensive centrilobular emphysema than panlobular emphysema (which involves predominantly lower lung zones). (**c**) Coronal reformatted image (2.0-mm section thickness) demonstrates emphysema mainly in upper lung zones (*arrows*), but also lung bases (*open arrows*). (**d**) High-magnification (×200) photomicrograph of surgical biopsy specimen from a different patient discloses emphysematous areas (*arrows*), destroyed centrilobular alveolar walls, and enlargement of respiratory bronchioles and associated alveoli

## Symptoms and Signs

The most common manifestation of α1-antitrypsin deficiency is early-onset (patients in their 30s and 40s) emphysema and bronchiectasis [42]. Cough, dyspnea, and wheezing are the frequently described symptoms. Extrapulmonary features of liver disease (chronic hepatitis and cirrhosis), skin disease (panniculitis), and vasculitis can be associated.

## CT Findings

Panacinar emphysema involves all portions of the acinus and secondary pulmonary lobule more or less uniformly. It manifests as a generalized decrease in lung parenchymal attenuation with a decrease in the caliber of pulmonary vessels in the affected lungs [43] (Fig. 23.9).

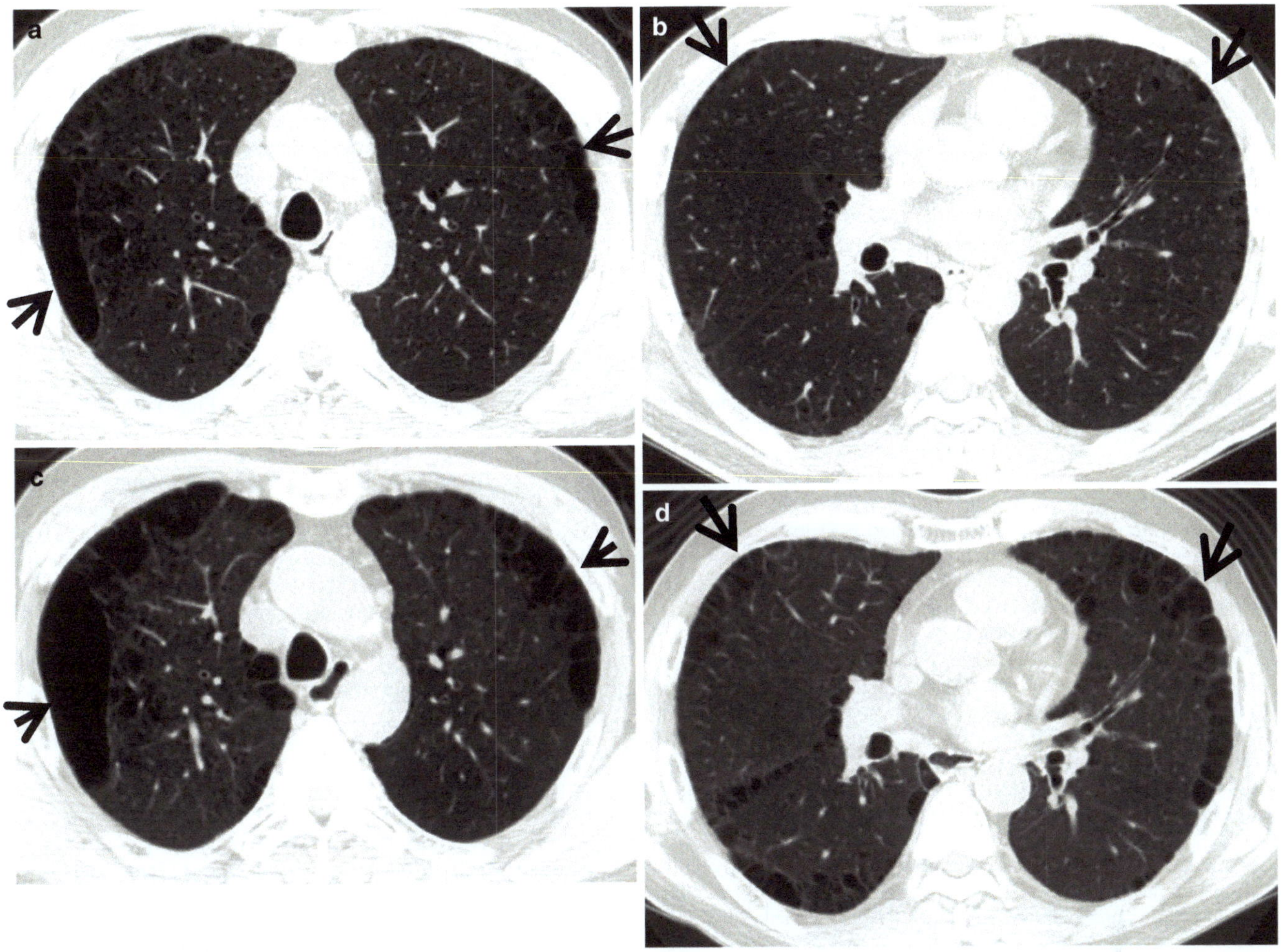

**Fig. 23.8** Paraseptal (distal acinar, bullous) emphysema showing evolution in a 50-year-old smoker man. (**a**, **b**) Lung window images of thin-section (1.0-mm section thickness) CT scans obtained at levels of aortic arch (**a**) and right bronchus intermedius (**b**), respectively, show paraseptal emphysema (*arrows*) involving mainly upper lung zones. (**c**, **d**) Fifty-month follow-up CT scans obtained at similar levels to **a** and **b**, respectively, demonstrate much increased extent of paraseptal emphysema (*arrows*) in both lungs

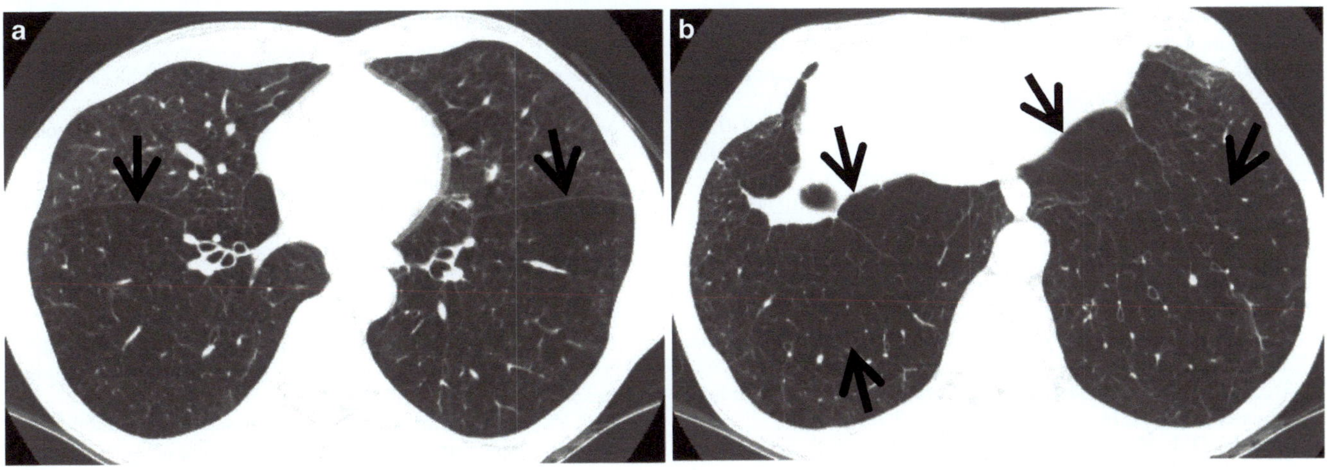

**Fig. 23.9** Panlobular emphysema in a 55-year-old man. (**a**, **b**) Lung window images of thin-section (1.0-mm section thickness) CT scans obtained at levels of right inferior pulmonary vein (**a**) and liver dome (**b**), respectively, show extensive areas of emphysema in lower lung zones. Please note whole secondary pulmonary lobules (*arrows*) are involved with emphysematous processes

## Patient Prognosis

The most common causes of death are respiratory failure and liver cirrhosis. Beyond the usual treatment of COPD, specific treatment consists of the infusion of purified pooled human plasma α1-antitrypsin, known as intravenous augmentation therapy. It has shown a clear efficacy in randomized, double-blind, placebo-controlled trials.

## References


1. Kulwiec EL, Lynch DA, Aguayo SM, Schwarz MI, King Jr TE. Imaging of pulmonary histiocytosis X. Radiographics. 1992;12:515–26.
2. Aberle DR, Gamsu G, Lynch D. Thoracic manifestations of Wegener granulomatosis: diagnosis and course. Radiology. 1990; 174:703–9.
3. Remy-Jardin M, Remy J, Cortet B, Mauri F, Delcambre B. Lung changes in rheumatoid arthritis: CT findings. Radiology. 1994;193:375–82.
4. Davis SD. CT evaluation for pulmonary metastases in patients with extrathoracic malignancy. Radiology. 1991;180:1–12.
5. Iwasaki Y, Nagata K, Nakanishi M, et al. Spiral CT findings in septic pulmonary emboli. Eur J Radiol. 2001;37:190–4.
6. Kim HJ, Lee KS, Johkoh T, et al. Pulmonary Langerhans cell histiocytosis in adults: high-resolution CT-pathology comparisons and evolutional changes at CT. Eur Radiol. 2011;21:1406–15.
7. Seo JB, Im JG, Goo JM, Chung MJ, Kim MY. Atypical pulmonary metastases: spectrum of radiologic findings. Radiographics. 2001;21:403–17.
8. Case records of the Massachusetts General Hospital. Weekly clinicopathological exercises. Case 10–2001. A 53-year-old woman with arthritis and pulmonary nodules. N Engl J Med. 2001;344: 997–1004.
9. Antin-Ozerkis D, Evans J, Rubinowitz A, Homer RJ, Matthay RA. Pulmonary manifestations of rheumatoid arthritis. Clin Chest Med. 2010;31:451–78.
10. Capobianco J, Grimberg A, Thompson BM, Antunes VB, Jasinowodolinski D, Meirelles GS. Thoracic manifestations of collagen vascular diseases. Radiographics. 2012;32:33–50.
11. Kobayashi T, Satoh K, Ohkawa M, Satoh A. Multiple rheumatoid nodules with rapid thin-walled cavity formation producing pneumothorax. J Thorac Imaging. 2005;20:47–9.
12. Kitamura A, Matsuno T, Narita M, Shimokata K, Yamashita Y, Mori N. Rheumatoid arthritis with diffuse pulmonary rheumatoid nodules. Pathol Int. 2004;54:798–802.
13. Chaudhuri MR. Cavitary pulmonary metastases. Thorax. 1970;25: 375–81.
14. Hirakata K, Nakata H, Nakagawa T. CT of pulmonary metastases with pathological correlation. Semin Ultrasound CT MR. 1995;16: 379–94.
15. Murata K, Takahashi M, Mori M, et al. Pulmonary metastatic nodules: CT-pathologic correlation. Radiology. 1992;182:331–5.
16. Hansell DM, Bankier AA, MacMahon H, McLoud TC, Muller NL, Remy J. Fleischner Society: glossary of terms for thoracic imaging. Radiology. 2008;246:697–722.
17. Beddy P, Babar J, Devaraj A. A practical approach to cystic lung disease on HRCT. Insights Imaging. 2011;2:1–7.
18. Seaman DM, Meyer CA, Gilman MD, McCormack FX. Diffuse cystic lung disease at high-resolution CT. AJR Am J Roentgenol. 2011;196:1305–11.
19. McCormack FX. Lymphangioleiomyomatosis: a clinical update. Chest. 2008;133:507–16.
20. Traweek T, Rotter AJ, Swartz W, Azumi N. Cystic pulmonary metastatic sarcoma. Cancer. 1990;65:1805–11.
21. Kumasaka T, Seyama K, Mitani K, et al. Lymphangiogenesis in lymphangioleiomyomatosis: its implication in the progression of lymphangioleiomyomatosis. Am J Surg Pathol. 2004;28: 1007–16.
22. Johnson SR, Cordier JF, Lazor R, et al. European Respiratory Society guidelines for the diagnosis and management of lymphangioleiomyomatosis. Eur Respir J. 2010;35:14–26.
23. Muller NL, Chiles C, Kullnig P. Pulmonary lymphangiomyomatosis: correlation of CT with radiographic and functional findings. Radiology. 1990;175:335–9.
24. McCormack FX, Inoue Y, Moss J, et al. Efficacy and safety of sirolimus in lymphangioleiomyomatosis. N Engl J Med. 2011;364: 1595–606.
25. American Thoracic S, European RS. American Thoracic Society/European Respiratory Society International Multidisciplinary Consensus Classification of the Idiopathic Interstitial Pneumonias. This joint statement of the American Thoracic Society (ATS), and the European Respiratory Society (ERS) was adopted by the ATS board of directors, June 2001 and by the ERS Executive Committee, June 2001. Am J Respir Crit Care Med. 2002;165: 277–304.
26. Tian X, Yi ES, Ryu JH. Lymphocytic interstitial pneumonia and other benign lymphoid disorders. Semin Respir Crit Care Med. 2012;33:450–61.
27. Johkoh T, Muller NL, Pickford HA, et al. Lymphocytic interstitial pneumonia: thin-section CT findings in 22 patients. Radiology. 1999;212:567–72.
28. Ichikawa Y, Kinoshita M, Koga T, Oizumi K, Fujimoto K, Hayabuchi N. Lung cyst formation in lymphocytic interstitial pneumonia: CT features. J Comput Assist Tomogr. 1994;18: 745–8.
29. Kim AY, Lee KS, Han J, Kim H, Kim K, Baek CH. Cystic pulmonary metastasis in a patient with scalp angiosarcoma: a case report. J Korean Soc Radiol. 2011;65:143–6.
30. Garcia Clemente M, Gonzalez Budino T, Escobar Stein J, Seco Garcia AJ, Celorio Peinado C, Rodriguez RJ. Metastatic pulmonary angiosarcoma. An Med Interna. 2004;21:27–30.
31. Park SI, Choi E, Lee HB, Rhee YK, Chung MJ, Lee YC. Spontaneous pneumomediastinum and hemopneumothoraces secondary to cystic lung metastasis. Respiration. 2003;70:211–3.
32. Thurlbeck WM, Muller NL. Emphysema: definition, imaging, and quantification. AJR Am J Roentgenol. 1994;163:1017–25.
33. Foster Jr WL, Gimenez EI, Roubidoux MA, et al. The emphysemas: radiologic-pathologic correlations. Radiographics. 1993;13: 311–28.
34. Madani A, Zanen J, de Maertelaer V, Gevenois PA. Pulmonary emphysema: objective quantification at multi-detector row CT–comparison with macroscopic and microscopic morphometry. Radiology. 2006;238:1036–43.
35. Zaporozhan J, Ley S, Eberhardt R, et al. Paired inspiratory/expiratory volumetric thin-slice CT scan for emphysema analysis: comparison of different quantitative evaluations and pulmonary function test. Chest. 2005;128:3212–20.
36. Gelb AF, Schein M, Kuei J, et al. Limited contribution of emphysema in advanced chronic obstructive pulmonary disease. Am Rev Respir Dis. 1993;147:1157–61.
37. Park YS, Seo JB, Kim N, et al. Texture-based quantification of pulmonary emphysema on high-resolution computed tomography: comparison with density-based quantification and correlation with pulmonary function test. Invest Radiol. 2008;43:395–402.

38. Matsuoka S, Yamashiro T, Washko GR, Kurihara Y, Nakajima Y, Hatabu H. Quantitative CT assessment of chronic obstructive pulmonary disease. Radiographics. 2010;30:55–66.
39. Mets OM, de Jong PA, van Ginneken B, Gietema HA, Lammers JW. Quantitative computed tomography in COPD: possibilities and limitations. Lung. 2012;190:133–45.
40. The definition of emphysema. Report of a National Heart, Lung, and Blood Institute, Division of Lung Diseases workshop. Am Rev Respir Dis. 1985;32:182–5.
41. Foster Jr WL, Pratt PC, Roggli VL, Godwin JD, Halvorsen Jr RA, Putman CE. Centrilobular emphysema: CT-pathologic correlation. Radiology. 1986;159:27–32.
42. Stoller JK, Aboussouan LS. A review of alpha1-antitrypsin deficiency. Am J Respir Crit Care Med. 2012;185:246–59.
43. Spouge D, Mayo JR, Cardoso W, Muller NL. Panacinar emphysema: CT and pathologic findings. J Comput Assist Tomogr. 1993;17:710–3.

# 24 Decreased Opacity without Cystic Walls

## Mosaic Attenuation, Vascular

### Definition

Please refer to section "Mosaic Attenuation" Chap. 13.

### Diseases Causing Vascular Causes of Mosaic Perfusion

Vascular causes of mosaic perfusion include chronic pulmonary thromboembolism and pulmonary arterial hypertension.

### Distribution

Areas of mosaic perfusion in chronic thromboembolism or pulmonary arterial hypertension are typically segmental or subsegmental in distribution [1].

### Clinical Considerations

Pulmonary arterial hypertension may be idiopathic or arise in association with chronic pulmonary thromboembolism; pulmonary embolism caused by tumor cells, parasitic material, or foreign material; parenchymal lung disease; liver disease; vasculitis; human immunodeficiency virus infection; or a left-to-right cardiac shunt [1].

> **Key Points for Differential Diagnosis**
> Please refer to section "Mosaic Attenuation" Chap. 13.

## Mosaic Attenuation, Obstructive Airway Disease

### Definition

Please refer to section "Mosaic Attenuation" Chap. 13.

### Airway Diseases Causing Mosaic Attenuation

Mosaic attenuation can be seen in a variety of airway diseases including bronchiectasis, cystic fibrosis, allergic bronchopulmonary aspergillosis (ABPA) (Fig. 24.1), *asthma* (Fig. 24.2), and constrictive bronchiolitis.

### Distribution

In patients with mosaic attenuation secondary to airways disease, lobular areas of low attenuation are common.

### Clinical Considerations

Inciting causes of asthma include environmental allergens, viral infections, exercise, analgesics, air pollution, weather changes, cigarette smoke, occupational sensitizing agents, and irritants [2]. Conditions associated with constrictive bronchiolitis include heart–lung or lung transplantations, chronic allograft rejection, allogeneic bone marrow transplantation with chronic graft-versus-host disease, and collagen vascular diseases, especially rheumatoid arthritis [3].

> **Key Points for Differential Diagnosis**
> Please refer to section "Mosaic Attenuation" Chap. 13.

K.S. Lee et al., *Radiology Illustrated: Chest Radiology*, Radiology Illustrated,
DOI 10.1007/978-3-642-37096-0_24, © Springer-Verlag Berlin Heidelberg 2014

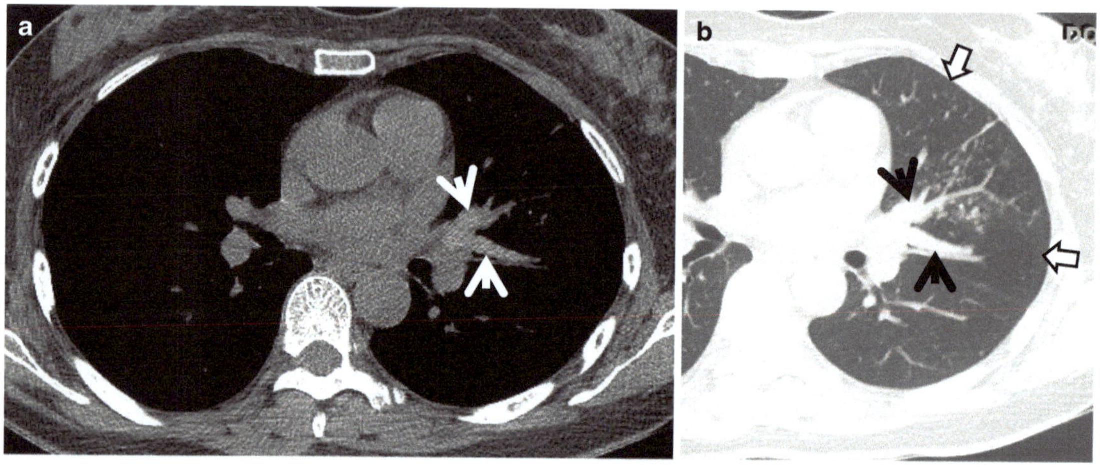


**Fig. 24.1** Allergic bronchopulmonary aspergillosis in a 56-year-old asthmatic woman. (**a**) Mediastinal window image of CT scan (2.5-mm section thickness) obtained at level of right middle lobar bronchus shows allergic mucin (*arrows*) exhibiting high-attenuation tubular lesions and filling lingular divisional bronchus and its branches. (**b**) Lung window image obtained at same level to (a) demonstrates mosaic perfusion area (*open arrows*) as well as allergic mucin (*arrows*)

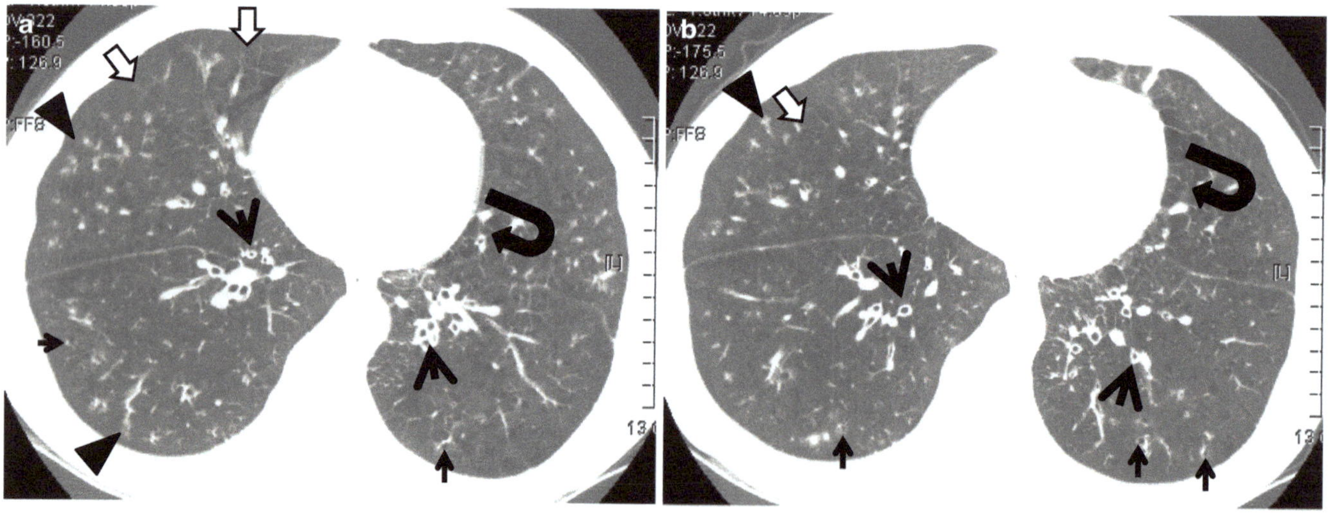


**Fig. 24.2** Status asthmaticus in a 45-year-old man. (**a**, **b**) Lung window images of thin-section (1.5-mm section thickness) CT scans obtained at levels of segmental bronchi (**a**) and subsegmental bronchi (**b**), respectively, show areas of mosaic perfusion (*open arrows*), emphysema (*curved arrows*), and tree-in-bud signs (*arrowheads*). Also note marked bronchial wall thickening (*arrows*) and dilatation (*small arrows*) in both lungs

## Asthma

### Pathology and Pathogenesis

The airway lumen is compromised of the accumulation of mucus and an exudate of eosinophils and desquamated epithelial cells mixed with components derived from the plasma but not including fibrin. Three major processes appear to contribute to the airway narrowing: increased amounts of mucus, inflammatory edema, and muscular hypertrophy. These are found principally in bronchi but may also be found in smaller airways, including bronchioles. The inflammation may even involve alveoli. The mucus commonly has a concentric or spiral pattern in cross section with many eosinophils and desquamated epithelium. There is goblet cell hyperplasia in the surface epithelium and the bronchial glands are enlarged, but not as much as in chronic bronchitis. The bronchioles may also contain mucous plugs and mucus may even be seen in alveolar ducts [4].

### Symptoms and Signs

Patients typically present with symptoms such as episodic breathlessness, wheezing, chest tightness, and cough. Unlike COPD, asthma is episodic and reversible from the standpoint of symptoms and lung function impairment. Asthma attack is frequently associated with environmental or occupational exposure to allergen or dust and upper respiratory tract viral infection.

## CT Findings

The most common CT findings of asthma are the thickening and narrowing of the medium-sized and small bronchi [5, 6] (Fig. 24.2). Other CT findings include mucoid impaction, cylindrical bronchiectasis, centrilobular small nodules, and multifocal and patchy areas of mosaic perfusion due to air trapping, emphysema, and rarely, cysts (Fig. 24.2).

## CT–Pathology Comparisons

Thickening and narrowing of the bronchi on CT is related to airway inflammation. The bronchi are thickened by the combination of edema and an increase in the amount of smooth muscle and in the size of mucous glands. Recurrent inflammation and airway remodeling result in bronchiectasis. Multifocal and patchy areas of mosaic perfusion are due to air trapping caused by constrictive bronchiolitis [6]. Centrilobular small nodules reflect the presence of mucus stasis in the bronchioles and peribronchiolar inflammation. Emphysematous change is secondary to cicatricial peribronchial fibrosis and cystic changes may result from overinflating distal to chronic inflammatory bronchiolitis.

## Patient Prognosis

Environmental control and avoidance of occupational exposure to allergen is important for asthma control. Since asthma is a chronic airway inflammatory disorder, inhaled corticosteroids are the principal therapy, with the use of bronchodilator to improve the symptoms.

## References


1. Grosse C, Grosse A. CT findings in diseases associated with pulmonary hypertension: a current review. Radiographics. 2010;30: 1753–77.
2. Rodrigo GJ, Rodrigo C, Hall JB. Acute asthma in adults: a review. Chest. 2004;125:1081–102.
3. King Jr TE. Overview of bronchiolitis. Clin Chest Med. 1993;14:607–10.
4. Roche WR. Inflammatory and structural changes in the small airways in bronchial asthma. Am J Respir Crit Care Med. 1998;157:S191–4.
5. Park CS, Muller NL, Worthy SA, Kim JS, Awadh N, Fitzgerald M. Airway obstruction in asthmatic and healthy individuals: inspiratory and expiratory thin-section CT findings. Radiology. 1997;203:361–7.
6. Silva CI, Colby TV, Muller NL. Asthma and associated conditions: high-resolution CT and pathologic findings. AJR Am J Roentgenol. 2004;183:817–24.

# 25 Decreased Opacity without Cystic Airspace: Airway Disease

## Definition

Please refer to section "Airway Disease (Bronchiectasis and Bronchiolectasis)" in Chap. 13.

## Diseases Causing Bronchiectasis and Bronchiolectasis

Diffuse form of bronchiectasis occurs in variety of genetic abnormalities, especially those with abnormal mucociliary clearance or structural abnormalities of the bronchus or bronchial wall (*cystic fibrosis* [Fig. 25.1], dyskinetic cilia syndrome, Williams–Campbell syndrome). Nontuberculous mycobacterial disease is the most common infectious causes of diffuse bronchiectasis. Noninfectious causes include allergic bronchopulmonary aspergillosis and asthma. Also note section "Airway Disease (Bronchiectasis and Bronchiolectasis)" in Chap. 13.

## Distribution

Please note section "Airway Disease (Bronchiectasis and Bronchiolectasis)" in Chap. 13.

## Clinical Considerations

Please note section "Airway Disease (Bronchiectasis and Bronchiolectasis)" in Chap. 13.

**Key Points for Differential Diagnosis**

| | Distribution | | | | | | | | Clinical presentations | | | Others |
|---|---|---|---|---|---|---|---|---|---|---|---|---|
| | Zones | | | | | | | | | | | |
| Diseases | U | M | L | SP | C | R | BV | R | Acute | Subacute | Chronic | |
| Cystic fibrosis | + | | | | + | | | | | | + | Bronchial wall thickening, peribronchial interstitial thickening, mucus plugging |
| Dyskinetic cilia syndrome | | | + | | + | | | | | | + | Situs inversus totalis, sinusitis |
| Williams–Campbell syndrome | + | + | + | | + | | | | | | + | Varicose and cystic bronchiectasis limited to 4th-, 5th-, 6th-generation bronchi |
| Nontuberculous mycobacterial disease | | + | + | + | | + | | + | | | + | With centrilobular nodules |
| Allergic bronchopulmonary aspergillosis | + | | | | + | | | | | | + | Centrilobular nodules, high attenuation mucus plugging |

*Note*: *U* upper, *M* middle, *L* lower, *SP* subpleural, *C* central, *R* random, *BV* bronchovascular

K.S. Lee et al., *Radiology Illustrated: Chest Radiology*, Radiology Illustrated,
DOI 10.1007/978-3-642-37096-0_25, 

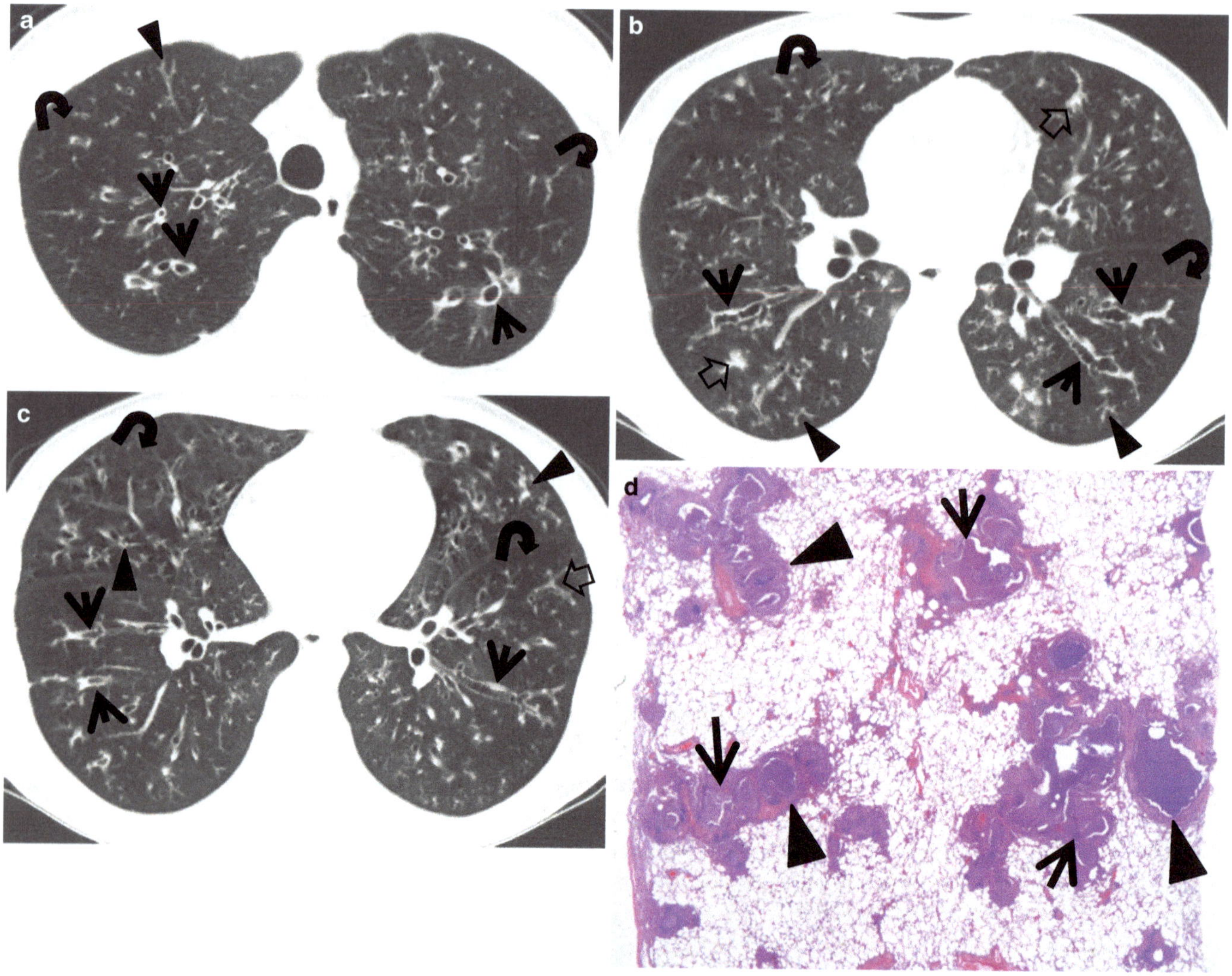


**Fig. 25.1** Cystic fibrosis in a 23-year-old man. (**a–c**) Lung window images of CT scans (2.5-mm section thickness) obtained at levels of great vessels (**a**), lower lobar bronchi (**b**), and inferior pulmonary veins (**c**), respectively, show areas of bronchiectasis (*arrows*), tree-in-bud signs (*arrowheads*), and mucus plugging (*open arrows*). Also note mosaic perfusion areas (*curved arrows*). (**d**) Low-magnification (×4) photomicrograph of surgical biopsy specimen discloses bronchiolar dilatation (*arrows*) owing to luminal impaction of mucus and inflammatory exudates. Also note bronchiolar wall thickening (*arrowheads*) with chronic inflammation and fibrosis

## Cystic Fibrosis

### Pathology and Pathogenesis

Cystic fibrosis is an autosomal recessive disease with the mutation of cystic fibrosis transmembrane conductance regulator gene and multisystem involvement. Patients have abnormal transport of chloride and sodium across the respiratory epithelium, resulting in thickened airway secretions and susceptibility to recurrent infections. Gross pathologic findings for end-stage disease show widespread bronchiectasis (more severe in upper lobe) with thick mucus plugs, pleural fibrosis or adhesions, pneumonic consolidation, and lobar atelectasis. Microscopically, there are acute and chronic inflammation involving the large and small airways associated with bronchial gland and goblet cell hyperplasia, squamous metaplasia, and mucostasis [1] (Fig. 25.1).

### Symptoms and Signs

Since cystic fibrosis is a genetic disease resulting in complications in multiple organs, especially involving the lungs and pancreas, it mimics a number of other diseases. Usual respiratory presentations in adults include cough, sputum, wheezing dyspnea, recurrent respiratory tract infection, and cor pulmonale if advanced. Usual gastrointestinal presentations in adults are recurrent abdominal pain, biliary cirrhosis with portal hypertension, and recurrent pancreatitis. Infertility may occur.

## CT Findings

The predominant HRCT finding in early stage of cystic fibrosis is a mosaic perfusion due to air trapping related to small airway disease. Other typical CT features include bronchiectasis and peribronchial thickening, mainly involving the upper lobes, and centrilobular nodules or a tree-in-bud pattern and atelectasis or consolidation secondary to mucous plugs [2, 3] (Fig. 25.1). Bronchiectasis is most often cylindrical, but varicose and cystic bronchiectasis can be seen in advanced cases.

## CT–Pathology Comparisons

Cystic fibrosis causes abnormal mucous gland secretions and subsequent effect of inflammation and infection on airways [2]. The earliest and most universal pathologic lesion of cystic fibrosis is mucous obstruction of bronchioles and small bronchi. A mosaic perfusion, which is the predominant early HRCT findings of cystic fibrosis, is caused by air trapping related to mucous obstruction and inflammation of bronchioles and small bronchi. The elicited inflammatory response damages the normal structure of the airways, and bronchiectasis develops. Upper lobe predominance of bronchiectasis and peribronchial thickening may reflect an effect of gravity on the elastin-damaged parenchymal tissue. Obstruction of airways by mucous plugs results in centrilobular nodules or a tree-in-bud pattern and atelectasis or consolidation on HRCT.

## Patient Prognosis

Treatment consists of control of mucus retention and chronic infection in the lungs, replacement of pancreatic enzymes, and nutritional therapy. New therapeutic approaches, including pharmacologic interventions and gene transfer, offer hope for further advances [4]. Lung transplantation has become an accepted therapy for respiratory failure secondary to cystic fibrosis. The outcome is highly variable, but 50 % of patients can now be expected to survive beyond 37 years.

## References


1. Oppenheimer EH, Esterly JR. Pathology of cystic fibrosis review of the literature and comparison with 146 autopsied cases. Perspect Pediatr Pathol. 1975;2:241–78.
2. Wood BP. Cystic fibrosis: 1997. Radiology. 1997;204:1–10.
3. Brody AS, Klein JS, Molina PL, Quan J, Bean JA, Wilmott RW. High-resolution computed tomography in young patients with cystic fibrosis: distribution of abnormalities and correlation with pulmonary function tests. J Pediatr. 2004;145:32–8.
4. Mogayzel Jr PJ, Naureckas ET, Robinson KA, et al. Cystic fibrosis pulmonary guidelines. Am J Respir Crit Care Med. 2013;187:680–9.

# Part III

# Application of Disease Pattern and Distribution, and Radiologic Signs to the Differentiation of Various Lung Diseases

# 26 Pneumonia

Pulmonary infection can also be classified into several radiologic and pathologic patterns according to its morphologic features. The three most common patterns are lobar pneumonia, bronchopneumonia, and interstitial pneumonia. Less common forms of infection include cellular bronchiolitis, septic embolism, miliary infection, and lung abscess. Because less common forms of infectious condition have been dealt in previous other chapters, the three most common patterns only are described in this chapter.

## Lobar Pneumonia

Lobar pneumonia is characterized histopathologically by filling of alveolar airspaces by an exudate of edema fluid and neutrophils. This filling is usually uniform within the affected lung and typically extends across pulmonary segments. The consolidation usually begins in the periphery of the lung adjacent to the visceral pleura and spreads via inter-alveolar pores and small airways centripetally, sometimes to involve the entire lobe. Bronchi that remain filled with gas and become surrounded by the expanding inflammatory exudate are often seen as air bronchograms on CT scans. The most common causative organisms are *Streptococcus pneumoniae*, *Klebsiella pneumoniae* (Fig. 26.1), and *Legionella pneumophila*.

On CT scans, homogeneous airspace consolidation involving adjacent segments of a lobe is the predominant finding. On HRCT, areas of ground-glass opacities (GGO) denoting incomplete filling of alveoli can be seen adjacent to the airspace consolidation [1]. The consolidation typically extends across lobular and segmental boundaries.

Segmental or lobar form of tuberculous pneumonia may occur in adults; in AIDS or non-AIDS immunocompromised patients including pregnant women, elderly, diabetics, alcoholics, and transplanted patients. Multiple small cavities may be shown within the consolidative lesion [2, 3] (Figs. 26.2 and 26.3).

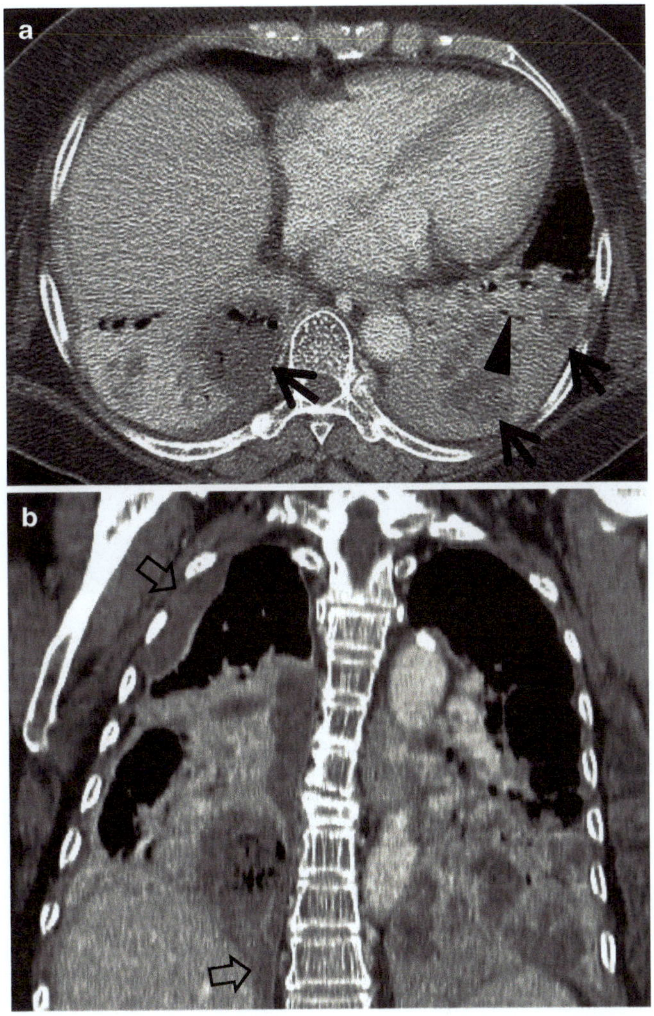


**Fig. 26.1** *Klebsiella* pneumonia in a 62-year-old woman. (**a**) Mediastinal window of enhanced CT scan (2.5-mm section thickness) obtained at level of liver dome shows dense lobar consolidation in both lower lobes containing multifocal areas of necrotic low-attenuation areas (*arrows*). Also note CT air-bronchogram signs (*arrowhead*) within consolidative lesions. (**b**) Coronal reformatted image demonstrates necrotic lobar consolidation involving both lower lobes. Also note right pleural effusion (*open arrows*)

K.S. Lee et al., *Radiology Illustrated: Chest Radiology*, Radiology Illustrated,
DOI 10.1007/978-3-642-37096-0_26, © Springer-Verlag Berlin Heidelberg 2014

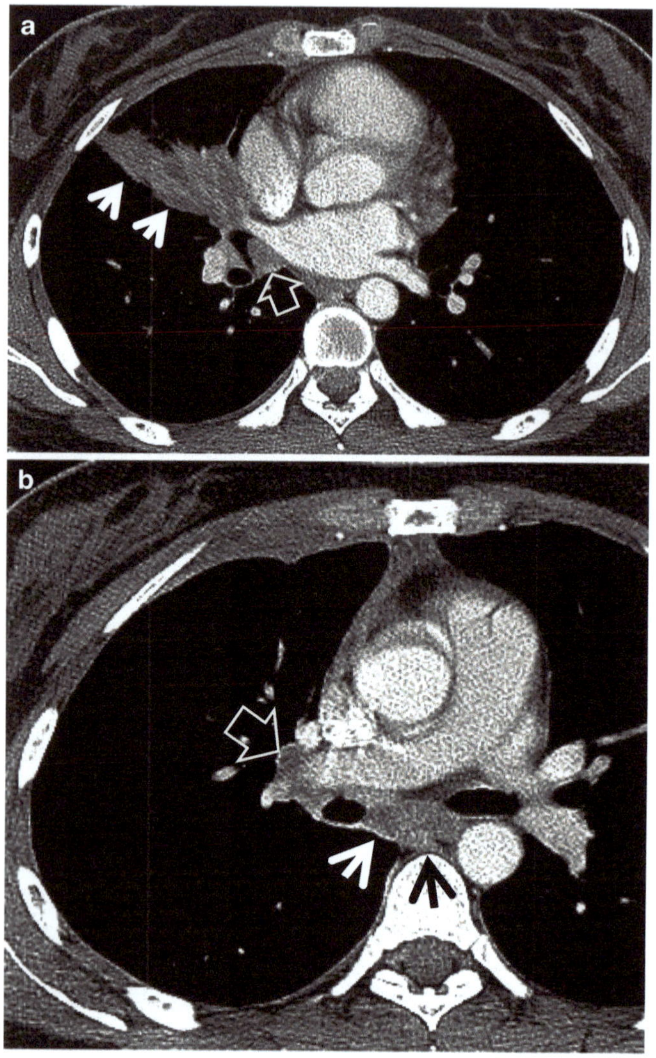


**Fig. 26.2** Tuberculous pneumonia manifesting as segmental consolidation in a 26-year-old woman. (**a**) Mediastinal window of enhanced CT scans (5.0-mm section thickness) obtained at level of basal trunk shows segmental consolidation (*arrows*) in right middle lobe. Also note enlarged right hilar lymph node (*open arrow*). (**b**) CT scan obtained at level of distal left main bronchus demonstrates enlarged and necrotic subcarinal lymph node (*arrows*) and right hilar node (*open arrow*)

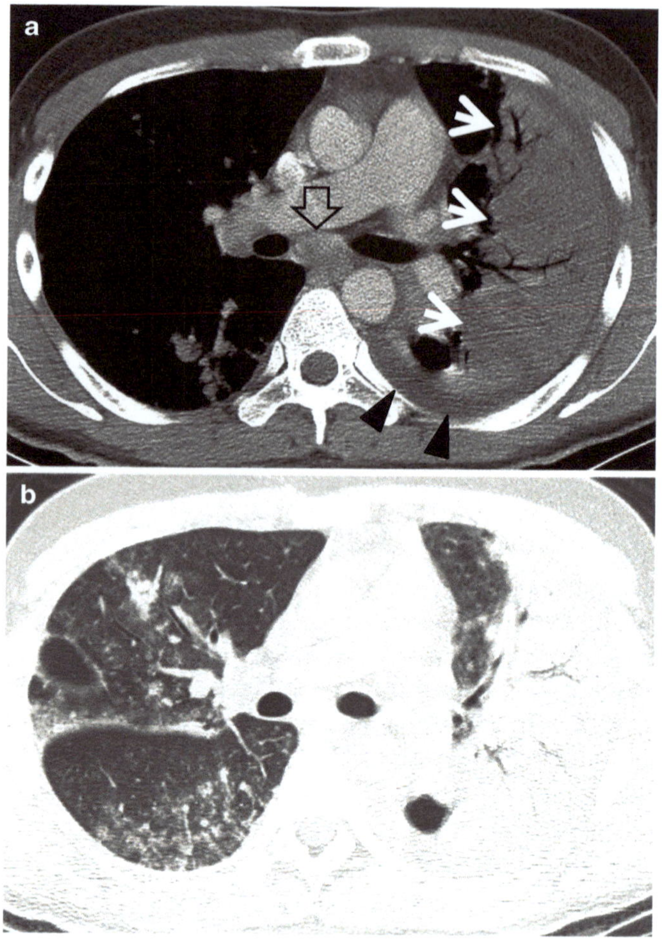


**Fig. 26.3** Lobar consolidation as a manifestation of pulmonary tuberculosis in a 24-year-old man. (**a**) Mediastinal window of enhanced CT scans (5.0-mm section thickness) obtained at level of main bronchi shows lobar consolidation (*arrows*) in left upper lobe. Some parenchymal lesions are also seen in right lung. Note enlarged subcarinal lymph node (*open arrow*) and left pleural effusion (*arrowheads*). (**b**) Lung window image obtained at the same level to **a** demonstrates adds findings of tree-in-bud signs and small nodules in contralateral right lung suggestive of bronchogenic spread of tuberculous pneumonia

## Bronchopneumonia

Bronchopneumonia is characterized pathologically by patchy, predominantly peribronchiolar inflammation. The reason why this localization is different from lobar pneumonia is unclear but may be related to relatively less abundant edema formation (associated with more difficult spread of infection within the lung) and more virulent organisms (resulting in greater tissue destruction) in bronchopneumonia. Although initially patchy, progression of disease may result in lobular and segmental consolidation (Fig. 26.4). The main causative organisms are *Staphylococcus aureus*, *Haemophilus influenzae*, *Pseudomonas aeruginosa*, and anaerobic bacteria.

Characteristic findings on HRCT include centrilobular small nodules and branching linear structures, airspace nodules, and multifocal lobular consolidation or GGO [1] (Fig. 26.5). The small nodules and branching linear opacities result in an appearance resembling a tree-in-bud and are related to the presence of the inflammatory exudate in the lumen and walls of membranous and respiratory bronchioles and the lung parenchyma immediately adjacent to them (Fig. 26.6). This appearance is similar to cellular bronchiolitis caused by viruses, *Mycoplasma pneumoniae* and *Chlamydia* [1, 4]. Unlike the latter (atypical pneumonias), however, the tree-in-bud pattern in bacterial bronchopneumonia usually comprises only a small proportion of the

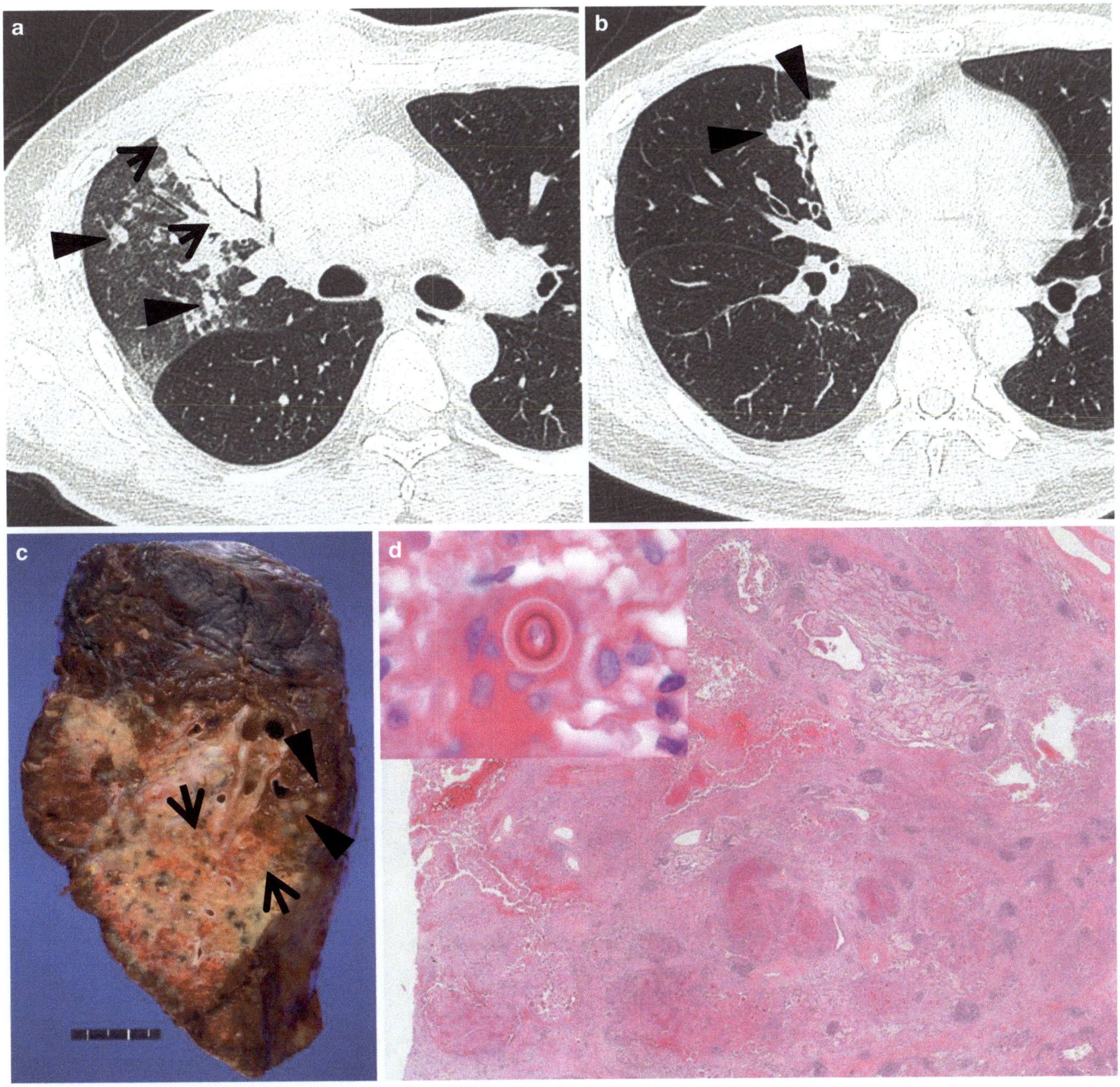


Fig. 26.4 Pulmonary blastomycosis manifesting as morphologic bronchopneumonia in a 45-year-old man. (**a**) Lung window image of thin-section (1.5-mm section thickness) scan obtained at level of main bronchi shows combination of subsegmental consolidation (*arrows*), acinus-sized small nodules (*arrowheads*), smaller nodules, and ground-glass opacity in right upper lobe. (**b**) CT scan obtained at level of basal trunk demonstrates nodular clustering (*arrowheads*) in right middle lobe. (**c**) Gross pathologic specimen obtained with right upper lobectomy depicts mainly consolidative lesion, but also small nodular lesions (*arrowheads*). Lesion has multifocal areas of small abscess (*arrows*). (**d**) Low-magnification (×4) photomicrograph discloses suppurative granulomatous inflammation. *Inset*: double-walled yeast in cytoplasm of multinucleated giant cell consistent with blastomycosis

HRCT abnormalities. In addition, thickening of bronchovascular bundles is more frequently observed in atypical pneumonia, in which individual opacity tends to be distributed at the inner zone in addition to the middle and outer zones and be recognized smaller than those of bacterial pneumonias [1] (Fig. 26.5).

Pulmonary tuberculosis also presents with prototypical morphologic dense bronchopneumonia. On CT, the lesion consists of tree-in-bud pattern, acinar nodule, lobular consolidation, and cavitating or noncavitating nodules or subsegmental or segmental consolidation. Bronchial wall thickening may be associated [2] (Fig. 26.6).

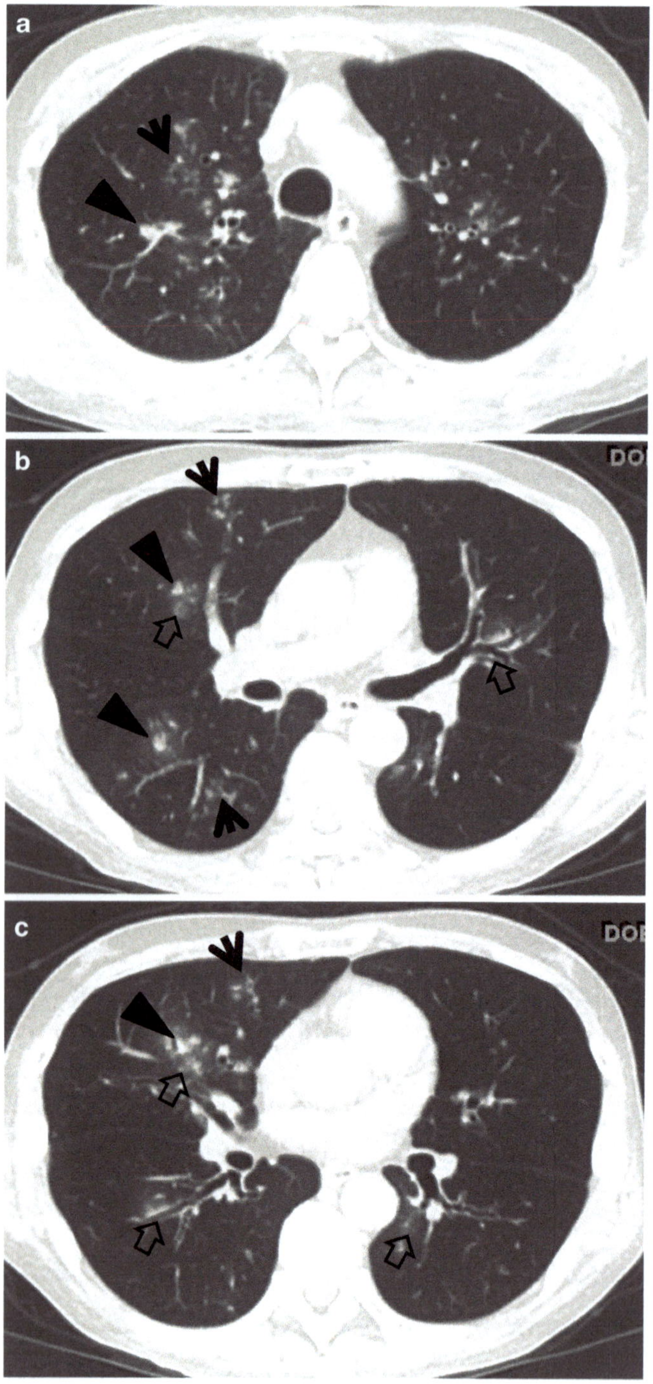


**Fig. 26.5** *Mycoplasma pneumoniae* pneumonia in a 29-year-old man who received hematopoietic stem cell transplantation owing to acute myeloid leukemia. (**a–c**) CT scans (2.5-mm section thickness) obtained at levels of aortic arch (**a**), bronchus intermedius (**b**), and basal trunks (**c**), respectively, show lung abnormalities comprising tree-in-bud signs (*arrows*), small nodules (*arrowheads*) and ground-glass opacity lesions (*open arrows*) in both lungs. Please note involvement of both central and peripheral portions of lungs

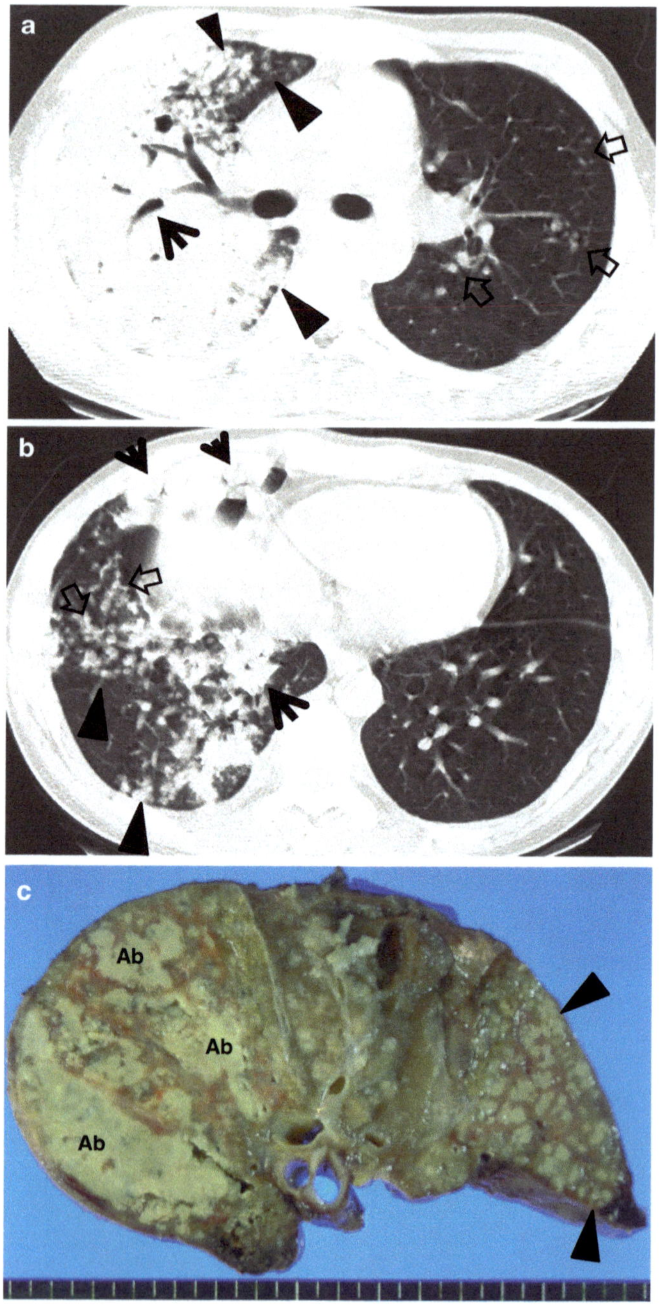


**Fig. 26.6** Bronchopneumonia in tuberculous infection in a 26-year-old man. (**a**) Lung window image of CT scan (5.0-mm section thickness) obtained at level of right upper lobar bronchus shows extensive bronchopneumonia consisting of cavitary consolidation (*arrow*), variable-sized nodules (*arrowheads*), and dilated bronchi in right upper lobe. Also note bronchogenic spread of infection to contralateral left lung (*open arrows*). (**b**) CT scan obtained at level of liver dome demonstrate less extensive bronchopneumonia involving right lower and middle lobes. Abnormality contains lobular consolidation (*arrows*), variable-sized nodules (*arrowheads*), and tree-in-bud signs (*open arrows*). (**c**) Gross pathologic specimen obtained with right pneumonectomy discloses tuberculous abscess (*Ab*) of yellow creamy necrotic materials seen as consolidation on CT scan, consolidation, variable-sized nodules, and nodular branching structures (*arrowheads*) shown as tree-in-bud signs at CT

## Interstitial Pneumonia

Interstitial pneumonia is characterized histologically by a mononuclear inflammatory cell infiltrate in the alveolar septa and interstitial tissue surrounding small parenchymal vessels (Figs. 26.7 and 26.8). The most common causes are *Mycoplasma pneumoniae*, viruses, and *Pneumocystis jiroveci*. Because *Mycoplasma pneumonia*e pneumonia and *Pneumocystis* pneumonia were described in other chapters, focused descriptions on viral pneumonias are rendered in this chapter.

The following are common pathologic findings in viral pneumonia: viruses can result in several pathologic forms of lower respiratory tract infection including tracheobronchitis, cellular bronchiolitis, and pneumonia. Because viral organisms replicate within tissue cells, the most prominent histologic changes are observed in the epithelium and adjacent interstitium. In tracheobronchitis, airway walls are congested and lumen contains mononuclear cell infiltrates. Degeneration and desquamation of the epithelial cells are seen. Cellular bronchiolitis, particularly important in children, appears with epithelial necrosis, neutrophilic exudate in the airway lumen, and predominantly mononuclear infiltrates in its wall. Parenchymal involvement, the pneumonia, starts with the involvement of the lung adjacent to the terminal and respiratory bronchioles; however, extension throughout the lobule may occur (Fig. 26.7). Rapidly progressive pneumonia may occur particularly in the elderly and in

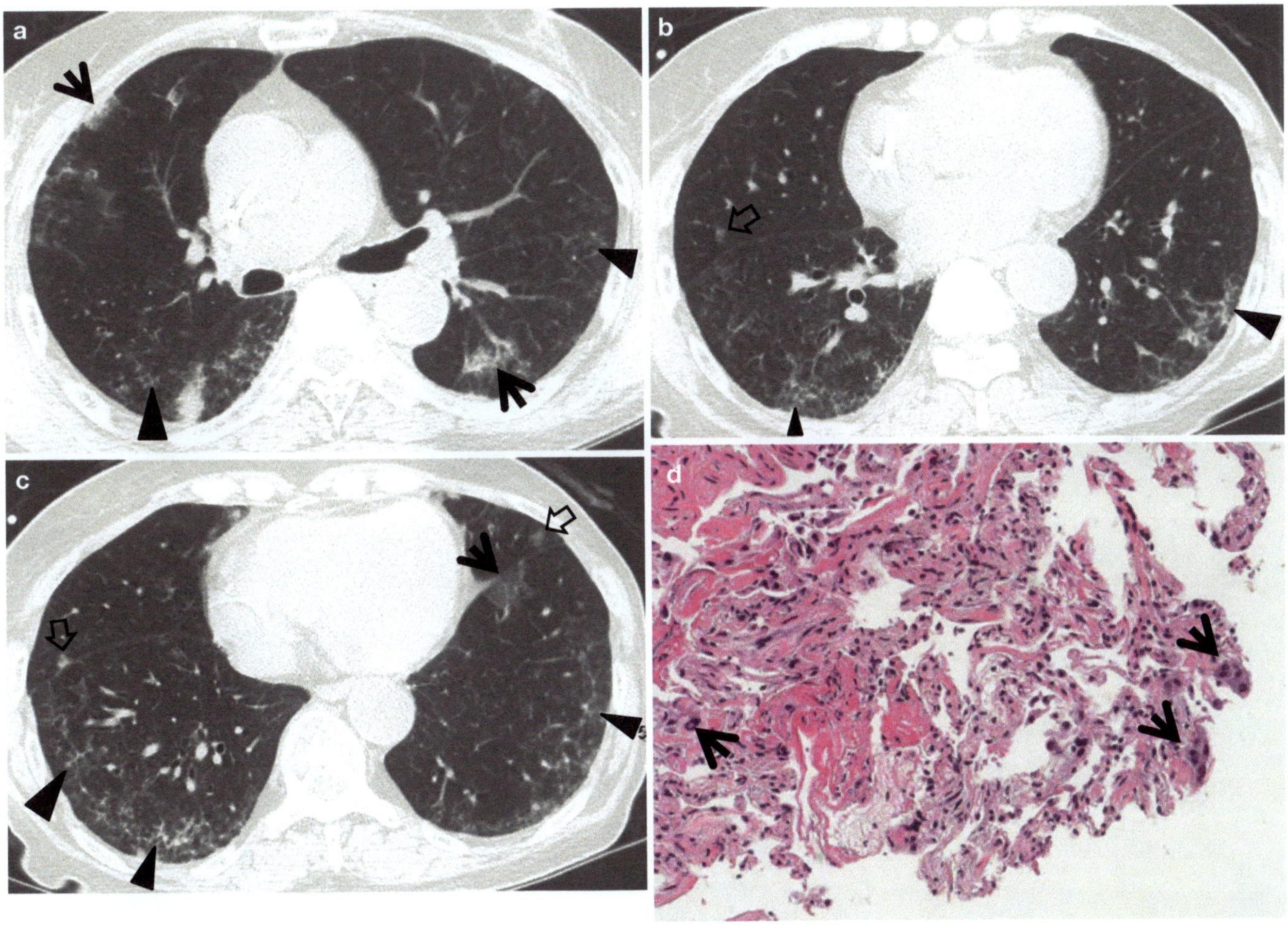


**Fig. 26.7** Cytomegalovirus pneumonia over a follow-up period of 3 weeks in a 68-year-old woman with diffuse large B-cell lymphoma. (**a**–**c**) Lung window images of CT scans (2.5-mm section thickness) obtained at levels of distal main bronchi (**a**), right inferior pulmonary vein (**b**), and cardiac ventricles (**c**), respectively, show bilateral bronchopneumonia pattern of lung abnormality comprising parenchymal opacity (*arrows*), tree-in-bud patterns (*arrowheads*), and variable-sized nodules (*open arrows*). (**d**) High-magnification photomicrograph of pathologic specimen obtained with transbronchial lung biopsy from left lower lobe discloses diffuse alveolar damage with fibrinous exudate and interstitial fibroblastic proliferation. Note suspicious viral inclusion (*arrows*) in atypical pneumocytes. (**e**) High-magnification (×400) photomicrograph reveals a pneumocyte harboring intranuclear large viral inclusion (*arrow*), which is single, basophilic, and round to oval with peripheral halo. *Inset*: immunohistochemical staining (ABC methods, ×200) for cytomegalovirus showing many infected pneumocytes

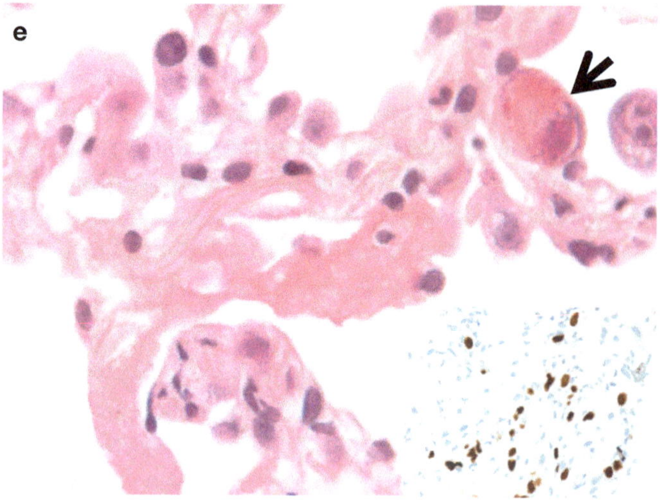


Fig. 26.7 (continued)

immunocompromised patients where the lungs histologically show diffuse alveolar damage comprising interstitial lymphocyte infiltration, airspace hemorrhage, edema and fibrin, type 2 cell hyperplasia, and hyaline membrane formation [5] (Figs. 26.7 and 26.8).

Viral pneumonia manifest radiologically as poorly defined nodules (airspace nodules of 4–10 mm in diameter) and patchy areas of peribronchial GGO and airspace consolidation. Because of the associated cellular bronchiolitis, hyperinflation is commonly present [5–7]. Progressive pneumonia shows the rapid confluence of consolidation leading to diffuse alveolar damage, consisting of homogeneous or patchy unilateral or bilateral airspace consolidation and GGO or poorly defined small centrilobular nodules [5] (Figs. 26.7 and 26.8).

CT parenchymal lung abnormalities may be classified into three main patterns according to the distribution and patterns of

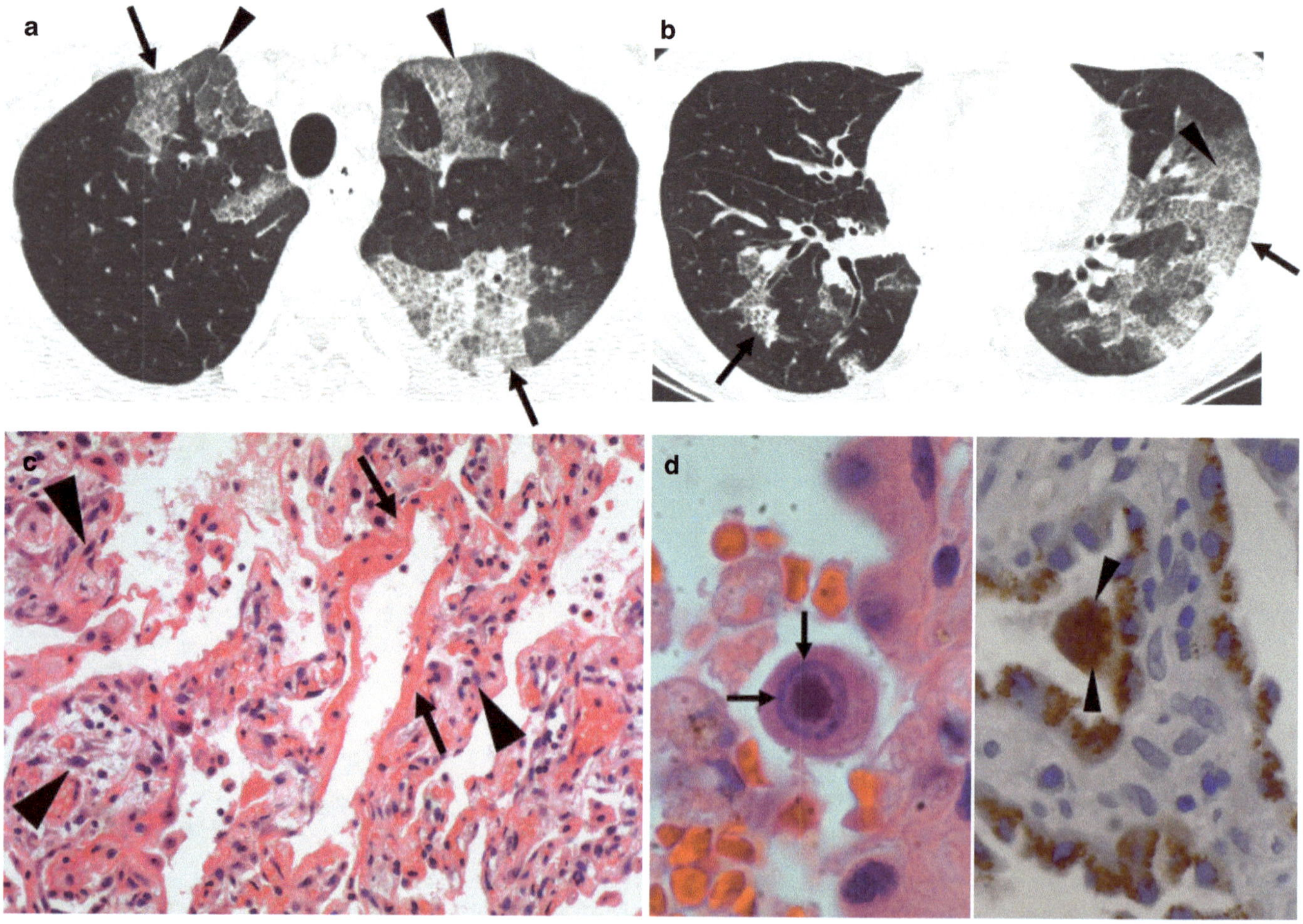


Fig. 26.8 Adenovirus pneumonia in a 35-year-old woman with non-Hodgkin's lymphoma who underwent hematopoietic stem cell transplantation 1 year ago. (**a**, **b**) Lung window images of thin-section (1.0-mm section thickness) CT scan obtained at levels of great vessels (**a**) and right inferior pulmonary vein (**b**), respectively, show extensive and patchy areas of ground-glass opacity (*arrows*) associated with interlobular septal thickening (*arrowheads*) and intralobular reticulation, forming so-called crazy-paving appearance in both lungs. (**c**) High-magnification photomicrograph obtained with surgical lung biopsy from left lower lobe displays intra-alveolar fibrinous exudate forming hyaline membrane (*arrows*) and interstitial fibroblastic proliferation (*arrowheads*) suggestive of mixed exudative and proliferative phase of diffuse alveolar damage (Reprinted from [11] with permission) (**d**) Photomicrographs of pathologic specimen (*left*, ×1,000) and after immunohistochemical staining for adenovirus (*right*, ×100) show alveolar lining cells with intranuclear inclusions (*arrows*, *left*) and poorly demarcated smudges (*arrowheads*, *right*) within nucleus, indicating positivity for adenovirus infection

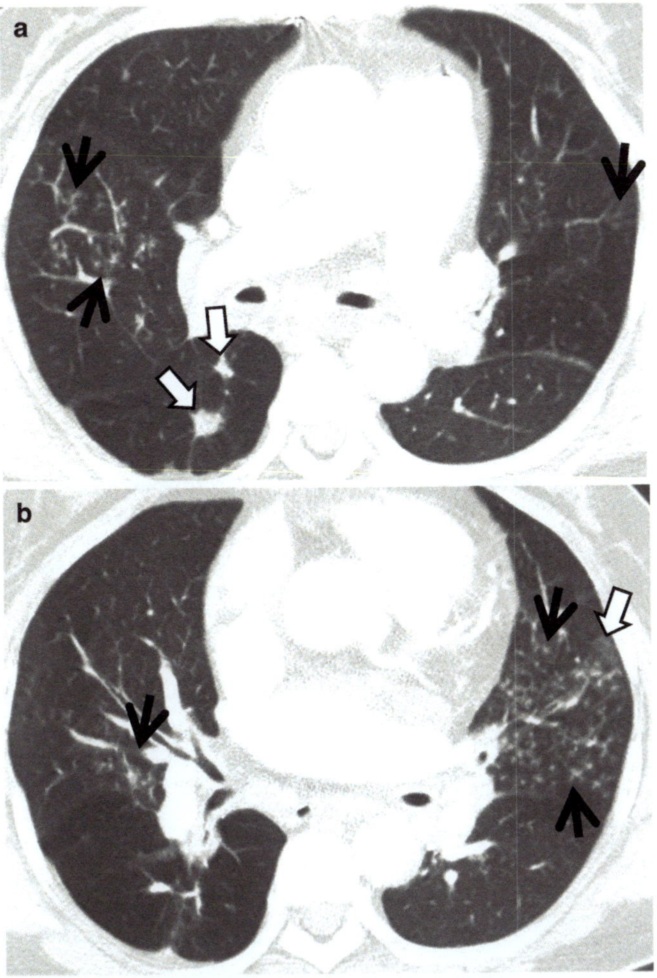

Fig. 26.9 Influenza A (H1N1) pneumonia showing bronchopneumonia pattern in a 68-year-old woman with previous aortic valve replacement. (**a**) Lung window image of CT scan (2.5-mm section thickness) obtained at level of right bronchus intermedius shows multifocal areas of tree-in-bud signs (*arrows*) and lobular consolidation or poorly defined nodules (*open arrows*) in both lungs. Enlarged calcified and ruptured lymph nodes were seen in the bilateral hila and mediastina, indicating possible anthracofibrosis of airways on mediastinal window image. (**b**) CT scan obtained at level of right middle lobar bronchus demonstrates multifocal areas of tree-in-bud sign (*arrows*) and lobular area of ground-glass opacity (*open arrow*) in both lungs (Reprinted from Kang et al. [8] with permission)

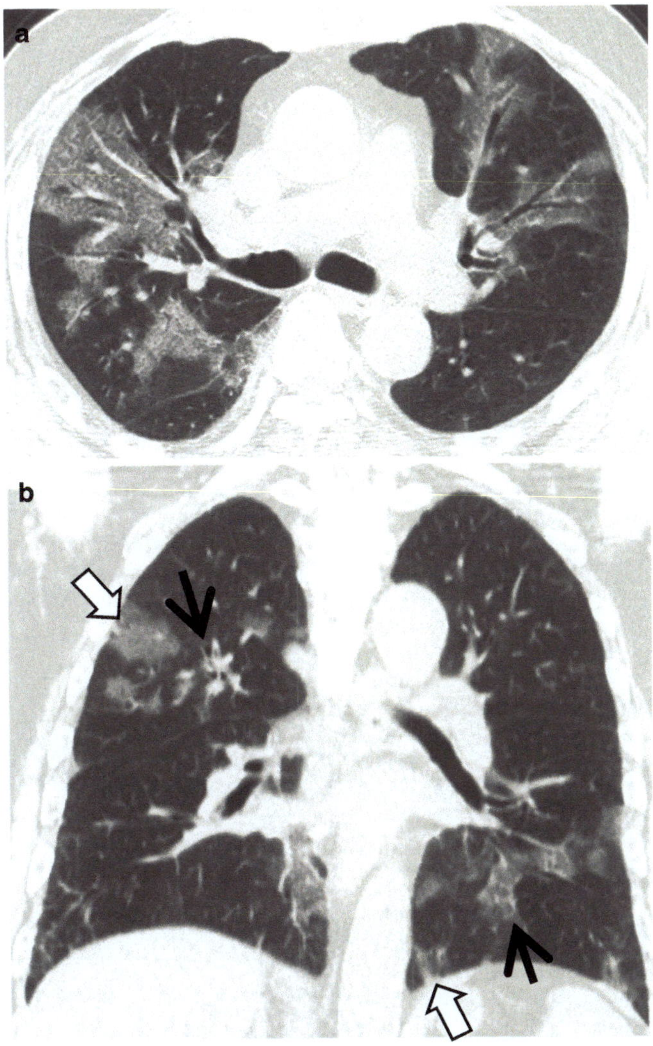

Fig. 26.10 Influenza A (H1N1) pneumonia showing cryptogenic organizing pneumonia pattern in a 66-year-old man. (**a**) Lung window image of CT scan (2.5-mm section thickness) obtained at level of right upper lobar bronchus shows patchy areas of ground-glass opacity distributed mainly along bronchovascular bundles in both lungs. (**b**) Coronal reformatted (2.0-mm section thickness) CT scan also demonstrates parenchymal opacity lesions distributed along bronchovascular bundles (*arrows*) or subpleural (*open arrows*) lungs (Reprinted from Kang et al. [8] with permission)

the lung abnormalities: cryptogenic organizing pneumonia (COP), acute interstitial pneumonia (AIP), and bilateral extensive bronchopneumonia (Figs. 26.9, 26.10, and 26.11). This classification may help stratify patients with viral pneumonia in terms of their prognoses. In a particular viral pneumonia (influenza A [H1N1] pneumonia), patients with bronchopneumonia pattern have a tendency to belong to the mild illness group, whereas patients with AIP pattern show more severe clinical course in their outcome [8]. According to one study, CT findings in patients having a mild pneumonia course consist mainly of inflammatory lesions involving large or small airways with focal centrilobular small nodules with tree-in-bud sign and bronchiolar wall thickening [9]. Fatal cases of the same pneumonia present as areas of consolidation with or without GGO on CT scans (AIP pattern) and the abnormalities are pathologically correlated with diffuse alveolar damage [10]. Therefore, it seems that pattern and extent of lung lesions observed at CT in viral pneumonias may be a determining factor for predicting patient's clinical course and prognosis [8].

The radiologic findings of adult viral pneumonias are variable and overlapping (Table 26.1). Specific organism diagnosis of a viral pneumonia cannot be made on the basis of imaging features alone. Clinical features such as patient age, immune status, time of year, illness in other family members, community outbreaks, onset, severity, duration of symptoms, and the presence of a rash remain as important aids in diagnosing viral causes of both atypical pneumonia and pneumonia in immunocompromised patients [5].

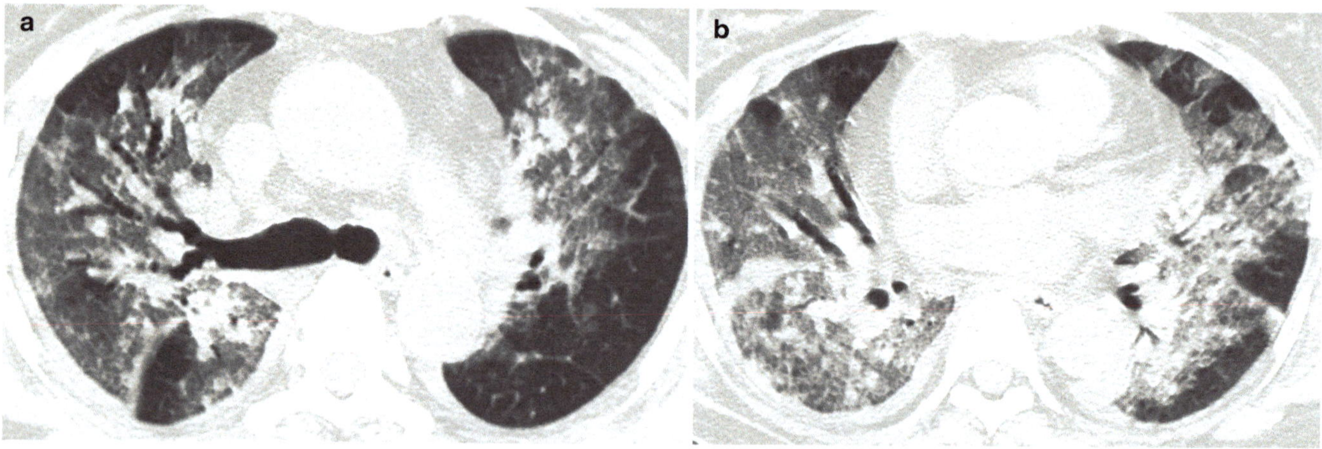


**Fig. 26.11** Influenza A (H1N1) pneumonia showing acute interstitial pneumonia pattern in a 58-year-old woman with multiple myeloma. (**a**, **b**) Lung window images of CT scan (2.5-mm section thickness) obtained at level of right upper lobar bronchus (**a**) and lower lobar bronchi (**b**), respectively, show patchy and extensive parenchymal opacity lesions without specific zonal predominance in both lungs. Additionally, traction bronchiectasis is noted in right upper lobe, suggesting proliferative phase of diffuse alveolar damage. Lesions progressed on follow-up chest radiographs and patient died of the disease in following 6 days (Reprinted from Kang et al. [8] with permission)

**Table 26.1** Summary of CT findings in viral pneumonias

| | Centrilobular nodules | GGO with lobular distribution | Segmental consolidation | Thickened interlobular septa | Diffuse GGO |
|---|---|---|---|---|---|
| Influenza | +++ | +++ | | | + |
| Measles | ++ | + | + | + | + |
| Hantavirus | | | ++ | + | +++ |
| Adenovirus | ++ | + | +++ | | |
| HSV | + | +++ | +++ | | + |
| VZV | +++ | + | | | |
| CMV | ++ | ++ | + | + | ++ |
| EBV | + | + | + | | + |

Reprinted from Kim et al. [5] with permission

*Note*: *HSV* herpes simplex virus, *VZV* varicella-zoster virus, *CMV* cytomegalovirus, *EBV* Epstein–Barr virus, *GGO* ground-glass opacity

## Referen ces


1. Tanaka N, Matsumoto T, Kuramitsu T, et al. High resolution CT findings in community-acquired pneumonia. J Comput Assist Tomogr. 1996;20:600–8.
2. Lee JY, Lee KS, Jung KJ, et al. Pulmonary tuberculosis: CT and pathologic correlation. J Comput Assist Tomogr. 2000;24:691–8.
3. Ikezoe J, Takeuchi N, Johkoh T, et al. CT appearance of pulmonary tuberculosis in diabetic and immunocompromised patients: comparison with patients who had no underlying disease. AJR Am J Roentgenol. 1992;159:1175–9.
4. Reittner P, Muller NL, Heyneman L, et al. Mycoplasma pneumoniae pneumonia: radiographic and high-resolution CT features in 28 patients. AJR Am J Roentgenol. 2000;174:37–41.
5. Kim EA, Lee KS, Primack SL, et al. Viral pneumonias in adults: radiologic and pathologic findings. Radiographics. 2002;22(Spec No):S137–49.
6. Han BK, Son JA, Yoon HK, Lee SI. Epidemic adenoviral lower respiratory tract infection in pediatric patients: radiographic and clinical characteristics. AJR Am J Roentgenol. 1998;170:1077–80.
7. Moon JH, Kim EA, Lee KS, Kim TS, Jung KJ, Song JH. Cytomegalovirus pneumonia: high-resolution CT findings in ten non-AIDS immunocompromised patients. Korean J Radiol. 2000;1:73–8.
8. Kang H, Lee KS, Jeong YJ, Lee HY, Kim KI, Nam KJ. Computed tomography findings of influenza A (H1N1) pneumonia in adults: pattern analysis and prognostic comparisons. J Comput Assist Tomogr. 2012;36:285–90.
9. Kim SY, Kim JS, Park CS. Various computed tomography findings of 2009 H1N1 influenza in 17 patients with relatively mild illness. Jpn J Radiol. 2011;29:301–6.
10. Marchiori E, Zanetti G, Fontes CA, et al. Influenza A (H1N1) virus-associated pneumonia: high-resolution computed tomography-pathologic correlation. Eur J Radiol. 2011;80:e500–4.
11. Chong S, et al. Adenovirus pneumonia in adults: radiographic and high-resolution CT findings in five patients. AJR Am J Roentgenol. 2006;186:1288–93.

# Drug-Induced Lung Disease

# 27

Drug-induced lung injury is seen as a wide variety of histologic reaction patterns and thus as diverse CT findings. The most common are interstitial pneumonia and fibrosis (either usual interstitial pneumonia [UIP] or nonspecific interstitial pneumonia [NSIP]), eosinophilic pneumonia (including DRESS syndrome; drug reaction with eosinophilia and systemic symptoms), cryptogenic organizing pneumonia (COP), diffuse alveolar damage (DAD), and hypersensitivity pneumonia [1, 2]. Other reactions such as granulomatous pneumonitis, vasculitis, alveolar proteinosis, obliterative bronchiolitis, and veno-occlusive disease are uncommon [2]. None of these histologic patterns is specific for either drug reaction in general or the reaction to a particular drug. Consequently, the diagnosis of drug-induced lung disease is based on a combination of radiologic, clinical, and histologic (when imperative) findings in a patient who has received a drug known to cause the abnormalities.

## Interstitial Pneumonitis and Fibrosis

One of the most common forms of drug-induced pneumonitis is nonspecific interstitial pneumonia (NSIP) [1, 2] (Fig. 27.1). This is characterized histologically by homogeneous alveolar wall thickening by fibrous tissue and mononuclear inflammatory cells. The reaction is seen most commonly in association with methotrexate, amiodarone, or carmustine toxicity (Table 27.1). The corresponding thin-section CT (TSCT) findings usually consist of patchy or diffuse areas of ground-glass opacity (GGO) (Fig. 27.1). With progression, there may be evidence of fibrosis, including reticulation, traction bronchiectasis, and honeycombing. The abnormalities show typically lower lung zone predominance. In some patients, the fibrosis is patchy in distribution and predominantly peribronchovascular; fibrotic NSIP pattern, commonly in patients receiving nitrofurantoin [3].

The second most common histologic form of drug-induced interstitial pneumonitis is usual interstitial pneumonia (UIP) (Fig. 27.2). This is characterized histologically by a heterogeneous pattern of chronic inflammation and fibrosis, with foci of dense and loose (fibroblastic) connective tissue being present in the same lobule. Progression of the interstitial disease leads to obliteration of alveolar airspaces by mature fibrous tissue associated with dilatation of residual transitional airways (honeycombing). This pattern of injury occurs most commonly in association with cytotoxic chemotherapeutic agents such as bleomycin, busulfan, methotrexate, doxorubicin, and carmustine. Noncytotoxic drugs such as nitrofurantoin, amiodarone, gold, and penicillamine also result in this reaction occasionally.

The predominant findings on TSCT are those of fibrosis with or without associated areas of consolidation. The fibrosis is characterized by the presence of irregular reticular opacities, honeycombing, architectural distortion, and traction bronchiectasis (Fig. 27.2). On TSCT, the abnormalities are usually bilateral and symmetric, with predominant lower lung zone involvement. A peripheral and subpleural distribution of abnormalities is common [1, 4].

## Eosinophilic Pneumonia

Eosinophilic pneumonia is characterized histologically by the accumulation of eosinophils in the alveolar airspaces and infiltration of the adjacent interstitial space by eosinophils and variable numbers of lymphocytes and plasma cells. Peripheral eosinophilia is present in up to 40 % of patients. As a drug reaction, it is seen most commonly in association with methotrexate, sulfasalazine, para-aminosalicylic acid, nitrofurantoin, and nonsteroidal anti-inflammatory drugs.

DRESS syndrome, standing for drug reaction (rash) with eosinophilia and systemic symptoms, is caused by exposure to certain medication, which may cause a rash, fever, inflammation of internal organs, lymphadenopathy, and characteristic hematologic abnormalities such as eosinophilia, thrombocytopenia, and atypical lymphocytes [5].

K.S. Lee et al., *Radiology Illustrated: Chest Radiology*, Radiology Illustrated,
DOI 10.1007/978-3-642-37096-0_27, © Springer-Verlag Berlin Heidelberg 2014

TSCT exhibits bilateral airspace consolidation, which tends to involve mainly the peripheral lung regions and the upper lobes [6, 7] (Fig. 27.3).

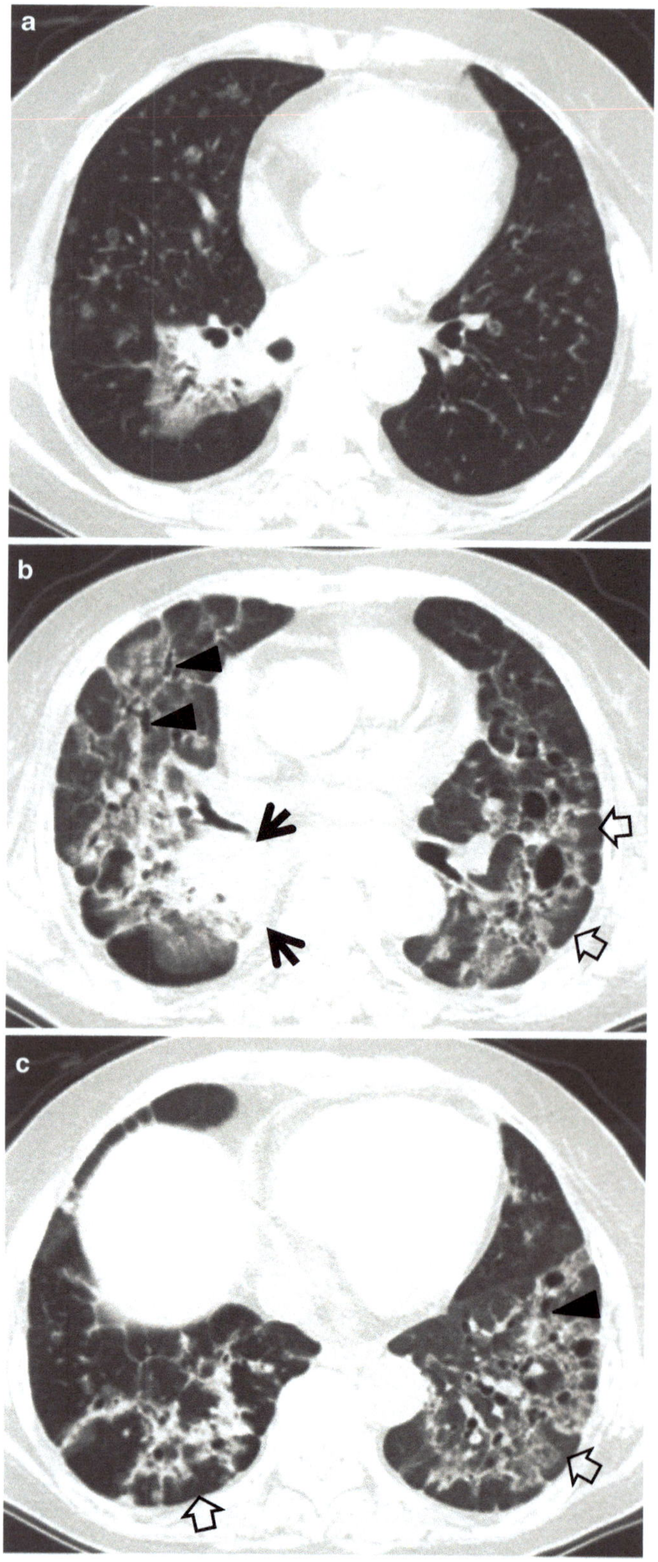


Fig. 27.1 Iressa (gefitinib)-associated pulmonary fibrosis of nonspecific interstitial pneumonia pattern of pulmonary fibrosis in a 75-year-old woman with lung adenocarcinoma. (**a**) Lung window image of CT scan (2.5-mm section thickness) obtained at level of right inferior pulmonary vein shows a 59-mm-sized mass in superior segment of right lower lobe and innumerable small cavitating and noncavitating nodules in both lungs (suggestive of pulmonary metastases). Patient received Iressa (gefitinib) chemotherapy. (**b**, **c**) Eighteen-month follow-up CT scans obtained at levels of right middle lobar bronchus (**b**) and liver dome (**c**), respectively, demonstrate still visible mass (*arrows* in **b**) in right lower lobe. Please also note ground-glass opacity, reticulation, traction bronchiectasis (*arrowheads*), and cystic lung changes in both lungs. Subpleural sparing (*open arrows*) and lung fibrosis of deep central involvement are noticed

Table 27.1 CT patterns of drug-induced lung disease and drugs causing such patterns of lung abnormality

| CT patterns | Associated drugs |
|---|---|
| Interstitial pneumonia and fibrosis (UIP or NSIP) | Methotrexate, amiodarone, carmustine, nitrofurantoin, bleomycin, busulfan, cyclophosphamide, doxorubicin, gold, penicillamine, gefitinib, sorafenib |
| Eosinophilic pneumonia | Methotrexate, sulfasalazine, para-aminosalicylic acid (PAS), nitrofurantoin, nonsteroidal anti-inflammatory drugs (NSAID) |
| Cryptogenic organizing pneumonia | Methotrexate, cyclophosphamide, carmustine, gold, nitrofurantoin, amiodarone, bleomycin, busulfan, erlotinib, sorafenib |
| Diffuse alveolar damage | Bleomycin, busulfan, cyclophosphamide, methotrexate, amiodarone, aspirin, narcotics, gefitinib |
| Hypersensitivity pneumonia | Nitrofurantoin, gefitinib, erlotinib |

*Note*: *UIP* usual interstitial pneumonia, *NSIP* nonspecific interstitial pneumonia

## Cryptogenic Organizing Pneumonia

Cryptogenic organizing pneumonia (COP) is characterized by parenchymal interstitial infiltration by mononuclear inflammatory cells and obliteration of the lumens of respiratory bronchioles, alveolar ducts, and (usually to a lesser extent) alveoli by fibroblastic tissue. The reaction has been reported most frequently in association with methotrexate, cyclophosphamide, gold, nitrofurantoin, amiodarone, bleomycin, and busulfan. On thin-section CT, the areas of consolidation often have a predominantly peripheral or peribronchovascular distribution [2, 8] (Fig. 27.4).

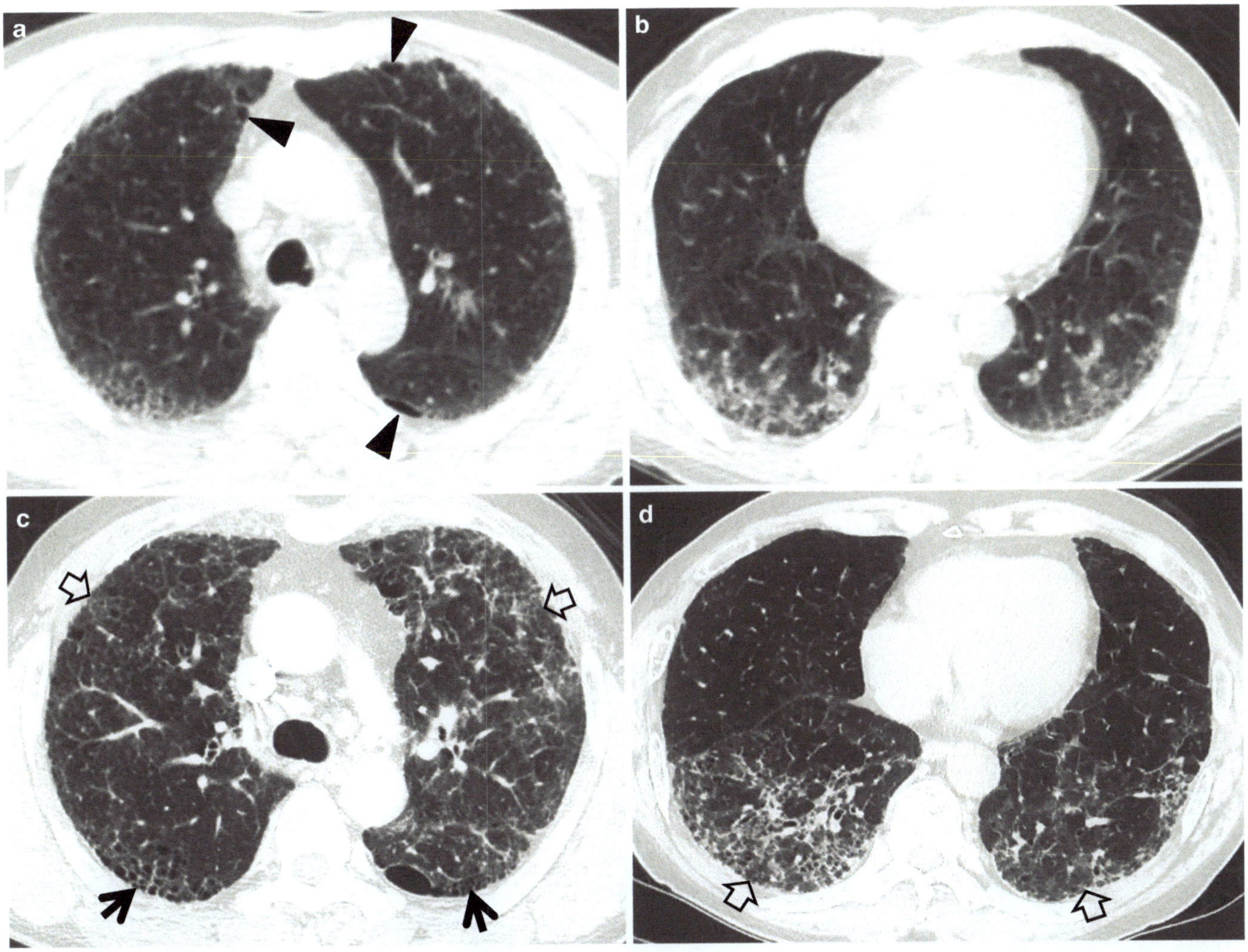


**Fig. 27.2** Gemcitabine-induced pulmonary fibrosis of usual interstitial pneumonia pattern in a 69-year-old man with pancreas head cancer. (**a**, **b**) Lung window images of CT scans (5.0-mm section thickness) obtained at levels of azygos arch (**a**) and cardiac ventricle (**b**), respectively, show combined pulmonary emphysema (*arrowheads*) and fibrosis (ground-glass opacity and reticulation) in both lungs. (**c**, **d**) Two-month follow-up CT scans obtained at similar levels to (**a**) and (**b**), respectively, demonstrate progressive pulmonary fibrosis with new appearance of honeycomb cysts (*arrows*) and increased extent of reticulation (*open arrows*)

## Diffuse Alveolar Damage

Diffuse alveolar damage (DAD) is characterized by the presence of alveolar airspace and interstitial edema, hyaline membrane formation, and proliferation of type II pneumocytes. In relation to drug-induced pulmonary disease, it occurs most commonly in association with cytotoxic agents such as bleomycin, aspirin, and narcotics. The corresponding radiologic features are those of adult respiratory distress syndrome (ARDS). TSCT demonstrates extensive bilateral areas of GGO and dependent airspace consolidation [9] (Fig. 27.5).

## Hypersensitivity Pneumonia

Hypersensitivity pneumonitis (HP) is a relatively uncommon manifestation of drug-induced lung toxicity. HP is histologically characterized by the presence of cellular bronchiolitis, peribronchiolar noncaseating granulomas, and lymphocytic interstitial pneumonia. On TSCT scans, HP is shown as small, poorly defined centrilobular nodules or widespread areas of GGO. TSCT images obtained at the end of maximal expiration may exhibit lobular areas of decreased attenuation and vascularity, representing air trapping. Conditions of HP may occur after gefitinib or erlotinib treatment [10] (Fig. 27.6).

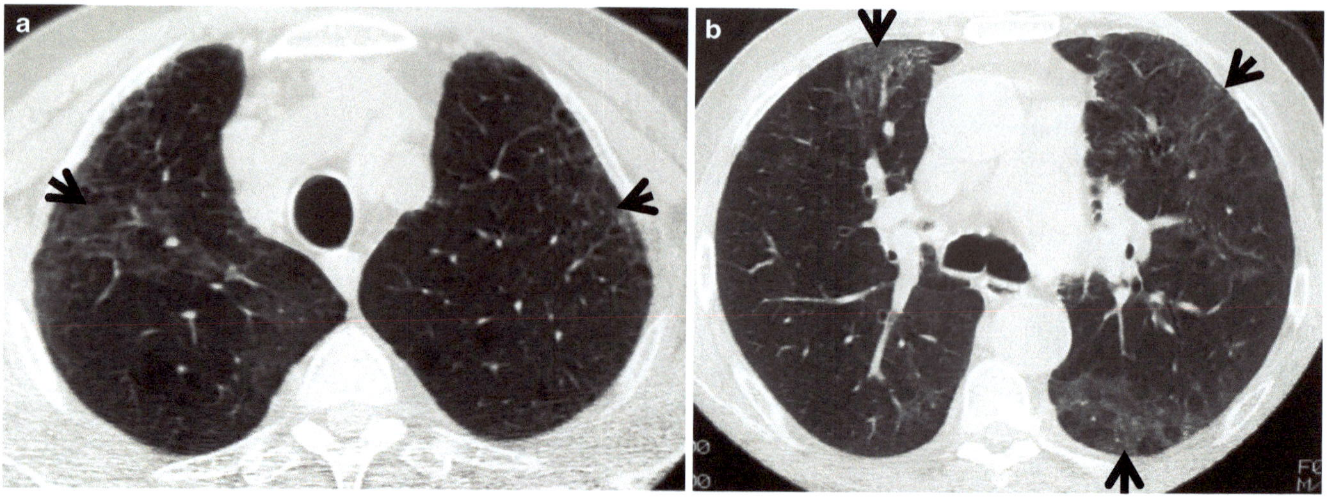


**Fig. 27.3** Methotrexate-associated eosinophilic lung disease in a 50-year-old man with Crohn's disease. (**a**, **b**) Lung window images of CT scans (5.0-mm section thickness) obtained at levels of great vessels (**a**) and main bronchi (**b**), respectively, show patchy areas of ground-glass opacity (*arrows*) in both lungs. Also note several areas of emphysema in upper lung zones. His peripheral blood eosinophil count was abnormally high and parenchymal opacity disappeared after cessation of methotrexate therapy

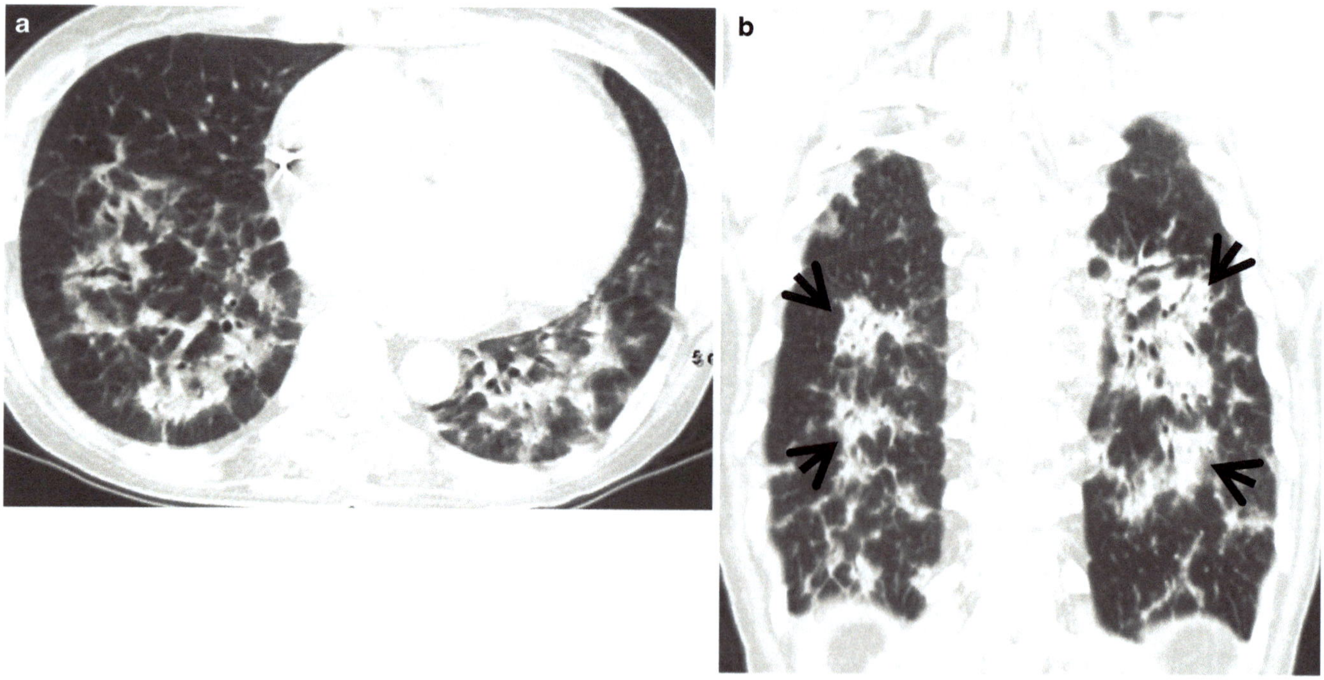


**Fig. 27.4** Amiodarone-induced interstitial lung disease of cryptogenic organizing pneumonia pattern in a 60-year-old man with arrhythmia. (**a**) Lung window image of CT scan (5.0-mm section thickness) obtained at level of cardiac ventricle shows patchy areas of consolidation in both lower lobes. (**b**) Coronal reformatted image (2.5-mm section thickness) demonstrates multifocal areas of consolidation (*arrows*), distributed mainly along bronchovascular bundles

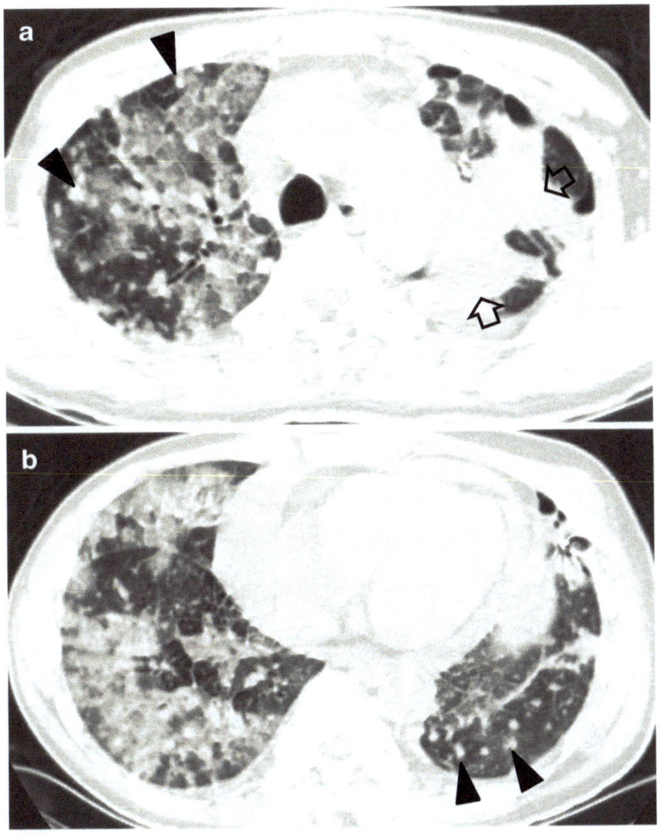


**Fig. 27.5** Iressa (gefitinib)-associated lung disease of acute interstitial pneumonia (diffuse alveolar damage) pattern in a 40-year-old man with lung adenocarcinoma (primary tumor in left lung, lung-to-lung and extrathoracic metastases). (**a**, **b**) Lung window images of CT scans (5.0-mm section thickness) obtained at levels of aortic arch (**a**) and cardiac ventricle (**b**), respectively, show patchy, extensive, and mixed areas of parenchymal consolidation and ground-glass opacity in both lungs. Also note primary cancer (*open arrows*) and lung-to-lung metastatic nodules (*arrowheads*). Patient took Iressa for 3 months

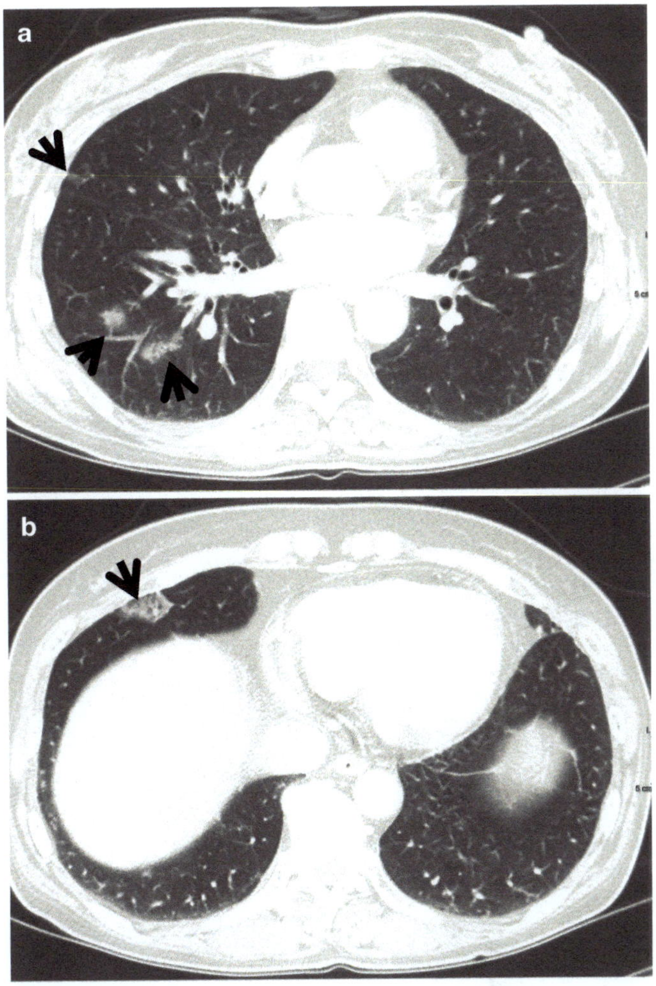


**Fig. 27.6** Iressa (gefitinib)-induced hypersensitivity pneumonia in a 53-year-old woman with lung adenocarcinoma and lung-to-lung metastases. (**a**, **b**) Lung window images of CT scans (5.0-mm section thickness) obtained at levels of inferior pulmonary veins (**a**) and liver dome (**b**), respectively, show patchy areas of parenchymal ground-glass opacity (*arrows*) in both lungs. The lesions disappeared spontaneously without any treatment

## References


1. Min JH, Lee HY, Lim H, et al. Drug-induced interstitial lung disease in tyrosine kinase inhibitor therapy for non-small cell lung cancer: a review on current insight. Cancer Chemother Pharmacol. 2011;68:1099–109.
2. Rossi SE, Erasmus JJ, McAdams HP, Sporn TA, Goodman PC. Pulmonary drug toxicity: radiologic and pathologic manifestations. Radiographics. 2000;20:1245–59.
3. Pietra GG. Pathologic mechanisms of drug-induced lung disorders. J Thorac Imaging. 1991;6:1–7.
4. Padley SP, Adler B, Hansell DM, Muller NL. High-resolution computed tomography of drug-induced lung disease. Clin Radiol. 1992;46:232–6.
5. Bocquet H, Bagot M, Roujeau JC. Drug-induced pseudolymphoma and drug hypersensitivity syndrome (drug rash with eosinophilia and systemic symptoms: DRESS). Semin Cutan Med Surg. 1996;15:250–7.
6. Cooper Jr JA, White DA, Matthay RA. Drug-induced pulmonary disease. Part 2: noncytotoxic drugs. Am Rev Respir Dis. 1986;133:488–505.
7. Searles G, McKendry RJ. Methotrexate pneumonitis in rheumatoid arthritis: potential risk factors. Four case reports and a review of the literature. J Rheumatol. 1987;14:1164–71.
8. Rosenow 3rd EC, Myers JL, Swensen SJ, Pisani RJ. Drug-induced pulmonary disease. An update. Chest. 1992;102:239–50.
9. Ellis SJ, Cleverley JR, Muller NL. Drug-induced lung disease: high-resolution CT findings. AJR Am J Roentgenol. 2000;175:1019–24.
10. Silva CI, Muller NL. Drug-induced lung diseases: most common reaction patterns and corresponding high-resolution CT manifestations. Semin Ultrasound CT MR. 2006;27:111–6.

# 28 Interstitial Lung Disease in Collagen Vascular Disease

Collagen vascular diseases (CVDs) showing features of interstitial lung disease (ILD) pattern include systemic lupus erythematosus (SLE), rheumatoid arthritis (RA), progressive systemic sclerosis (PSS), dermatomyositis (DM) and polymyositis (PM), ankylosing spondylitis (AS), Sjögren's syndrome, and mixed connective tissue disease (MCTD). Histopathologically, interstitial lung diseases associated with CVD are diverse and include nonspecific interstitial pneumonia (NSIP), usual interstitial pneumonia (UIP), cryptogenic organizing pneumonia (COP), apical fibrosis, diffuse alveolar damage (DAD), and lymphoid interstitial pneumonia (LIP) patterns (Tables 28.1 and 28.2). NSIP accounts for large proportion, especially in PSS, DM and PM, and MCTD. More favorable prognosis in interstitial pneumonia associated with CVDs than in idiopathic interstitial pneumonias (IIPs) may be explained by the larger proportion of NSIP pattern than UIP pattern. Thin-section CT (TSCT) seems to help characterize and determine the extent of ILD in CVDs [1].

## Systemic Lupus Erythematosus (SLE)

Pleuropulmonary involvement occurs in approximately 50–60 % of SLE patients [1]. Most involvements are pleural diseases. In one prospective study including 1,000 patients, lung involvement was identified only in 3 % at the onset of the disease; an additional 7 % developed lung disease over the period of observation [2]. Pulmonary manifestations of SLE comprise both acute and chronic lesions. Acute disease includes pulmonary hemorrhage, acute lupus pneumonitis (Fig. 28.1), and pulmonary edema. Chronic disease such as interstitial pneumonitis and fibrosis is less common in SLE than in other connective tissue disorders [3].

Acute lupus pneumonitis occurs in 1–4 % of patients. Histopathologic findings of acute lupus pneumonitis include alveolar wall damage and necrosis leading to inflammatory cell infiltration, hemorrhage, edema, and hyaline membrane formation. Thrombi in small vessels, associated with an interstitial pneumonitis, have been well documented, although this is an unusual feature of acute lupus pneumonitis [3].

Diffuse interstitial pneumonitis and fibrosis is uncommon; in one series of 120 patients, only 5 (4 %) showed the interstitial lung disease [4]. Pathologic findings in these cases are those of UIP or NSIP pattern (Fig. 28.2). A few cases of COP pattern have been reported [1].

Radiographic evidence of interstitial fibrosis, consisting of a reticular pattern involving mainly the lower lung zones, is seen in only about 3 % of patients who have SLE. By contrast, interstitial abnormalities are seen in approximately 30 % of patients on TSCT [5, 6]. These include interlobular septal thickening (33 %), irregular linear opacity (33 %), and architectural distortion (22 %). Such abnormalities are usually mild and focal; diffuse disease occurs in only 4 % of patients [4]. Honeycombing (HC) is uncommon. Ground-glass opacity (GGO) and consolidation on TSCT may reflect the presence of interstitial pneumonitis and fibrosis, acute lupus pneumonitis, hemorrhage or, occasionally, COP pattern of lung abnormality.

**Table 28.1** Frequency of involvement of interstitial pneumonia and other pulmonary diseases in various collagen vascular diseases

| | SLE | RA | PSS | DM/PM | Sjögren's syndrome | MCTD |
|---|---|---|---|---|---|---|
| UIP | + | ++ | ++ | ++ | + | ++ |
| NSIP | + | + | ++++ | ++++ | + | +++ |
| DAD | ++ | + | + | + | | |
| BOOP | + | | + | ++ | + | |
| LIP | | | | | +++ | + |
| Hemorrhage | +++ | | | | | |
| Airway disease | | ++ | | | ++ | |

Reprinted from Kim et al. [1] with permission

*Note*: *UIP* usual interstitial pneumonia, *NSIP* nonspecific interstitial pneumonia, *DAD* diffuse alveolar damage, *BOOP* bronchiolitis obliterans organizing pneumonia, *LIP* lymphocytic interstitial pneumonia, *SLE* systemic lupus erythematosus, *RA* rheumatoid arthritis, *PSS* progressive systemic sclerosis, *DM* dermatomyositis, *PM* polymyositis, *MCTD* mixed connective tissue disease

K.S. Lee et al., *Radiology Illustrated: Chest Radiology*, Radiology Illustrated,
DOI 10.1007/978-3-642-37096-0_28, © Springer-Verlag Berlin Heidelberg 2014

**Table 28.2** Most common pathologic and radiologic findings of idiopathic interstitial pneumonias

| Histologic pattern | Pathology | Radiologic findings: Common radiographic findings | Distribution on CT | Usual CT findings |
|---|---|---|---|---|
| UIP | Architectural destruction, fibrosis with HC, fibroblastic foci; alternating areas of normal lung, inflammation, fibrosis, and honeycombing (temporally heterogeneous) | Reticular abnormality with volume loss, basal | Peripheral, subpleural, basal | Irregular linear opacity, HC, traction bronchiectasis/bronchiolectasis, architectural distortion, focal ground-glass opacities |
| NSIP | Varying proportion of interstitial inflammation and fibrosis, divided into cellular (inflammation) and fibrosing (fibrosis) patterns; patchy with intervening normal lung; temporally uniform | GGO and reticular opacity, basal | Peripheral, subpleural, basal, symmetric | GGO, irregular linear opacities, consolidation |
| COP | Intraluminal organizing fibrosis in distal airspaces; patchy; preservation of lung architecture; temporally uniform; mild chronic interstitial inflammation | Patchy bilateral consolidation | Subpleural and/or peribronchovascular | Patchy consolidation and/or nodules |
| DAD | Alveolar edema, hyaline membrane, fibroblastic proliferation with little mature collagen; diffuse; temporally uniform | Progressive diffuse GGO or consolidation | Diffuse | Consolidation, GGO, often with lobular sparing; traction bronchiectasis later |
| LIP | Infiltration of T lymphocytes, plasma cells, and macrophages; lymphoid hyperplasia; diffuse; predominantly septal | Reticular opacities, nodule | Diffuse | Centrilobular nodules, GGO, septal and bronchovascular thickening, thin-walled cysts |

Reprinted from Kim et al. [1] with permission

*Note*: *UIP* usual interstitial pneumonia, *NSIP* nonspecific interstitial pneumonia, *COP* cryptogenic organizing pneumonia, *DAD* diffuse alveolar damage, *LIP* lymphocytic interstitial pneumonia, *HC* honeycombing, *GGO* ground-glass opacity

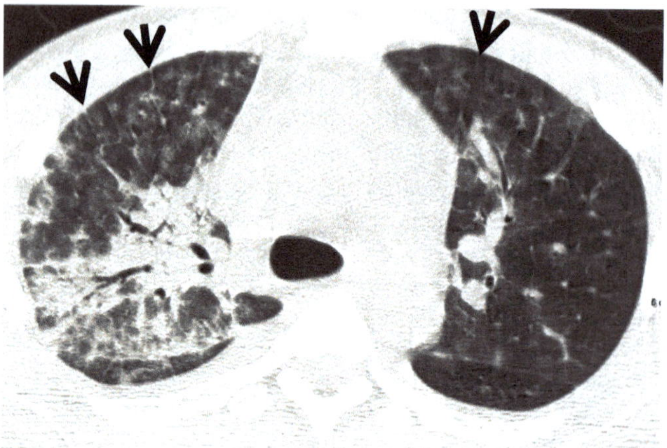

**Fig. 28.1** Acute lupus pneumonitis in a 47-year-old woman with systemic lupus erythematosus. Lung window image of CT scan (2.5-mm section thickness) obtained at level of azygos arch shows patchy and extensive areas of parenchymal opacity in upper lung zones. Also note mild and smooth thickening of interlobular septa (*arrows*)

## Rheumatoid Arthritis (RA)

Pleuropulmonary complications in rheumatoid arthritis (RA) are common and include interstitial pneumonitis and fibrosis, rheumatoid (necrobiotic) nodules, COP pattern of lung abnormality (Fig. 28.3), bronchiectasis, bronchiolitis obliterans, follicular bronchiolitis, and pleural effusion or thickening [1]. Interstitial pneumonitis and fibrosis are the most common pulmonary manifestation of RA (Fig. 28.4). Evidence of interstitial fibrosis is seen on chest radiographs in approximately 5 % of patients with RA [7] and on TSCT in 30–40 % [8]. The complication is seen most frequently in men between 50 and 60 years of age [9].

The majority of patients who have interstitial fibrosis associated with RA have UIP pattern of lung abnormality (Fig. 28.4); a small percentage has histologic findings of NSIP pattern [1]. Nodular aggregates of lymphocytes may be prominent in both the parenchymal interstitium and in the interstitial tissue in bronchiolar walls and interlobular septa (follicular bronchiolitis). According to a report, a wide variety of histopathologic features were seen in open lung biopsy from patients with rheumatoid lung disease [10]. Five different groups based on histologic patterns were identified: pulmonary rheumatoid nodules, UIP pattern, COP pattern, lymphoid hyperplasia, and cellular interstitial infiltrates (NSIP pattern). Few cases of DAD have been reported [11].

The predominant abnormality on TSCT consists of reticulation caused by a combination of intralobular lines and irregular thickening of interlobular septa [12]. HC is seen, most markedly near the diaphragm. According to a study [13], three predominant CT patterns were identified in 29 patients: reticulation with or without HC ($n=19$),

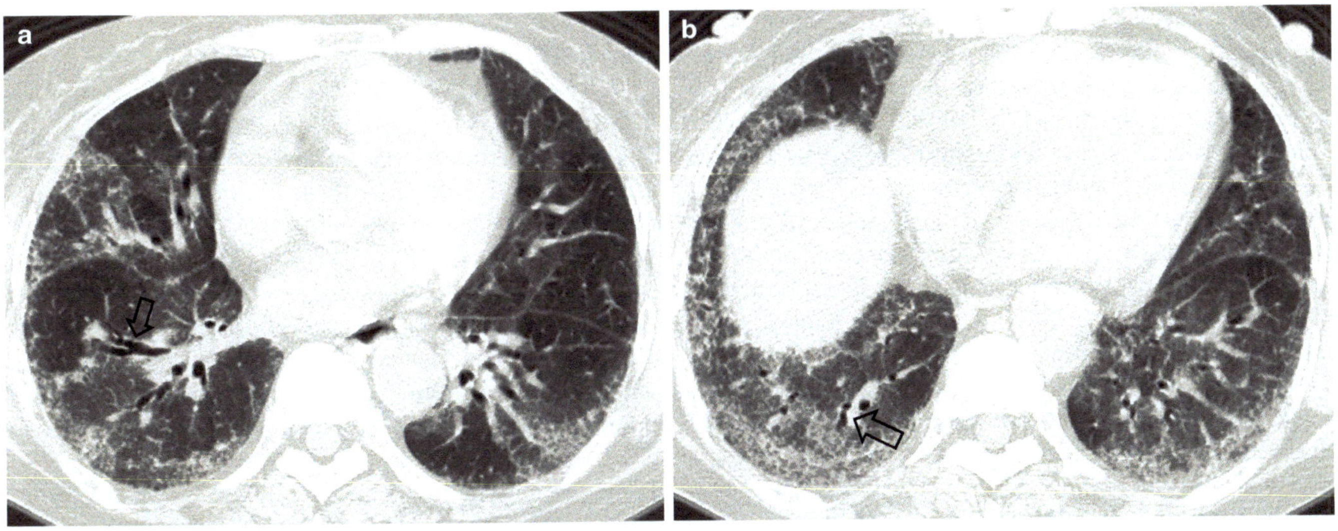


**Fig. 28.2** Pulmonary fibrosis of nonspecific interstitial pneumonia pattern in a 37-year-old woman with systemic lupus erythematosus. (**a**, **b**) Lung window of CT scans (2.5-mm section thickness) obtained at levels of inferior pulmonary veins (**a**) and liver dome (**b**), respectively, show patchy areas of ground-glass opacity and reticulation in subpleural lungs and along bronchovascular bundles in both lungs. Also note traction bronchiectasis (*open arrows*)

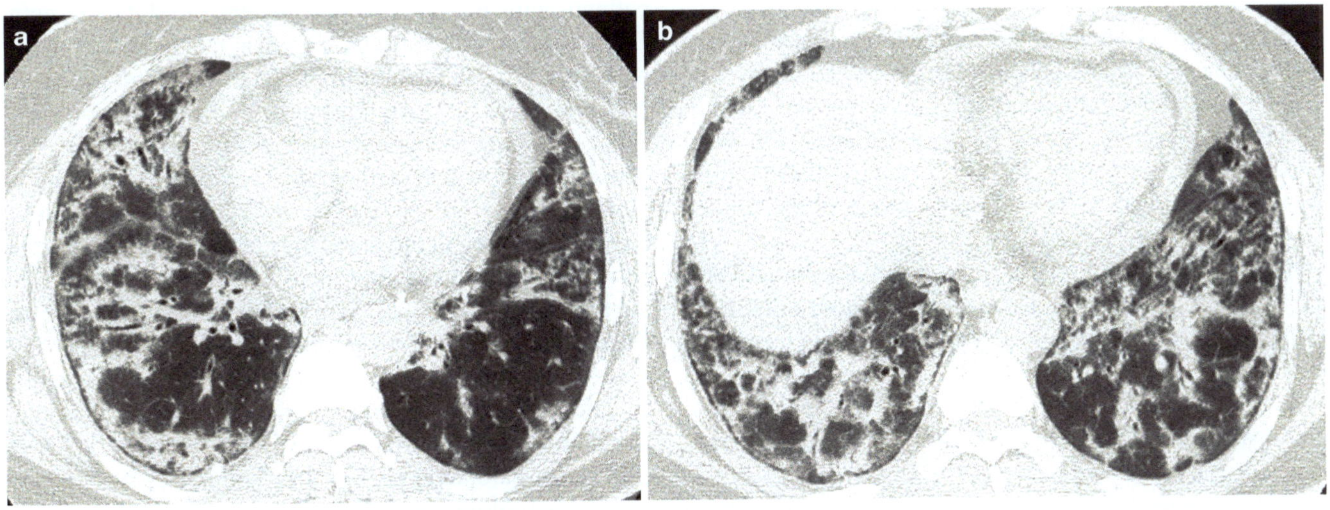


**Fig. 28.3** Interstitial pneumonia of cryptogenic organizing pneumonia pattern in a 48-year-old woman with rheumatoid arthritis. (**a**, **b**) Lung window of CT scans (2.5-mm section thickness) obtained at levels of inferior pulmonary veins (**a**) and liver dome (**b**), respectively, show patchy areas of consolidation in both lungs, distributed along bronchovascular bundles or along subpleural lungs

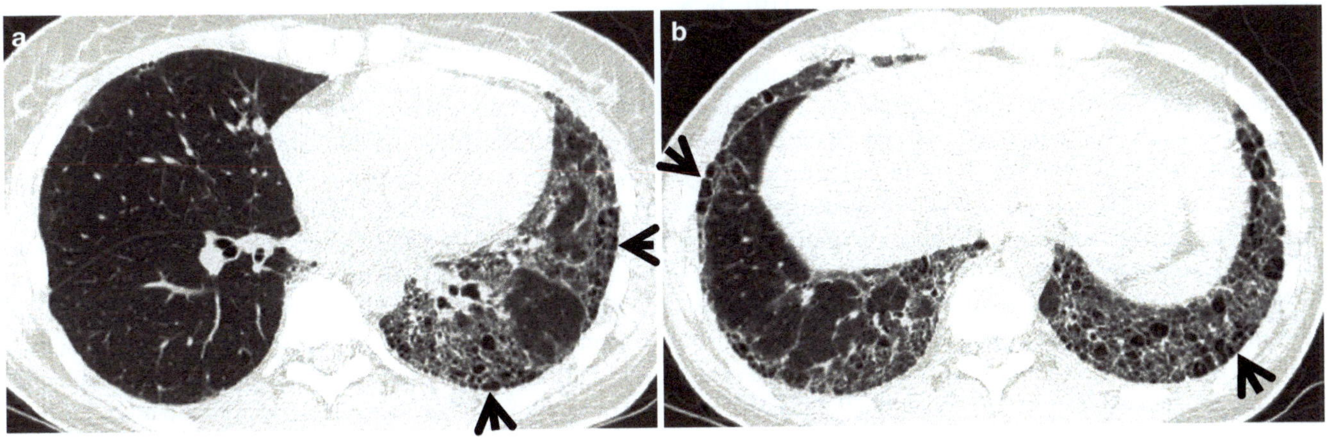


**Fig. 28.4** Interstitial fibrosis of usual interstitial pneumonia pattern in a 35-year-old woman with rheumatoid arthritis. (**a**, **b**) Lung window of CT scans (2.5-mm section thickness) obtained at levels of inferior pulmonary veins (**a**) and liver dome (**b**), respectively, show patchy areas of reticulation in both lungs. Also note honeycomb cysts (*arrows*)

centrilobular branching linear structures with or without bronchial dilatation ($n=5$), and consolidation ($n=5$). Reticulation and centrilobular branching linear structure corresponded histopathologically to UIP and bronchiolitis obliterans, respectively. Consolidation corresponded to COP with or without findings of coexistent chronic eosinophilic pneumonia. Reticulations deteriorate rapidly especially when they are associated with the new appearance of multifocal areas of GGO. Centrilobular branching linear structures show a tendency to progress to bronchiectasis. Consolidation shows a tendency to improve in one half of patients and to evolve into HC in the remaining half at serial CT.

Interstitial lung changes are frequent and independent of disease duration. Interstitial changes are more frequent and severe in rheumatoid factor-positive patients and in patients with more severe joint involvement [14].

## Progressive Systemic Sclerosis (PSS)

Pulmonary involvement is more common and more severe in PSS than in other types of collagen vascular disease. The most common pulmonary manifestations are interstitial fibrosis, which occurs in approximately 80 % of patients [15]. Pulmonary fibrosis is equally likely in limited and diffuse diseases but is less severe in the limited form [16].

At autopsy, some degree of parenchymal interstitial fibrosis is frequent. The histologic features are those of NSIP or UIP pattern (Fig. 28.5). Follicular bronchiolitis is seen occasionally. Although COP pattern may be associated with a variety of CVDs, there are rare reports of bronchiolitis associated with scleroderma [1]. DAD has often been recognized rarely in association with PSS [17].

TSCT frequently demonstrates the evidence of interstitial pneumonitis and fibrosis in patients who have normal or questionable radiographic findings [18]. The abnormalities involve mainly the lower lung zones and have a predominant peripheral and posterior distribution [19]. In a recent study by Kim et al. [20], serial TSCT findings were correlated with the results of pulmonary function tests in 40 patients with PSS and interstitial pneumonia. The overall extent of disease and extents of HC and GGO increased significantly on follow-up CT. Both forced vital capacity and forced expiratory volume in 1 s decreased significantly in the follow-up examination. The increase in the extent of HC on CT correlated significantly with the decrease in diffusing capacity for carbon monoxide. The rate of progression of HC in patients with idiopathic UIP is a mean of 0.4 % of lung volume in a month [21]. According to a study [20], the progression rate of HC in PSS is 0.07 % of lung volume in a month.

## Polymyositis (PM) and Dermatomyositis (DM)

The thorax is commonly affected in PM or DM, generally in one or more of three forms: (a) hypoventilation and respiratory failure as a result of involvement of the respiratory muscles; (b) interstitial pneumonitis (usually with a histologic pattern of UIP or NSIP) (38); and (c) aspiration pneumonia secondary to pharyngeal muscle weakness (probably the most common pulmonary complication) [1, 22].

Interstitial lung disease associated with PM–DM has a wide spectrum of histopathologic features. Three major groups can be identified on the basis of histologic patterns: COP, UIP/NSIP (Fig. 28.6), and DAD (Fig. 28.7) patterns. Histologic appearance is useful for determining patient prognosis. Patients with DAD or UIP pattern show poor prognosis with only a 33 % survival rate at 5 years [1, 23]; however, patients with COP pattern have excellent prognosis. Patients with NSIP pattern have good prognosis.

Initial TSCT findings of pulmonary involvement in patients with PM–DM are prominent interlobular septa, GGO, patchy consolidation, parenchymal bands, irregular peribronchovascular thickening, and subpleural lines. HC may be seen in up to 16 % of patients who have abnormal chest radiographs or pulmonary function [24]. Areas of consolidation with or without GGO correspond histopathologically to COP or organizing DAD pattern. Patchy consolidation, parenchymal bands, and irregular peribronchovascular thickening improve on sequential CT, becoming pleural irregularities and prominent interlobular septa, GGO, and subpleural lines on follow-up CT scans [25]. Therefore, consolidation with patchy and subpleural distribution, parenchymal bands, and irregular peribronchovascular thickening are reversible. Occasionally, areas of GGO with parenchymal bands or subpleural lines representing pathologic area of UIP pattern may progress to HC [26].

## Sjögren's Syndrome

The most common thoracic complications of Sjögren's syndrome are LIPs (Fig. 28.8) and airway abnormalities such as follicular bronchitis, bronchiectasis, and bronchiolitis. Less common complications include interstitial pneumonitis and fibrosis (Fig. 28.9), COP, lymphoma, pulmonary hypertension, and pleural effusion or fibrosis [27].

Pathologically, LIP is characterized by a diffuse, usually bilateral, interstitial infiltration of lymphoplasma cells [1]. It is usually most prominent in relation to bronchioles and their accompanying vessels but can be seen in the alveolar interstitium. Fibrosis is usually mild [28].

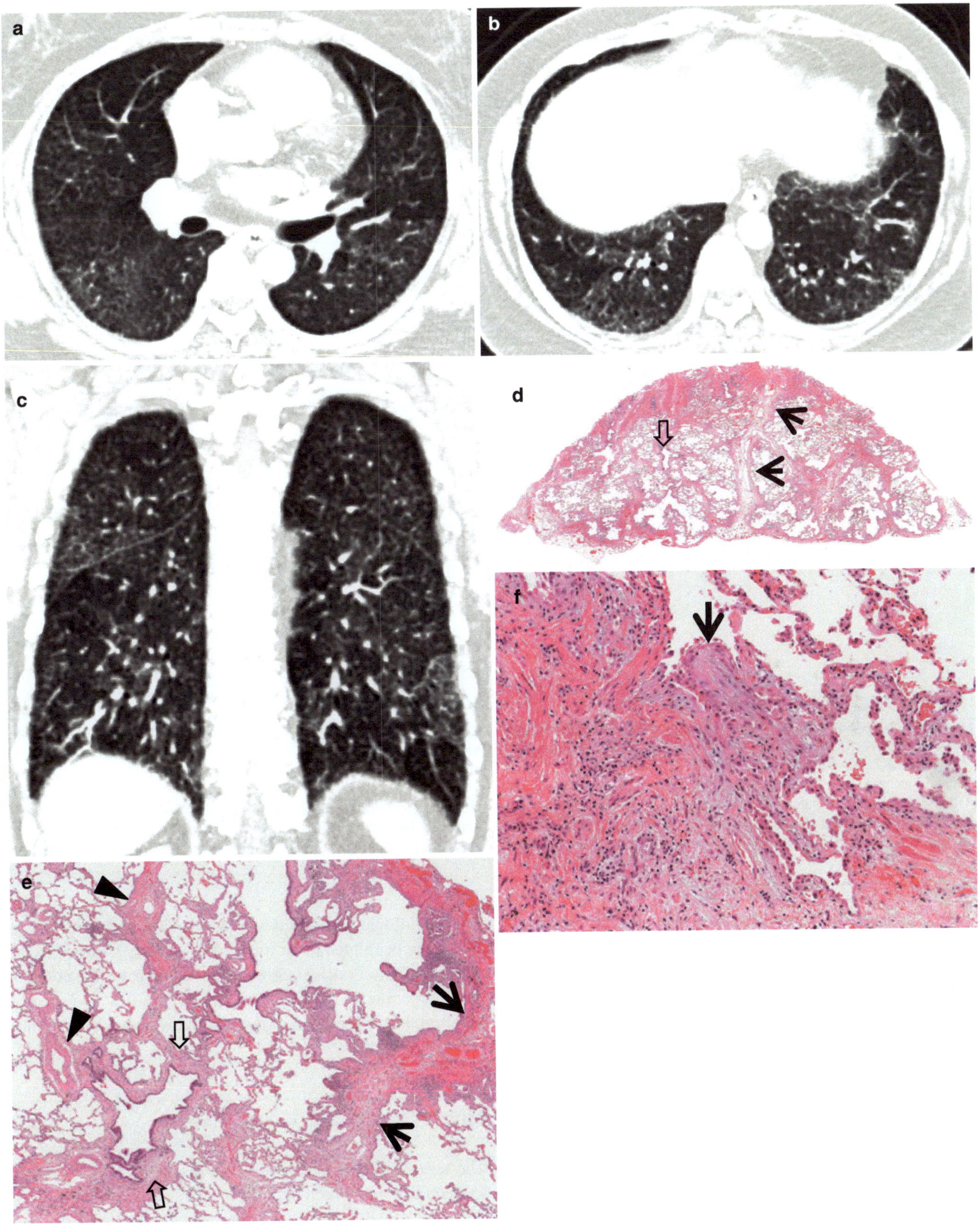


**Fig. 28.5** Interstitial fibrosis of usual interstitial pneumonia pattern in a 59-year-old woman with progressive systemic sclerosis. (**a**, **b**) Lung window of CT scans (3.0-mm section thickness) obtained at levels of bronchus intermedius (**a**) and liver dome (**b**), respectively, show patchy and extensive areas of reticulation and ground-glass opacity in both lungs. (**c**) Coronal reformatted image (3.0-mm section thickness) demonstrate similar pattern of reticulation and ground-glass opacity extensively in both lungs. (**d**) Low-magnification (×4) photomicrograph of surgical lung biopsy specimen obtained from right lower lobe exhibits dense fibrosis along interlobular septum (*arrows*) and around bronchiole (*open arrow*). (**e**) High-magnification (×100) photomicrograph depicts dense fibrosis in interlobular septum (*arrows*) and around bronchiole (*open arrows*). Also note thick fibrotic vessel wall (*arrowheads*). (**f**) High-magnification (×200) photomicrograph discloses area of focal active fibrosis (*arrow*)

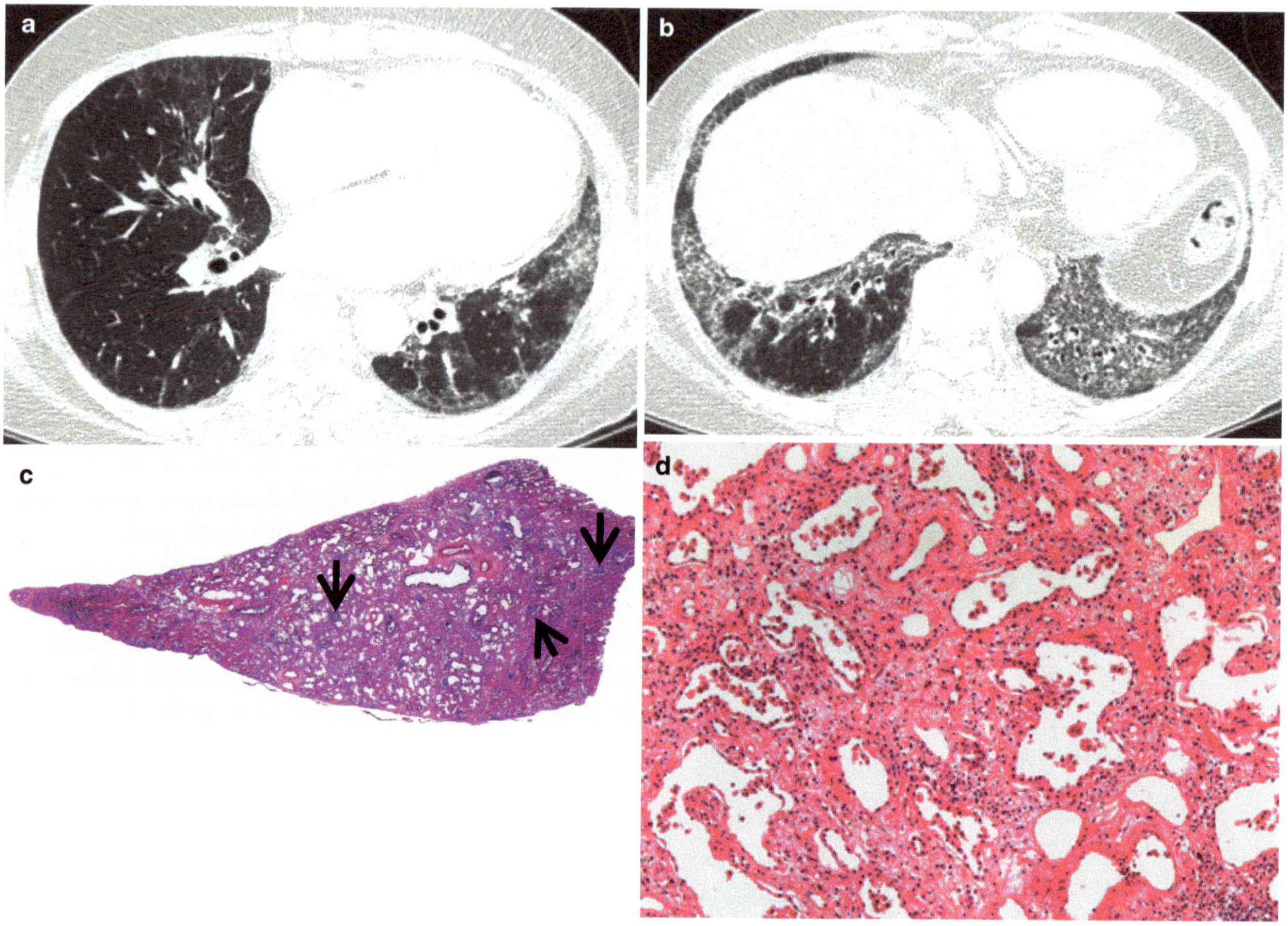


**Fig. 28.6** Pulmonary fibrosis of nonspecific interstitial pneumonia pattern in a 48-year-old woman with polymyositis (*PM*)–dermatomyositis (*DM*). (**a**, **b**) Lung window of CT scans (2.5-mm section thickness) obtained at levels of right inferior pulmonary vein (**a**) and liver dome (**b**), respectively, show patchy areas of mixed ground-glass opacity and reticulation in bilateral lower lung zones. (**c**) Low-magnification (×4) photomicrograph of surgical lung biopsy specimen obtained from right lower lobe demonstrates temporally and regionally homogeneous pulmonary fibrosis and chronic inflammatory cell infiltration with uniform alveolar wall thickening. There is no architectural distortion. Also note interstitial aggregates of lymphoid follicle (*arrows*). (**d**) High-magnification (×100) photomicrograph discloses diffuse uniform widening of interstitium due to fibrosis and chronic inflammatory cell infiltration. Also note absence of architectural distortion

In a prospective study [29] dealing with TSCT findings of lungs in 50 consecutive patients, lung abnormalities were detected in 17 patients (34 %) on CT as compared with in 7 (14 %) patients on chest radiographs. The most common findings consisted of bronchiolectasis and poorly defined centrilobular small nodular or branching linear opacities (seen in 11 patients), areas of GGO (in 7), and HC (in 4). Areas of HC or both HC and GGO suggesting pulmonary fibrosis were bilateral and asymmetric and present almost exclusively in the periphery of the lower lobes [30]. A characteristic pattern of extensive areas of GGO with scattered thin-walled cysts is seen in approximately 50 % of patients with LIP [28, 31]. Similar findings have been described in LIP not associated with Sjögren's syndrome [28]. Interstitial peribronchiolar lymphoplasmacytic infiltrates associated with overinflation of the secondary pulmonary lobule in histopathologic specimens suggest that at least some of the cysts may be related to air trapping secondary to bronchiolar stenosis [32]. Poorly defined centrilobular small nodules and thickening of the bronchovascular bundles also seen in LIP represent expansion of the interstitial tissue by lymphoplasma cell infiltration [28].

## Mixed Connective Tissue Disease

The term "mixed connective tissue disease" (MCTD) refers to a condition in which patients have mixed features of SLE, PSS, and PM. Respiratory involvement has been described in 20–80 % of patients. Common pulmonary abnormalities include interstitial pneumonitis and fibrosis, pulmonary hypertension, and pleural effusion.

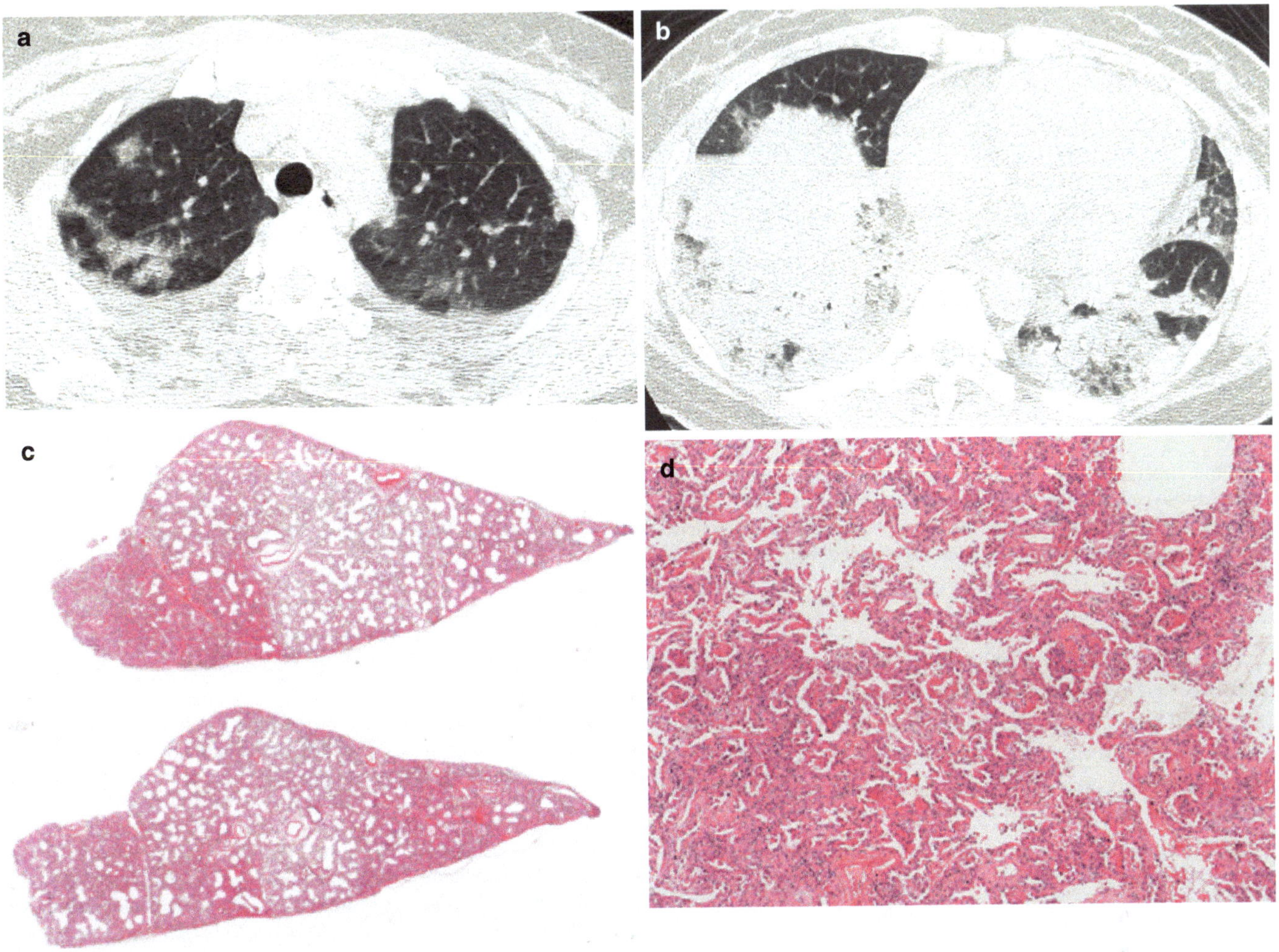


**Fig. 28.7** Diffuse alveolar damage in a 43-year-old woman with polymyositis–dermatomyositis. (**a, b**) Lung window of CT scans (2.5-mm section thickness) obtained at levels of aortic arch (**a**) and liver dome (**b**), respectively, show patchy areas of consolidation in both lungs. Also note bilateral pleural effusions. (**c**) Low-magnification (×4) photomicrograph of surgical lung biopsy specimen obtained from left lower lobe demonstrates diffuse widening of alveolar walls and edematous thickening of interlobular septa. (**d**) High-magnification (×100) photomicrograph highlights alveolar wall thickening with interstitial fibroblastic proliferation. Note some intra-alveolar fibrin and few inflammatory cells

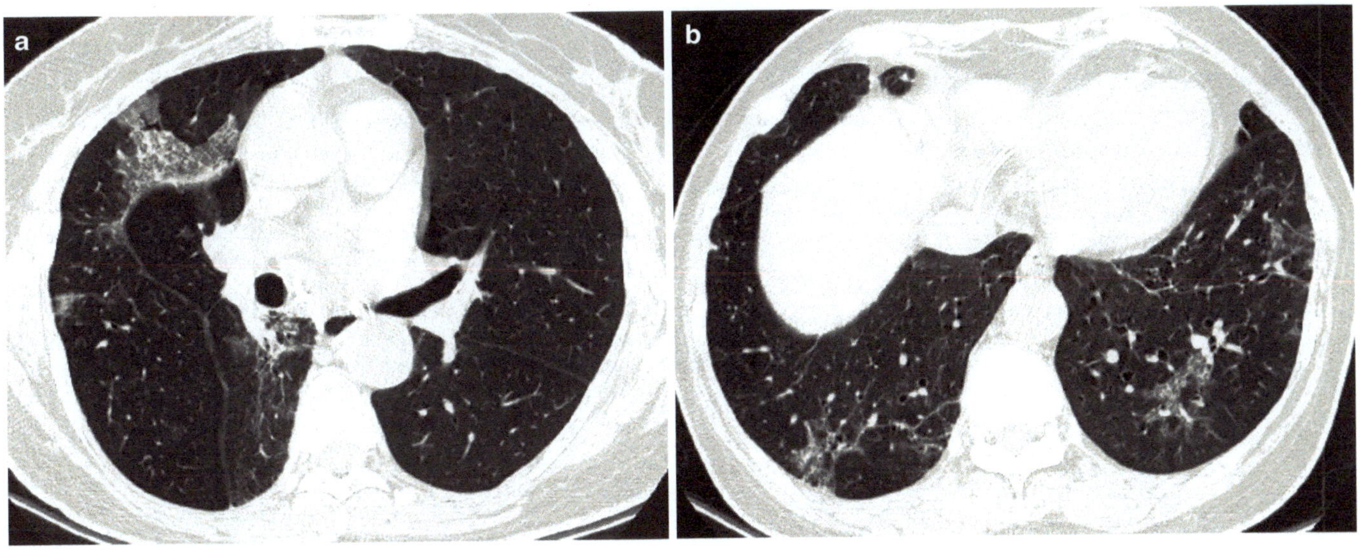


**Fig. 28.8** Lymphocytic interstitial pneumonia in a 63-year-old woman with Sjögren's syndrome. (**a, b**) Lung window of CT scans (2.5-mm section thickness) obtained at levels of bronchus intermedius (**a**) and liver dome (**b**), respectively, show patchy areas of ground-glass opacity harboring internal reticulation. Surgical biopsy specimen disclosed interstitial lymphocytic infiltration, finding compatible with lymphocytic interstitial pneumonia in Sjögren's syndrome

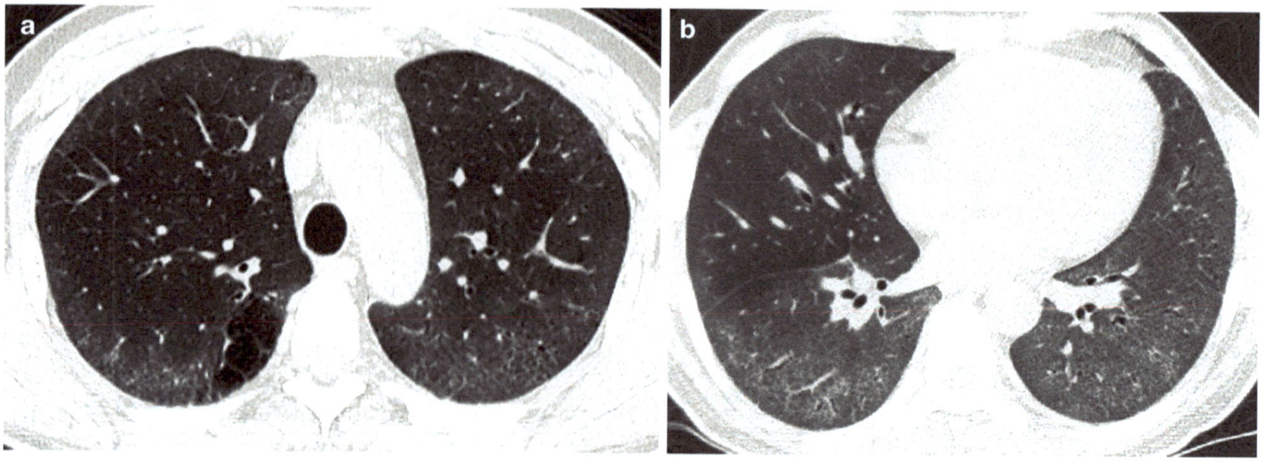


**Fig. 28.9** Interstitial fibrosis of nonspecific interstitial pneumonia pattern in a 49-year-old man with Sjögren's syndrome. (**a, b**) Lung window of CT scans (2.5-mm section thickness) obtained at levels of aortic arch (**a**) and inferior pulmonary veins (**b**), respectively, show patchy and extensive areas of ground-glass opacity and fine reticulation in both lungs. Surgical biopsy specimen disclosed uniform interstitial fibrosis, compatible with fibrotic nonspecific interstitial pneumonia

Pathologic findings of pulmonary involvement of MCTD are classified into interstitial fibrosis and vascular changes. Interstitial fibrosis has the appearance of UIP or NSIP pattern. Typical vascular changes consist of bland intimal proliferation of the lung arterioles, plexogenic angiopathy, and chronic pulmonary emboli [33].

TSCT scans show a predominant subpleural distribution of fibrosis. Other radiologic abnormalities include areas of parenchymal consolidation that may be related to COP pattern of lung abnormality [34].

## Ankylosing Spondylitis

Ankylosing spondylitis is a chronic inflammatory disease affecting mainly the joints of the axial skeleton (sacroiliac, costovertebral, and apophyseal joints). It affects mainly men (male to female ratio 10:1). Approximately 1–2 % of patients develop pleuropulmonary complications [35].

Pathologic findings of interstitial lung disease in ankylosing spondylitis include prominent interstitial fibrosis with hyaline and elastic degeneration of collagen, especially in the apices of the lungs. Chronic inflammatory cell infiltrations have also been reported [36].

A variety of abnormalities can be seen on TSCT, including evidence of apical fibrosis, paraseptal emphysema, bronchiectasis, interstitial fibrosis, mediastinal lymph node enlargement, and tracheal dilatation [37].

## References

1. Kim EA, Lee KS, Johkoh T, et al. Interstitial lung diseases associated with collagen vascular diseases: radiologic and histopathologic findings. Radiographics. 2002;22(Spec No):S151–65.
2. Cervera R, Khamashta MA, Font J, et al. Systemic lupus erythematosus: clinical and immunologic patterns of disease expression in a cohort of 1,000 patients. The European Working Party on Systemic Lupus Erythematosus. Medicine (Baltimore). 1993;72:113–24.
3. Mayberry JP, Primack SL, Muller NL. Thoracic manifestations of systemic autoimmune diseases: radiographic and high-resolution CT findings. Radiographics. 2000;20:1623–35.
4. Haupt HM, Moore GW, Hutchins GM. The lung in systemic lupus erythematosus. Analysis of the pathologic changes in 120 patients. Am J Med. 1981;71:791–8.
5. Bankier AA, Kiener HP, Wiesmayr MN, et al. Discrete lung involvement in systemic lupus erythematosus: CT assessment. Radiology. 1995;196:835–40.
6. Fenlon HM, Doran M, Sant SM, Breatnach E. High-resolution chest CT in systemic lupus erythematosus. AJR Am J Roentgenol. 1996;166:301–7.
7. Jurik AG, Davidsen D, Graudal H. Prevalence of pulmonary involvement in rheumatoid arthritis and its relationship to some characteristics of the patients. A radiological and clinical study. Scand J Rheumatol. 1982;11:217–24.
8. Gabbay E, Tarala R, Will R, et al. Interstitial lung disease in recent onset rheumatoid arthritis. Am J Respir Crit Care Med. 1997;156:528–35.
9. Anaya JM, Diethelm L, Ortiz LA, et al. Pulmonary involvement in rheumatoid arthritis. Semin Arthritis Rheum. 1995;24:242–54.
10. Yousem SA, Colby TV, Carrington CB. Lung biopsy in rheumatoid arthritis. Am Rev Respir Dis. 1985;131:770–7.
11. Aratake K, Eguchi K, Migita K, et al. An autopsy case of rheumatoid arthritis accompanied with acute exacerbation of interstitial pneumonia. Nihon Rinsho Meneki Gakkai Kaishi. 1998;21:129–36.

12. Remy-Jardin M, Remy J, Cortet B, Mauri F, Delcambre B. Lung changes in rheumatoid arthritis: CT findings. Radiology. 1994; 193:375–82.
13. Akira M, Sakatani M, Hara H. Thin-section CT findings in rheumatoid arthritis-associated lung disease: CT patterns and their courses. J Comput Assist Tomogr. 1999;23:941–8.
14. Muller-Leisse C, Bussmann A, Meyer O, Vorbruggen W, Genth E, Gunther RW. Pulmonary manifestations in rheumatoid arthritis: high-resolution computed tomography in correlation with the skeletal changes and the laboratory chemical changes. Rofo. 1996;165:438–44.
15. Minai OA, Dweik RA, Arroliga AC. Manifestations of scleroderma pulmonary disease. Clin Chest Med. 1998;19:713–31; viii–ix.
16. Arroliga AC, Podell DN, Matthay RA. Pulmonary manifestations of scleroderma. J Thorac Imaging. 1992;7:30–45.
17. Muir TE, Tazelaar HD, Colby TV, Myers JL. Organizing diffuse alveolar damage associated with progressive systemic sclerosis. Mayo Clin Proc. 1997;72:639–42.
18. Warrick JH, Bhalla M, Schabel SI, Silver RM. High resolution computed tomography in early scleroderma lung disease. J Rheumatol. 1991;18:1520–8.
19. Remy-Jardin M, Remy J, Wallaert B, Bataille D, Hatron PY. Pulmonary involvement in progressive systemic sclerosis: sequential evaluation with CT, pulmonary function tests, and bronchoalveolar lavage. Radiology. 1993;188:499–506.
20. Kim EA, Johkoh T, Lee KS, et al. Interstitial pneumonia in progressive systemic sclerosis: serial high-resolution CT findings with functional correlation. J Comput Assist Tomogr. 2001;25:757–63.
21. Akira M, Sakatani M, Ueda E. Idiopathic pulmonary fibrosis: progression of honeycombing at thin-section CT. Radiology. 1993;189:687–91.
22. Tazelaar HD, Viggiano RW, Pickersgill J, Colby TV. Interstitial lung disease in polymyositis and dermatomyositis. Clinical features and prognosis as correlated with histologic findings. Am Rev Respir Dis. 1990;141:727–33.
23. Schwarz MI. The lung in polymyositis. Clin Chest Med. 1998;19:701–12; viii.
24. Ikezoe J, Johkoh T, Kohno N, Takeuchi N, Ichikado K, Nakamura H. High-resolution CT findings of lung disease in patients with polymyositis and dermatomyositis. J Thorac Imaging. 1996;11:250–9.
25. Mino M, Noma S, Taguchi Y, Tomii K, Kohri Y, Oida K. Pulmonary involvement in polymyositis and dermatomyositis: sequential evaluation with CT. AJR Am J Roentgenol. 1997;169:83–7.
26. Akira M, Hara H, Sakatani M. Interstitial lung disease in association with polymyositis-dermatomyositis: long-term follow-up CT evaluation in seven patients. Radiology. 1999;210:333–8.
27. Cain HC, Noble PW, Matthay RA. Pulmonary manifestations of Sjogren's syndrome. Clin Chest Med. 1998;19:687–99; viii.
28. Johkoh T, Muller NL, Pickford HA, et al. Lymphocytic interstitial pneumonia: thin-section CT findings in 22 patients. Radiology. 1999;212:567–72.
29. Franquet T, Gimenez A, Monill JM, Diaz C, Geli C. Primary Sjogren's syndrome and associated lung disease: CT findings in 50 patients. AJR Am J Roentgenol. 1997;169:655–8.
30. Koyama M, Johkoh T, Honda O, et al. Pulmonary involvement in primary Sjogren's syndrome: spectrum of pulmonary abnormalities and computed tomography findings in 60 patients. J Thorac Imaging. 2001;16:290–6.
31. Meyer CA, Pina JS, Taillon D, Godwin JD. Inspiratory and expiratory high-resolution CT findings in a patient with Sjogren's syndrome and cystic lung disease. AJR Am J Roentgenol. 1997;168: 101–3.
32. Ichikawa Y, Kinoshita M, Koga T, Oizumi K, Fujimoto K, Hayabuchi N. Lung cyst formation in lymphocytic interstitial pneumonia: CT features. J Comput Assist Tomogr. 1994;18:745–8.
33. Prakash UB. Lungs in mixed connective tissue disease. J Thorac Imaging. 1992;7:55–61.
34. Prakash UB. Respiratory complications in mixed connective tissue disease. Clin Chest Med. 1998;19:733–46; ix.
35. Lee-Chiong Jr TL. Pulmonary manifestations of ankylosing spondylitis and relapsing polychondritis. Clin Chest Med. 1998;19:747–57; ix.
36. Casserly IP, Fenlon HM, Breatnach E, Sant SM. Lung findings on high-resolution computed tomography in idiopathic ankylosing spondylitis–correlation with clinical findings, pulmonary function testing and plain radiography. Br J Rheumatol. 1997;36:677–82.
37. Fenlon HM, Casserly I, Sant SM, Breatnach E. Plain radiographs and thoracic high-resolution CT in patients with ankylosing spondylitis. AJR Am J Roentgenol. 1997;168:1067–72.

FSC
www.fsc.org
MIX
Papier | Fördert gute Waldnutzung
FSC® C083411

Kolibri 360 GmbH
Ferdinand-Jühlke-Straße 7
99095 Erfurt, Deutschland
produktsicherheit@kolibri360.de